Human Sexuality and Its Problems

John Bancroft MD FRCP FRCPsych
MRC Reproductive Biology Unit, Edinburgh

SECOND EDITION

CHURCHILL LIVINGSTONE
EDINBURGH LONDON MELBOURNE AND NEW YORK 1989

CHURCHILL LIVINGSTONE
Medical Division of Longman Group UK Limited

Distributed in the United States of America by
Churchill Livingstone Inc., 1560 Broadway, New
York, N.Y. 10036, and by associated companies,
branches and representatives throughout the world.

First published 1983
Second edition 1989
  Reprinted 1990

ISBN 0-443-034559

British Library Cataloguing in Publication Data
Bancroft, John, *1936*–
    Human sexuality and its problems. — 2nd ed.
    1. Man. Sexuality
    I. Title
    612'.6

Library of Congress Cataloging-in-Publication data
Bancroft, John.
    Human sexuality and its problems/John Bancroft;

    Includes index.
    1. Sexual disorders.   2. Sex (Psychology)   3. Sex
(Biology)
    I. Title.
    [DNLM: 1. Sex.   2. Sex Behavior.   3. Sex
Disorders.   WM 611
    B213h]
    RC556.B333 1989
616.85'83 — dc19

Produced by Longman Singapore Publishers (Pte) Ltd.
Printed in Singapore

Human Sexuality and Its Problems

This volume is dedicated to Frank Beach.

Contents

Acknowledgements

Beth Alder, Judy Bury, Derek Chiswick, Alan Dixson, Judy Greenwood, Philip Myerscough and Pam Warner read through drafts of the revised chapters and made useful comments. Alan Dixson drew a diagram of a sagittal section of the brain for me. Cynthia Graham did much of the proof reading. I very much appreciate their help.

I am also grateful to D T Baird, C Carati, W C de Groat, J Gillis, H G Forest, J Forrest, A McInnis, S Ratcliffe, R Green, T F Lue, A McNeilly, J C van Wieringen and G Wagner for their kind permission to reproduce photographs or figures.

1

Introduction

The thread of sexuality is woven densely into the fabric of human existence. There are few people for whom sex has not been important at some time and many for whom it has played a dominant part in their lives.

Sex is a motive force bringing two people into intimate contact. They may have nothing in common except mutual sexual interest. Their encounter may be brief or it may lead on to the principal relationship in their lives. This is important not only at an individual, personal level, but also socially and politically. The nature of the relationships between men and women is crucial to our social and political systems. The dominance of men over women is one important dimension of the more general issue of dominance of one group over another. Sex is a political issue in another sense. The sexual values of a society are clearly identified with the establishment, and rejection of sexual value has always been one expression of political revolt or alienation. Perhaps only recently has such sexual revolt figured in political theory.

Sex and gender are inter-related in complex ways. Sex permeates our symbolism and much of our art. In many languages, inanimate objects arc endowed with gender.

The quality of sexual attractiveness has a wide influence. In a materialistic society it is used to impart appeal to non-sexual objects — the commercial exploitation of sex is all around us. This stems from the powerful link between sexual attractiveness and self-esteem. For many, sexual appeal will be or will be seen to be the most powerful asset they possess.

And beneath all this is some biological substrate, ill understood except for its clear link with reproduction. The biological quality of sexuality is perhaps that aspect of human behaviour which reminds us most strongly of our place amongst the animal kingdom. In spite of this, comparative study of human and animal sexuality has been limited. There are a few notable exceptions (e.g. Ford & Beach 1952) which are rewarding and informative. They indicate that in addition to some striking universals of sex amongst animals, including humans, there are many species differences. Perhaps the characteristic of human sexuality which sets it most clearly apart from that of most other animals is its relative separation from reproduction. Sex has obviously come to play a much wider sociobiological function than the production of offspring. We see this to some extent in other animals, particularly certain primates. In the chimpanzee, for example, sex may have a socially cohesive role (see Chapter 2) which is perhaps organised in a way which reduces tension in male groups. More commonly, when sexual selection operates, and male competes with male for the female, we see sexually related intermale aggression which may be instrumental in determining the dominance hierarchy of the male group. In such circumstances we also see the associated development of male physical supremacy over the female with various patterns of male dominance evolving (see Chapter 4). The physically dominant, exploitative male is by no means a uniquely human phenomenon! Thus we can see how evolution of the sexual process can have major repercussions on other aspects of an animal's existence.

But in few if any other species has fertility and population growth reached such a level that fertility control becomes a major biological need for proper survival of the species. It is therefore not surprising that it is only in the human species that the reproductive aspect of sexual behaviour has ceased to be of primary significance (see chapter 12).

If human sexuality has a wider function than in most other species, it is because there are fewer biological constraints. Hence the need for social constraints. Human sexuality is, in my view, an enigma or riddle. After 25 years of studying the sexual behaviour of humans it has lost none of this mystery for me. I suspect that the essence of this riddle is that whilst there are uniquely human difficulties in containing our sexuality, it is far from certain that the consequences would all be beneficial if those difficulties were resolved. There is a tension or conflict between our identities as rational, civilised beings and our sexual identities and less rational sexual drives. Our sexuality endows us with an absurd quality which gives some immunity against pomposity and excess dignity. On the other hand, our sexual vulnerabilities have become incorporated into some of our least attractive or most questionable characteristics. Our sex role stereotypes, for example, institutionalise the sexual irresponsibility of the male, whilst assuming sexual responsibility and other less enviable virtues in the female.

And of course, our basic vulnerability is not confined to sex. Human beings are constantly showing themselves capable of the most appalling inhumanities to each other when placed in certain circumstances. If sex stops us getting too pompous, then our inherent and it would appear universal potential for inhumanity should stop us from becoming too self-righteous.

But the riddle remains. If we were to become sexually controlled, biologically and socially tidy in our sexual expression, what sort of people would we be?

Given this complexity and the conflictual nature of human sexuality, we should not be surprised to find that sexual problems of various kinds are common. Animals are not immune to sexual difficulties. Prize bulls may become impotent. It is difficult to judge how much their self-esteem is affected, or how much distress they experience; with the economic consequences of their plight, the distress of their human owners is more obvious. In many species male may sexually mount male, or female female. Apart from the temporary irritation that this may cause the recipient, there is no evidence that such animals become socially stigmatised because of such behaviour. In general humans are more vulnerable to sexual problems.

USING THIS BOOK

This book is primarily intended for health professionals who are especially interested in working with sexual problems. But it also has a wider purpose, that is, to emphasise the broad variety of factors and the complexity of their interactions which must be taken into account when attempting to understand human sexuality. In an age when scientific disciplines are becoming increasingly specialised, it is more and more difficult to bring together new knowledge in a manner that helps us comprehensively to understand the human condition. Sexuality is a prime example of the growing need for such a synthesis, and there are many others. For the medical profession, sex provides as good a model of psychosomatic relationships as one can find. But still medical thought tends to evade the complexities of mind–body interaction, perhaps to a large extent because of the intellectual discomfort of doing otherwise. A proper understanding of human sexuality *demands* a truly psychosomatic approach.

Bringing together and integrating ideas from the wide variety of disciplines which impinge on sexuality is a formidable challenge, and a never-ending one. The possibilities for pursuing relevant lines of enquiry are almost limitless. It has therefore been difficult to know how to structure a book of this kind. My method has been somewhat idiosyncratic. I have aimed to discuss, and hopefully clarify, those areas of knowledge I have found important in my own understanding of human sexuality, and to dwell on those aspects I regard as particularly difficult or fundamental. That is the explanation for the somewhat arbitrary selection of basic biological issues in Chapter 2. I have given extra emphasis to those issues which are central to my own research — in particular hormone–behaviour relationships — though I also believe that such issues are central to a psychosociobiological approach. This book inevitably contains a very personal selection. There are some areas of knowledge, such as molecular biology, which are expanding at a phenomenal rate and on which I have scarcely touched. There are other areas which are not new, but my interest in them has developed only relatively recently, such as social history and social anthropology; these subjects have received greater attention in this second edition. I have paid more attention to marriage and love, but there are many other areas which remain more or less neglected (e.g. prostitution). It is my hope that these inadequacies will be rectified in further editions. Clearly each reader will need to be selective in his or her use of this book. I hope experts in each area will be understanding and tolerant when I have oversimplified their special knowledge, though I expect no mercy if I have misinterpreted it.

I have retained the overall structure of the first edition, whilst substantially rewriting the text. Chapter 2 is considerably expanded to deal with recent advances in our knowledge of sexual biology. Sexual development has been dealt with more extensively and now follows the basic biological chapter. I have been more adventurous in proposing my own theoretical ideas about development. There is a new brief chapter on sexuality and ageing (Chapter 5), reflecting increasing knowledge in this area as well as the author's increasing age. I have also formed a separate chapter on the assessment of sexual problems (Chapter 8), allowing detailed consideration of the many new developments in the investigation of sexual dysfunction, especially in the male. In Chapter 12 I have included a section on pregnancy and the puerperium to balance the contraceptive and infertility aspects.

Compared with most other areas of human behaviour, the study of sex has lacked scholarship. There are some exceptions, the most notable in the English language being Havelock Ellis and Alfred Kinsey. Freud obviously comes to mind and one cannot dispute his major influence. But he and his followers have brought to the subject the style of thought, characterising psychoanalytic psychology, which is outside the mainstream of conventional scientific scholarship and which, in my view, has erected as many barriers to scientific progress as it has dismantled.

There are obvious reasons for the shortage of scientific endeavour in this field. There has been widespread and powerful opposition to any objective enquiry. This has not only discouraged scholars from venturing into the field but has often had an adverse affect on those who have. Masters & Johnson, two other major influences, are often and justly criticised for their lack of conventional scientific method and their idiosyncratic approach. But it nevertheless seems likely that they were encouraged on to this path by the medical and scientific community's inability to apply the same level of dispassionate and objective appraisal which would have been given to most other areas of enquiry. The situation has changed since their first book was published in 1966. An increasing volume of scientific research is now being subjected to the usual procedures of peer group criticism when results are published in reputable scientific journals. Obstacles to such research are still substantial but for reasons discussed later in this introduction, we are entering an era when human sexuality is being actively reappraised on many levels; the next 10 years may be very different from the last in the opportunities for research that may arise.

As the resistance to objective enquiry lessens, other adverse reactions take place. The scientist who aims to present scientifically rigorous objective findings in this field will fall prey to criticism that he is reducing sex to physiological or mechanical absurdities. There is a strong resistance in many quarters to scientific expertise in such an emotive area of human behaviour. Obviously some of this criticism has been justified. The intellectual vacuum that has been created by these various obstacles has been partially filled by people with less than intelligent ideas. The expanding field of sex therapy has been readily exploited in this way. If there has been a bias of ethical values amongst sexologists and sex educators, good or bad, it has been towards the radical, permissive, liberated end of the spectrum, providing further fuel for reaction.

One lesson to be learnt from all this is the need, when discussing emotive issues such as human sexuality, to take both objective fact and personal values into consideration. Whatever your intentions, a discourse on human sexuality will rarely be accepted by others as morally or emotionally neutral. It is not possible to give a lecture on sexual anatomy or physiology without conveying, unwittingly or otherwise, some additional message about sexual values. Because these are more likely to be misinterpreted if communicated unwittingly, it is therefore advisable to present them explicitly after proper consideration. The reader will therefore find this author's personal values made clear at various points in this book, as well as more systematically in the next section.

A PERSONAL STATEMENT

To help the reader judge to what extent the presentation of evidence in this book is influenced by my personal prejudices, I will provide here an explicit statement of my sexual values. In fact, at the time of writing, sexual values are being vigorously debated and reappraised as a consequence of two dramatic developments in our society: the AIDS epidemic and the apparent increase in child sexual abuse. It is therefore timely for me to offer a more detailed and considered comment than I gave in the introduction to the first edition.

It should be self-evident, since I am the author of this book, that I regard sex as a profoundly important aspect of human existence. I see it as a force working for both good and bad, with much of the good stemming from its potential for causing harm. But first, without going into philosophical niceties, I will explain how I attempt to judge the good and bad in human behaviour.

I do not believe that we are provided with a fundamental morality which is beyond our questioning or doubt. Hence I have little in common with those who resort to the Scriptures on the assumption that this fundamental morality is in some sense written on tablets of stone, presumably by God. The Scriptures provide us with many interesting and useful accounts of moral analysis which need to be interpreted in their historical context.

It is becoming apparent how variable such interpretation can be by modern theologians, let alone theological thinkers across history. On the other hand, I am not a simple utilitarian — not because I regard basing one's moral standards on the consequences of one's actions as inherently wrong, but because I believe it is impossible to have sufficient awareness of the consequences to make moral decisions on purely rational grounds. In other words I accept that a priori judgements about morality are inevitable. Such judgements, however, require every now and then to be reappraised and sometimes modified. In medicine at the present time an increasing number of situations of a completely novel kind confront us with new moral challenges. In vitro fertilisation and antenatal screening are two recent powerful examples. Confronted with such issues it is not possible, in my view, to resolve them on the basis of some given immutable moral principle. There is no alternative to working out a moral position to suit the new situation. In doing so we must not be surprised if we sometimes get it wrong or if we need to modify our position in the light of experience or new evidence. There is a need for moral humility.

Sexuality presents us with several such challenges. In judging sexual morality I look for the functions or purposes of sexual behaviour (see Chapter 3). But it seems to me inescapable that sexuality has evolved in the human species to serve more than the reproductive function. As mentioned earlier, such non-reproductive functions of sex have sometimes emerged in other subhuman primates. These non-reproductive functions include pair-bonding and fostering intimacy, providing pleasure, bolstering self-esteem, asserting masculinity or femininity, anxiety or tension reduction, the expression of hostility, and material gain. I find I am comfortable with some of these functions but not others. I approve of the way that sex can bind a couple and foster intimacy. I have no problem with sex as a source of pleasure, providing that the pleasure is mutual. I am not comfortable with the use of sex as a way of asserting one's masculinity or femininity. Perhaps if I had lived 200 years ago I might have reached a different conclusion on that point. But at this stage in our social development I regard the nature of relationships between men and women, and the need to reduce the exploitation of one sex by the other, to be of the utmost importance for the successful continuation of our species. Hence, any way in which sex is used to reinforce old stereotypes of masculine dominance and exploitation, even those from our biological heritage, cause me concern. This is not an entirely straightforward issue. It may be that for both men and women to get the real benefits of being sexual some distinction between 'maleness' and 'femaleness' will continue to be necessary, at least as far as heterosexual sex is concerned.

My particular view of the binding effect of sexuality is somewhat idiosyncratic. Experience of sexual pleasure may be seen as a potentially uncomplicated positive consequence, particularly when shared by two people. But more important, in my view, is the binding effect of sexual *in-*

timacy, which in turn depends on the vulnerability inherent in the sexual situation. To enjoy sex requires us to let go, to become abandoned to a degree, undefended. In such a state we are vulnerable. For many species this vulnerability is probably an important reason why sexual behaviour is controlled and limited to the minimum time required for the purposes of reproduction. Otherwise the animals would be exposing themselves to undue danger. For humans, it is not physical but psychological or emotional attack which is most likely — risk of being exploited, rejected or humiliated. These are some of the bad consequences of sex. But to be able to expose oneself to such a risk and yet remain safe reinforces the feelings of security in a relationship, and has a binding effect. Few would disagree that if sex works well it strengthens a relationship, whilst if it goes badly it may weaken it. But opinions may vary as to whether this beneficial effect is a consequence of the sexual pleasure or the emotional security which is involved. I would emphasise the latter. To a considerable extent, the emotional security of a sexual relationship is undermined when sex is used for other purposes such as asserting masculinity or dominance, or bolstering self-esteem.

Thus I judge my sexual values on two levels. One concerns 'good use': whether, in my view, sex is being used constructively for the benefit of a relationship between two people. Sex which is simply recreational is not necessarily immoral, but is unlikely to serve the purposes of intimacy and security which I espouse. It is therefore, in my value system, 'wasted sex'.

On the second level, I regard sexual behaviour as immoral when it is used by one person to exploit the vulnerabilities, either psychological or physical, of another, whether for sexual pleasure, the bolstering of self-esteem, or other self-directed benefits.

On this basis, I have no problem in accepting that homosexual intimacy can be as valid as heterosexual. There is plenty of 'wasted sex', in my terms, in the homosexual world, and no shortage of immoral sex. The main difference from the heterosexual world, in this respect, is that the homosexual is living in a society which rejects his or her sexuality however it may be expressed, regarding any overt expression as sinful. Some of the evolution of homosexual behaviour in modern society therefore needs to be understood as a reaction to this rejection, and a rejection, in turn, of the values of heterosexual society. This has led in some respects to a celebration of casual uncommitted sex, much of which, in my view, comes into the category of 'wasted sex' and with recent developments in sexually transmitted disease, has to be seen increasingly as 'dangerous sex'. But it has served other purposes. The homosexual world has in recent times been exploring sexual relationships unfettered by conventional restraints and with an almost frantic intensity. There are many thoughtful gay men and women for whom this has provided important lessons about human sexuality. There is much that the heterosexual community can learn from these homosexuals if we are prepared to listen. (see Chapter 6 for a fuller discussion). The reaction of the gay community to the spectre of AIDS provides us with another tragic but powerful learning opportunity. One of the most poignant lessons of the AIDS epidemic is the vivid evidence it provides of the love which exists between many gay couples as they contend with the disease. Anyone who has doubted that homosexual love can be of the highest order should doubt no longer.

It is thus my belief, crucial to my sexual value system, that homosexual love and intimacy can be as valid as heterosexual love, and that the rejection of homosexuality, regardless of the nature of the homosexual relationship, is as unjustifiable as the acceptance of heterosexuality whatever form it takes.

I have been privileged to have my views on this matter subjected to theological analysis and criticism. In October 1982 the Pope John Center in St Louis, Missouri, USA, organised a meeting of scientists and Catholic theologians to discuss issues of sex and gender, with a particular emphasis on homosexuality. I was one of the scientists invited and each scientist's paper was published in a book arising from the conference (Schwartz et al 1983). Each scientific paper was followed by a theological cum philosophical critique. Mine was provided by Prof. W. A. Frank of the Benedictine College, Atchison, Kansas, who expressed the view, presumably representative of Catholic thought, that I was wrong in my basic assumption that homosexual love can be as valid as the heterosexual variety. He based this on the belief that sexuality is ineradicably linked with fertility, even if the fertile aspect is only symbolic, and that homosexual sexuality is essentially sterile.

I suspect that the Roman Catholic Church has difficulty in accepting sexual behaviour in any form (reluctance to accept the absurd and undignified passion of sexual excitement has a long history, at least in European religious thought) but sexuality clearly cannot be entirely rejected. So it is accepted by the Church, providing it is linked in some sense with reproduction, the one inescapable part of God's plan.

I react to the reproductive consequence of sex in a rather different way. It confronts us with another balancing act between good and bad; this choice is probably our most important task as sexually responsible individuals. The fact that a third person may be created by such activity leads us to some extremely complex moral issues. I reject the view that the responsibility for the creation of a third person is in the hands of God rather than the individuals concerned, and believe most strongly that one of our principal moral obligations is to avoid the creation of life when we are not in a position to ensure, to the best of our ability, the well-being of the new person. To assume that all that is required is that the two people should be married is missing the moral point. And to advocate that the responsibility should be met by avoiding all sexual contact is not only hopelessly unrealistic, but, with the availability of effective methods of fertility control, unnecessarily rejecting the considerable advantages of sex.

A morality that requires a married couple to believe that voluntary child-lessness is morally unacceptable is an influence which our seriously over-crowded human race could do without. These are issues which are not only relevant to the sexual morality of the individual but also to the collective responsibility and benefit of society.

Hypocrisy abounds in social attitudes to sexuality and has, I believe, very destructive effects. I include under this heading a tendency to accept un-wanted pregnancies amongst teenagers rather than be seen to condone sexual activity by giving them access to contraception.

Much of conventional sexual morality emphasises the key role of the parents and family in guiding the sexuality of the emerging adolescent. Attempts to provide teenagers with sex education or counselling outside the family are frequently condemned. The recent dramatic increase in awareness of the extent of child sexual abuse within the family is there-fore particularly ironic. The complex social reaction to child sexual abuse tells us something about our confused attitudes to childhood sexuality, and this subject will be discussed further in Chapter 13. But such abuse is, in my view, a clear example of 'immoral sex' and its occurrence emphasises the importance of providing children, especially adolescents, with the op-portunity to discuss their emerging sexuality with responsible adults other than their parents. I discuss in Chapter 3 the difficulties that the majority of parents have in dealing comfortably with the sexuality of their teenage children. I do believe that parents provide the most important influence on the sexual development of the *young* child, but they are not the best people to provide sexual guidance for the teenager.

The double standard is another form of hypocrisy which I reject. This, in essence, attributes responsibility for sexual behaviour to the female and in so doing gives men licence for irresponsibility which I believe has far-reaching effects. The issue is explored more fully in Chapter 5.

The conflicts of opinion and values surrounding human sexuality reflect the inherent complexity of the issues — the riddle I alluded to earlier. In stating my own views I must acknowledge the uncertainty which accompanies them, and the fact that they have changed and will no doubt continue to change as I gain further experience, undergo important changes in my personal circumstances or simply get older. It has often concerned me that my views, and those of others, about sexual morality may be determined not only by which point in the life cycle we have arrived at, but where we fall on the spectrum of sexual drive or appetite. Is it easier for an individual with a relatively low sexual appetite to adopt a restric-tive attitude to sex? Does it become easier as we get older and our sexual appetites lose their edge? Is it easier to advocate monogamy when the op-portunities for alternative sexual lifestyles have largely gone? I am sure it is important to take individual variability of sexual responsiveness into ac-count when aiming for any value system of general relevance.

I nevertheless acknowledge the need to reappraise our values and assumptions about sexual permissiveness in relation both to long-term sexual relationships or marriage, and to the sexual maturation of our teenagers. It is not that I feel any deep-rooted moral objection to a lack of sexual exclusiveness in long-term relationships. It is rather that I am increasingly aware of the difficulties that the vast majority of humans have in coping with it. The ideal of the open marriage seems to me to be a fine one. In addition to the central primary relationship, it recognises other less permanent, sexual or non-sexual relationships, which may in themselves be mutually rewarding and self-fulfilling. But few primary relationships can survive such apparent if unintended challenges. The essential security of the dyad is weakened, and further undermined by the ravages of jealousy. In addition to the psychological hazards, we are entering a new era of physical hazard lurking behind sexual activity — not just AIDS and other sexually transmitted diseases, but also the link between early sexual experience and cervical cancer (see p. 584).

As these points of view gain importance I find myself moving towards a less permissive position regarding both premarital and extramarital sexuality. But I certainly have no wish to return to the hypocrisy which permeated so much of our earlier sexual restrictions. I hope and regard as possible that out of this moral dialectic will arise some fresh, more honest form of sexual constraint that will not only steer our teenagers away from sexual danger without spoiling their unfolding joy of sexual intimacy, but also help us to avoid much of the distress and bitterness that accompanies marital breakdown these days. This, I hope, will be combined with a generally more responsible attitude to parenthood so that children will not be born because 'that is the normal thing to do' or because no suitable alternative role to parenthood is available, or because taking precautions would indicate an unacceptable degree of sexual intention, but because two people have a genuine and shared desire to experience parenthood.

Finally, I make no apology for placing so much emphasis on help or treatment for those with sexual problems. The distress and unhappiness caused by such problems is considerable and the cost in disturbed or broken families substantial. Although somatic aspects are important, many of these problems result from or are aggravated by the distorted and hypocritical attitudes to sex which have prevailed in our society. Whilst it may be true, as we shall see, that treatment and the therapists providing it can add to these distortions, such effects are largely outweighed by the benefits. There are important problems to be resolved in the field of sex therapy, not least those of ethical significance. But by continuing efforts and self-criticism the field of sex therapy should make an important contribution to a sexually healthier society in the future.

REFERENCES

Ford C S, Beach F A 1952 Patterns of sexual behaviour. Eyre & Spottiswoode, London
Masters W, Johnson V E 1966 Human sexual response. Churchill Livingstone, London
Schwartz M F, Moraczewski A S, Monteleone J A 1983 Sex and gender: a theological and scientific inquiry. Pope John Center, St Louis, Missouri

2

The biological basis of human sexuality

THE PSYCHOSOMATIC CIRCLE

The biological characteristics of an essentially sexual experience include changes in our genitalia, in particular erection of the penis and tumescence and lubrication of the vagina, heightened awareness of pleasurable erotic sensations, and changes in our subjective state which we call sexual excitement and which involve some form of central neurophysiological arousal. This is linked with cognitive processes attending to the sexual meaning of what is happening, either by focusing on external events or internal processes such as imagery. It is through this cognitive component that the whole gamut of social and interpersonal influences impinge upon our sexuality. In a proportion of occasions orgasm, perhaps the quintessence of the sexual experience, will occur.

The whole body is involved in this interplay of psychological and somatic processes. The sexual experience is par excellence psychosomatic. The genital responses, as we shall see, depend on specific local vascular mechanisms, but sexual excitement is accompanied by a more generalised cardiovascular response which is manifested in blood pressure and heart rate changes and increased blood flow to the skin. Orgasm, still largely a neurophysiological mystery, involves both central processes in the brain and widespread peripheral effects experienced as acute increases in the intensity of erotic sensation and muscle contractions which are largely involuntary.

I find it helpful to simplify this complex system using the psychosomatic circle shown in Figure 2.1. We can introduce some sequential order in this way, recognising links between (1) cognitive processes which influence (2) the limbic system and other parts of the brain, providing the neurophysiological substrate for our sexuality. This system in turn influences the periphery via (3) the spinal cord and reflex centres within it, which, via peripheral somatic and autonomic nerves, control (4) genital responses as well as (5) other peripheral manifestations of sexual excitement. Perception, awareness and cognitive processing of these peripheral and genital changes complete the circle. Fitting somewhat uncertainly in this schema is (6) the orgasm which has been given a central position in the diagram as much for

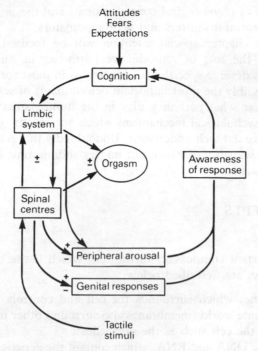

Fig. 2.1 The psychosomatic circle of sex.

symbolic as physiological reasons, though the orgasm does seem to involve mechanisms within both the brain and the spinal cord.

Because of the circularity of this system we can break into it at any point. Somewhat arbitrarily I will start at the genitalia.

Before moving on to these crucial components of sexuality it is appropriate first to consider some basic processes. The field of cellular and molecular biology and biochemistry is developing at a phenomenal rate and an aspiring sexologist cannot possibly expect to keep up with such developments in any detail whilst remaining in contact with all the other developments impinging on this field. Nevertheless it is helpful to have a passing acquaintance with the most fundamental mechanisms so that we can more easily comprehend new developments in the field of drug and hormone action, both of which are of growing importance to sexual medicine. A complex biological system of this kind involves specialised cellular mechanisms such as smooth muscle contraction and relaxation, which play a crucial role in the vascular changes leading to erection; changing sensitivity of sensory structures, and in a more general sense, increased levels of cellular activity which presumably underlie the central state of sexual excitement. In addition, the psychosomatic circle relies on communication and feedback between different parts of the system; it is often failure in these areas that leads to sexual difficulties. So we must pay some attention to new concepts of physiological control systems and the inter-related roles of hormones, neurotransmitters and neuromodulators.

Later in this chapter special attention will be focused on two other aspects: firstly, the role of reproductive hormones in human sexuality. These hormones deserve special consideration as in most subhuman species they provide possibly the most important determinants of sexual behaviour. We must be clear what part they play in the human situation. Secondly, I will discuss psychological mechanisms which act on our sexual responses in ways which are not well understood. Undoubtedly this is one of the main areas of human sexuality of which our understanding must be improved in the next few years.

BASIC CONCEPTS

THE CELL

The most important components of the cell, which is the basic functional unit of the body, are described below:

1. cell membrane, which surrounds the cell and controls its relationship with the outside world (membranes also surround other important structures within the cell such as the organelles);
2. nucleic acids, DNA and RNA, which contain the genetic message of the cell and have the capacity to manufacture protein;
3. a variety of other intracellular substances and structures.

Whilst there are many different types of specialised cells with specific functions, various basic mechanisms of cellular function which deserve brief consideration are to be found in most systems.

Electrical activity

All cells show transmembrane electropotential. Thus an electrode placed inside the cell will show a potential 50–80 mV more negative than an electrode placed outside the cell. Inside the cell the concentration of potassium (K^+) ions is high while that of sodium (Na^+) is low. The reverse applies in the extracellular space. But as the K^+ ion is smaller than the Na^+ ion there is, as a result of the concentration gradient, a diffusion of K^+ out of the cell without any compensatory shift inwards of Na^+. Therefore a negative charge builds up inside the cell to the point at which it prevents further K^+ loss. The cell in this stabilised state is said to be polarised.

Most cells, if they are subjected to a depolarising current, react by losing the transmembrane potential and becoming electrically neutral until the negative charge builds up again. But certain cells, called excitable, react in a different way to depolarisation. The loss of the negative charge overshoots zero, resulting in a brief self-limiting positive potential within the cell, which is called an action potential. This excitable response depends on special ion channels opening in the cell membrane due to conformational changes in membrane structure. This allows Na^+ ions to rush in and K^+ ions to rush out. The original negative potential is then restored by a rapid elimination of Na^+ ions.

This excitable response is a characteristic of cells such as neurons and muscle cells. Depolarisation and the production of the action potential may result from chemical opening of ion channels, which occurs at nerve endings, or by passage of the action potential across from one cell to another, which occurs between adjoining smooth muscle cells.

Receptor mechanisms

Specialised receptor molecules exist both within the cell membrane and within the cytoplasm. These combine with specific agents (i.e. agonists) such as hormones or drugs, and the agonist–receptor complex then triggers a sequence of biochemical events which results in the specific effect of that cell. Such triggering may:

1. open ion channels, as described above, and lead to an action potential or changes in other ions, such as Ca^+, which are important for influencing intracellular processes.
2. release a second messenger such as cyclic AMP or cyclic GMP which then initiates a cascade of further biochemical processes.
3. interact with the nucleic acids when the agonist–receptor complex moves through the cytoplasm to bind with specific acceptor sites on the chromatin. This results in transcription of the genetic message to messenger RNA and the initiation of protein synthesis.

CONTROL SYSTEMS

As our psychosomatic circle implies, the various types of specialised cell functions in the body are co-ordinated by a variety of control systems. These largely depend on chemical messengers which are released by one cell to affect another. Much of the body's control depends on the nervous system, in which the continuing links between neuronal cells provide the equivalent of an electrical wiring system between one part of the body and another. Nevertheless most of the communication between these neuronal cells depends on chemicals called neurotransmitters and neuromodulators. Chemical messengers may also be carried from one part of the body to another by the blood stream and this is the classical concept of the hormone. But as we shall see there are many hormone-like substances which act by diffusing from one cell to affect neighbouring cells without having to enter the blood, and others which also function as neurotransmitters or modulators between nerve cells. As our understanding of these functions increases the traditional distinction between hormone and neurotransmitter becomes increasingly blurred and we are having to revise many of our basic concepts. As Burnstock (1986) has pointed out:

> the philosophy of the evolutionary biologist would be more appropriate than the physical scientist in developing this new framework. We need to recognize the variety of mechanisms that are available and to enjoy seeing how nature utilizes various combinations of mechanisms to solve the particular problem encountered by different organs in different species.

The work of Burnstock and others (e.g. Höckfelt et al 1986) has also shown us not only that chemical messengers can act in various ways in different parts of the bodies, but that nerve transmission, previously understood to depend on single transmitter mechanisms, often depends on the action of more than one cotransmitter released by the same neuron.

THE NEURON, THE SYNAPSE AND NEUROTRANSMITTERS

The neuron is the basic cell of the nervous system. It consists of a cell body to which are attached short branches or dendrites which act as the receiving stations from other neurons, and one long branch or axon which transmits the signal onto the next neuron or other effector cell, often over long distances. The junction between the end of the axon and the dendrite of the next cell is called the synapse, or, when the axon is connecting with a muscle cell, the neuromuscular endplate. The signal is transmitted along the axon by means of a rapidly moving action potential. The duration of such signals is so short that they can be repeated several hundred times a second. When the electrical signal reaches the synapse or endplate, transmission to the next cell then depends on the release of the appropriate neurotransmitters.

Some understanding of what happens at the synapse is necessary if we are to grasp the physiological mechanisms and pharmacological influences on sexual response which will be discussed later in this chapter. A schematic representation of a synapse is shown in Figure 2.2. In the endplate or synaptic button are found small vesicles which contain neutrotransmitters. The arrival of the action potential at the synaptic button releases the transmitters from these vesicles into the synaptic gap where they make contact with the post-synaptic receptor on the receiving dendrite. The transmitter–receptor complex then initiates an action potential in the receiving cell, often by opening ion channels. This synaptic transmission is controlled in subtle and complex ways. The neurotransmitter binds only momentarily with the post-synaptic receptor. Once it is re-released three things may happen. The neurotransmitter may:

1. be destroyed by the appropriate enzyme (e.g. monoamine oxidase);
2. be reabsorbed by the synaptic button and recycled (i.e. re-uptake) or
3. bind to a receptor on the synaptic button, i.e a presynaptic receptor.

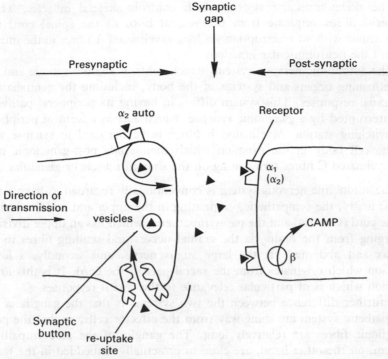

Fig. 2.2 Schematic noradrenergic synapse (adapted from Deakin & Crow 1986).
▲ = Noradrenaline transmitter.

These presynaptic receptor–transmitter complexes act as autoregulators or feedback control of the synaptic transmission, e.g. the complex may inhibit further release of the transmitter. Hence the confusing array of pharmacological effects which must be taken into account — drugs which block the destroying enzyme (e.g. monoamine oxidase inhibitors), block re-uptake of the neurotransmitter (e.g. tricylic antidepressants) or stimulate autoreceptors and hence inhibit neurotransmitter release (e.g. alpha$_2$ agonists) or act as antagonists, blocking post-synaptic receptors and preventing the transmitter action. (An antagonist is an agent which binds with the receptor without provoking the agonist–receptor complex effects, and which, by its binding, prevents an agonist from acting.)

STRUCTURE OF THE NERVOUS SYSTEM

Structural organisation of the brain is a highly complex subject which is beyond the scope of this book, though some brain structure–function relationships underlying sexuality will be considered later in this chapter. The control of the rest of the body by the central nervous system depends on two parallel networks of neurons:

1. The skeletomuscular system which controls skeletal muscles. These nerve fibres originate from the ventral horn of the spinal cord and continue without interruption via long myelinated A fibres to the muscle and the neuromuscular junction.
2. The autonomic nervous system, which controls smooth muscle and the remaining organs and systems of the body, including the genitalia and sexual responses. This system differs in having its peripheral pathways interrupted by a ganglionic synapse, which acts as a form of peripheral switching station. Myelinated B fibres leave the cord to synapse with the cell body in the ganglion which then sends post-ganglionic non-myelinated C fibres terminating on the smooth muscle or glandular cell.

The autonomic nervous system is conventionally regarded as having two parts: firstly, the sympathetic, originating in the upper and middle sections of the cord (C to L4) and the parasympathetic, which has an upper division, emerging from the brain via the cranial nerves and sending fibres to the thorax and abdomen via the large vagus nerve, and secondly, a lower division which originates from the sacral part of the cord. It is this lower division which is of particular relevance to the sexual responses.

A further difference between the two systems is that the ganglia of the sympathetic system are some way from the effector cells, so that the post-ganglionic fibres are relatively long. The ganglia of the parasympathetic system, on the other hand, are close to or actually embedded in the target organ, so that post-ganglionic fibres are very short (and the preganglionic fibres consequently longer).

The traditional model of the autonomic nervous system depicts the sympathetic and parasympathetic pathways exerting counterbalancing control on the target organs, each with its own particular neurotransmitter — acetylcholine in the parasympathetic and noradrenaline in the sympathetic, with acetylcholine acting as neurotransmitter at the ganglionic synapse in both systems. Hence the parasympathetic system is called cholinergic and the sympathetic, adrenergic. This has been shown to be a misleading oversimplification.

Adrenergic transmission involves two types of receptor, alpha and beta, based on specific pharmacological effects. Each type is further subdivided into alpha$_1$ or beta$_1$ and alpha$_2$ or beta$_2$. Beta receptors are usually inhibitory (i.e. relaxing) in their effects on smooth muscle, but have an excitatory effect on cardiac muscle. Beta$_1$ receptors are mainly found in cardiac muscle and beta$_2$ receptors in the bronchial, intestinal and vascular smooth muscle. Thus, stimulation of beta$_2$ receptors in vascular smooth muscle results in dilatation of blood vessels.

Alpha$_1$ receptors are generally excitatory, leading to constriction of the smooth muscle relaxed by beta$_2$ receptors. Alpha$_1$ receptor mechanisms are probably Ca^{2+} ionophore in type, i.e. they open up Ca^{2+} channels in the cell membrane. Beta receptors function by activating the second messenger cyclic AMP pathway.

Most alpha$_2$ receptors are functionally quite distinct. They provide the presynaptic autoregulation mechanism described above. Thus, stimulation of an alpha$_2$ receptor inhibits the release of noradrenaline at the synapse and therefore has an effect comparable to blocking either alpha$_1$ or beta receptors post-synaptically (Fig. 2.2). It is possible that alpha$_2$ receptors may also act as autoregulators in cholinergic transmission, allowing cross-talk between the adrenergic and cholinergic systems (Burnstock 1986). The picture is also complicated by the fact that some alpha$_2$ receptors are found post-synaptically; their function is not yet clear.

In the light of recent evidence, this classical model of autonomic nerve transmission must now be modified further. It is now clear that more than two neurotransmitters are involved. In addition to cholinergic and adrenergic, we have purinergic (involving a purine nucleotide, probably adenosine triphosphate (ATP), peptidergic (peptides such as vasoactive intestinal polypeptide (VIP), substance P, enkephalin, neuropeptide Y and several others) and aminergic (amino acids such as gamma-aminobutyric acid (GABA) and dopamine). Furthermore it is now apparent that more than one neurotransmitter may be operating within one synapse, resulting in various patterns of co-transmission. Burnstock (1986), for example, has described the co-transmission of noradrenaline and ATP in sympathetic nerves and acetylcholine and VIP in parasympathetic nerves. This more complex picture may account for some of the previous anomalies and inconsistencies in the pharmacological evidence, such as failure to block all cholinergic effects with atropine. A schematic model of co-transmission at

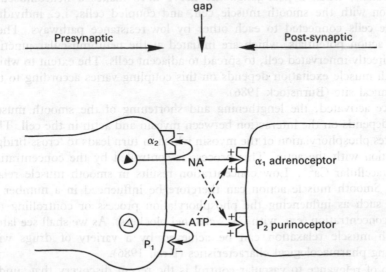

Fig. 2.3 Schematic synapse showing co-transmission by noradrenaline (NA) and adenosine triphosphate (ATP) in the sympathetic nervous control of some blood vessels. Thus each substance acts as a neurotransmitter and neuromodulator. (adapted from Burnstock 1986)

sympathetic synapses controlling vascular smooth muscle is shown in Figure 2.3. The two transmitters have different primary effects. ATP acts on purino-receptors of the smooth muscle to initiate a rapid excitatory junction potential (EJP). Noradrenaline acts on alpha$_1$ receptors to produce a slower second phase of contraction. It is also likely that each transmitter acts as a neuromodulator of the other, inhibiting release by autoregulation and enhancing effects at the post-synaptic receptor (Burnstock 1986).

This concept of co-transmission will be seen to be relevant when we consider some of the pharmacological effects on sexual response later in this chapter.

So far we have considered transmission at synapses and neuromuscular junctions in the periphery. Neurotransmission in the brain follows the same basic principles, though dopamine and 5-hydroxytryptamine play a much greater role in central transmission than they do in the periphery and we will be considering the relationship between central neurotransmission and sexual response in more detail later.

SMOOTH MUSCLE

Contraction and relaxation of smooth muscle is the basic mechanism of the vascular changes underlying genital responses. Many of the drugs which are becoming important in sexual medicine exert their effects on smooth muscle. Closer consideration of smooth muscle function is therefore warranted.

Stimulation of smooth muscle cells depends on two mechanisms: direct innervation, when a post-ganglionic nerve fibre makes a neuromuscular junction with the smooth muscle cell, and coupled cells, i.e. individual muscle cells connected to each other by low-resistance pathways. These allow action potentials, which are initiated at the neuromuscular junction of a directly innervated cell, to spread to adjacent cells. The extent to which smooth muscle excitation depends on this coupling varies according to the anatomical site (Burnstock 1986).

Once activated, the lengthening and shortening of the smooth muscle fibre depends on the interaction between myosin and actin in the cell. This requires phosphorylation of the myosin which in turn leads to 'cross-bridge' formation with the actin. This process is controlled by the concentration of intracellular Ca^{2+}. Low concentration results in smooth muscle relaxation. Smooth muscle action can therefore be influenced in a number of ways, such as influencing the phosphorylation process or controlling the Ca^{2+} concentration (e.g. with Ca^{2+} channel blockers). As we shall see later, smooth muscle relaxation can be achieved by a variety of drugs with differing pharmacological characteristics (Krall 1986).

Also of relevance to vascular control is the recent discovery that, under the influence of agents such as acetylcholine the endothelium or lining of blood vessels, releases a specific smooth muscle relaxing substance (endothelium-derived relaxing factor (EDRF)). This is of potential importance in understanding the relevance of arterial disease such as atheroma to sexual dysfunction. Thus a damaged artery may be not only mechanically obstructed by atheromatous plaque but may also be less capable of dilating when stimulated.

THE NATURE OF HORMONES

A hormone is a form of chemical messenger which typically travels from its cell of origin to its target cell via the blood stream. Some hormones are broken down so quickly by local or circulating enzymes that their effects are confined close to their site of origin. Prostaglandins, for example, are rendered inactive as they pass through the lungs. These are called *local hormones*. Other substances circulating in the blood are inactive until altered chemically in the vicinity of the target cell. These *prehormones* also allow the site of hormone action to be selective.

There are two main chemical types of hormone to be considered: steroids (e.g. oestradiol, testosterone) and peptides (e.g. gonadotrophins, prolactin). Steroid hormones, although produced in various tissues, are to some extent stored in the blood since they are bound to plasma proteins. Testosterone, for example, is present in three forms in the plasma: bound firmly to a specific globulin, called sex hormone binding globulin (SHBG; in the male 30–60% of total testosterone is in this form); bound more loosely to albumin (40–70% in this form), and unbound or free (2.5%). It is the free and to some extent relatively available albumin-bound fractions which are biologically active (Manni et al 1985), whereas the firmly bound SHBG fraction, which is in dynamic equilibrium with the other fractions, is protected from metabolic clearance and provides a store of steroid.

Peptide hormones, on the other hand, are stored in the cell or gland which makes them and released when required, often in a pulsatile fashion. Consequently, in contrast to steroids, their level in the blood may fluctuate considerably or may only be detectable for a brief period after release. It is the peptides that are likely to be found in the role of neurotransmitter as well as hormone. Some of them function principally as *releasing hormones*, i.e. releasing other peptides from their cells of origins (e.g. luteinising hormone-releasing hormone (LHRH)). Most have been found to be widely distributed in the body, suggesting that they arose at a primitive stage of development and have been adapted to serve specialised functions in some cases and in others to be involved in more varied processes. A number of these peptides will need further consideration in relation to the hormonal control of reproduction.

Most cells will only be affected by a hormone if they contain its specific receptor. Receptors for steroids lie within the cytoplasm and when activated lead to the unique steroid pattern of protein synthesis, described earlier. There is evidence that some steroids also act at the cell membrane to alter excitability of the cell. Oestradiol has an excitatory and progesterone an inhibitory effect (Dufy & Vincent 1980). Receptors for peptides are mainly found in the cell membrane, and involve a variety of second messenger pathways, such as cyclic AMP.

HORMONES AND THE REPRODUCTIVE SYSTEM

The principal hormone system concerned with reproduction and sexual behaviour is the anterior pituitary–gonadal system which we will look at more closely. The anterior pituitary–adrenal cortex system is also relevant, though it is concerned with a much wider range of functions than the reproductive or sexual. The adrenal cortex produces a proportion of the steroids related to sex, and it is partly through this pathway that acute stress may influence sex steroid levels.

The posterior pituitary releases two peptide hormones; vasopressin (or antidiuretic hormone) and oxytocin. Oxytocin causes milk ejection in the suckling woman, but it is its second effect, the contraction of uterine muscle, that is most relevant to sexual behaviour and we will consider this hormone briefly at a later stage. Both of these hormones are of interest as they are synthesised in the brain (the paraventricular and supraoptic nuclei of the hypothalamus) and then transported along the axons of the supra-opticohypophyseal nerve tract to the posterior pituitary where they are stored, bound to a specific protein, until they are released in pulsatile fashion into the blood. The posterior pituitary is thus merely a storage extension of the hypothalamus.

The local hormones of most reproductive significance are the various prostaglandins, which, though widespread in the body, do have a special and as yet incompletely understood role in the reproductive system.

THE ANTERIOR PITUITARY–GONADAL SYSTEM

The main components of this system are shown schematically in Figure 2.4. Let us look more closely at the various levels involved.

Hypothalamus

This mediates control of the system by other parts of the brain such as the cortex and pineal gland. The hypothalamus itself directly influences the system by means of controlling hormones, which it secretes and transports through the blood–brain barrier to the anterior pituitary gland by means of special blood vessels called the hypophyseal portal system. There are two controlling hormones which concern us: LHRH and prolactin-inhibiting factor (PIF).

LHRH is a short-chain polypeptide hormone which stimulates the baso-

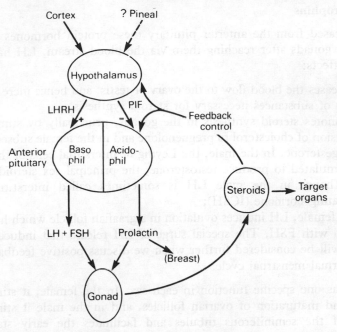

Fig. 2.4 Main components of the anterior pituitary-gonadal system. LHRH = luteinising hormone-releasing hormone; PIF = prolactin-inhibiting factor; FSH = follicle-stimulating hormone.

philic cells of the anterior pituitary to produce LH. There is still disagreement whether the same hormone also stimulates release of the other principal gonadotrophin, follicle stimulating hormone (FSH), or whether there is a slightly different releasing hormone for this purpose. Let us assume for simplicity that there is only one hormone, called LHRH. This is released in a pulsatile fashion from the ventromedial and anteromedial areas of the hypothalamus (see Fig. 2.4) which produces sharp pulsatile release of LH and rather more gradual release of FSH into the blood. LHRH is an example of a local hormone which is broken down rapidly in the blood and probably does not reach the general circulation in detectable amounts. Receptors for LHRH, or a very similar peptide, are found in other parts of the body, and, in particular, in the ovary and testis. Therefore LHRH may also serve some function in those areas either as a result of local production or by small amounts from the hypothalamus, circulating in the blood.

PIF is a dopaminergic substance, probably dopamine itself. It has an inhibitory effect on the acidophilic cells of the anterior pituitary, which without such inhibition would continue to produce prolactin. There are therefore two types of control: one stimulatory, the other inhibitory.

Gonadotrophins

Once released from the anterior pituitary these protein hormones in turn affect the gonads after reaching them via the blood stream. LH has three distinct effects:

1. It increases the blood flow to the ovary or testis, and hence increases the supply of substances necessary for steroid synthesis;
2. It promotes steroid synthesis in the gonads, principally by stimulating conversion of cholesterol to pregnenolone and in the female subsequently to progesterone. In the male, the Leydig or interstitial cells of the testis are stimulated to produce testosterone, the principal sex steroid in the male (hence in the male LH is sometimes called interstitial cell-stimulating hormone (ICSH);
3. In the female, LH induces ovulation in a graafian follicle which has been primed with FSH. The special surge of LH release that induces ovulation will be considered further when we discuss positive feedback and the normal menstrual cycle.

FSH has one specific function in each sex. In the female, it stimulates growth and maturation of ovarian follicles, and in the male it stimulates growth of the seminiferous tubules and facilitates the early stages of spermatogenesis.

The endogenous opioids are a relatively recent addition to the list of peptides. They are called opioid because they share affinity for receptors with morphine-like substances. Their discovery caused great excitement as it was thought possible that they were the 'natural analgesic'. However their effects are very widespread and they are probably best understood as peptide neurotransmitters. They undoubtedly play an important part in the hypothalamic pituitary–gonadal system, probably modulating the feedback effects of steroids on the hypothalamus and pituitary.

Prolactin remains a mystery peptide. As its name implies, it has a definite function in stimulating growth and activity of the milk-secreting system of the breast. But it probably has other effects which are less well understood. A certain amount seems to be necessary for normal steroid synthesis in the ovary, whereas too much is associated with inhibition of both ovarian and testicular function. Part of the difficulty in understanding prolactin function is that, as a hormone, it is uniquely controlled by an inhibitory substance, PIF or dopamine, which is itself a central neurotransmitter of widespread significance. Anything which leads to a reduction of dopaminergic activity in the hypothalamus will result in increased prolactin secretion. It then becomes difficult to distinguish between the effects of the raised prolactin itself and other possible effects of reduced dopaminergic activity. In other words, prolactin may simply be a marker hormone in such situations. The function of prolactin is especially obscure in the male, though as we shall see, high levels of prolactin are usually associated with impaired sexual function in men.

Inhibin is a peptide hormone of which the structure has only been described very recently, though its existence has been assumed for some time. It is produced in very small quantities by both the ovary and the testis and is believed to exert negative feedback on the hypothalamic pituitary system, specifically reducing the release of FSH. Now that it can be synthesised its precise function in reproduction may become clear in the next few years.

Steroid hormones

Sex steroids (oestrogens, progestagens and androgens) are produced principally by the gonads and the adrenal cortex. They have a wide variety of metabolic effects, but have a particular role in reproduction. They are responsible for most of the development of secondary sexual characteristics at puberty and are necessary for the establishment and maintenance of pregnancy and lactation in the female, and spermatogenesis in the male. It is their possible effects on sexual appetite and response, or arousability, that is of importance for this book, and we will therefore need to consider these steroids in some detail.

Before doing so, we should consider the next crucial step in the control of the hypothalamic pituitary–gonadal system — the feedback effects of steroids on the hypothalamus. As far as we know most of the principal sex steroids exert a negative feedback effect, probably both on the release of LHRH and the response of the anterior pituitary to LHRH. This provides a homeostatic mechanism in both the male and the female in which any rise in circulating steroid is followed by a decreased LH release (FSH is affected in a comparable way).

However, we must allow for the additional and mysterious feedback mechanism that appears to be confined to the female. In certain circumstances, as the level of oestrogen and possibly progesterone rises, the negative feedback switches into a positive feedback on either the hypothalamus, anterior pituitary or both. This explains the characteristic LH surge which precedes ovulation and which will be considered in more detail when we discuss the normal menstrual cycle.

The three principal types of sex steroid, oestrogens, progestagens and androgens, all have a common basic structure which is similar to cholesterol. There is considerable interconversion between different steroids, with a number of intermediate stages which may be present in the blood but are relatively inactive until further conversion (i.e. prehormones). The principal steroids and their intermediates are shown in Figure 2.5. Sex steroids are also closely related chemically to adrenocortical steroids. 17α-OH progesterone, for example, is a precursor of hydrocortisone and aldosterone.

The principal oestrogens are oestradiol-17β and oestrone; oestrone probably depends on conversion to the former for most of its oestrogenic activity. In the female the ovary is the principal source of oestradiol. Some

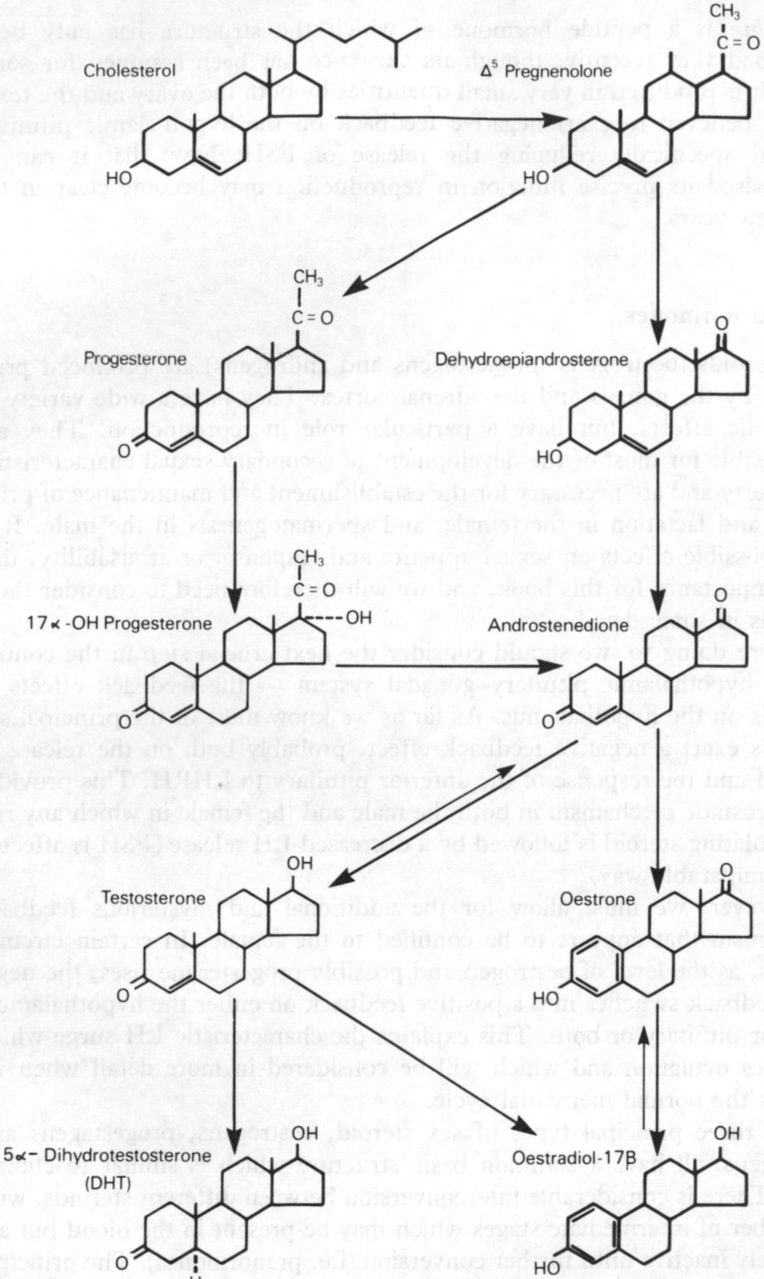

Cholesterol

Δ⁵ Pregnenolone

Progesterone

Dehydroepiandrosterone

17α -OH Progesterone

Androstenedione

Testosterone

Oestrone

5α- Dihydrotestosterone
(DHT)

Oestradiol-17β

Fig. 2.5 Sex steroids and their intermediate stages.

oestrogens are produced by the adrenal cortex, and in both men and post-menopausal women, peripheral conversion of either androstenedione or testosterone is an important source of oestrogen.

Progesterone, the principal progestagen, is produced mainly by the corpus luteum of the ovary, though it occurs as an intermediate stage in the production of other steroids by both the gonads and the adrenal cortex. It is present in the circulation of the male in negligible amounts.

The principal androgens are testosterone, dihydrotestosterone (DHT) and androstenedione. In women, androstenedione is the androgen which is present in largest amounts in the blood, and it is converted into testosterone and DHT in the tissues. Approximately 50% of a woman's androstenedione comes from the ovary; the other half comes from the adrenal cortex. In the male, the main circulating androgen is testosterone, which is mainly produced by the testes, although negligible amounts come from the adrenals. Circulating DHT comes from both sources but is mainly produced peripherally in the tissues.

The binding of testosterone and oestradiol to SHBG has already been mentioned as a method of protecting the steroid from metabolic breakdown. Other steroids such as androstenedione, oestrone and progesterone are only weakly bound, mainly to albumin. Steroids are metabolised mainly by the liver and kidney to water-soluble conjugates of sulphuric and glucuronic acid. These are then excreted in the urine. Conjugates of both oestrone and oestradiol appear in the urine and can be measured as such, thus providing an index of the daily production of oestrogens. The main urinary products of testosterone arc androsterone and aetiocholanolone, and of progesterone, pregnanediol.

FUNCTIONS OF SEX STEROIDS

The functions of sex steroids are complex and varied; few systems are immune to their metabolic effects. We can list their main sites of action which concern us under three headings;

1. Reproductive tract and genital organs;
2. Secondary sexual characteristics;
3. Central nervous system, particularly those parts of the limbic system which subserve sexual behaviour.

We will briefly consider the first two headings now. The third, the effects on the central nervous system and behaviour, will be dealt with more fully later in this chapter.

Effects of steroids on the reproductive tract and secondary sexual characteristics

Androgens

The fundamental part androgens play in sexual differentiation and early anatomical development will be considered in Chapter 3. In the male, the increases in these hormones which occur at puberty are responsible for the enlargement of the penis, scrotum and possibly testes as well as for the greater responsiveness of these tissues to tactile stimulation (see Fig. 2.19, p. 37). Androgens also determine the characteristic pattern of masculine body hair growth, which is not usually fully expressed until well into adult life. They affect the larynx, resulting in deepening of the voice, which is characteristic of male puberty. The sweat and sebaceous glands are activated, sometimes leading to the acne which is so common at this age. Androgens promote increased muscle bulk and influence bone growth in a way which is not completely understood. The adolescent growth spurt in boys probably depends on low levels of testosterone characteristic of pre- and early puberty. As higher levels develop they lead to epiphyseal closure and cessation of the growth spurt.

In the post-pubertal male, testosterone is necessary for normal spermatogenesis and secretory activity of the prostate gland and seminal vesicles.

In the female the somatic function of androgens is less well understood. Androgens obviously contribute to body hair growth and sebaceous gland activity. They may be necessary in small amounts for the normal pubertal development of the external genitalia, especially the labia majora and clitoris which are the embryological counterparts of the scrotum and penis. We know that high doses of exogenous androgens may produce enlargement and increased sensitivity of the clitoris in adult women, but this may not be a physiological effect. Androgens may also contribute to epiphyseal closure in the female, though the levels involved are much smaller.

Oestrogens

In the pubertal girl oestrogens cause enlargement of the breasts. They also influence pubertal growth of the uterus and fallopian tubes, vagina and vulva and are largely responsible for the adolescent growth spurt in girls (Short 1980a). Of particular importance to normal sexual response is the effect oestrogens have on the vaginal epithelium. They appear to be necessary for the normal vaginal transudate which follows erotic stimulation, though the mechanism involved is not understood.

Oestrogens may influence pubic and axillary hair growth, though this is not certain. They stimulate the endometrium to proliferate and they indirectly provoke ovulation; these effects will be considered in more detail when we deal with the menstrual cycle.

The functions of oestrogens in the male are not understood. They may be responsible for the slight and transient breast enlargement that occasionally occurs at puberty (gynaecomastia of puberty). They may also play an important part in the control of normal bone growth and epiphyseal closure in the male.

Progestagens

Progesterone, as its name implies, has a special function in maintaining pregnancy which will be considered further below. In the non-pregnant woman it is mainly produced by the corpus luteum. In most of its effects it acts synergistically with other hormones, in particular oestrogens. It acts both on breast tissue that has been primed with oestrogen to promote the growth of alveoli and subsequent milk production. In the endometrium, the proliferative state produced by oestrogens in the first half of the menstrual cycle is changed into the secretory endometrium by the addition of progesterone.

Some synthetic progestagens have androgenic effects which are considered later. With progesterone, the naturally occurring progestagen, these effects are probably negligible.

BIOLOGICAL RHYTHMS AND NORMAL PATTERNS OF HORMONAL CHANGE

An important source of information about hormonal effects on behaviour in humans stems from the patterns of hormone change which normally occur. These include the various biological rhythms as well as the changes that occur predictably through the life span associated in particular with puberty and ageing. We will consider the nature of these basic patterns before using them to further our understanding of human sexuality.

Of the various endocrine rhythms or cycles in the human the most important is the menstrual cycle. Others are the diurnal rhythm and a possible seasonal rhythm (see p. 99).

The menstrual cycle

This fascinating aspect of endocrine function is fundamental not only to our reproduction, but also to the state of womanhood, being, apart from anatomy, the most distinct female characteristic. At a time when methods are available for controlling or stopping the menstrual cycle, its biological and psychological significance become of great topical interest. As yet there are still many mysteries surrounding this phenomenon, though the gaps in our knowledge are gradually being filled.

By convention the first day of menstruation is regarded as the first day of a new cycle. This is the beginning of the follicular or proliferative phase — the first term referring to the growth of a new follicle in the ovary, the second to the proliferation of the endometrium which accompanies it. From the beginning there is a gradual rise in levels of FSH and LH due to an increase in the frequency of pulsatile release of these hormones from the pituitary. This leads to the development of a new graafian follicle and secretion of steroids (oestradiol-17β, androstenedione and 17α-hydroxy-progesterone, a precursor) by the theca interna cells. As the oestradiol rises so the FSH level starts to fall because of negative feedback. The LH does not fall as one might expect; instead when the oestradiol reaches a certain level

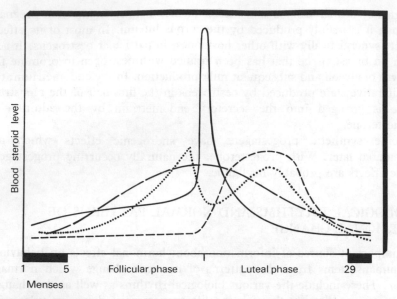

Fig. 2.6 Hormone changes during the menstrual cycle. ——— = luteinising hormone;
. . . . . . = oestradiol; - - - - - = progesterone; ——— ——— = testosterone.

it triggers the characteristically female positive feedback response, which produces the preovulatory surge of LH. This then provokes ovulation from the by now ripe follicle, a mature ovum being released into the fallopian tube. Once this takes place the follicle becomes a corpus luteum which secretes large amounts of progesterone as well as oestradiol. There is thus a peak of oestrogen in the late follicular phase, followed by the LH peak, followed by ovulation, a rise in progesterone and a second rise in oestrogen. These are shown in Figure 2.6. After ovulation we enter the second phase of the cycle, called luteal (i.e. dependent on the corpus luteum) or secretory, referring to the further change in the endometrium induced by the combination of progesterone and oestrogen. This prepares the endometrium for implantation of the ovum if it is fertilised. The corpus luteum has a limited life and when it starts to regress the progesterone and oestrogen levels fall, followed by spasm of the endometrial arteries and the consequent shedding of the endometrial lining, called menstruation. This brings us to the beginning of the next cycle.

How this system switches from negative to positive feedback in the case of LH, and what produces the luteal regression are the two principal mysteries of the menstrual cycle.

Pregnancy

The pregnant condition has special endocrine characteristics, largely due to the presence of an additional endocrine gland, the placenta. The endocrine function of this organ does depend however on its 'collaboration' with both the mother and the fetus. It relies on a maternal supply of cholesterol for steroid synthesis and on fetal liver enzymes for some of the later stages of steroid production, in particular that of oestriol, the oestrogen of pregnancy. It is also capable of producing huge quantities of progesterone. The placenta is also unusual in being apparently autonomous, i.e. not controlled by either negative or positive feedback.

The earliest and still mysterious phenomenon of pregnancy is the recognition by the mother's reproductive system that fertilisation or implantation has occurred. This in some way prevents the usual monthly regression of the corpus luteum and hence allows continued production of progesterone which is essential for the continuation of pregnancy. In the human female the self-protective effect of the conceptus is probably due to the action of human chorionic gonadotrophin (HCG)), a peptide hormone produced by it; a second peptide hormone (human chorionic somatomammotrophin (HCS)) may act together with HCG to form the luteotrophic complex. HCG is very similar in structure to LH and is produced in large quantities by the trophoblastic layer of the placenta early in pregnancy, providing the basis for the usual forms of pregnancy test. When injected into non-

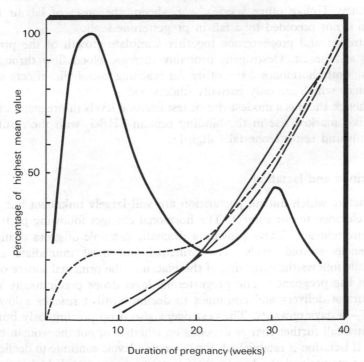

Fig. 2.7 Plasma hormone concentrations during pregnancy and their relation to placental weight. ——— = human chorionic gonadotrophin; ----- = progesterone; ——— ——— = total oestrogens; ——— = placental weight. (Heap & Flint 1984)

pregnant women or men it acts like LH. In the pregnant woman, in addition to maintaining the corpus luteum of pregnancy, it probably stimulates steroid synthesis by the placenta itself. HCS has many of the properties of a mixture of growth hormone and prolactin. It is also produced in large quantities, although it reaches its peak later rather than earlier in pregnancy (Fig. 2.7). In addition to its luteotrophic action it promotes growth of the breast, and may have other functions which are as yet not understood.

In the human, the essential role of the corpus luteum of pregnancy is short-lived because by the 20th week the placenta takes over and its production of progesterone and oestrogens continues to rise enormously until the end of pregnancy, reflecting the lack of any regulation by the hypothalamic pituitary system (see Fig. 2.7).

As previously mentioned, progesterone usually acts synergistically with other hormones, especially oestrogen. Understanding its effects is complicated by the fact that this synergism varies with the progesterone:oestrogen ratio, probably being maximal when the ratio is approximately threefold. As the ratio declines the effects of the two steroids tend to become mutually antagonistic.

Progesterone reduces the excitability of the myometrium and its responses to oxytocin and this may play an important part in maintaining pregnancy. Unlike other species, e.g. sheep, the onset of labour in the human is not preceded by a fall in progesterone level.

Oestrogen and progesterone together stimulate growth of the pregnant uterus and breast. Oestrogens probably increase blood flow through the uterus. Both hormones have other far-reaching metabolic effects during pregnancy which are only partially understood.

Although there is a modest rise of testosterone levels in pregnant women, there is a marked rise in the binding protein SHBG, with the result that free unbound testosterone falls slightly.

Parturition and lactation

The factors which initiate parturition are still largely unknown but are of little relevance to our subject. The hormonal changes following parturition are more relevant. These provide a dramatic example of gross changes in endogenous steroid levels. The principal and most immediate change obviously follows the expulsion of the placenta, the principal source of steroids in late pregnancy. The progesterone level drops precipitously within 24 hours of delivery and continues to decline until it reaches a low level from 7–14 days onwards. The oestrogens also drop precipitously but after the initial fall further change depends on whether or not the woman breast-feeds. If lactation is established, the oestrogen levels continue to decline and are then maintained at a low level. If lactation is not established oestrogens rise to more normal levels from the third post-partum week, until normal menstruation resumes. Prolactin, which is at a high level in late pregnancy, dips only slightly during the early stages of breastfeeding, whereas in the non-lactating woman it declines to within the normal range by the end of the third week (Fig. 2.8).

Thus the hormonal pattern continuing during the puerperium depends on whether lactation is established. We see the ingenious way in which parturition allows lactation to start in the well prepared but previously non-lactating breast. During pregnancy, the placenta, as already mentioned, acts autonomously and produces large quantities of oestrogen. This acts synergistically with progesterone and prolactin to produce full development of the milk-secreting mechanism but the oestrogens also inhibit actual milk production. In addition they have a positive feedback effect on the acidophilic cells of the anterior pituitary, stimulating prolactin production. Once the placenta is expelled, oestrogen production is largely dependent on the ovary which of course is always susceptible to external control. Part of this control is by prolactin or at least the changes in the dopaminergic system related to prolactin, which inhibit oestrogen production, whilst being maintained by the reflex effects of suckling. Consequently prolactin levels are maintained whilst oestrogen levels fall, allowing milk production and release to ensue. It may be the maintenance of prolactin levels during lactation and the consequent ovarian suppression that underlies the amenorrhoea and infertility of the lactation woman (see Chapter 12). This effect weakens, however, as lactation continues. After the 10th week or so prolactin levels gradually fall and ovulation may occur in spite of continued breastfeeding (Bonnar et al 1975). The frequency of suckling may be an important factor. The return to ovulatory cycles is most likely to occur after there has been a substantial drop in suckling frequency and the introduction of supplementary feeds (Howie et al 1982).

HORMONE LEVELS DURING CHILDHOOD AND ADOLESCENCE

The post-natal period

At birth the male infant has circulating levels of testosterone which are approximately half that of the normal adult (i.e. approximately 240 mg/100 ml), whereas the levels in the female infant are similar to those in the adult, and much lower than in the male (i.e. approximately 30 mg/100 ml). In both sexes there is a dramatic drop within the first few days, presumably due to the withdrawal of HCG. Oestrogen levels also drop to prepubertal levels in both sexes (see Fig. 2.9).

The sensitivity of the hypothalamus to negative feedback has still not reached its maximum at birth, so that with the withdrawal of HCG there is a further rise in LH and FSH.

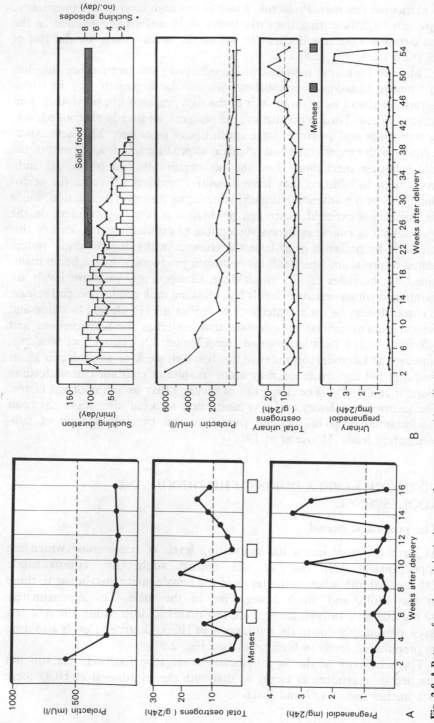

Fig. 2.8 A Return of ovarian activity (urinary total oestrogens > 10 ug/24 h) in a bottlefeeding mother. **B** Delayed return of ovarian activity and ovulation (urinary pregnanediol > 1 mg/24 h) in the early puerperium in a breastfeeding mother. (Courtesy of A S McNeilly; Howe & McNeilly 1982)

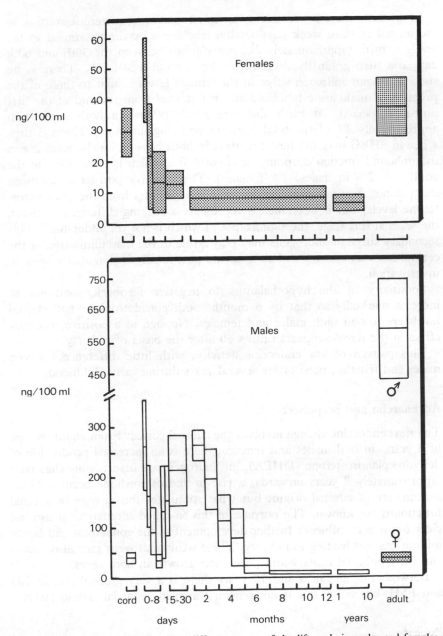

Fig. 2.9 Plasma testosterone levels at different stages of the life cycle in males and females — means and s.d. (From Forest et al 1976)

In the male there is secondary rise in circulating testosterone starting in the second or third week post-natally, reaching a maximum similar to the levels at birth (approximately 260 mg/100 ml) between the 30th and 60th day, and then gradually declining to low prepubertal levels. There is no such post-natal androgen surge in the female; levels similar to those of the prepubertal male are established and maintained from the end of the first post-natal period. At birth they are relatively low in both sexes with approximately 3% of the total testosterone being unbound. There is then a rise in SHBG over the next few days in both boys and girls, resulting in the unbound fraction dropping to about 0.7%, which is lower than in the adult (i.e. 2% in males, 1% females). The effective post-natal androgen surge is not therefore quite as dramatic as it appears from the total testosterone levels, but it nevertheless represents a striking difference between the sexes at this stage, the significance of which is not yet understood. This secondary surge of androgens may play a role in the masculinisation of the central nervous system, and as it occurs post-natally is potentially open to investigation.

Sensitivity of the hypothalamus to negative feedback continues to increase markedly so that by 6 months both gonadotrophins and steroid levels are low in both males and females. No sign of a positive feedback effect in the female appears until well after the onset of puberty.

This pattern of low endocrine activity, with little difference between males and females, persists for several years during early childhood.

Adrenarche and prepuberty

The next endocrine change involves the adrenal cortex. From about the age of 6 years, in both males and females, there is an increased production of dehydroepiandrosterone (DHEA), an androgen precursor; somewhat later (approximately 8 years onwards) a rise in androstenedione occurs. These steroids are of adrenal origin, but what stimulates this change in adrenal function is not known. The purpose of this so-called adrenarche is also not clear but it may influence further development of the gonadostat and hence initiate changes leading to puberty. These weak androgens may also stimulate early pubertal axillary and pubic hair growth in both sexes.

Between the ages of 6 and 10 years there is a very gradual rise in LH and FSH, but as yet this is not reflected in rising gonadal steroid levels.

Puberty

The precise mechanism controlling the onset of puberty is still uncertain. It probably depends on a change in the production and release of LHRH, but whether this results from a decrease of an inhibitory signal or increase in stimulatory drive is not yet clear. This change is associated with a progressive reduction in the sensitivity of the hypothalamus to negative feedback, resulting in a more substantial rise in gonadotrophins and steroids until a new gonadostat level is set. (Cameron et al 1989; Hopwood et al 1989). The possible effects of adrenal steroids have already been mentioned. Other hormonal factors may also be involved. The response of the testis to HCG administration has been shown to increase closer to puberty, indicating that some maturation of the testis is also involved. The pituitary response to LHRH administration also increases. However the rise in gonadotrophins also occurs in individuals without gonads. Obviously more is involved than a reduction of negative feedback. Presumably some maturational process in the hypothalamus is taking place.

The earliest signs of pubertal endocrine changes are nocturnal surges of gonadotrophins before there is any noticeable change in daytime levels.

Puberty in the male

In the male it is not until a bone age of approximately 12 years is reached that there is any increase in testosterone production. Thereafter it rises steeply until the age of 15 to 17 years, after which there is a further slight rise to adult levels by the early or mid 20s. The LH and FSH levels, having risen at puberty, decline in late adolescence until they reach lower adult levels, presumably reflecting the increased steroidogenic and spermatogenic potential of the fully grown testis. There is also a fall in SHBG during adolescence to adult levels.

Oestrogens in the male are predominantly in the form of oestrone. Though the testis secretes oestradiol and small amounts of oestrone, the majority of oestrogen comes from the peripheral conversion of androgens to oestrone.

The development of the secondary sexual characteristics accompanying the hormonal change of puberty is varied in its timing. The earliest change is accelerated growth of the testes and scrotum (9.5–13.5 years). Shortly after this pubic hairs begin to appear. About a year later the penis starts to grow (10.5–14.5 years) accompanied by development of the internal structures, the seminal vesicles and prostate (see Fig. 2.19). About a year after the start of penile growth the first ejaculation occurs. The growth spurt in boys starts between 10.5 and 16 years with deceleration of growth starting about 18 months later. The voice starts to break and deepen towards the end of the growth spurt (Marshall & Tanner 1970). About one-third of boys show noticeable enlargement of the breasts around the middle of puberty which normally recedes after about a year.

The considerable difference in timing and speed of these pubertal changes contributes to the uncertainty about body image that adds to the adolescent's problems. The age of onset of puberty has also declined over the past 200 years. Daw (1970) in a study of J. S. Bach's choir in Leipzig, found that the average age at which boys' voices changed from treble to alto was 17 to $17\frac{1}{4}$ years. In London today it is 13.3 years.

Puberty in the female

The timing of pubertal changes in girls is well documented. Breast development and growth of pubic hair usually starts between the ages of 9 and 13 years, whilst menarche occurs normally between $11\frac{1}{2}$ and $15\frac{1}{4}$ years (Marshall & Tanner 1969). The mean age at menarche has declined about 1 year between the beginning of this century and the late 1970s to about 12.5 years (MacMahon 1973). The growth spurt starts about 2 years earlier in girls than in boys. The girls' growth therefore ends earlier, contributing to the sex difference in size. The relationship between these events and hormonal changes is less well documented. Brown et al (1978) found that breast development coincides with a rise of oestrogen from earlier childhood levels and that oestrogen levels then start to fluctuate, often irregularly at first, causing bleeding when levels are high enough. Probably the commonest sequence of events is a series of anovulatory cycles before a full ovulatory cycle occurs, though the time between onset of menstruation and ovulation must be very variable (see Chapter 5, section on adolescent infertility).

Once normal regular cycles are established — and this may take several months — they usually continue in a predictable way, normally interrupted only by pregnancy and lactation. A proportion of women have irregular cycles and unpredictable ovulation.

SEXUAL RESPONSES

HUMAN SEXUAL ANATOMY

At a time when biological differences between men and women are being questioned and challenged, the anatomical differences of the genitalia remain incontrovertible, in spite of common embryological origins (see Chapter 3).

The woman

The appearance of the vulva or external genitalia of a nulliparous woman is shown in Figure 2.10. Only the labia majora are visible. These are well endowed with fat and covered, together with the mons, by pubic hair with a characteristically female distribution, with the appearance of an inverted triangle with its base as a straight line across the mons. (The male distribution is rhomboidal with hair typically spreading up the midline towards the navel.) To observe the other structures it is necessary to separate the

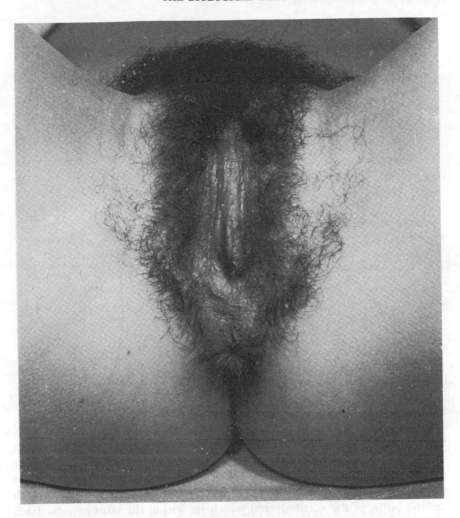

Fig. 2.10 The external genitalia of the female.

labia (Fig. 2.11) when the glans of the clitoris, labia minora and urethral and vaginal openings come into view.

The clitoris

The clitoris is a much more extensive structure than its visible part, the glans, would suggest. Although it is primarily a sensory organ with an intensive sensory nerve supply in its glans, its deeper structures do fulfil other functions. Like the penis, it has a body formed from two corpora cavernosa and a single corpus spongiosum. It is firmly anchored to the underlying bone by the attachment of the diverging crura or roots of the corpora cavernosa. These erectile structures thus form a resilient padding along

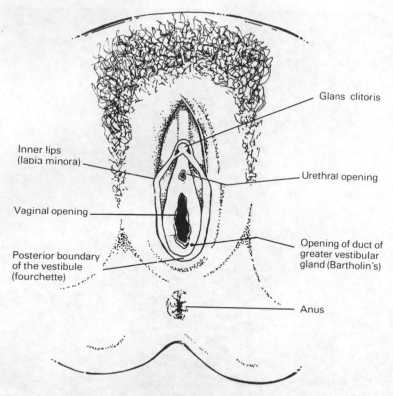

Fig. 2.11 The external genitalia of the female with the labia drawn apart.

the bony margins of the arch, not only promoting the woman's comfort during penile thrusting, but also providing erotic stimulation to the deeper parts of the clitoris. The corpus spongiosum is formed by fusion above the urethral orifice of two sausage-shaped masses of erectile tissue, which are the bulbs of the vestibule and which lie within the labia majora. Each bulb is invested by a thin layer of muscle, the bulbospongiosum. We would therefore underline the anatomical continuity and functional link between these deeper parts of the clitoris and the vagina, which is effectively lengthened anteriorly by the swelling of these erectile structures during sexual arousal (Fig. 2.12).

The vulva

Also flanking the vaginal opening are the labia minora, which are folds of skin much thinner than the labia majora, devoid of fat but also highly vascular. Anteriorly, as the labia minora converge towards the clitoris, they each bifurcate into two smaller folds, the inner of which merge together in the midline to form the frenulum of the glans of the clitoris. The outer folds form a fold of skin or prepuce enveloping the clitoris near its tip.

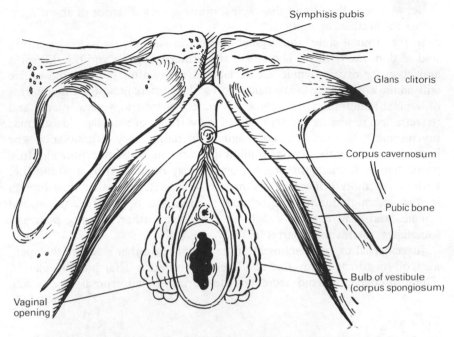

Fig. 2.12 Deep erectile structures of the clitoris. Homologous erectile structures, which in the male are incorporated into the body of the penis, are in the female displaced around the vaginal opening. The corpora cavernosa provide a cushion in their attachment to the pubic bone whereas the corpora spongiosa (divided in the female) form the deep erectile tissues underlying the labia majora.

Posteriorly the labia minora are joined behind the vaginal opening by a sharp fold of skin, the fourchette. The area bounded by the clitoris, labia minora and fourchette is termed the vestibule and is normally moist. During sexual arousal not only do the erectile tissues of the deeper clitoral structures become engorged, but so do the labia minora which consequently become a little everted, exposing their inner moist surfaces and further preparing the vestibule for entry of the penis. If penile entry is attempted in the sexually unaroused female, the flaccid labia minora may be carried into the vaginal opening, causing discomfort. In the aroused woman, reciprocal movement of the engorged labia minora during penile thrusting serves to stimulate the body and glans of the clitoris.

In multiparous women, the vascular engorgement of the labia minora which occurs during pregnancy and childbirth leads to a permanent enlargement due to a degree of varicosity of the contained vasculature. As a result, the labia minora are often visible between the labia majora, even in the unaroused state. This accounts for the considerable variability in external appearance of the vulva in different women, many of whom are self-conscious about this appearance and may be reassured to learn that such variation is usual after childbearing.

Between the clitoris and the vaginal opening — a distance of about 2 cm — lies the urethral opening.

In the virginal state, the vaginal opening is partially occluded by a thin fold of skin, the hymen. The size of the hymeneal orifice and the thickness and elasticity of the hymen are variable. Usually after puberty the orifice will admit a finger. In a woman who has had intercourse (or other forms of vaginal penetration) the hymen is generally torn in several places and its retracted remnants are represented by a fringe of skin tags (carunculae myrtiformes) surrounding the vaginal opening. Very occasionally, the hymen is sufficiently elastic to allow penetration without rupturing. In a proportion of women, the original hymen may be divided by a strand (i.e. with two or more orifices). This may become stretched rather than broken so that although intercourse or tampon insertion is possible, the strand remains and may become caught or stretched further, causing pain and sometimes vaginismus (Sarrel 1976).

Just external to the attachment of the hymen, on either side, are the openings of the ducts from the two greater vestibular (Bartholin's) glands. These discharge mucoid secretion late during sexual arousal (see p. 62).

The vagina

The vagina is a tube which, in the non-aroused state, is collapsed with a cross-section shaped like the letter H. It is usually 10–11 cm in length to the depth of the posterior fornix. The lumen of the vagina, when distended, is like an inverted flask. This is because the upper two-thirds are lax and capacious, whereas the lower third is closely invested by the surrounding pelvic floor muscles. The strongest of these muscles is the levator ani, the fibres of which form a U-shaped sling around the posterior and lateral vaginal wall at the junction of the lower and middle third. Intense spasm of this muscle in a nulliparous woman can virtually occlude the vagina (see discussion of vaginismus, pp. 381–3; Fig. 2.13). Poor tone in these muscles, or the inability to contract them voluntarily, has been blamed for loss of sexual pleasure and even orgasmic difficulties (Graber 1982) (see p. 381).

In the non-aroused woman, the vagina is normally curved backwards over the pelvic floor (see Fig. 2.13) and is not straight, as is often portrayed in anatomical texts. The vaginal wall includes a thick rugose lining of squamous epithelium, layers of longitudinal and circular plain muscle, and a very extensive plexus of veins, especially on the lower part. There is a rich arterial blood supply.

The uterus

The uterus, a pear-shaped organ with a thick muscular wall, has a narrow lower part, the cervix or neck, which protrudes into the anterior wall of the

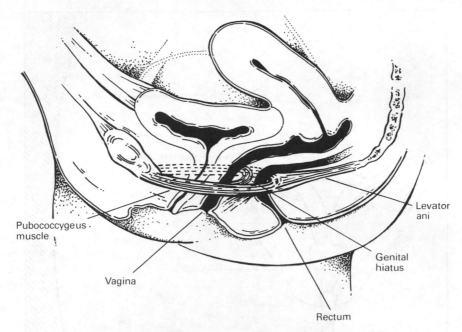

Pubococcygeus
muscle

Levator
ani

Genital
hiatus

Vagina

Rectum

Fig. 2.13 The muscular supports of the vagina. This diagram shows the sling of muscle fibres surrounding the urethra, vagina and rectum, running from the pubic bone to the coccyx. The levator plate formed by these fibres supports the rectum and the vagina in its non-aroused horizontal position.

vagina near its upper limit. The narrow cervical canal linking the vagina with the uterine cavity is lined by mucus-secreting glands. The recesses at the upper end of the vagina surrounding the cervix are called the fornices.

Usually, the uterus inclines forwards from its attachment to the upper vagina, forming an acute angle anteriorly, when it is said to be anteverted. In a minority of women the uterus is retroverted. The cervix then points downwards and forwards into the vagina, and the body of the uterus lies immediately above the posterior fornix. The upper parts of the vagina and the cervix are tethered to the side walls of the pelvis by a radiating mesh of connective tissue, the parametrium, which contains smooth muscle fibres.

The ovaries

The fallopian tubes (oviducts) enter the upper part of the uterus on each side. The ovaries lie lateral to the uterus below the fallopian tubes (see Fig. 2.14). Each contains ova (egg cells) surrounded by a cluster of cells forming a follicle. Every month a single follicle ripens and the ovum is discharged to be collected by the fimbria of the fallopian tube and transported down its length to the uterine cavity.

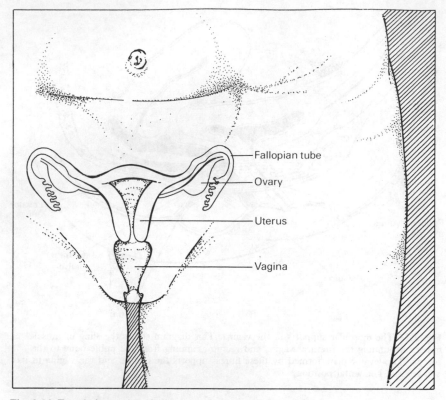

Fig. 2.14 Female internal genitalia.

The man

The penis

The shaft or body of the penis is formed principally by a fused pair of corpora cavernosa, cylinders of tough fibrous tissue, the tunica albuginea, filled with a sponge-like lattice of vascular spaces or erectile tissue which inflates with blood during erection. The detailed structure of this erectile tissue is of fundamental importance to the mechanism of erection, and will be considered in more detail on p. 53. The bulk of this tissue consists of vascular spaces or sinusoids containing smooth muscle in their walls. Beneath the two fused corpora cavernosa lies another erectile column, the corpus spongiosum which envelops the urethra in its course along the lower surface of the penis (Figs. 2.15, 2.16). Engorgement of the corpus spongiosum occurs in such a way that the urethral lumen avoids occlusion by compression and remains sufficiently patent for the rapid ejaculation of seminal fluid. This patency is partly maintained by specialised surrounding fibrous architecture. But in any case, the pressures in the spongiosum during erection are much lower than those found in the corpora

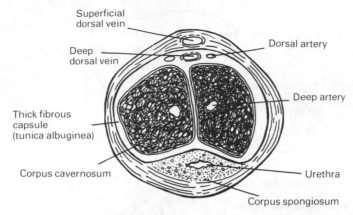

Fig. 2.15 Cross-section of the body of the penis, showing erectile spaces and principal blood vessels.

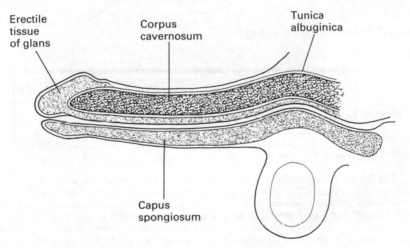

Fig. 2.16 Erectile tissues of the penis. Each crus of the corpora cavernosa is inserted into the pubic bone.

cavernosa which are consequently the most important structures in the fully erect penis. At the root of the penis the corpora cavernosa diverge to be firmly attached to the pelvic bones. The corpus spongiosum expands around the dilated part of the urethra to form the bulb of the urethra (see Fig. 2.16).

Near the root of the penis, the outer surfaces of the erectile columns are invested by layers of muscle, the bulbospongiosus and ischiocavernosus muscles which contract rhythmically during orgasm and also semi-voluntarily during the development of erections (see Figs. 2.17, 2.18). Contraction of these muscles may contribute to the development of the high pressures within the corpora cavernosa; however their role in this respect has not been established (see below).

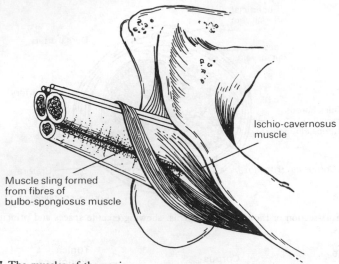

Fig. 2.17 The muscles of the penis.

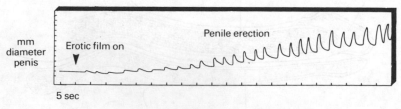

Fig. 2.18 Rhythmic contractions of the penile muscles (bulbospongiosus and ischiocavernosus) during the development of an erection. About one in four men tested in the laboratory show this pattern. Most are aware of these contractions and can prevent them if asked. In the case illustrated here, the subject was unable to stop them and the contractions were also observed during his nocturnal erections. Their functional significance is not known, but some men try to 'pump up' their erection in this way. It is not yet clear whether this helps or hinders the erection. With a full erection such contractions produce transient dramatic increases in intracavernosal pressure which increase the rigidity of the erect penis. (See p. 59)

Near the tip of the penis, the corpus spongiosum expands to form the glans, a cushion-like expansion of the penile shaft, separated from it by a shallow groove. In the uncircumcised male, the glans is covered by a hood of lax skin, the prepuce or foreskin which is wholly or partially removed in those males who have been circumcised (Fig. 2.19). On the lower surface, the prepuce is attached to the glans by a longitudinal fold of skin, the frenum. The separation of the foreskin from the underlying glans is sometimes incomplete in the neonate and normally requires androgens for its completion. During erection of the penis, the foreskin is partially retracted by tension of the skin along the elongated penile shaft, exposing the tip of the glans and the urethral orifice. During coital thrusting, the foreskin is

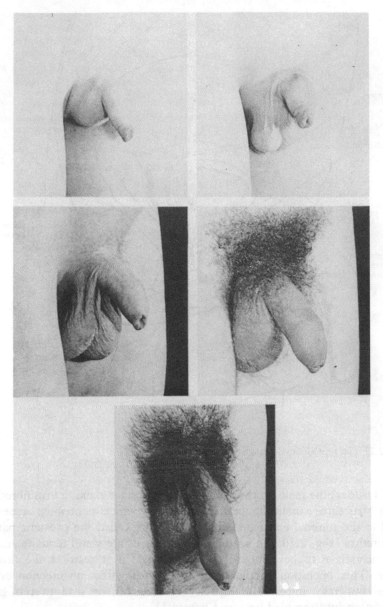

Fig. 2.19 Normal male genitalia showing the five stages of development of genitals and pubic hair as defined by Marshall & Tanner (1970). (From van Wieringen et al 1971)

intermittently retracted further by friction with the vaginal walls, exposing the glans completely. If however the mobility of the preputial skin is restricted, difficulty and discomfort may result during intercourse (see p. 379).

Beyond the dilated urethral bulb, and before its junction with the uri-

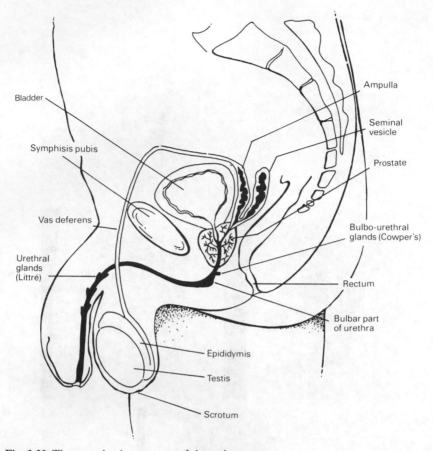

Fig. 2.20 The reproductive anatomy of the male.

nary bladder, the male urethra traverses the prostate gland, a firm fibromuscular structure containing branching glands which contribute accessory fluid to the seminal ejaculate. This is therefore called the prostatic part of the urethra (Fig. 2.20). In ageing males the prostate gland tends to enlarge and may have to be removed (prostatectomy) if it restricts the flow of urine. This operation should have no physical effect on erection or orgasm, but may impair the capacity to ejaculate or lead to retrograde ejaculation into the bladder (see Chapter 11).

The testes

The male gonads or testes lies in a superficial pouch of skin and muscle, the scrotum. The testes develop during fetal life in the abdominal cavity and migrate down into the scrotum during the latter part of fetal development. This 'externalisation' of the testes provides them with a cooler environmental temperature which is essential for normal spermatogenesis. In boys in whom there is a failure of testicular descent, i.e. undescended testes or cryptorchidism, damage to the testes both in their germinal and endocrine functions will result unless the condition is treated. Within the scrotum, the level of the testes is controlled by two muscles, the dartos which can corrugate and shrink the scrotal wall, and the cremaster muscle which forms a sling encircling the testis and spermatic cord within the scrotum.

The testes contain two principal types of cells, the interstitial (Leydig) cells which produce steroid hormones, principally testosterone, and the tubular cells from which spermatozoa are derived. The sperm pass from the seminal tubules into a long convoluted tubule which forms the epididymis of the testis. The structure is linked on each side to the urethra by a long fibromuscular tube, the vas deferens, which at its upper end expands to form the ampulla of the vas. This is a storage chamber for sperm, lying behind the bladder.

The seminal vesicles are two elongated sacs which also lie behind the bladder and prostate gland. They secrete a significant volume of accessory fluid which is discharged along the ejaculatory duct together with the contents of the ampullae of the vas, into the prostatic part of the urethra. Further secretion during sexual arousal comes from the bulbourethral (Cowper's) glands which lie on each side of the urethra near its bulbous portion and the urethral glands along the penile part of the urethra. This can lead to discharge of fluid before ejaculation occurs, and in many men at a relatively early stage of sexual arousal. The fluid is clear and viscous and varies considerably in amount between men. Some 22% of Kinsey's subjects reported no such secretion whereas about 18% normally experienced fairly excessive secretion, sufficient to drip from the penis Gebhard & Johnson 1979). In some men this is a source of embarrassment. The function of this fluid is not known, but it has sometimes been found to contain a few sperm.

The blood supply

The blood supply of the penis is important since disease in these vessels may be an important cause of erectile failure (see Chapter 11). Although there is considerable variation (Ginestie & Romieu 1978), the commonest arrangement is as follows. The internal pudendal artery, which is one of the two terminal branches of the anterior trunk of the internal iliac artery, passes round the side of the pelvis until it reaches the inner side of the lower part of the pubic bone. Close to the midline, just before its pierces the perineal membrane, the internal pudendal artery gives off a large-calibre but short branch to supply the bulb of the corpus spongiosum. The main artery then divides into the deep artery of the penis, which runs through the corpus cavernosum and the dorsal artery of the penis which

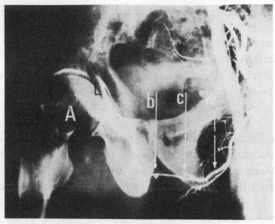

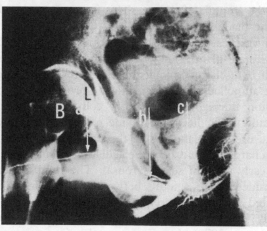

Fig. 2.21 Selective internal iliac arteriography in a normal 31-year-old man, showing the left side of the arterial supply to the penis. A Contrast medium has reached the area where the single arteries to the penis branch off. b) Left deep penile artery where it pierces the crus of the left corpus cavernosum. c) Proximal part of the bulbar artery before it enters the spongiose body. d) Distal segment of the internal pudendal artery (also called the penile artery) around the passage of the urogenital diaphragm.
B Some seconds later. The contrast medium has now filled the left dorsal artery (a) all the way to the glans. b) The deep penile artery pierces the tunica albuginea, and the contrast medium fills a large part of the cavernous body (the cloudy area below the dorsal artery). The bulbar part of the corpus spongiosum is also visible as a solid white structure, supplied by the bulbar artery, c). (Courtesy of Gorm Wagner and Richard Green)

runs along the dorsum of the penis within the loose fibrous tissue surrounding the tunica to the glans where it divides into two branches. Along its length it may give off small branches which penetrate the fibrous sheath of the corpus cavernosum and anastomoses with the deep artery of the penis. When the penis is flaccid, the penile arteries are tortuous, straightening as an erection develops (Figs. 2.21, 2.22).

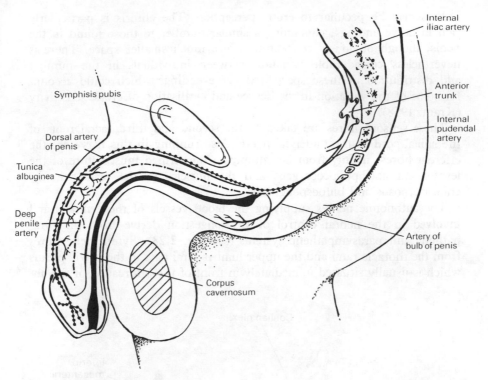

Fig. 2.22 Arterial supply of erectile tissues of penis. The dorsal artery, which supplies the erectile tissue of the glans and distal part of the corpus spongiosum, also sends fine branches through the tunica albuginea into the corpus cavernosum.

Venous drainage of the foreskin and skin of the penile shaft is via the superficial dorsal vein which, noticeable on the surface of the penis, turns either to the right or left before joining the external pudendal vein, a tributary of the long saphenous vein. Drainage of the glans penis and the corpora cavernosa is mainly via the deep dorsal vein. The small emissary veins from within the corpora cavernosa empty into 5–10 sets of circumflex veins which run round the outside of the tunica albuginea before joining the deep dorsal vein, which itself eventually drains into the prostatic plexus.

Nerve supply

Peripheral

The genitalia of both men and women are richly supplied with sensory nerve endings. Many of them are specialised in type though their precise function is not always understood. Some are concentrated around blood vessels and may be important in monitoring vasocongestion (Levin 1980).

Others may be peculiar to erotic perception. The clitoris is particularly rich in nerve endings, containing a similar number to those found in the penis, though obviously concentrated in a much smaller space. There is nevertheless considerable variation between individuals in the number and distribution of these specialised nerve endings which could account for some of the variation in the degree and localisation of erotic sensitivity (Krantz 1958).

These sensory fibres are taken to the second and third sacral roots of the spinal cord in the pudendal nerve. Also running in this nerve are the efferent fibres, mainly from S4, supplying the striped musculature of the levator ani and pubococcygeus and the muscles of the penis, the ischiocavernosus and bulbospongiosus.

The autonomic nerves supplying the blood vessels of the genitalia and involved in the neural control of vasocongestion derive from the sympathetic and parasympathetic systems (see Fig. 2.23). Sympathetic fibres from the thoracic rami and the upper lumbar rami pass to the pelvic plexus which is usually situated immediately in front of the bifurcation of the ab-

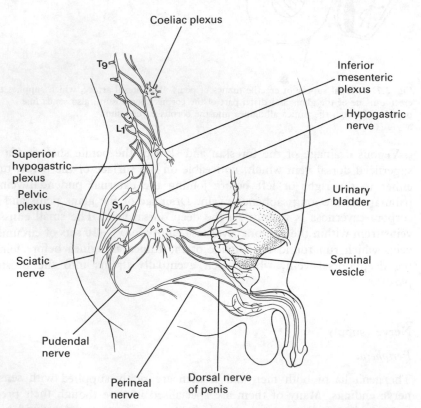

Fig. 2.23 Autonomic innervation of the urinary bladder and male genitalia. (modified from de Groat & Booth 1984)

dominal aorta. From there, fibres run to the genitalia as well as other pelvic viscera, including the bladder. They may be organised in discrete nerves or scattered as a complex network of fibres and so may pass to the genitalia within the pudendal nerve. The anatomical distribution is quite variable, posing a problem for the surgeon operating in this area who endeavours to avoid damaging them.

The parasympathetic supply is from the sacral outflow, S2, 3 and 4, and these fibres run to the genitalia via the pelvic splanchnic nerves which are usually more discrete and predictable in position than their sympathetic counterparts. The branches supplying the penis or the clitoris are called the nervi erigentes. The functional significance of these sympathetic and parasympathetic fibres will be considered further below.

PHYSIOLOGICAL RESPONSES OF THE MALE GENITALIA

The changes in the genitalia of both the male and the female mainly result from localised vasocongestion. These local vascular changes can occur within 10 to 30 seconds of the onset of sexual stimulation, whether psychic (i.e. mediated via the brain) or reflexive (i.e. via reflex pathways in the spinal cord), and before any other discernible physiological changes have occurred.

In the male the principal effect is erection of the penis. This is the most crucial of the genital responses, often the subject of much concern and self-observation, and its failure is the most important form of sexual dysfunction reported by men. We will therefore consider this response in considerable detail.

In addition to penile erection, the testes become elevated due to retraction of the spermatic cords and contraction of the associated cremaster muscle. The wall of the scrotum becomes thicker and tighter, due in part to local vasocongestion but also to contraction of the dartos muscle in its wall. If stimulation is prolonged or intensified the testes are pulled up to the perineal floor and increase in size. The purpose of these changes is not clear. Masters & Johnson (1966) have suggested that elevation of the testes is necessary if the full force of ejaculation is to occur, though it is not clear why this should be so. Contraction of the scrotum may serve to support the elevated testes. The purpose of the testicular enlargement, if any, is not understood.

Penile erection

The function of penile erection in the male is obvious. Adequate entry of the penis into the vagina, and consequent deposition of semen, is relatively difficult without full erection. The erect penis also acts to stimulate the genitalia of the female, whilst serving as the main tactile erotic input for the male.

The stiffness of an erect penis depends on the filling with blood of the erectile tissues within the corpora cavernosa and the increase in intracavernosal pressure to around systolic levels. The tough fibrous tunica albuginea surrounding the corpora cavernosa contains the increased pressure, and the integrity of the resulting hydraulic system produces the rigidity. Vascular engorgement of the glans and corpus spongiosum also occurs during erection but does not contribute to the crucial rigidity of the organ.

This much is clear and generally agreed. However, supplying an explanation for this remarkable feat of biological engineering is much more controversial. Over the years various attempts have been made to explain the physiological mechanisms of erection. In the past decade there has been a dramatic increase in the amount of related physiological and clinical research, stimulated by the recent increase in surgical and pharmacological treatments of erectile failure. There is much new evidence to consider, but unfortunately, there remains a fair amount of uncertainty. Much of this recent evidence is from animal studies and we should not lose sight of the many species differences in both structure and physiology, and we should be cautious in generalising from one species to another.

Traditional physiological textbooks have, perhaps out of a sense of propriety, shown scant attention to the phenomenon of erection, usually describing the process as simply one of increased arterial inflow to the penis resulting from parasympathetically induced arterial dilatation. The sympathetic nervous system, it is assumed, causes reversal of erection or detumescence. For some time this has been considered an inadequate explanation by many physiologists and anatomists. Contraction of the ischiocavernosus and bulbospongiosus muscles has been suggested as a method of increasing intracavernosal pressure but it is unlikely that this would be persistent enough to explain a sustained erection. To produce the pressure necessary for rigidity, reduced emptying as well as increased filling of the erectile tissues is obviously required.

What is the mechanism involved in this reduction of venous outflow? Various explanations have been offered. In the 1900s Ebner and other anatomists described specialised muscular valves or 'polsters' which, it was suggested, produced sudden changes both in venous outflow and arterial inflow (Dickinson 1949). The existence of such valves has been challenged in recent years (Newman & Northup 1981). Entrapment of the blood by compression of the veins beneath the tunica albuginea as intracavernosal pressure increases has also been a favoured explanation. Whilst this may contribute to hydraulic efficiency of the system it is unlikely to be a sufficient explanation. Reduction in venous outflow can be observed early in the development of an erection, before any appreciable increase in intracavernosal pressure will have occurred (see Fig. 2.27). The importance of substantially reducing venous outflow has been further emphasised in recent years by the discovery that erectile failure is sometimes caused by venous 'leaks' in the system.

Deysach (1939), commenting on the histological difference between erectile tissue of animals with an os penis (i.e. most mammals and primates) and those without (e.g. humans) described 'sluice channels' in the human-type penis which, he suggested, diverted blood into the erectile spaces during erection. Other specialised vascular structures have been described by Wagner et al (1982) who, studying plastic injection casts of post-mortem specimens, found vessels passing from the corpora cavernosa through the tunica into the spongiosum. It was postulated that these act as shunts allowing large quantities of blood to pass quickly through the erectile spaces in the flaccid condition. Closure of the muscular walls of these vessels then diverts blood into the corpora cavernosa in response to erotic stimulation. There is as yet no physiological evidence to support this model.

There has also been evidence for many years that the sympathetic pathways carry fibres which are involved in the development of erection as well as in detumescence (Bancroft 1970). In the cat, the lower part of the sympathetic chain is responsible for psychic erections, with the sacral, parasympathetic outflow controlling reflexive responses (Root & Bard 1947). There is some suggestion of a similar division of function in men from studies of paraplegic patients (Bors & Comarr 1960; Kuhn 1950).

Further problems have arisen in establishing which neurotransmitters are involved. Although electrical stimulation of the nervi erigentes does lead to arterial dilatation and increased blood flow, in most species studied this effect is not blocked by atropine, making a simple cholinergic mechanism unlikely (Brindley 1983). Human erections in response to erotic stimuli are also unaffected by atropine (Wagner & Brindley 1980). Active searching for other possible neurotransmitters is currently underway in a number of laboratories. Vasoactive intestinal polypeptide (VIP), a neuropeptide, has attracted considerable attention and is undoubtedly present in the erectile tissues, its concentration increasing as an erection develops (Virag et al 1982). However, in several species it also increases with simple handling of the penis without erection (Dixson et al 1984) and as yet injection of VIP into the cavernosal spaces has been disappointing in producing erection (Ottesen et al 1984).

A recent development has been the recognition of the large amount of smooth muscle within the corpora cavernosa, mainly within the walls of the sinusoids. A number of reports of the effects of drugs and neurotransmitters on strips of such smooth muscle tissue have appeared in the literature, providing a useful in vitro method for studying pharmacological effects (Benson 1983). It has also been shown that both cholinergic and adrenergic receptors are present in cavernosal tissue but the latter are mainly in the smooth muscle walls of the sinusoids and are about 10 times more frequent than the former (Benson et al 1980) with a greater proportion of alpha than beta receptors (Levin & Wein 1980).

Perhaps the most important new source of evidence relating to the physiology of erection has been the studies of drugs injected into the corpora cavernosa in human subjects. Brindley (1983) and Virag et al (1982) have pioneered this technique, initially as a method of investigating erectile failure, but more recently as a possible means of treatment. The diagnostic and therapeutic implications will be discussed later in this volume. A variety of drugs have now been shown by this method to produce erection in men (Table 2.1), though with varying duration of erections resulting. Pharmacologically this is a heterogeneous group of compounds but they do all share in common the capacity for relaxing smooth muscle — some by adrenergic blockade (e.g. phenoxybenzamine), some by calcium channel blocking (e.g. verapamil), others by as yet unknown mechanisms (e.g. papaverine). We thus have to incorporate these findings into any explanatory model of erectile function.

Table 2.1 Effects of intracavernosal injections of drugs (from Brindley 1984)

Producing full erection	Duration
Phenoxybenzamine	1–6h
Papaverine	2–2.5h
Phentolamine	5–10min
Verapamil	2–2.5min
Thymoxamine	1–2.5min
Causing swelling of penis but never full erection	
Guanethidine	
Naftidrofuryl oxalate	
Causing shrinkage of erectile tissue	
Metaraminol	
Imipramine	
Clonidine	
Causing little or no effect	
Atropine	
Neostigmine	
Morphine	
Dextromoramide	
Lignocaine	
Hydralazine	
Idazoxan	

A current theoretical model of erection

Combining these various sources of information we can now piece together a 'most likely' explanatory model, though still largely hypothetical (Lue 1986). The crucial components of erection, according to this model, are as follows:

1. Relaxation of the smooth muscle in the sinusoidal walls. These are normally constricted by an active process of adrenergic tone. *Reduction of*

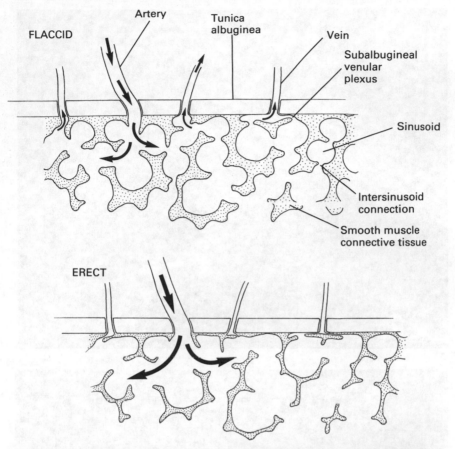

Fig. 2.24 Relaxation of the smooth muscle in the sinusoidal walls of the erectile tissue or the corpora cavernosa. These are normally constricted by an active process of adrenergic tone. *Reduction* of this tone and consequent relaxation then results in filling and enlargement of the spaces with blood, and reduced venous drainage. (modified from Fournier et al 1987)

this tone and consequent relaxation then results in filling and enlargement of the spaces with blood (Fig. 2.24).

2. Passive compression of the venules running between the sinusoidal spaces, impeding venous outflow and further increasing sinusoidal filling (Figs. 2.25, 2.26).

3. Dilatation of arteries and resulting increased inflow. It is not yet clear whether this precedes, accompanies or follows the sinusoidal relaxation.

4. The possibility of some additional active reduction of venous outflow has not yet been excluded.

The combination of these processes, it is assumed, leads to an effective sealing off of the corpora cavernosa and a build-up of intracavernosal

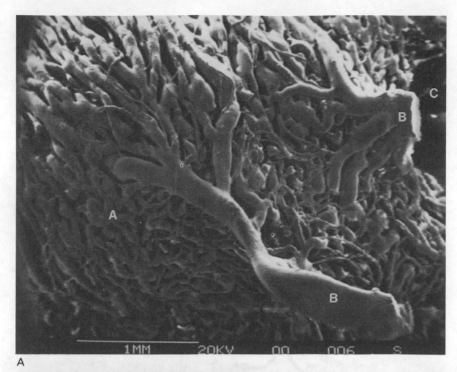

A

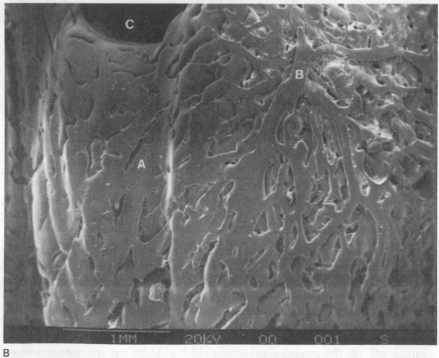

B

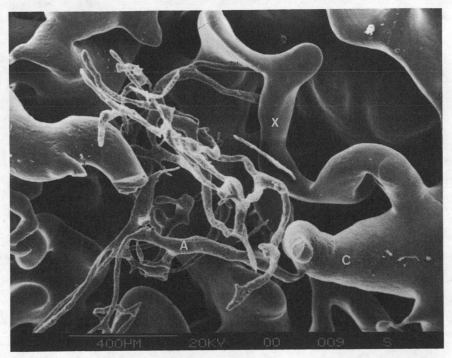

C

Fig. 2.25 A Scanning electron micrograph (×29) of hilar portion of non-papaverine-injected corpus of dog. Note extensive venular plexus (A) coalescing into two veins (B), which rise from surface to traverse tunica albuginea (dissolved in this corrosion cast). Corporeal artery penetrates surface at (C).
B Papaverine-injected corpus of dog. Note flattened appearance of entire venular plexus (A) and subalbugineal portion of vein (B). C = the arterial hiatus.
C Scanning electron micrograph (×55) of human penile corrosion cast (cadaveric). Note venular structure (A) anastomosing with the sinusoids (C). Venule found at midshaft. (X = intersinusoidal connection.) Courtesy of T. F. Lue (Fournier et al 1987)

pressure to levels around systolic. This is probably sufficient to produce rigidity.

5. Additional stiffening may result from transient contraction of the ischiocavernosus and bulbospongiosus muscles which has been shown to produce grossly elevated intracavernosal pressure. This mechanism could be elicited by the bulbocavernosus reflex. During neurological examination this reflex is elicited by squeezing the glans penis (see p. 425. It is possible that contact of the erect penis with the vaginal introitus also elicits this reflex, resulting in a further stiffening and easier entry. When erectile responses are measured in the laboratory it is common to find these contractions occurring as a semi-voluntary attempt to 'pump up' an erection (see Fig. 2.18).

What are we to conclude about the neurotransmitters involved? First we

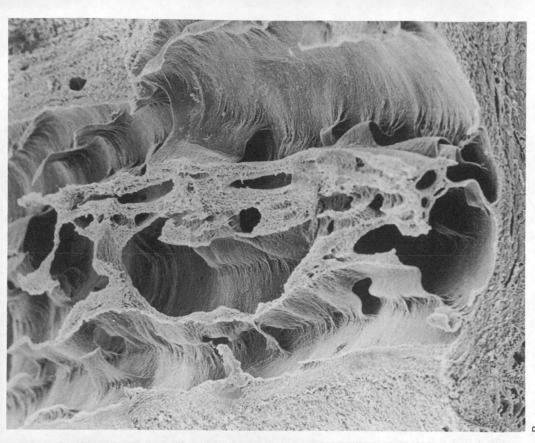

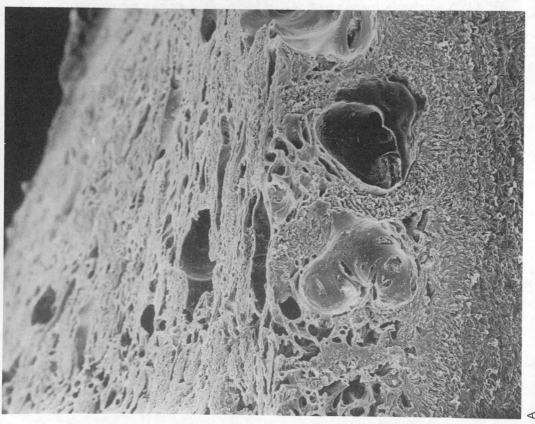

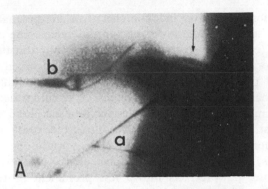

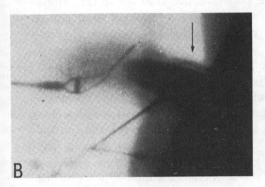
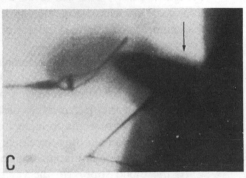

Fig. 2.27 Infusion cavernosography with simultaneous measurement of changes in penile circumference and intracavernous pressure in a normal 29-year-old man. **A** Flaccid penis. Arrow points to contrast medium in the dorsal venous drainage system. a = Double lumen needle; b = mercury-in-rubber strain gauge. **B** Early erection (in response to erotic film). There is a slight increase in the length of the cavernous bodies. Arrow points to slight narrowing of the medium in the dorsal venous drainage system. **C** Fuller erection. Contrast medium in the drainage system has disappeared. The intracavernous pressure is 35 mmHg. Reduction of venous drainage is thus occurring at an early stage of erection. (Courtesy of Gorm Wagner and Richard Green)

should acknowledge that *reduction* in adrenergic tone may play a crucial role. Secondly the failure to demonstrate that either acetylcholine (ACH) or VIP are clearly responsible may be because, as discussed on p. 19, autonomic control of penile vasculature involves a subtle co-transmission with both ACH and VIP. If so, our pharmacological techniques may have been too crude to simulate such processes.

This remains a fascinating area of vascular physiology and it is to be hoped that in the next few years many of the remaining uncertainties will be resolved. The possibility of a major breakthrough in the pharmacological treatment of erectile failure remains a tantalising possibility.

PHYSIOLOGICAL RESPONSES OF THE FEMALE GENITALIA

The consequences of erotically induced local vasocongestion in the female are more extensive and complex than in the male. The venous plexus which surrounds the lower part of the vagina, the erectile bulbs of the vestibule (equivalent to the corpus spongiosum) and the deeper structures or corpora cavernosa of the clitoris become engorged (see Fig. 2.12). A turgid cuff thus forms which narrows and elongates the outer third of the coital canal. If stimulation continues or is intensified, reaching the phase preceding orgasm, which Masters & Johnson (1966) call the plateau phase, congestive swelling of the vulva causes reddening and 'pouting' of the labia minora.

The clitoris, which erects to a variable degree in the earlier stages of sexual response, now retracts into a less prominent attitude against the symphisis pubis. This can result in apparent reduction in size of the clitoris as arousal increases; this change is sometimes misinterpreted as a sign of lessening arousal. In fact retraction rather than reduction in size is occurring.

In the deeper parts of the female genital tract, the uterus also becomes engorged and increases in size, at the same time rising in the pelvis. This displacement probably results from contraction of the smooth muscle fibres within the parametrial tissues supporting the uterus and upper vagina. This also seems to elongate and causes the upper two-third of the vagina to 'balloon'. Slow irregular contractions of the vaginal vault may occur as sexual stimulation continues.

As the blood supply to the vaginal wall increases a fluid appears on the vaginal epithelium (usually at an early stage), quickly forming a lubricating coat, which was likened by Masters & Johnson (1966) to a sweating response. The characteristics of this fluid indicate that it is a modified plasma transudate (Levin 1980). It is important to remember that the lining of the vagina is squamous epithelium; it contains no mucous glands. Although mucus secretion from the endocervix does occur, varying in amount according to the stage of the menstrual cycle, this apparently makes little difference to the amount of fluid secreted during sexual response, and vaginal lubrication is largely unaffected following hysterectomy and removal of the cervix. Mucus secretion from the greater vestibular (Bartholin's) glands also occurs but this is late during sexual arousal and modest in amount. Sharp pain in the region of these glands (see Fig. 2.11) occurring during the late stages of sexual response can be an indication of a Bartholin's retention cyst.

As erection of the penis in the male facilitates entry into the vagina, so do the genital changes in the female. The congested and 'pouting' labia and more patent introitus invites entry of the penis, whilst the vaginal transudate lubricates the vaginal barrel in readiness. The narrowing of the outer third of the vagina, the so-called 'orgasmic platform' adds to the stimulation of the penis. The function of the ballooning of the inner third of the vagina is not clear, though, together with the orgasmic platform, it may aid conception by encouraging the formation of a seminal pool near the cervix and reducing drainage of semen out of the vagina. The elevation of the uterus effectively pulls the cervix out of the way of the deeply thrusting penis; buffeting of the cervix can cause discomfort. It follows that if vaginal entry is attempted without these genital responses having occurred, discomfort or pain may be experienced.

The vaginal transudate, by its effects on electrolyte content and pH of the vagina, may make the vaginal milieu more favourable to sperm, though the relative importance of this is still disputed.

The sole function of the clitoris, or at least the visible part of it, the glans, is to provide the principal source of erotic stimulation for the female. It is exquisitely sensitive, and may contain as many nerve endings as are normally found in the glans penis, though the number does vary considerably from woman to woman (Krantz 1958).

Less attention has been paid to the vascular mechanisms and neural control involved in the female response than in the case of the male. It is possible that similar specialised vascular mechanisms are involved, though obviously there is no functional equivalent of the hydraulic system of the penile corpora cavernosa. The same neurotransmitters may also be involved. Atropine also fails to block the female response (Wagner & Levin 1980) and VIP is found in the vaginal wall as well as in the penis (Levin 1980).

The mechanism underlying vaginal transudation is not understood. It presumably depends on increased blood flow through the vaginal wall, though this remains to be demonstrated, and the porosity of the vaginal epithelium may be dependent on normal levels of oestrogen acting locally. It is a remarkable fact that if an artificial vagina is surgically created in a woman with congenital absence of the vagina, the tube of epidermis used for the purpose will eventually form vaginal transudate in response to sexual stimulation, apparently similar to that of the normal vagina (Masters & Johnson 1966).

THE CENTRAL NERVOUS SYSTEM AND SEXUALITY

Sensory mechanisms

Smell

Olfactory stimuli are of considerable importance in the sexual behaviour of most non-human mammals (Keverne 1978). The word 'pheromone' is often used to describe such olfactory cues, though the term was originally used to describe a chemical attractant in insects and there is nothing of comparable specificity or potency in the mammalian world. Two types of olfactory effect must be considered:

1. olfactory priming, by which an olfactory stimulus has some gradual effect on the physiology of the recipient over a period of time; an example of such an effect is alteration of the timing of menstruation;

2. olfactory signalling, by which olfactory stimuli have a more immediate effect on the behaviour of the recipient. Urinary and vaginal odours, indicating that the female is in oestrus and hence 'attractive', act in this way.

How important are such mechanisms in human sexuality? It is worth noting that most mammals have a dual olfactory system. One originates from the olfactory bulbs and communicates with the cortex. The other starts at the vomeronasal organ and communicates via the vomeronasal nerve with the limbic system. The exceptions to this dual system are the higher primates and humans who do not have the vomeronasal system, and hence no obvious direct contact with the limbic system. Therefore it might be expected that differences would be found in the function of olfaction in such primates.

In spite of this more limited olfactory system there is some evidence that human females synchronise their menstrual cycles with one another, presumably via olfactory priming (McClintock 1971; Graham & McGrew 1980). Sleeping with a male partner also increases the incidence of ovulation (Veith et al 1983). This is not necessarily dependent on sexual activity and it has been suggested that it is an effect of axillary odours from the male. Cutler and her colleagues (1986) claim that the application of male axillary secretions to women tends to make their menstrual cycles more regular.

Signalling pheromones play an important role in primate sexual behaviour, in particular vaginal odours. These result from aliphatic acids produced by bacterial action in the vagina which varies according to the amount of oestrogen and the phase of the ovarian cycle. These odours inform the male that the female is in oestrus, receptive and hence 'attractive'. However, once a female is identified as attractive these olfactory signals are not necessary for sexual activity to be maintained (Keverne 1978). Such responses are not stereotypical however; they vary in importance considerably from male to male. It is also possible that the signalling effect is acquired as the result of learning (i.e. experience of previous females in oestrus) rather than an innately programmed response.

Similar aliphatic acids are present in the vaginae of women and vary in a similar way with the menstrual cycle (Michael et al 1974). As yet no sexual signalling with these cues has been demonstrated in humans. There are other observations of possible relevance. Women vary through the menstrual cycle in their ability to perceive odours, with maximal sensitivity around ovulation. Women are more likely than men to smell androstenol, a steroid emitted by the boar which elicits a sexually receptive posture in the oestrous sow. But an attempt to render men more attractive to women using this odour was unsuccessful (Black & Biron 1982). Similarly, synthetic aliphatic acids, similar to those in the vagina, failed to influence sexual attractiveness or interaction between human pairs (Morris & Udry 1978).

It is nevertheless difficult to exclude the importance of olfaction in human sexuality. Our apocrine glands, which produce body odour, are well developed. Oral−genital contact is widespread. There is a substantial market for scents, perfumes and deodorants, though this may be as much concerned with masking unattractive odours as exploiting attractive ones. Anecdotal evidence suggests that for some people olfactory cues are extremely important, not only in initial attraction to a sexual partner but also in the maintenance of a stable relationship. But we do not know the proportion of people affected in this way or whether there is a sex difference in such sensitivity. This is an area where more research is required.

Visual signals

These are clearly important sexual stimuli for both human and subhuman primates. There is a striking capacity for both men and women, monitored in the laboratory, to respond to films of sexual activity with some degree of genital response, even if they do not find the film pleasant or agreeable (see p. 686 for further discussion of the interaction between such external erotic stimuli and cognitive processes). Later in this chapter we will consider evidence suggesting that our responsiveness to such stimuli may involve different mechanisms or pathways to those associated with spontaneous sexual appetite or genital response during sleep. In Chapter 4, we will consider further the role of visual signals in sexual attractiveness.

Tactile sensation

Touch is obviously an important source of erotic stimulation. The sensory pathways from the genitalia are described on p. 51. There are dramatic changes in the erotic tactile sensitivity of the genitalia during vasocongestive responses such as erection. This may be secondary to structural changes, induced by the tumescence, which alter the sensory mechanism so that ordinary cutaneous sensations become erotic in quality. Hart & Leedy (1985) have described structural characteristics of the genital sense organs consistent with this explanation.

In animal studies, sectioning of the dorsal nerve of the penis, which supplies much of the sensory area of the penis, appears to prevent erection and ejaculation in various species, indicating how important this sensory input is for normal genital response (Hart & Leedy 1985). In humans this becomes relevant in those cases of peripheral nerve damage affecting the genitalia (e.g. multiple sclerosis) where loss of sensation may be contributing to erectile failure.

But clearly erotic touch is not confined to the genitalia. In the right circumstances tactile stimulation of many parts of the body can be intensely erotic. This reminds us that the input of sensory stimulation from the periphery has to be processed centrally and can be substantially influenced at this stage. An interesting and basically unexplained phenomenon occurs in many individuals with transection of the spinal cord. Having lost all sensation below the level of the injury, they may find that the skin region just *above* the level of sensory loss develops an erotic sensitivity which it did not previously possess. Some reorganisation of the perception of tactile stimuli has presumably taken place (see p. 577). On a more dynamic level, central processes can influence whether genital stimulation is perceived as erotic. In some instances erotic anaesthesia seems to develop in spite of non-erotic sensation being intact. The underlying mechanisms for such a pattern are not understood but presumably inhibition of erotic sensory input is taking place at some central level in the cord or above.

Spinal pathways

The spinal centres for reflexive erection (and presumably for the comparable vasocongestive responses in the female) are situated somewhere in the sacral part of the cord. The localisation of these centres has been more precise in some animal species (see Fig. 2.28) but we have no comparable evidence for humans.

The localisation of the fibre tracts as they ascend and descend in the cord is also uncertain. Men who have received bilateral anterolateral cordotomies, usually at an upper thoracic level for the relief of intractable pain, often report loss of erection and ejaculation, though their ordinary tactile two-point discrimination and vibration sense in the penis is unchanged. This suggests that close to the spinothalamic pathways for pain and

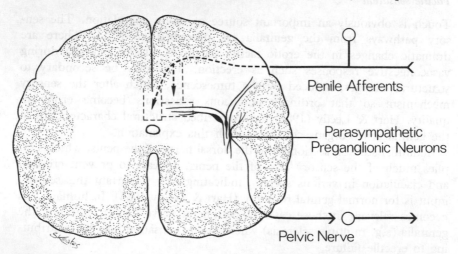

Fig. 2.28 The spinal centres for reflexive erection (and presumably for the comparable vasocongestive responses in the female) are situated somewhere in the sacral part of the cord. The localisation of these centres has been more precise in some animal species such as the cat, shown in this figure but we have no comparable evidence for humans. (modified from Nadelhaft et al 1980; Courtesy of W. C. de Groat)

temperature run fibres either from above, involved in the central control of erection, or from the periphery, involved in the specifically erotic components of genital sensation (Brindley 1982).

Localisation in the brain

Our knowledge of central localisation of sexual function is limited and almost entirely dependent on animal data. There is evidence from a variety of sources that the limbic system is the neural substrate of sexuality as it is for other appetitive functions (Maclean 1976). Studies with implanted electrodes in anaesthetised male squirrel and rhesus monkeys have demonstrated that there are a number of sites, not necessarily contiguous, where stimulation produces either erection or ejaculation. These include

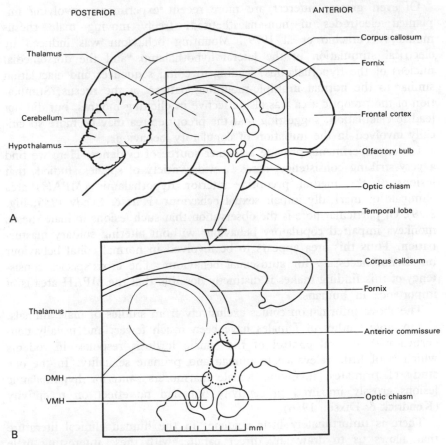

POSTERIOR   ANTERIOR

Thalamus

Corpus callosum

Fornix

Cerebellum

Frontal cortex

Hypothalamus

Olfactory bulb

Optic chiasm

Temporal lobe

A

Corpus callosum

Fornix

Thalamus

Anterior commissure

DMH

VMH

Optic chiasm

mm

B

Fig. 2.29 A Sagittal section of the brain of the rhesus monkey showing hypothalamic area. **B** Enlarged view of the hypothalamic area; the dotted line indicates the medial preoptic area (MPOA) in which lesions produce disruption of sexual behaviour (see text). Drawing by Dr Alan Dixson.

the preoptic region, lateral hypothalamus, tegmentum and anterior part of the cingulate gyrus. In contrast, stimulation is consistently ineffective in the hippocampus, fornix, mammillary bodies, posterior cingulate gyrus, caudate nucleus, ansa lenticularis and the genital receiving area of the post-central gyrus. (Maclean & Ploog 1962; Robinson & Mishkin 1968; Fig. 2.29). These studies have also demonstrated the existence of both excitatory and inhibitory mechanisms affecting the peripheral response of erection, illustrating the point that the parallel functioning of excitation and inhibition is fundamental to much of neurophysiology and important to our understanding of sexual dysfunction. The existence of a normal level of inhibitory erectile tone from higher centres is suggested by the common finding that transection of the spinal cord is followed by lowering of threshold for reflexive erection, as though the spinal centres for erection have been released from higher control.

Of even greater interest are more recent experiments involving implanted electrodes in non-anaesthetised, freely moving male rhesus monkeys (Perachio et al 1979). Mounting behaviour was induced by electrical stimulation of the lateral hypothalamus and the dorsomedial nucleus of the hypothalamus, leading to coital sequences and ejaculation similar to the normal multiple-mounting pattern of the rhesus. Stimulation of the preoptic area was also effective in eliciting mounts, but did not lead to ejaculation, suggesting that the preoptic area may be more specifically involved in the initiation of copulatory behaviour.

Lesion experiments provide a further source of evidence. Here we find a very striking consistency, across a wide variety of species studied, that lesions of the medial preoptic—anterior hypothalamic (MPAH) area eliminate or markedly impair sexual behaviour (Hart & Leedy 1985; Fig. 2.29). Of particular note is the observation that such lesions in male rhesus monkeys impaired copulatory behaviour without altering solitary masturbation. Thus this area appears to be involved in normal coital behaviour but is not necessary for autosexual behaviour. The cross-species consistency of this finding makes it distinctly possible that the MPAH area is of importance in humans.

The above information comes exclusively from studies of male animals. Comparable studies of females have been much fewer, and usually concerned with central control of the female lordosis response in rodents which is of little relevance to human and primate sexuality. In the one study of primates, involving female marmosets, anterior hypothalamic lesions grossly impaired proceptivity but had no effect on receptivity (Kendrick & Dixson 1986).

There is unfortunately little evidence in the human clinical literature that allows us to draw any direct parallel with these interesting male primate data, and we should be cautious in extrapolating from these studies to man. So far there have been no reports of erection produced by stimulation during the course of stereotaxic operations in men (Brindley 1982).

Stimulation of most parts of the human neocortex has never elicited responses of a sexual nature (Penfield & Jasper 1954); presumably the erotic quality of an experience is imposed somewhere else in the brain.

Unilateral lesions in the brain have been made in attempts to treat sexual criminals by neurosurgical means. Such lesions have been placed in areas extending from the ventromedial nucleus of the hypothalamus rostrally to the medial preoptic area (Muller et al 1973; Dieckman & Hassler 1976). The recipients were reported to have experienced a reduction of sexual interest. In the literature on animals, however, unilateral lesions have been ineffective and it is not possible to conclude that these extraordinary and ethically extremely questionable surgical procedures are producing direct effects on human sexual behaviour. Meyers (1961, 1962) has reported interesting changes following lesions to the ansa lenticularis carried out to relieve abnormal motor signs. This resulted in complete loss of sexual interest and erectile failure. The relevant sites of these lesions were not entirely clear.

An area situated close to the MPAH is of interest for another reason. This is the sexually dimorphic nucleus. The function of this nucleus is not known but its characteristic is that it is substantially larger in the male brain than in the female. First described in the rat by Gorski (1978), it has also been identified in the human brain (Swaab & Fliers 1985) where it is 2.5 times larger in the male. It decreases in size with increasing age. Lesions of this nucleus of the rat do not interfere with sexual behaviour. It contains cells that stain for vasopressin but as yet the functional significance of this is not known.

As yet we must be very tentative in suggesting localisation of sexual function within the human male brain and we can say virtually nothing about such localisation in women.

SEXUAL AROUSAL

Although 'sexual arousal' is a widely used term, its precise meaning is seldom clear, covering a variety of psychological and physiological states, some difficult to describe or measure. And yet for an adequate understanding of human sexual responses and how they fail, sexual arousal needs to be clearly defined.

This point may be served by an analogy. A state comparable to sexual arousal is hunger. A hungry person experiences a subjective state called 'appetite', which motivates him to obtain food and focuses his attention on that goal. Accompanying this subjective experience, and in part contributing to it, are various physiological changes, many of which are in preparation for impending food intake. Our appetite for food increases (up to a point) the longer we have been without it. To some extent this mechanism depends on biochemical processes, e.g. hypoglycaemia. But psychological processes are also involved; we learn to feel hungry at certain times and in certain situations, and for some people this learning can have a powerful effect on appetite. Our appetite is also increased by the sight or smell of attractive food — unless we are sated, when even the most delicious food loses its appeal.

The similarity with sexual arousal is obvious. We experience a sexual appetite which motivates us to seek sexual stimulation. The effect of sexual abstinence on sexual appetite is probably more complex than in the case of food. But there are also biological and psychological factors which interact to influence sexual appetite or 'drive'. A wide variety of external stimuli, including sights, sounds or smells, as well as internal imagery or fantasy, can have this effect. One of the most powerful sexual stimuli, however, is touch, especially of the erogenous areas of the body. Thus if our initial appetite is sufficient to manifest itself in sexual behaviour involving such touch, sexual arousal in all its forms may become markedly enhanced. The system is a self-amplifying one; as genitalia respond in preparation for sexual activity such as coitus, they become even more sensitive to touch, with a consequent escalation of arousal. Sexual stimuli are sometimes divided into two types, those dependent on the brain, such as visual, auditory, olfactory and internal imagery, known as psychic stimuli, and those dependent on touch, called reflexive, because they can be effective without the brain, as following spinal cord transection. Obviously they interact with one another; psychic stimuli will increase the sensitivity to reflexive stimuli and vice versa. And whilst they may vary in relative strength, their effects are much the same. But their effects on genital responses may involve different central and peripheral nerve pathways or neurotransmitters, and therefore the distinction between psychic and reflexive is of potential clinical importance.

As with food, our sensitivity to these different external stimuli varies with some internal state which may be biochemically or hormonally determined. Thus with a high degree of this intrinsic arousability we may respond strongly to minimal external stimulation, whereas in other instances considerable external stimulation and perhaps only direct touch will succeed in producing sexual responses. Our understanding of this intrinsic state of arousability is very limited at the present time but will be considered later in relation to hormone action.

Kinsey and his colleagues (Kinsey et al 1953) fostered the unitary concept of sexual arousal, seeing it as a state incorporating a variety of phenomena, each varying in intensity with the total state. In other words, with slight arousal there is a slight degree of each of the components, e.g. genital response, cardiovascular changes, central excitement, increased tactile sensitivity and so on. Masters & Johnson (1966) added to this model the concept of an inevitable *sequence* of physiological events: a unitary concept of arousal of both incremental and sequential kind. They described the four phases of excitement, plateau, orgasm and resolution. The criteria for distinguishing between excitement and plateau seem unclear and somewhat arbitrary. Orgasm, and particularly ejaculation, can occur in association with very variable degrees of excitement.

Although we can readily see how this line of thinking has developed, it must now be regarded as unhelpful. It implies too many assumptions about the inter-relationships of these various phenomena which may inhibit their further clarification. It is particularly important to keep an open mind on this issue when we consider the various types of sexual dysfunction.

Kaplan (1979) introduced the triphasic concept. According to this, human sexuality has three phases: sexual desire, excitement and orgasm. 'These three phases are physiologically related but discrete. They are interconnected but governed by separate neurophysiological systems'. She may eventually be proved right in this assertion but as yet there is no evidence to support her view and in addition the conceptual distinction between desire and excitement needs more careful scrutiny before one can begin to postulate discrete underlying neurophysiological mechanisms.

To examine these concepts more closely let us consider sexual arousal under two headings:

1. Sexual appetite or desire.
2. Central and peripheral arousability.

Sexual appetite or desire

Of the various aspects of the human sexual experience, sexual desire remains perhaps the most resistant to conceptual analysis. The task has not been helped by the use of ill defined or undefinable concepts such as 'libido' or 'drive' (Peters 1960) and there are advantages, at our present level of understanding, in using terms like 'desire', 'interest' or 'appetite' which serve a descriptive rather than explanatory function.

As with hunger, what we experience as sexual desire or appetite is a complex interaction between cognitive processes, neurophysiological mechanisms and the prevailing affect or mood.

Some state of central arousability is involved, determining the individual's capacity for reacting to an appropriate stimulus with a sexual response. Obviously the presence and potency of external stimuli depend on many factors, but mediating between the individual's arousability and the stimuli in his or her environment is a tendency to seek out stimuli as well as cognitive processes influencing his or her interpretation of these stimuli. In addition there is the important capacity to produce internal images, creating his or her own sexual stimuli in fantasy.

These processes are set against and influenced by the mood of the moment. In a depressed mood we are less likely to interpret experiences in pleasant sexual terms. A mood of inertia reduces the likelihood that we will initiate overt sexual behaviour.

These interactions are complex. Do we have sexual thoughts because we have sexual desire or is it the other way round? Is a sexual fantasy a sexual stimulus or a response? Both versions may be correct in each case. Some authorities, especially those who view human sexuality from a psychosocial standpoint, play down the contribution of physiological determinants. In my view it is as unhelpful to deny the importance of biological factors as it is to minimise the sociological factors. We cannot evade the uncomfortable complexity of sociobiological interactions.

Consequently, when we investigate sexual desire we should not expect to reduce it to its basic ingredients. The best we can do at the present time is to look at this complex process through various 'windows'. Through the cognitive window we can ask questions about sexual thoughts and fantasies. In their current research into disorders of sexual desire Schiavi & Schreiner-Engel (personal communication) use the following definition of sexual desire.

1. The spontaneous occurrence of sexual thoughts.
2. Awareness of an interest in initiating sexual activity (or accepting it if initiated by one's partner).
3. The recognition and seeking out of sexual cues.

These aspects can all be measured. 'Sexual thoughts' is however a broad term. It includes various types of internal imagery which can have quite a powerful sexual stimulus effect, leading to excitement and genital response. The role of cognitive processes, sexual imagery or fantasy and the effects of mood will be considered in more detail later in this chapter.

There are obviously many factors in our environment which will increase or decrease the likelihood of our thinking about sex, not all of them primarily sexual in character. But that aspect of the neurophysiological substrate which responds to sexual thoughts with increased central arousal and genital response may be influenced by other non-cognitive factors leading in turn to a secondary increase in sexual thoughts. Thus 'high arousability' of this system may result in an increased likelihood of responding to *external* stimuli with central excitement and genital responses, leading to an increase in sexual thoughts and the experience of increased sexual desire. An interesting window into this state of arousability, when it is relatively independent of the effects of the environment or cognitive processes, is provided by the genital responses that occur during sleep, which we will consider in more detail in the next section.

We should therefore see sexual desire as an experiential and not a neurophysiological concept, and for operational purposes seek to identify and measure the three obvious dimensions of this experience — the cognitive, in terms of thoughts and internal imagery; the affective, in terms of mood or other emotional states, and the neurophysiological, in terms of central arousability. We should also remember not only that these three dimensions interact with each other, but that each is subject to a particular class of influences — our cognitive processes are subject to socio-psychological, our neurophysiological processes to biochemical and hormonal influences and our mood to both psychological and biochemical factors.

In the next section we will consider ways of looking through the physiological window.

The physiological window: central and peripheral arousability

We have little problem at a subjective level in recognising a state of sexual arousal or excitement. We may not only be aware of genital responses, but also of other bodily changes and a totally subjective sense of excitement which comes to our attention. To be objective about such states is another matter. We can measure a variety of peripheral responses, mostly under the control of the autonomic nervous system, and use these as indicators of peripheral arousal. But the subjective state of excitement is more elusive. It no doubt has physiological correlates in the form of measurable electrocortical arousal, but as yet we have very little evidence of such changes. Studies of cortical-evoked potential (Lifshitz 1966) and of the 'expectancy wave' of the electroencephalogram (EEG) or 'contingent negative variation' (Costell et al 1972) in response to visual erotic stimuli have been reported. We have possible evidence of EEG changes associated with orgasm but, as has already been implied, orgasm is a neurophysiological event which should be considered separately. For the person who is becoming sexually excited subjectively and experiencing genital responses, we have no evidence of any accompanying electrocortical activity.

As yet, we should not assume, as the theoretical models of arousal have encouraged us to do in the past, that central arousal and peripheral arousal are linked manifestations of the same process. They are clearly related, but in a potentially complex way. One individual may respond to awareness of peripheral changes with increased excitement, another may interpret changes inappropriately and react with fear. The two processes, whilst inter-related, are potentially independent of one another.

A wide variety of peripheral changes accompanying sexual stimulation have been recorded. Most are cardiovascular, e.g. raised blood pressure, altered heart rate, skin temperature or skin colour changes. Respiratory changes, pupillary dilatation and alterations in electrodermal activity may also occur. Probably the most predictable response accompanying genital changes is a rise in systolic and diastolic blood pressure, but this may only be transient (Fig. 2.30).

The important conclusion from the various laboratory studies is that no particular pattern of peripheral non-genital responses characterises a sexual response. Most of the observed changes can be seen in response to other types of arousing but non-sexual stimuli (Zuckerman 1971; Bancroft

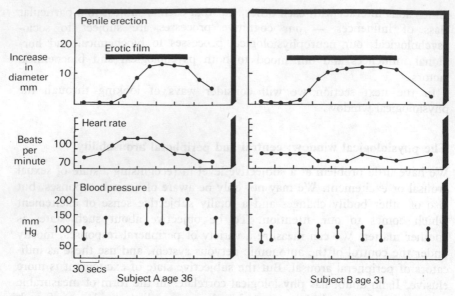

Fig. 2.30 Blood pressure rise during sexual arousal in two normal men. Subject A shows a marked rise associated with an increased heart rate. Subject B shows a very slight rise with an associated decrease in heart rate. The blood pressure response is variable between subjects but in 12 normal men tested in this way the average increase in blood pressure was 24.7 (±17.4) mmHg systolic and 15.2 (±10.8) mmHg diastolic. (Bancroft & Bell 1985)

1980a). It is possible that erection of the nipple in both men and women and enlargement of the breasts in women may be specifically sexual responses (Masters & Johnson 1966) but as yet we cannot be certain on this point.

THE RELATIONSHIP OF GENITAL RESPONSES TO SEXUAL AROUSAL

We have already considered the peripheral mechanisms involved in genital responses. How are they related to other components of sexual arousal? Genital responses following erotic stimulation can be readily measured in the laboratory in both men and women. In the male changes in circumference or volume of the penis and changes in amplitude of the penile arterial pulse can be measured (see Fig. 9.9, p. 436). In the female, pulse amplitude or oxygen tension changes in the vaginal wall or temperature changes in the labia have been used as measures of genital vasocongestion. We will be considering these techniques and how they can be used for diagnostic purposes in more detail in Chapter 9. At this stage it is sufficient to point out that such measurement, in parallel with measures of other non-genital responses, has shown that genital responses are not necessarily accompanied by other peripheral evidence of arousal (Figs 2.30, 2.31).

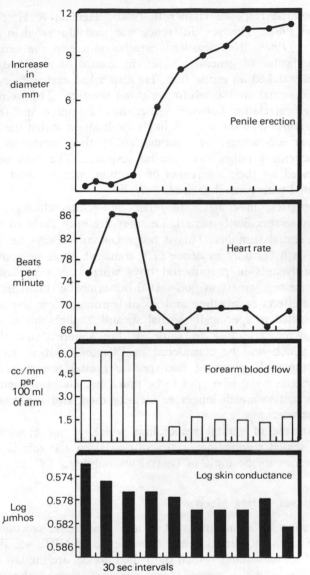

Fig. 2.31 Sexual response (i.e. erection) associated with a decrease in peripheral arousal in a normal male. (Bancroft & Mathews 1971)

We cannot conclude therefore that the occurrence of a genital response is an indication of sexual arousal in a more general sense. This has been a considerable cause of confusion, particularly in the male. Erection of the penis is often equated with sexual arousal ('I have an erection therefore I am aroused'). This leads to high correlations between measurement of erection and self-ratings of arousal. In contrast, women, who are less aware of their genital responses, show lower correlations between subjective ratings and genital response (Bancroft 1980a; Heiman & Hatch 1981; Steinman et al 1981). This sex difference was well illustrated in an early study by Levi (1969). He measured catecholamines in the urine, as a biochemical indicator of general arousal, in groups of men and women after they had watched an erotic film. He also asked each subject to rate their degree of sexual arousal whilst watching the film. The women gave a much higher correlation between self-ratings of arousal and their urinary catecholamines than the men. A likely explanation is that the women, in making their self-ratings, were influenced by their awareness of cues of general excitement rather than genital response. The men would be mainly influenced by their awareness of erection, which would itself be poorly correlated with general arousal.

Genital responses, in contrast to other non-genital changes, can be regarded as more specifically sexual, i.e. they are only likely to occur in response to a sexual stimulus. This is not necessarily always the case. In Chapter 3 we will consider evidence of a transient phase of non-specific erectile responsiveness in prepubertal boys when they experience erections in response to a variety of non-sexual but arousing situations. Before long, with the effects of labelling and social learning, these responses become discriminated to specifically sexual stimuli, though this discrimination can go wrong, leading to some of the abnormalities of sexual development which will be considered in Chapter 3. It is not known whether a comparable phase of non-specific genital responsiveness occurs in prepubertal girls, who tend to be much less aware of their genital responses and to take much longer to identify them and appreciate their sexual significance.

Another example of genital responding which is not necessarily associated with sexual stimulation occurs during sleep and this is of great potential relevance to the topic of central arousability.

Genital responses during sleep

It has been known for some time that men normally have erections at intervals during sleep (nocturnal penile tumescence or NPT; see Fig. 9.3, p. 432). Erections on waking, which most men notice, are the last of these nocturnal responses which precede and continue beyond the point of waking. (They are not, as is often supposed, the result of having a full bladder.)

There are now substantial normative data on these responses, showing them to be almost universal amongst normal males, though varying in important ways through the life cycle. The frequency, duration and degree of these nocturnal erections increase during childhood to reach a peak in adolescence and thereafter gradually decline. Elderly men will still get sleep erections but they will be less frequent and less strong. There is a close association between sleep erections and phases of rapid eye movement (REM) sleep, though they are to some extent independent and the changing patterns through the life cycle are different for these two phenomena (Karacan et al 1976; see p. 434).

What is the likely relationship between these sleep responses and sexual arousability? We now know that sleep erections are not only impaired in men with loss of sexual desire but also in states of depression (when sexual desire is also likely to be reduced) and with androgen deficiency when sexual desire is also specifically affected (see p. 93). Sleep erections are often accompanied by sexual dreams, which raises the question whether they are a response to the sexual stimulating effect of the dream. The association with dreams is not invariable however, and, particularly in view of the evidence from women (see below), it is thought most likely that the sexual dreams are in response to the erections. Two recent studies have shown that the EEG hemispheric asymmetry, which occurs typically as a correlate of sexual arousal in the waking state, also occurs in association with NPT, suggesting that other manifestations of central arousal are occurring (Hirshkowitz et al 1984; Rosen et al 1986).

Thus it seems possible that this objectively measurable response gives us a 'window' into the central arousability system which is relatively unaffected by cognitive processes of the waking state. The theoretical and research implications of this possibility will be considered more fully later in this chapter.

Episodes of increased vaginal blood flow, physiologically comparable to penile erection, occur during sleep in women. They are as frequent as sleep erections, but have a less predictable association with REM sleep. Also the vascular changes occurring are as great as those recorded during full response to orgasm in the waking state (Fisher et al 1983). Of interest was the finding that the episodes associated with REM sleep were unlikely to be associated with sexual dreams.

ORGASM

Of all the various sexual responses, orgasm remains the most mysterious and the least well understood. It is difficult to define because it is such a subjective experience occurring often at a time when one's powers of observation are impaired, if not suspended. For the post-pubertal male the event is clearly marked by the occurrence of ejaculation. For the female, no such unequivocal event occurs (see later for further discussion of this point) and it is therefore more common for a woman than for a man to be uncertain whether an orgasm has happened.

And yet the orgasm is endowed with considerable importance. Its occurrence is often regarded as the goal of sexual activity and the natural conclusion; the pleasure and reduction of tension associated with it are important reinforcers in the learning of sexual behaviour; lack of orgasm is a cause of concern in many people.

Kinsey et al (1953) regarded an orgasm as an 'explosive discharge of neuromuscular tension' and described it as follows: 'as the individual approaches the peak of sexual activity he or she may suddenly become tense, momentarily maintain a high level of tension, rise to a new peak of maximum tension — and then abruptly and instantaneously release all tensions and plunge into a series of muscular spasms or convulsions through which he or she returns to a normal or even subnormal physiologic state'. There are many other definitions in the literature but they have in common a peak of tension which is then dramatically reduced. But such a definition begs several questions — what sort of tension? How could it be measured? Clearly this is definition by analogy and is not descriptive in a scientifically adequate sense.

As with sexual arousal, orgasm is a complex experience composed of a variety of phenomena. These include:

a. objective changes in the genitalia;
b. changes in skeletal muscle tone and semi-voluntary movements;
c. general cardiovascular and respiratory changes;
d. somatic sensory experiences, and
e. altered consciousness.

Orgasm is also characterised by its inevitable sequal — the post-orgasm phase — when most of these changes revert to normal, but with a speed which suggests an active rather than passive process. Let us consider these various types of change and how they differ in males and females.

Genital responses during orgasm

The male

Usually before any of the other phenomena of orgasm occur the male becomes aware that ejaculation is imminent — the point of so-called 'ejaculatory inevitability', when ejaculation follows inevitably within 1–3 seconds. Ejaculation means forceful expulsion of semen from the urethra, sometimes propelled for a distance of 50 cm or more. If semen drains from the urethra without this force it is called emission. The processes underlying this response are complex and not fully understood. Masters & Johnson (1966) divide it into two stages. In stage I, smooth muscle contraction occurs in the vas efferens of the testis, the epididymis, vas deferens, together with the seminal vesicle, prostate and ampulla. A substantial part of the seminal fluid comes from the prostate. Accumulation of fluid builds up in the prostatic urethra, whilst the urethral bulb dilates in anticipation. Retrograde passage of the fluid into the bladder is prevented by closure of the internal sphincter, which also prevents urine from joining the semen. Stage II starts with a relaxation of the external bladder sphincter, allowing the pent-up fluid into the urethral bulb. The semen is then propelled along the penile urethra by rhythmic contractions of the bulbospongiosus and ischiocavernosus muscles, the sphincter urethrae and the urethral bulb.

The volume of semen ejaculated varies considerably, usually between 1 and 6 ml. With repeated ejaculations over a short period the volume and sperm content becomes progressively less. Usually the largest volumes occur after relatively long periods of ejaculatory abstinence.

The female

The duration of the orgasmic experience varies considerably among women, though Levin & Wagner (1985), measuring duration in the laboratory, reported a mean of 20 seconds. A few seconds after the onset of the subjective experience of orgasm there is an initial spasm of the muscles surrounding the outer third of the vagina (the 'orgasmic platform'), followed by a series of rhythmic contractions, usually five to eight in number. Synchronous contractions of the anal sphincter occur in some women (Bohlen et al 1982). Uterine contractions may also occur but are less rhythmic than those in the vagina.

Masters & Johnson consider these vaginal contractions to be the essence of the female orgasm, comparable physiologically to the rhythmic contractions which subserve ejaculation in the male. It has been contested that women may experience 'orgasm' without these vaginal contractions (Bohlen et al 1982) and this issue is still disputed. Inadequate tone in these muscles has been suggested as a cause for orgasmic dysfunction in women (Graber & Kline-Gaber, 1979), but Chambless et al (1982) found no relationship between the strength of the levator ani (pubococcygeus) muscle contraction and orgasmic responsiveness.

General muscular responses during orgasm

The pattern of general skeletal muscle activity during non-orgasmic sexual arousal varies considerably, though there is no obvious sex difference in this respect. Much of this motor activity is voluntary and depends on the body position involved. As excitement increases, certain motor responses become more predictable and less voluntary, especially pelvic thrusting and contraction of the rectus abdominus muscles, sternomastoid and facial musculature, and sometimes carpopedal spasm. During orgasm spasm of these various muscle groups is maximal, and muscle tension declines rapidly once orgasm has passed. Not only the extent but also the intensity of these spasms, which have both tonic and clonic phases, vary considerably and in their most extreme forms resemble generalised convulsions, leading Kinsey and his colleagues to liken such an orgasm to an epileptic fit. The possibility that these two types of neurophysiological event may indeed have some features in common is considered further below.

Cardiovascular and respiratory responses associated with orgasm

As already described, changes in heart rate and blood pressure, together with other peripheral vascular responses, may occur during sexual excitement, though to a very variable degree. With orgasm, however, there is a predictable though short-lived rise in both heart rate and blood pressure which starts shortly before the orgasm occurs.

According to Littler et al (1974) rises in blood pressure during the excitement phase are inconsistent because of compensatory baroreceptor-induced bradycardia. This compensatory mechanism appears to be over-ruled at the time of orgasm. Increases in heart rate at this time range from 20 to 80 beats/min, systolic blood pressure from 25–120 mmHg and diastolic pressure from 25 to 50 mmHg (see p. 564 for further evidence).

Respiration rate, which also shows variable changes during the excitement phase, predictably shows hyperventilation shortly before orgasm. Masters & Johnson (1966) cite rates of around 40 breaths/min. One wonders whether any of the carpopedal spasms occurring at this time may be due to hyperventilation tetany. Singer (1973) emphasises a characteristic respiratory pattern of apnoea accompanying certain types of female orgasm. Physiological evidence of this pattern is given by Fox & Fox (1969). A characteristic 'sex flush', an erythematous rash affecting the skin of the trunk, occurs shortly before orgasm in a proportion of women and men. The incidence of this phenomenon is not known, though of Masters & Johnson's laboratory subjects, 75% of the women and 25% of the men showed it.

The somatic sensations of orgasm

The somatic feelings experienced during orgasm are to some extent determined by the specific genital responses. Thus the sensation of ejaculation is a characteristic part of the male's and vaginal or uterine contractions of the female's experience. But apart from these sensations, the experience is felt or at least described in very different ways. The sensation may be confined to the perineum or spread over part or all of the body. Subjective descriptions are so varied that any attempt to describe a typical orgasmic experience would be misleading. Vance & Wagner (1976) obtained written descriptions from a group of men and women, and when the obviously sex-linked features were removed, it was not possible to distinguish between male and female accounts.

The following are examples from this study:

'An orgasm . . . located (originating) in the genital area, capable of spreading out further . . . legs, abdomen. A sort of pulsating feeling — very nice if it can extend itself beyond the immediate genital area.'

'Begins with tensing and tingling in anticipation, rectal contractions starting series of chills up spine. Tingling and buzzing sensations grow suddenly to explosion in genital area, some sensation of dizzying and weakening — almost loss of conscious sensation, but not really. Explosion sort of flowers out to varying distance from genital area, depending on intensity'.

'A heightened feeling of excitement with severe muscular tension especially through the back and legs, rigid straightening of the entire body for about 5 seconds, and a strong and general relaxation and very tired relieved feeling'.

'I really think it defies description by words. Combination of waves of very pleasurable sensations and mounting of tensions culminating in a fantastic sensation and release of tension'.

'Often loss of contact with reality. All senses acute. Sight becomes patterns of colour, but often very difficult to explain because words were made to fit in the real world'.

'Stomach muscles get "nervous" causing a thrusting movement with hips or pelvis. Muscular contractions all over the body'.

Altered consciousness

Some of the descriptions given above imply altered consciousness. At its quietest, an orgasm may leave the subject completely in control; at its most extreme, there may be virtual loss of consciousness and certainly loss of control, similar to certain types of epileptic fit in both its convulsive quality and its alteration of consciousness. Although many of the sensory and motor components of orgasm may reflect spinally mediated mechanisms, this altered consciousness strongly suggests some central neurophysiological event. We will return to this point when considering underlying mechanisms.

After the orgasm: the refractory period

A characteristic of orgasm is the state of calm that follows it. There is a fairly rapid return of the various physiological manifestations of arousal and vasocongestion to normal, together with a subjective feeling of calm. Without orgasm, these changes take much longer to resolve, especially in the woman where congestion of the pelvic organs may remain for several hours, sometimes with a sense of discomfort, if no orgasm occurs.

The male following orgasm usually remains unresponsive to further sexual stimulation for a period of time known as the 'refractory period'. In the young male this may be a matter of minutes, whereas in the older male it may be many hours. Women, on the other hand, may be able to experience repeated multiple orgasms in a short period, and many have been observed to do so by Masters & Johnson in their laboratory investigations.

These workers therefore regard the refractory period as a uniquely male phenomenon. This conclusion should not be too readily accepted. There are females who describe a definite refractory period and this may be associated with certain types of female orgasm, possibly not the type that is likely to occur in a laboratory setting. Kinsey et al (1953) reported only 14% of their female sample as being multiply orgasmic on a regular basis. There may be many women who fail to realise their potential in this respect, though a higher percentage who do might be found if Kinsey's survey were repeated now. Nevertheless, it is highly likely that the women in Masters & Johnson's study were not representative of women in general. The refractory period is not inevitable in the male either. Kinsey et al (1948) found that prepubertal boys who masturbated to orgasm were able to repeat orgasm within a few minutes, and nearly a third were able to achieve five or more orgasms in rapid succession (at this age, unaccompanied by ejaculation). This ability becomes markedly reduced with advancing age, although the most noticeable change occurs at the onset of puberty and the first ejaculation. By contrast, the occurrence of multiple orgasms in women remains relatively constant throughout their lifespan. Although we should challenge Masters & Johnson's assertion on this point there are undoubtably important male—female differences in this respect.

Types of female orgasm

One of the most intriguing debates in the field of human sexuality has concerned the nature of the female orgasm. This started with Freud's doctrine that the continued reliance of a woman on clitoral stimulation in order to experience orgasm is a sign of immaturity, a failure of the 'clitoral–vaginal transfer' which signals sexual maturity. The battle has raged ever since, fuelled in part by those large numbers of women who question whether they should be regarded as immature on these grounds. Kinsey et al (1953) emphasised the insensitivity to touch of the vaginal wall in contrast to the clitoris and labia minora, and hence concluded that vaginal as distinct from clitoral orgasms were a 'biological impossibility'. They may have underestimated the importance of pressure rather than touch as a vaginal stimulus. Masters & Johnson (1966) developed this theme, claiming that either direct or indirect stimulation of the clitoris is always necessary for orgasm, and that the physiological changes accompanying it are the same whatever the method of stimulation. This has led to the conclusion that instead of two types of female orgasm (clitoral and vaginal) there is only one. Evidence to the contrary continues to accumulate. The women in Fisher's study (Fisher 1973) described fundamentally different types of orgasmic experience, often in the same individual. Fox & Fox (1969) have physiological correlates of different types occurring in one particular woman. Bentler & Peeler (1979) found that young female students distinguished quite clearly between orgasm experienced during vaginal intercourse, and those resulting from direct clitoral stimulation, whether with their partners or alone. Singer (1973) considered the evidence and reached the conclusion that there are at least two basic patterns which may combine — he calls these 'vulval' and 'uterine'. The vulval orgasm depends on clitoral stimulation, occurring either directly or indirectly during coitus or petting, and manifested by vaginal contractions. The uterine experience, he suggests, is characterised by more marked emotional reactions, by apnoea and without vaginal contractions. He speculates that this may depend on uterine or visceral buffeting which occurs with deep vaginal penetration during coitus. It is this type of orgasm, which is more emotionally fulfilling, that he associates with a female refractory period. He explains the apparent absence of this type of orgasm from the observations of Masters & Johnson in the laboratory as being due to the difficulty in obtaining the necessary psychological conditions in that setting. The vulval orgasm, he suggests, is more mechanical and hence easier to produce. If so, evidence of this kind of orgasm must be confined to careful verbal reporting or more private physiological investigation as carried out by Fox & Fox in their own home.

This controversy remains largely unresolved, except that there is now general agreement that Freud's attribution of immaturity to clitoral orgasm is untenable. Masters & Johnson have done women a service in that respect. Findings from Fisher's (1973) study even suggest the opposite. Women who had a definite preference for vaginal orgasms were more prone to anxiety. He suggested that reliance on vaginal intercourse, rather than direct clitoral stimulation, could serve to avoid more intense sexual excitement which these women find threatening, perhaps because they are generally less comfortable about somatic changes in their own bodies. He also pointed out that vaginal intercourse might be a more acceptable form of behaviour for these women than stimulation, which has masturbatory connotations. Hite (1976) in her survey found a substantial majority of women who required clitoral stimulation in order to experience orgasm and this has been found in a number of surveys (see Chapter 4). The continuing debate of these various aspects of female orgasm is a fascinating one in several respects, as it is not just a matter of sexual physiology. Doris Lessing (whose description of several types of female orgasm in her novel *The Golden Notebook* is often quoted in sexological texts), wrote the following: 'There can be a thousand thrills, sensations, etc. but there is only one real female orgasm and that is when a man, from the whole of his need and desire, takes a woman and wants all her response. Everything else is a substitute and a fake and the most inexperienced woman feels this instinctively'. At a time when many women are reacting against traditional forms of male dominance and female dependence, such a description is like to provoke a mixed reaction in women. It is easy to see how the physiological issues can become obscured. The latest chapter in this controversy concerns female ejaculation and the 'G' spot.

The 'G' spot and female ejaculation

Two more recent and related controversies have concerned the existence of a localised zone of erotic sensitivity within the vagina called the 'G' spot, and the female's capacity for ejaculation.

The 'G' spot, so-called after Grafenburg (1950) who first described it, is said to be a small area of exquisite erotic sensitivity on the anterior wall of the vagina; orgasm is produced by stimulation of it. This type of orgasm has been linked with the ejection of fluid from the urethra, called female ejaculation. These two ideas conflict with conventional wisdom and have generated considerable debate. Much of this has been fuelled by the somewhat sensational presentation of these ideas, with obvious commercial implications. The discovery and description of a 'new erotic zone' in women is a saleable idea — many women were keen to find out if they owned such a previously undisclosed source of erotic pleasure — whereas the notion of female ejaculation adds a novel twist to the on-going controversy about the biological as distinct from socially contrived differences between men and women. Obviously it is important not to reject a new idea simply because it has been commercially exploited. What should we conclude from the available evidence, and how new, in fact, are these ideas?

As mentioned earlier, Kinsey concluded, partly on the basis of studies he had performed in collaboration with Dickinson, that the walls of the vagina were insensitive to touch. The concept of the 'G' spot suggests that at least in some women certain parts of the vaginal wall are highly sensitive. Hoch (1980) has for some time described an erotic sensitivity of the anterior vaginal wall in some women, though he disputes that this is localised to a small area. The urethra runs close to the anterior vaginal wall for part of its course between the bladder and the vulva. For some individuals, men and women, the urethra does appear to be erotically sensitive, as evidenced by the tendency for some people to sexually stimulate themselves by inserting objects into the urethra. In his original description Grafenburg related this anterior vaginal wall sensitivity to the urethra and this is, in my view, the most likely explanation for the so-called 'G' spot: that in a proportion of women erotic sensitivity of the urethra is perceived through the anterior vaginal wall, where it runs closest to the vagina. The majority of women, it would seem, are not aware of any such localised sensitivity.

What of female ejaculation? There is no doubt that a small number of women are seriously worried by a tendency during orgasm to pass fluid, which they take to be urine. Probably in some cases urinary incontinence does occur. But are there other explanations? Such fluid has been reported to contain constituents, e.g. prostatic acid phosphatase, suggestive of prostatic secretion, raising the possibility that vestigial remnants of prostatic tissue may persist in some women and account for the fluid. Descriptions of some female 'ejaculators' include the development during sexual response of a swelling in the anterior vaginal wall close to the sensitive area, which disappears once 'ejaculation' has occurred. This is presumably the fluid collecting in the urethra at that point. It seems reasonable to conclude from the available evidence that a small proportion of women do produce fluid, which is not urine, from the urethra at the time of orgasm. Its ejection can in a literal sense be called ejaculation, but to what extent is the process homologous in physiological terms to male ejaculation, or in anatomical terms to the prostatic origin of male ejaculatory fluid?

As we shall see in Chapter 3, the prostate gland is derived embryologically from the wolffian duct system, which normally atrophies during female development. The female urethra is, however, surrounded by glandular tissue. In some women these glands are organised to feed into a paraurethral duct system, running along either side of the outer part of the urethra and opening just inside the urethral meatus. Such structures are normally called Skene's glands after the man who described them in 1880. Huffman (1948) in a more recent and detailed anatomical study found that these paraurethral duct systems were the exception rather than the rule. He found considerable variability between women in the extent and location of these glands, most of which open directly into the urethra along its course. That the embryological origin of these glands is similar or even homologous to that of prostatic tissue has been suggested for a long time. More recently these glands have been found to be immunologically similar to prostatic tissue and to secrete prostatic acid phosphatase (Pollen & Dreilinger 1984), though it should be pointed out that prostatic acid phosphatase is produced by tissues other than the prostate (e.g. the kidney). In addition, there are in the male comparable glands along most of the urethra. Although little attention has been paid to the anatomy and physiology of these male structures, it is probable that they (rather than Cowper's glands) are responsible for the pre-ejaculatory emission experienced by many men during sexual arousal. In the Kinsey survey (Gebhard & Johnson 1979) 78% of male subjects were aware of this pre-ejaculatory fluid, and although in the majority this only involved a drop or two, in nearly 20% there was sufficient fluid to drip from the penis, causing embarassment in some such men. It is possible that all the glandular structures along the urethra, including these periurethral glands and the prostate, have features in common. The comparable glands in the female may also share some features, including embryological origin, but there is little purpose in referring to them as the 'female prostate', any more than we call the periurethral glands in the male 'prostatic tissue'. If, however, the glands in the female do originate from the wolffian system, then we should expect to find them to be much more developed in a few women than is usual in the majority, accounting for the occasional woman who produces an unusual amount of fluid. It is also interesting to speculate whether such tissue of wolffian origin may respond to testosterone and therefore be more developed in women with relatively high androgen levels. Such tissue has been shown to be testosterone-dependent in female rodents (Korenchevsky 1937) but I know of no relevant data for women.

To what extent is ejection of such fluid homologous to male ejaculation? It is important to remind ourselves that ejaculation in the male has two components: the emission of fluid which depends on smooth muscle contraction passing fluid along both the vas and urethra, and the additional pumping effect of the rhythmic striped muscle contraction accompanying orgasm, which adds to the emission the forceful ejaculatory spurt. In a women who collects fluid, from whatever source, in her urethra, possibly contained during sexual stimulation by restriction of the perivaginal muscles, the onset of orgasm and the rhythmic muscle contractions which are basically similar to those in the male would lead to ejaculation of the fluid. Thus the ejaculatory process may be found in both cases, but the emission of fluid only in the male. In any case, rather more has been made of this issue than the subject warrants. What is of clinical importance is the recognition that some women do eject fluid during orgasm which is not necessarily urine. This information could be very reassuring to those women who are deeply embarrassed by what they assume is urinary incontinence.

The functions of orgasm

The reproductive function of orgasm in the male is obvious because of the associated ejaculation of semen. The pleasure experience during orgasm will also act as a motivator for further reproductive acts. In the female, the function is not so obvious. It has been suggested that orgasm enhances fertility by producing negative pressure in the uterus and hence suction of semen through the cervix. The evidence for this is disputed and Masters & Johnson found no such negative pressure. Nor is there any evidence linking orgasmic potential with fertility in the human female.

Orgasmic pleasure can have the same motivating effect in the female as in the male. Yet the situation remains paradoxical. Women, we have reason to believe, have greater orgasmic potential than men and yet a much higher proportion of women never experience orgasm. In other mammalian species it is difficult to know whether females experience orgasm at all, and it seems likely that it is at most an occasional event. If there is a basic difference between males and females in orgasmic potential it seems likely that this would be more evident in subhuman than in human mammals, on the grounds that most biologically determined differences become relatively obscured the higher up the mammalian tree. Yet it appears to be the other way round.

The refractory period in the male serves a spacing function — allowing a replenishment of sperm numbers and avoiding excessive sexual activity which could be biologically maladaptive. Females probably do not have this spacing device, or at least not to the same extent. Perhaps as a consequence, Sherfey (1966) has described the female as sexually insatiable and consequently has had her sexual activity contained by powerfully repressive social inhibitions; this is an intriguing if somewhat contentious point of view.

Mechanisms underlying orgasm

Semans & Langworthy (1938), following their study of sexual responses in cats, suggested the neurophysiological basis of emission and ejaculation which is usually accepted as relevant to the human male. They postulated an ejaculation centre in the lumbar cord which produces emission via the sympathetic outflow from the first two lumbar roots and ejaculation via the sacral parasympathetic outflow (S2–4), and presumably dependent on contraction of the ischiocavernosus, bulbospongiosus and contractor urethrae muscles. The evidence for this in man is lacking. Effects on sexual responses of sympathectomy involving different parts of the sympathetic chain were reported by Whitelaw & Smithwick (1951) and they proved to be variable and inconsistent. It was, however, relatively common for emission to be impaired when lumbar parts of the cord were removed, and unusual if only thoracic rami were affected.

Various drugs, especially anti-adrenergic compounds like guanethidine and certain tranquillisers such as thioridazine, sometimes lead to failure of ejaculation. Typically the man experiences orgasm without the sensation of emission or ejaculation — the so-called 'dry-run orgasm' (Money & Yankowitz 1967). This is commonly attributed to failure of control of the internal bladder sphincter leading to retrograde ejaculation into the bladder. Whereas this undoubtedly happens after certain kinds of prostatectomy and as an occasional consequence of diabetic neuropathy, there is no evidence that this is the explanation in the case of anti-adrenergic drugs. It thus seems possible that emission can be pharmacologically blocked without interfering with orgasm. In men with severe premature ejaculation, it is common for them to describe a minimal or absent orgasm and no ejaculatory component; the semen just oozes out of the urethra. These men would appear to be experiencing emission with no ejaculation and little or no orgasm. The relationship between these three components therefore remains obscure, except that they usually occur together. It seems probable however that the muscular contractions that produce ejaculation are part of the motor component of orgasm, whereas emission, a smooth muscle response, is distinct and separable; this would conform with the neural separation of the two processes described by Semans & Langworthy (1938) in the cat.

We have no evidence of the peripheral mediation of orgasm in the female, though it is usually assumed to be similar to the male.

Also obscure is the relationship between the refractory period and these various components of orgasm. In rats, the normal refractory period that occurs after coitus does not occur after electroejaculation (Beach et al 1966). Now that methods of electroejaculation are being developed for human males, mainly for paraplegic men, comparable evidence for the human may become available. In men with severe premature ejaculation, in whom, as already stated, emission may be the only discernible response, the refractory period is often unusually prolonged or severe. Multiple orgasms have been described in men, apparently obtained by a conscious inhibition of ejaculation (Robbins & Jensen 1978). The implication is that the refractory period depends upon the occurrence of emission rather than orgasm. But from the evidence presented, it is not clear that the orgasms reported were any more than peaks of excitement and arousal.

So far, we have considered mechanisms operating at a spinal level. But these uncertainties bring us to a fundamental question about orgasm. To what extent is it a spinal phenomenon, or to what extent does it depend on central events? In the squirrel monkey, when sites in the limbic system of the brain are stimulated erection or ejaculation is produced, followed by a state of quietude, when further erections are less likely to be elicited (MacLean & Ploog 1962; Robinson & Mishkin 1968). This sounds comparable to the refractory period after orgasm. Once again we lack comparable evidence for the female monkey. Kinsey, it will be remembered, likened the more intense orgasm to an epileptic fit. EEG changes resembling petit mal or the late stage of a grand mal seizure have been recorded during self-induced orgasm (Mosovich & Tallafero 1954). Heath (1972) recorded changes from implanted electrodes in a man and woman, both epileptic patients, and each showed localised discharges from the septal region associated with orgasm. These were similar to epileptiform changes but were localised and did not reach scalp electrodes. Cohen et al (1976) used a change in laterality of the EEG as an indicator of a significant cerebral neurophysiological event and found that this occurred in the majority of their normal subjects during orgasm. When it did not occur, the orgasms were of low intensity. In contrast, Graber et al (1985) failed to find any distinctive EEG changes in four men during masturbation and ejaculation; the authors concluded that changes reported by other workers were at least in part the result of movement artifact.

We remain uncertain therefore about the existence of a central phenomenon associated with orgasm. The considerable variation in intensity of orgasm could well be accounted for by variation in the intensity of such a central component, which when intense would not only lead to alteration of consciousness but could also influence the intensity of spinal responses. A further theoretical possibility is that two types of central event occur: one excitatory, the other inhibitory. The refractory period might be determined by the inhibitory component. In orgasm with prolonged refractory period, the inhibitory component may predominate, as in the man with severe premature ejaculation. With intensely pleasurable orgasms, the excitatory component may predominate and the refractory period may be consequently shorter. This hypothesis is open to empirical testing.

In most respects, however, we are only in a position to speculate about the neurophysiological basis of orgasm and the apparent male–female difference remains a particularly intriguing issue.

THE ROLE OF SEX HORMONES IN SEXUAL BEHAVIOUR

The sexual behaviour of most subprimates is very much under the control of hormones. The female of most species will only be sexually active at particular times of her hormonal cycle, usually known as the oestrus or 'heat'. If castrated, she will show no sexual activity at all. Her sexual behaviour is therefore largely dependent on ovarian hormones, though the pattern of hormones involved varies from species to species. Female carnivores (e.g. cats and dogs) require oestrogen alone; in rodents (e.g. rats, guinea-pigs) 'heat' is usually induced by oestrogen followed a few hours later by a large amount of progesterone. Ungulates (e.g. sheep) require oestrogen preceded by progesterone.

Beach, many years ago, pointed out how, with greater biological development, animals' sexual behaviour became less determined by hormones and more under the control of factors such as learning and environmental stimuli. In primates, however, the extent to which female sexual behaviour is under hormonal control and is restricted to a limited oestrus varies considerably from species to species and is more dependent on such factors as the level of sexual activity, social organisation or adaptation to the environment than on the degree of biological development. This variability is relevant to understanding hormones and human sexuality, as will be seen later.

In the male, hormonal determinants are rather less varied; sexual behaviour depends on androgens, and in particular testosterone, regardless of the species.

In general, when we consider the human evidence we will find that the male conforms with this cross-species generalisation. The human female presents another very complex story.

ORGANISATION VERSUS ACTIVATION

Hormonal effects on the central nervous system are of two fundamentally different kinds. The first, the organising effects of hormones on the sexual differentiation of the brain during early development, will be considered in Chapter 3. The second type is the activating effects of hormones in eliciting, facilitating or maintaining behaviour in the mature animal. For the first, hormones, mainly androgens, act at certain critical stages of development. For the second the effects depend on the continued or recurrent presence of the hormones. These two aspects of hormonal action are inter-related as the early organising effects of a hormone may influence the target organ response to later activating effects of the same hormone.

Our evidence for the activating effects comes from three principal sources.

1. The experimental manipulation of hormone levels in laboratory animals and the observed effects on behaviour; such laboratory studies have given us some as yet very incomplete evidence of the inter-relationships between sex steroids and neurotransmitters, such as cerebral amines.
2. The observed relationship between sexual activity and natural variations in sex hormone levels; we have some evidence from studying primates in their natural habitat and rather more from human studies.
3. The study of sexual behaviour associated with abnormal endocrine states and the therapeutic use of exogenous hormones or anti-hormones.

We will consider the evidence from these various sources in some detail.

HORMONES AND MALE SEXUALITY

Animal evidence

Although we must be cautious in extrapolating from subprimate data to man, many of the following points derived from the study of male subprimates are proving to be of considerable human relevance.

1. The male's sexual behaviour predictably declines following castration, with various components of copulatory behaviour being affected at different speeds. Thus ejaculation is the first to disappear, followed by intromission and eventually mounting. With androgen replacement, these responses are restored in the reverse order.
2. Although sexual decline after male castration is predictable, the speed and extent of that decline varies considerably from individual to individual within the same species. One animal may cease all sexual activity within a few days; another may still be ejaculating a year later. A fair proportion continue with a low level of mounting behaviour indefinitely. Ward (1977) has summarised some of the principal factors causing this variance as follows: 'It appears that the expression of masculine sexual patterns is more dependent upon the sensitivity or responsiveness of the central tissues on which androgens act than on minor fluctuations in adult steroid titres, provided that sufficient hormone is present to exceed the minimum threshold for behavioural activation. The sensitivity of the target tissue in turn is determined by genetic predisposition, the presence of androgens during fetal sexual differentiation, and adequate prepubertal socialisation.'
3. If the prepubertal androgen rise does not take place, the subsequent development of adult patterns of copulatory behaviour will be delayed

but not prevented, provided that androgen levels rise later. In other words, the timing of the pubertal androgen surge is not apparently critical.

4. The relevant sites of action of androgens in the male animal are at least of three kinds, which to some extent can be experimentally separated. These are the limbic system of the brain (especially anterior hypothalamus); the spinal cord (where reflexes serving erection and ejaculation are androgen-dependent) and the penis. In many animals, including many primates but not man, the penile glans and shaft are covered in small spines which in some way increase sensory input during direct tactile stimulation. These spines are androgen-dependent. The spinal reflex effects have been maintained in castrated males by localised injection of testosterone and the penile changes by means of dihydrotestosterone. But only if the *brain* is androgenised will a full and normal pattern of sexual activity arise.

With primates, the male has received much less attention than the female. Many species are seasonal, so that testicular activity and mating behaviour are confined to certain seasons of the year. Systematic studies of male hormone–sexual behaviour relationships have been confined to three species; the rhesus and stumptail macaques and the talapoin (Dixson 1983).

Effects of castration and anti-androgens are similar to those observed in other mammals, with ejaculation and intromission the most androgen-dependent components of the copulatory pattern. Not only is there individual variation of effects within species, as described above, but also there are some species differences, with the stumptail macaque being relatively less affected by hormonal manipulation than the other two species (Dixson 1983).

The human male

The role of androgens

Until recently the relevance of reproductive hormones to the sexuality of men remained controversial. Clinical endocrinologists, with their experience of treating hypogonadal states, had seldom expressed any doubts. However, in the absence of controlled and systematically collected data, and because of the inconsistencies reported, some authorities, such as Kinsey, concluded that hormones were largely redundant in human sexuality; such effects as do occur are mediated by non-specific changes in energy or mood (Kinsey et al 1953).

In recent years the greater readiness to analyse the complexity of human sexual interaction and the availability of modern methods of hormone assay has produced evidence which is steadily clarifying the picture as far as the human male is concerned. There are still some unanswered questions, but there has been a gratifying consistency across the various controlled studies and sources of evidence, despite the usually small numbers of subjects involved.

Sources of evidence include controlled studies of hormone replacement in hypogonadal men, the effects of anti-androgens and exogenous androgens in eugonadal men and correlational and developmental studies. There is also limited evidence of the effects of sexual activity or erotic stimuli on hormone levels.

Hormone replacement in hypogonadal men

The most crucial evidence comes from placebo-controlled evaluation of androgen replacement in hypogonadal men (Davidson et al 1979; Luisi & Franchi 1980; Skakkebaek et al 1981). These studies have shown conclusively that within 3 to 4 weeks of androgen withdrawal there is a decline in sexual interest and, eventually, in the capacity for seminal emission (Fig. 2.32). The effects on sexual activity are less predictable because of the confounding effect of the sexual partner but this effect tends to decline as a consequence of reduced sexual interest. These changes are reversed within 7 to 14 days of androgen replacement. The effect on sexual interest has been shown to be dose-related (Fig. 2.33; Davidson et al 1979; Salmimies et al 1982; O'Carroll et al 1985).

The effects of androgen withdrawal on mood have been more variable, and though there is little doubt that well-being and energy are often influenced, such effects are less predictable and less striking than those on sexual interest, making it unlikely that the sexual effects are secondary to non-specific mood effects (O'Carroll et al 1985).

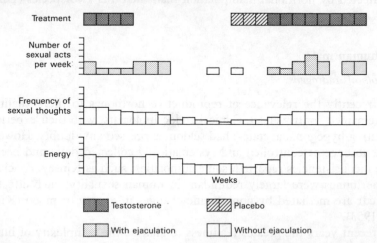

Fig. 2.32 The effects of testosterone replacement in a hypogonadal man aged 40, castrated one year earlier for testicular neoplasm. Sexual activity, ejaculation, sexual thoughts and energy all decline about 3 weeks after stopping testosterone treatment. There is no response to placebo, but a rapid response within one or two weeks of restarting testosterone treatment. (Skakkebaek et al 1981)

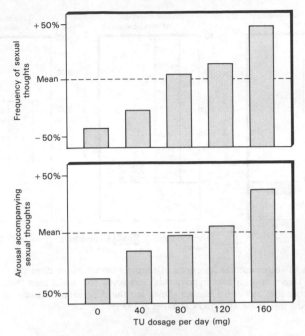

Fig. 2.33 Dose-response relationship between testosterone undecanoate (TU) and median standardised visual analogue ratings of frequency of sexual thoughts (top) and arousal accompanying sexual thoughts (bottom). Both relationships are significant ($p < 0.01$,) according to Page's test for ordered alternatives. (O'Carroll et al 1985)

The relationship between androgens and erectile function has proved to be more complex, and it is necessary to distinguish between erections during sleep (NPT) and erections in response to erotic stimuli. Hypogonadal men have impaired sleep erections (Cunningham et al 1982) and androgen replacement has been shown significantly to improve the frequency, magnitude and latency of NPT (Fig. 2.34, Kwan et al 1983; O'Carroll et al 1985) and a dose–response relationship with the frequency of erections on waking has been reported.

In contrast, erections in response to erotic films, measured in the laboratory, have been unaffected by androgen withdrawal and replacement, in spite of marked effects on sexual interest and behaviour (Fig. 2.35). In our study (Bancroft & Wu 1983) we found that erections in response to erotic fantasy did appear to be androgen-dependent, but support for this was not found by Kwan et al (1983).

Thus, whilst the central processes leading to spontaneous erection, such as during sleep, appear to be androgen-dependent, mechanisms leading to erection in response to certain types of external erotic stimuli (i.e. those mediated via the brain) remain intact despite androgen deficiency.

The role of androgens in the erectile response to tactile stimulation of the penis (i.e. external stimuli mediated via the spinal cord) is unclear. In men

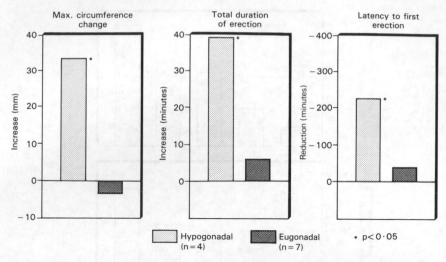

Fig. 2.34 Effects of intramuscular injections of testosterone esters on three parameters of nocturnal penile tumescence in four hypogonadal and seven eugonadal men (with probable psychogenic erectile dysfunction). Changes shown are the differences between recordings before and after the injections. (from O'Carroll et al 1985)

both tactile sensitivity of the penis (Newman 1970; Edwards & Husted 1976) and number of testosterone receptors in the penile skin (Deslypere & Vermeulen 1984) decline with age. Whether these two processes are causally related remains to be demonstrated.

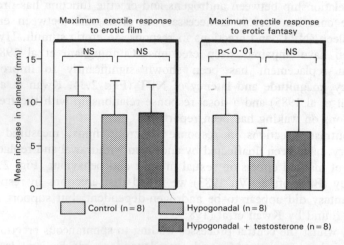

Fig. 2.35 Erectile response to erotic film and fantasy in hypogonadal men with and without testosterone replacement. The hypogonadal men did not differ from controls in their response to film. Their response to fantasy, however, was significantly lower than that of the controls when they were androgen-deficient and improved with testosterone replacement. Their latency of erectile response was significantly reduced after hormone replacement. (from Bancroft & Wu 1983)

The effects of anti-androgens

The limited amount of controlled evidence of the effects of anti-androgens is entirely consistent with the evidence from hypogonadal studies given above. In a group of sexual offenders both cyproterone acetate, an anti-androgen and ethinyloestradiol, an oestrogen reduced sexual interest and activity, slightly impaired the erectile response to erotic fantasies and slides but left the response to erotic film unaffected (Fig. 2.36; Bancroft et al 1974). NPT was not measured in this study.

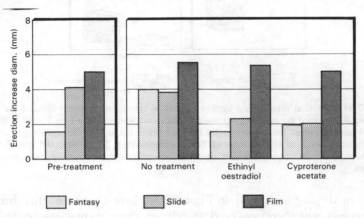

Fig. 2.36 Effects of cyproterone acetate (an anti-androgen) and ethinyloestradiol on erectile response to erotic stimuli in 12 sexual offenders (from Bancroft et al 1974). The reduction in response to fantasy and slide whilst taking the two treatments was significant; $P < 0.05$.

Studies of eugonadal men

How does the above evidence from hypogonadal studies relate to our knowledge of the man whose circulating testosterone levels are within the normal range? In younger men correlational studies of levels of circulating testosterone and measures of sexual interest or activity have shown no association (Raboch & Starka 1973; Kraemer et al 1976; Brown et al 1978b). In one study, measuring erections in response to erotic stimuli in young men, a correlation was found between testosterone levels and the latency but not the degree of erection (Lange et al 1980). The failure to find significant correlations between androgens and sexual behaviour in eugonadal men is perhaps not surprising. It is widely assumed that there is a threshold level of circulating testosterone above which level an increase will have no additional behavioural effect. It is also frequently assumed that such a threshold is close to the bottom of the laboratory normal range, though there is no evidence to support such a view. If such a threshold does exist it is likely to vary between individuals and may in many cases fall well within the normal range. But in any case we should not expect to find that variations in androgen levels are reflected in variations in sexual behaviour unless the hormonal variation is predominantly below the threshold. This

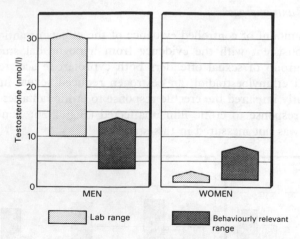

Fig. 2.37 Hypothetical relationship between levels of circulating testosterone and the behaviourally relevant range of testosterone in men and women. The Lab Range is the observed normal range; the behaviourally relevant range is the hypothetical range over which changing levels of testosterone would affect behaviour. It is postulated that the behaviourally relevant range is smaller than the laboratory normal range in men, but larger in women.

point is made diagramatically in Figure 2.37. Investigation of this threshold phenomenon will therefore need to rely on experimental manipulation of circulating testosterone. As yet there have been no such placebo-controlled studies in normal men, though in a World Health Organization (WHO) study of testosterone as a male contraceptive, some subjects reported 'increased libido' (WHO 1982).

In a placebo-controlled cross-over study of a group of eugonadal patients complaining of loss of sexual interest, two-weekly injections of testosterone

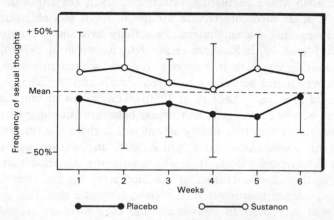

Fig. 2.38 Self-rating of sexual thoughts during testosterone (intramuscular Sustanon) and placebo treatment in 10 men complaining of reduced sexual interest. Individual scores have been standardised and expressed as variations from the overall mean in percentage of the range used. (from O'Carroll & Bancroft 1984)

esters produced a modest but significant increase in sexual interest (O'Carroll & Bancroft 1984; Fig. 2.38). And in four XXY men with androgen levels in the lower part of the normal range, oral testosterone undecanoate produced a significant increase in sexual interest when compared with placebo (Wu et al 1981). Evidence from older men will be presented in Chapter 5.

Effects of drugs on androgen levels

Further evidence comes from recent studies of male epileptics, who commonly report low sexual interest. In the past this has been attributed to the epileptic process, but recent studies have shown that, at least in some cases, this is associated with low free testosterone levels in the plasma (Toone et al 1983). Most anti-convulsants raise levels of SHBG in the blood by stimulating liver enzymes. This may result in low free testosterone in spite of raised or normal total testosterone levels. Reduced free T in such men has also been associated with impaired sleep erections (Fenwick et al 1986; see p. 93).

Hormone levels in men with sexual dysfunction

Much of the evidence in this category is of limited value because of a failure to distinguish between erectile dysfunction and loss of sexual interest. In groups of 'impotent' men undifferentiated in this way, testosterone levels have been normal (Lawrence & Swyer 1974; Schwartz et al 1980) or low (Raboch et al 1975).

In one report (Ismail et al 1970), men with loss of sexual interest and gradual onset of erectile failure were found to have low testosterone, but this was not the case in a further study (Raccy et al 1973). Men with erectile failure and normal sexual appetite have been found to have normal levels of testosterone and luteinising hormone (Pirke et al 1979). The response of 'impotent' men to both HCG and LHRH was found to be normal by Pirke and his colleagues (1979), whereas an impaired response to HCG was reported by Delitala et al (1977).

Evidence from treatment studies using hormones is also mostly confounded in a similar way. Two studies (Bruhl & Leslie 1963; Jakobovitz 1970) claim significant benefit from testosterone, but apart from the failure to assess separately problems of erection and sexual interest, the reports are too brief to allow proper evaluation. Cooper et al (1973) reported a small, transient effect with a low dose of a synthetic androgen, whereas Benkert et al (1979) reported negative results using oral testosterone undecanoate.

In our study (O'Carroll & Bancroft 1984), two groups of men, one with primary loss of sexual interest, the other with erectile dysfunction as their principal complaint, received injections of testosterone esters and placebo in a double-blind cross-over study. The men in the first group showed a significant increase in sexual interest, whereas the second group showed no improvement in erectile function (Fig. 2.38). This evidence, though limited, is consistent with the conclusion presented earlier that androgens are involved in sexual interest, but less so in erectile function.

Developmental studies

Precocious puberty in boys is most commonly due to the adrenogenital syndrome. Money & Alexander (1969) reported a series of such cases and found an early onset of sexual interest consistent with an androgen effect, though the sexual interest was expressed in a way that was consistent with the boys' social and emotional (i.e. chronological) age. Recently Udry et al (1985) studied the relationship between androgens and sexuality during normal pubertal development and found that the increase of sexual interest which occurred around puberty could be better accounted for by the increase in circulating testosterone levels than by the boys' stage of physical maturation. This is further evidence of the direct effects of androgens on the development of sexual interest and responsiveness (Fig. 2.39).

Whether there is a sensitive period of development when androgens have maximal effect on sexual development remains unclear. One way of answering this question is to look at cases of hypogonadism which became established before the onset of normal puberty and to see whether the age at which androgen replacement was started influenced the degree of sexual development. So far there is no conclusive evidence of this kind. Gooren (1988) has recently reported a study in which he compared the treatment of hypogonadism of hypergonadotrophic (i.e. secondary to testicular failure) and hypogonadotrophic (secondary to pituitary or hypothalamic failure) type in boys around the age of 15. He found that the first group responded

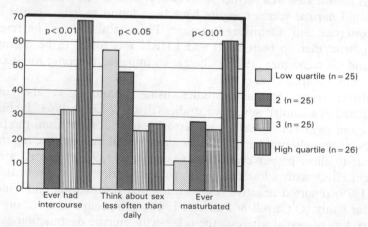

Fig. 2.39 The relationship between plasma free testosterone and measures of sexuality of boys in early adolescence. 101 boys were divided into four quartiles according to their free testosterone index. (Vory et al 1985)

better and more quickly to androgen replacement, suggesting that the hypothalamic deficiency was associated with a failure or delay in the developmental process.

Cyclical variation in androgens

Plasma testosterone shows a marked circadian (i.e 24-h) rhythm, though the timing of the rhythm varies on a seasonal basis. Reinberg & Lagoguey (1978) found no relationship between this circadian rhythm and sexual activity which, given that the behavioural effects of testosterone probably take days rather than hours to be expressed, is not surprising. There is limited evidence that seasonal variation in testosterone levels may be associated with seasonal peaks of sexual activity (Udry & Morris 1967; Smals et al 1976; Reinberg & Lagoguey 1978).

Prolactin and male sexual function

Hyperprolactinaemia in men is usually associated with sexual impairment, which is often corrected once the prolactin levels are reduced (Carter et al 1978; Franks et al 1978). Prolactin-secreting adenomas are the most likely cause of very high prolactin levels and these are rare in men. Buvat et al (1985) assessed the incidence of this cause by measuring plasma prolactin in 1053 clinically idiopathic cases of male sexual dysfunction. Among 850 cases of erectile dysfunction there were 10 cases (1.1%) of marked hyperprolactinaemia (i.e. above 35 ng/ml); six of these were found to have pituitary adenomas. Prolactin was normal in 51 cases of ejaculatory failure and 27 cases of reduced sexual interest without erectile failure.

The precise nature of this prolactin effect has remained obscure, in particular whether sexual interest and/or erectile function is primarily affected. NPT has been found to be impaired in hyperprolactinaemic men (Cunningham et al 1982) and to improve when the prolactin levels are reduced with bromocriptine (Marrama et al 1984).

Recently we reported a single case study involving a man who presented with loss of sexual desire and erectile failure. The erectile problem disappeared and his sexual relationship was much improved following a course of sex therapy involving him and his wife before it was discovered that he was grossly hyperprolactinaemic. Subsequently, placebo-controlled evaluation of bromocriptine treatment showed that lowering the prolactin resulted in a further increase in his level of sexual interest, but the change was small when compared to the impact of the sex therapy (Bancroft et al 1984). Schwartz et al (1982) have reported similar evidence from 12 men attending the Masters & Johnson Institute who were discovered to have been hyperprolactinaemic some time after completing sex therapy. Most showed improvement in erectile function following sex therapy, despite their continuing high prolactin levels, but there was an additional increase in sexual interest once the hyperprolactinaemic was treated.

It therefore seems probable that the primary effect of hyperprolacti-naemia is to reduce sexual interest, in a manner comparable to androgen deficiency. Erectile dysfunction in such cases is likely to be a psychogenic reaction to the loss of sexual interest and the consequent tension and conflicts within the sexual relationship. In a similar way, erectile failure may follow the loss of sexual interest in men with androgen deficiency.

LHRH and sexual behaviour

A direct effect of LHRH on mating behaviour, independent of its control of pituitary gonadotrophin release, has been convincingly demonstrated in a variety of species (Moss & Dudley 1982), although as yet there is only one comparable example from primates (the female marmoset; Kendrick & Dixson 1985) and none in humans. Two studies have investigated its use in the treatment of erectile dysfunction (Benkert et al 1975; Davies et al 1976), both with inconclusive results, at least partly due to inadequate definition and selection of cases. Mortimer et al (1974) treated men with hypopituitarism due to LHRH deficiency and found an increase in sexual interest following LHRH administration which apparently preceded the rise in testosterone. But this is anecdotal evidence and is not conclusive. Evans & Distiller (1979) measured erectile response to erotic stimuli after LHRH and placebo in six men and found no significant difference. Although LHRH analogues are now being used for a variety of conditions there are as yet no reports of them producing a positive effect on sexuality.

The effects of sexual stimulation on hormones in men

In those studies which have assessed the effects of sexual activity on hormones, the results have been somewhat inconsistent. Fox et al (1972) reported a rise in testosterone in one man both before and following orgasm. Purvis et al (1976), studying men producing semen samples, found a rise in testosterone following masturbation but there was no luteinising hormone rise to account for this response and no evidence of a rise in T during the anticipatory phase. This may reflect the lack of erotic quality in masturbating in such circumstances. In the first study, sexual activity involved the partner and may have been associated with some anticipatory arousal. In other studies there has been failure to find any hormonal change after both coitus and masturbation (Stearn et al 1973; Lee et al 1974).

Assessment of hormonal changes following exposure to visual erotic stimuli has also produced inconsistent results, including no change (Lincoln 1974), a somewhat delayed rise in plasma T (Pirke et al 1974) and a rapid though transient rise in luteinising hormone (LaFerla et al 1978). Important but unrecognised differences in experimental conditions may account for much of this difference, but there are clearly no simple predictable effects of sexual activity on hormonal levels in men.

Mechanisms of hormonal action in male sexuality

Biochemical aspects

How are the important effects of testosterone mediated? Do they depend on the direct effects of testosterone per se or is its reduction to 5-alpha-dihydrotestosterone (DHT) or aromatisation to oestradiol required? The somatic effects of androgens (e.g. on the prostate and seminal vesicles) largely depend on DHT, but what of the central nervous system?

In subprimates many effects of androgens on the brain depend on aromatisation, and although there are important species differences, androgenic behavioural effects can be reproduced by oestradiol implanted in appropriate sites in the brain. In ungulates (e.g. deer and sheep) oestrogens administered peripherally are as effective as testosterone, if not more so, in restoring androgen-dependent sexual behaviour in castrated males (Short 1979). DHT receptors are found in the brain (especially in the septal region and the pituitary) but are much less plentiful than oestradiol receptors (McEwen 1976) and it is still not clear whether there are receptors specific for testosterone. In most mammals DHT is ineffective on its own but may act synergistically with oestradiol (Whalen et al 1985). An exception to this, which may be relevant to man, is the rhesus monkey; in castrated males relatively high doses of DHT are effective in restoring sexual behaviour (Cochran & Perachio 1977).

In humans we have evidence that aromatisation of testosterone to oestradiol does occur in the hypothalamus (Naftolin et al 1975) but it is unlikely that the sexual effects of androgens depend on this process in view of the anti-androgenic and anti-sexual effects oestrogens have on male sexuality (Bancroft et al 1974). This is further supported by a failure to affect sexual interest or behaviour in normal men given either tamoxifen, an anti-oestrogen, or testolactone, an aromatase inhibitor (Gooren 1985).

The possibility that DHT is the mediating androgen in men is suggested by the finding that DHT undecanoate can replace testosterone undecanoate in the hormone replacement of hypogonadal men without affecting their sexuality (Gooren 1985). In contrast, it has been reported that men with 5-alpha-reductase deficiency experience 'normal' levels of sexual interest following puberty (Imperato-McGinley et al 1974).

Target organ responses to androgens

We have identified the principal sexual target of androgens as sexual interest or appetite. But further analysis of the concept of sexual interest will be required before our understanding progresses any further. Is the primary effect to alter the response or responsiveness of some arousal mechanism to cognitive or perceptual processes? Are fantasies directly influenced by androgens? The limited evidence we have reported (Bancroft & Wu 1983;

Bancroft et al 1974) raises the possibility that fantasies are androgen-dependent, at least in some individuals. Kwan et al (1983) have rejected this suggestion, but in my opinion the issue remains open.

Various ways in which androgens might influence fantasy have been suggested though none as yet with any conviction (Bancroft 1980b). It has been suggested that androgens influence persistence of attention which might in turn affect sexual behaviour (Andrew 1978). Visuospatial ability may be relevant to the visual imagery used in erotic fantasies. This ability is usually greater in men than in women, a sex difference which only becomes apparent at puberty, and which has not yet been explained. Testosterone, which increases at puberty much more in the male, could be involved. O'Carroll (1984) found that visuospatial skills did not change after androgen replacement in hypogonadal men, making it unlikely that a testosterone-dependent effect on such skills accounts for the behavioural changes observed.

Frequency of erotic fantasies has been seen as a measure of sexual appetite and it remains to be investigated whether variability in the use of erotic fantasies is correlated with circulating androgen levels in either men or women.

Davidson (1984) has suggested that in addition to maintaining sexual interest, testosterone may also influence sexual pleasure during sexual activity, possibly by enhancing sensory function. As yet the predictable enhancing effects of androgen replacement on sexual interest or thoughts in hypogonadism has not been found with self-ratings of sexual enjoyment (O'Carroll et al 1985). But specific testing of this possibility, particularly in relation to tactile sensitivity, awaits proper investigation.

Whilst it is now beyond dispute that spermatogenesis and semen production are androgen-dependent, the relationship of androgens to orgasmic capacity remains uncertain and requires further study. It is also not clear whether the virtual absence of ejaculation in the hypogonadal state is a result of lack of seminal fluid or a failure of the neurological process of seminal emission or both.

The distinction between sexual interest and erectile function has helped considerably to clarify the role of androgens in male function. The differential effects observed probably account for much of the confusion in the earlier literature about the effects of castration in men (e.g. Tauber 1940; Hamilton 1943) — a clear distinction between erectile response to erotic stimulation and spontaneous interest in sex was seldom made. But it is by now clear that to pursue such issues we should be constantly seeking to improve and refine our concepts — in particular our analysis of the various components of the sexual system which may be directly affected by hormones or pharmacological agents. The distinction which is beginning to emerge between spontaneous erections (e.g. during sleep) and those in response to erotic stimuli is of particular interest and will be considered further later in this chapter.

HORMONES AND FEMALE SEXUALITY

The subprimate evidence

In 1976 Beach introduced three concepts into the study of female sexuality.

1. attractiveness, which is some feature of the female which influences the male's behaviour. The more attractive the female, the more the male will approach and try to mount her. Attractiveness is therefore measured as the number of attempted mounts by the male, latency to first attempt or sometimes by bar pressing activity of the male to gain access to the female;
2. receptivity, which is the extent to which the female accepts the male's mounts, measured as the number of male mounts not rejected;
3. proceptivity, which is the extent to which the female takes the initiative by making some behavioural invitation (this can be seen as the female equivalent of male attractiveness, although it is seldom used in that sense).

This method of analysis has contributed substantially to our understanding of hormone–behaviour interactions, though as we shall see later these concepts do not transfer readily to the human situation and are problematic when applied to primates.

The original use of receptivity in the subprimate applied in particular to the lordosis response seen in the female rodent. This is a specific posture which facilitates mounting and intromission by the male. It is a complex reflex response which is highly dependent on oestrogen-sensitive mechanisms (Pfaff & Modianos 1985) and there is no counterpart in the primate or human female. Proceptivity and attractiveness have more general relevance. We will look at those concepts in more detail when considering primates.

Primate evidence

Although many primate species do not menstruate, the female's hormonal cycles are often similar to the menstrual cycle of the human female and hence evidence of periodic sexual activity related to particular stages of the cycle could be relevant to the human condition. To what extent do primates show oestrous behaviour and with what hormonal basis?

Whereas it is generally agreed that many of the more primitive primates, such as the lemurs, show fairly clearcut oestrous cycles, there is less consensus of opinion about the old and new world monkeys and the great apes. Probably the most widely held view is that most of the more developed primates do show some degree of oestrous cyclicity which is often obscured by social or environmental factors. This would account for the rather inconsistent evidence obtained both from observation of animals in the wild and in captivity (Rowell 1972). The potentially over-riding effect of social factors led Yerkes (1939) to propose that the extent that the sexual activity of a species was linked to the female hormonal cycle was inversely' related both to the degree of encephalisation and the degree of sexual dominance of the female by the male.

More recent evidence, both from the wild and from studies of captive animals, has shown Yerkes's hypothesis to be too simple. As we shall see, whilst the sexual dominance of the male is relevant, the degree of encephalisation is less important than the social structure of the species, the pattern of adaptation to the environment and food supply and the level of sexual drive of the male and possibly of the female. In some instances it has been clearly essential for reproduction to link sexual activity with ovulation; in others the frequency of sexual activity is sufficient to ensure optimum fertility so that the pattern of sexual activity can evolve to serve other biological purposes without jeopardising reproduction. Comparison of three of the great apes, the gorilla, orang-utan and chimpanzee, illustrates this point particularly well, as has been shown by Nadler (1980) and Short (1980b).

The male gorilla lives with a small harem of females. The huge size of the male is used to compete with other males to ensure access to such a group of females. But apart from his physical dominance, the male gorilla is a relatively sexless creature with a very small penis relative to his body size, and small testes. Sexual activity depends largely on the female taking the initiative. This she does around the time of ovulation, though for most of her adult life she will be in a state of lactational anoestrus. Even with a group of females there will be relatively long periods between occasions when one of the group is sexually receptive and proceptive. In between these times the male appears to be sexually disinterested. It is obviously essential in such circumstances that sexual activity occurs around the time of these occasional ovulations if the group is to reproduce. Thus we see a clear oestrous pattern of female proceptive behaviour which is basically similar in animals observed both in captivity and the wild.

The orang-utan has a very different social structure. These apes live predominantly in isolation presumably because of the constraints of their food supply. Adult males inhabit a territory which may overlap with that of one or more females. The male orang-utan is not only much bigger than the female but also, by comparison with the gorilla, highly sexed. If he comes across a female he is likely to copulate with her, raping her if she is not receptive. The females, who usually live with one or two dependent young, tend to keep clear of the males. As with the gorilla, their periods of fertility are widely spaced, presumably because of lactational anoestrus, but when they are once again fertile they will seek out a male and make themselves sexually available. The male indicates his position by his characteristic bellowing.

Nadler's studies of the captive orang-utan have been informative for a variety of reasons. In his earlier studies (Nadler 1977) he reported that pairing male and female orang-utans in the typical experimental setting led to copulation more or less every time and regardless of the phase of the female's menstrual cycle. He did find, however, that around the time of ovulation, copulation was more likely to be repeated and the female would be more receptive and needing less to be raped. In later experiments (Nadler 1980) he gave the female control over access to the male by putting her in an adjoining cage with a connecting opening large enough for her to pass through but too small for the male. Then he found that the female would visit the male and copulate with him around the time of ovulation. This is a parallel to the situation in the wild. This evidence illustrates clearly how a natural pattern can be obscured by studying behaviour in an unnatural setting. Thus we see that the female orang-utan shows a clear oestrous cycle, linked to ovulation, providing that she is able to control access to the male.

The chimpanzee is quite different, living in small social groups of both males and females. Whereas sexual activity may occur at any time of the female's cycle, it is undoubtedly maximal for a period of 10–16 days when there is considerable swelling of the female's external genitalia, clearly visible to males from some distance. During this phase there is frequent mating with most males in the group. This genital swelling is associated with the rising oestradiol levels of the follicular phase and ovulation occurs towards the end of this period of maximal swelling or early in the following phase of detumescence. Most of the copulation during this phase is therefore unlikely to lead to conception. It is possible that this pattern is serving the sexual needs of the males in the group without weakening group cohesion. It may also help the female to select a mate for reproductive purposes. There is a tendency, towards the end of the phase of maximal swelling, for the female to disappear from the rest of the group in the company of one particular male. According to Tutin (1980) conception is most likely to result from these temporary consortships. Here then we have an oestrous pattern of a different kind, much more extensive than is required for reproduction alone but possibly serving other needs of a social group of highly sexed animals.

Thus we can conclude that the combination of male physical dominance and high sexual drive will result in a less clear oestrous pattern if the male has access to the female. Social organisation, on the other hand, may either give the female more control of sexual activity, in which case the peri-ovulatory pattern will be more obvious, or lead to other patterns of sexual activity which are serving social as well as reproductive purposes.

Other differences between primate species, even within the same genus, can be marked. Thus with pig-tailed macaques approximately 60% of sexual interactions are initiated by the female; in the bonnet macaque the figure is almost 0% (Rosenblum personal communication). Does this reflect species differences in the constitutional levels of sexual appetite (e.g. has the bonnet male a much higher level of sexual appetite than the pig-tail male which makes female proceptivity unnecessary) or are we perhaps failing to observe some important but cryptic signals from the female bonnet to the male?

A further factor to be considered is novelty, which in itself enhances the attractiveness of a mate and may therefore obscure other determinants of attractiveness. Thus the marmoset pair, when first established, copulate fairly frequently regardless of the female's endocrine status. As they get used to one another mating becomes maximal in the late follicular phase of the cycle (Dixson & Lunn 1987). For primates who normally live in established pairs, novelty may therefore obscure the basic oestrous pattern.

If we accept that some form of oestrus exists in most primates, we are left with the question of which hormonal mechanism is responsible. In some instances, hormonally determined attractiveness of the female to the male may be the main factor. When cyclical change in female receptivity and/or proceptivity is involved we have to consider both central and peripheral mechanisms. The genital swelling of the chimpanzee (and gorilla), which is likely to be an oestrogen-dependent peripheral change, could affect the female's behaviour by making her more aware of her genitalia and hence more sexually aroused; no central hormonal effect need be involved. Alternatively sexual appetite or interest could be influenced by hormonal action in the hypothalamus or elsewhere in the brain. Direct effects of oestrogen or androgen, which both peak at mid-cycle, could be involved. Apart from excitatory effects, the cyclical pattern could depend on inhibitory effects of progesterone and periodic escape from this during the follicular phase. We do have some experimental evidence to guide us, though results from different laboratories are not always consistent and there are undoubtedly some major differences between primate species. In the experimental model used most commonly with primates, the female is castrated and her sex steroids are manipulated by means of injected exogenous supplies. She is then exposed to an intact male for a short period at a time (say 15 minutes) before both are returned to their solitary cages. Sexual activity during that period is then observed and recorded. Most such evidence relates to the rhesus macaque.

The attractiveness of the female rhesus is dependent on oestrogens. These probably act by influencing formation of vaginal odours (sometimes called pheromones; see p. 63) or by inducing colour changes and swelling in the vulva, all of which act as sexual signals to the male.

According to Herbert (1977) and his colleagues, proceptivity in the female rhesus is dependent on androgens. Once ovariectomised, her remaining source of endogenous androgens is the adrenal gland. The androgen levels can be almost eliminated either by surgical removal or dexamethasone suppression of the adrenal. Proceptivity declines markedly in such circumstances and can be restored with testosterone or androstenedione (but not dihydrotestosterone). Receptivity is affected to a lesser extent by removing androgens and seems less dependent on hormonal factors than the other two components.

The role of progestagens in this system is still somewhat obscure, but very small amounts given into the vagina, and without altering plasma levels, will apparently block the local oestrogen effect so that female attractiveness is reduced. In these circumstances, if her oestrogen levels in the central nervous system are normal, she will respond to the declining interest of the male by becoming increasingly proceptive. If, on the other hand, her attractiveness is reduced by a primary decrease in the oestrogen levels both centrally and peripherally, there will be no such compensatory increase in proceptivity. This evidence suggests that oestrogens are necessary but not sufficient for normal proceptive behaviour (Baum et al 1977).

Further evidence concerning the site of action of these hormones in the brain has shown that proceptivity can be restored by implanting testosterone into specific sites in the anterior hypothalamus of the female.

Whilst there is general agreement about the dependence of olfactory and visual cues of attractiveness on oestrogens in the female rhesus macaque, there is much less general agreement about the respective roles of androgens and oestrogens in female receptivity and proceptivity (Johnson & Phoenix 1976; Michael et al 1978). The inconsistent results from various studies and between different groups of workers are probably related to a number of methodological inconsistencies. In each laboratory very small numbers of animals are involved in these experiments and it is possible that an unwitting selection of animals that respond 'true-to-type' may have occurred. The differences between laboratories may then reflect genetic variation within the species. Goldfoot (personal communication) has demonstrated how much individual variation in behavioural responsiveness exists in rhesus females. There are also differences in the testing procedures and in the control of such factors as novelty which may serve to obscure more subtle hormone behaviour relationships. In addition it is difficult to know what relevance these highly artificial test situations have to the natural behaviour of these animals. There are also likely to be species differences even amongst macaques. Stump-tail macaques tested in this way show no obvious hormonal determinants of female sexuality. The marmoset is striking in that proceptivity, receptivity and attractiveness continue apparently unaffected after ovariectomy (Dixson 1987). When we turn to the human female therefore, there is no obvious or ideal primate model that we can use.

The human female

In comparison with men, women provide us with much greater opportunities to study the relationship between reproductive hormones and sexual behaviour. They experience menstrual cycles and pregnancies associated with predictable and recurrent hormonal changes. They undergo a relatively discrete cessation of ovarian function (i.e. the menopause) which has no direct parallel in men. Surgical castration is much more common amongst women than men. Enormous quantities of steroid hormones are administered to women either for contraception or hormone replacement. Endocrine abnormalities which have demonstrable behavioural effects in men, such as hyperprolactinaemia or primary hypogonadism, are far more common in women. Anti-hormones, such as anti-androgens, are used much more extensively. It is therefore truly remarkable that whereas the picture for men, as I have described already, is taking shape with gratifying consistency across studies and different types of evidence, the picture for women remains confused, with inconsistent and often contradictory results. As will be described later, it is my belief that this seemingly chaotic state of affairs is telling us something important about female sexuality and its hormonal basis.

The menstrual cycle in women

Evidence of the distribution of sexual activity and sexual interest during the menstrual cycle of women is conflicting, though the majority fails to support a mid-cycle or periovulatory peak. In a recent review of 32 such studies, 17 found increases premenstrually, 18 post-menstrually, 4 during menstruation and 8 around the time of ovulation (Schreiner-Engel 1980). Apart from the basic possibility that women vary in this respect, a number of methodological inconsistencies and inadequacies could account for these conflicting results. The method of identifying the appropriate hormonal phase of the cycle is likely to be crucial. Udry & Morris (1977) have shown that by varying the method of identifying the cycle phase one can produce a variety of behavioural patterns. There is little doubt that direct endocrine assessment of the cycle is necessary. Also few studies have satisfactorily distinguished between female proceptivity and spontaneous interest, and sexual activity which is initiated by the male partner. Adams et al (1978) made a bold attempt and reported a peak of female-initiated behaviour around mid-cycle. However, numbers were small and again no satisfactory method of marking the cycle phases was used.

Three recent studies throw light on this problem. In a study of 55 women with normal ovulatory cycles, each cycle was divided into six hormonally distinct phases by means of repeated assaying of plasma steroid levels (Sanders et al 1983). Distribution of sexual activity through the cycle in these women showed a significant peak in the mid-follicular (i.e. post-menstrual) rather than late follicular (periovulatory) phase (Fig. 2.40). Some of these women showed marked cyclical variation in their mood and energy with a peak in the middle third of the cycle and a marked decline premenstrually. It was found that a woman's rating of sexual interest would be affected by her general mood and energy state. Thus those women who felt markedly better in the middle third of the cycle were more likely to

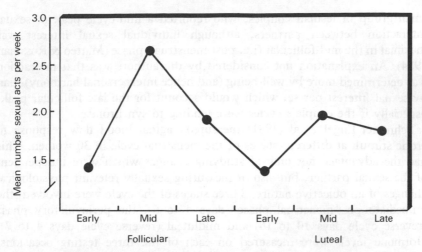

Fig. 2.40 Distribution of sexual activity in six phases of the cycle in 40 women with normal menstrual cycles. Analysis of variance showed a significant cycle effect, with peak in the mid-follicular phase. (Bancroft et al 1983)

express sexual feelings at that time. When these non-specific effects of mood and energy on self ratings of sexuality were controlled by statistical means, a pattern then emerged of peaks of sexual feelings in the mid-follicular (post-menstrual) and late luteal (premenstrual) phases. There was therefore no evidence of a periovulatory oestrous pattern, except for that superimposed in some women by non-specific mood changes (Bancroft et al 1983).

In a large scale retrospective study, several thousand women reported on the highs and lows of sexual interest and the peaks and troughs of well-being. The sexual interest was closely related to the well-being (Warner & Bancroft 1988; Fig. 2.41). This may be relevant to a recent study of a

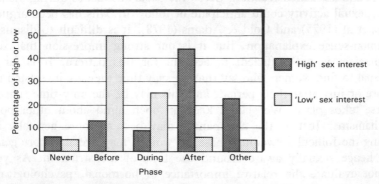

Fig. 2.41 The timing of 'highs' and 'lows' of sexual interest in 3252 women. They were asked to indicate whether the highs and lows occurred in the week before menses, during menses, the week after, other times of the cycle or never. 76% of these women reported their trough of well-being to be the week before, 13% during menses. 52% reported their peak of well-being the week after, 37% at other times. (Warner & Bancroft 1988)

small group of lesbian couples, who reported a mid-cycle peak of sexual interaction between partners, although individual sexual interest was maximal in the mid-follicular (i.e. post-menstrual) phase (Matteo & Rossman 1984). An explanation not considered by the authors was that interaction was determined more by well-being (and hence interpersonal harmony) than by sexual interest per se, which would account for the late follicular peak, especially if the couple's cycles were tending to synchronise.

Schreiner-Engel et al (1981) measured vaginal blood flow response to erotic stimuli at different stages of the menstrual cycle in 30 women. This had the advantage not only of studying changes which were independent of the sexual partner, but also of measuring sexually relevant physiological changes of an objective nature. Three stages of the cycle were involved; the immediate post-menstrual phase (days 4 to 6), the periovulatory phase (reverse cycle days 10 to 16) and midluteal (reverse cycle days 4 to 7). Hormone levels were measured on each of the three testing occasions. Vaginal responses were significantly lower during the periovulatory phase than the other two phases. These findings are consistent with those in our previous study (Sanders et al 1983).

As yet the hormonal basis of this pre- and post-menstrual pattern, if any, remains obscure. So far, in none of these studies is there any evidence of an oestrogen effect on cyclical change in sexual interest, though as we shall see later, minimal amounts of oestrogen may be required for normal sexuality. It is more difficult to be certain about progesterone. It remains possible that progesterone, at least at certain levels or certain ratios to oestradiol, may have an inhibitory effect on female sexuality. Escape from such a progesterone effect could account for either the late luteal or follicular increase in sexual interest. This must remain speculation until we have further evidence. The possible role of androgens will be discussed later.

There are other fairly obvious reasons for peaks of sexual activity just before and after menstruation. Given the usual abstinence during menstrual flow, sexual activity could anticipate or follow it. This has been argued by Spitz et al (1975) and Gold & Adams (1978). It is difficult to dismiss this common-sense explanation. But it is our strong impression that such a mechanism is not sufficient to account for this pattern. It is far from unusual to find women who say that the *only* time they are interested is just before or just after their period, and this may be the only time that intercourse takes place. We should keep an open mind about other possible mechanisms. Just as the chimpanzee may become more genitally aware during the follicular swelling phase, so women may become more genitally and hence sexually aware around the time of menstruation. As yet we cannot evaluate the relative importance of hormonal, psychological and peripheral somatic factors in the sexual cyclicity of women.

If, as seems increasingly likely, the basic sexual cycle of most women is perimenstrual rather than periovulatory, we may ask what is the evolutionary significance of such a pattern. The previous discussion about the various types of oestrous cycle in subhuman primates is now very relevant. Given that humans normally mate as established pairs and the human male is not only sexually assertive but also fairly sexed, there is no need for an ovulation-linked oestrous cycle. Optimum fertility will be achieved without it. The evolutionary process may therefore have become more concerned with the non-reproductive consequences of female sexuality. But why this should lead to a perimenstrual oestrous cycle remains to be resolved (Bancroft 1987).

Other rhythms

Circannual rhythms of androgens, which have been reported in men (see above) have not been demonstrated in women. A well tried method for studying seasonal variations in sexual activity is by following changes in conception rates. A number of studies in different countries and at different times have looked at this. These are well reviewed by Parkes (1976). Predictable patterns do occur with peaks being consistent in particular areas of the world but varying from one area to another. The patterns have survived the influence of modern fertility control and are similar in both legitimate and illegitimate births. In England and Wales there is a major peak for conception in the summer and a minor peak around Christmas and the New Year. Obviously the relationship between sexual activity and conception is unpredictable, but Parkes concludes that these conception peaks do reflect peaks of sexual activity and are influenced by such factors as environmental comfort (i.e. suitable temperature) and the festive or holiday seasons. However such peaks may be determined as much or more by the male.

Pregnancy and lactation

There are massive changes in hormone levels during pregnancy and the post-partum period. However, there are also other important changes, both physiological and psychosocial, which make the interpretation of the evidence less than straightforward.

The majority of women show a decline in sexual interest and activity as pregnancy continues. One of the earliest studies by Landis et al (1950) found that sexual interest could increase, decrease or stay the same, which might be the case if any group of women, pregnant or not, were followed over a period of a year or so. Masters & Johnson (1966) found that an increase in sexual responsiveness during the second trimester was quite common, though decline in the third trimester was normal. A decline in sexual interest during the first trimester was common in nulliparous women, but not in those who had had previous pregnancies. A number of studies have been reported recently and these are consistent in showing a predominant decline during pregnancy (Christensen & Hertoft 1980; De

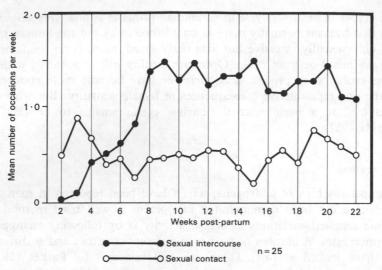

Fig. 2.42 Sexual behaviour recorded in weekly diaries by 25 primiparous women for 22 weeks post-partum; sexual intercourse and other forms of sexual contact. (from Alder & Bancroft 1983)

Aloysio et al 1980; Herms et al 1980; Robson et al 1981). So far there is no evidence linking these changes to hormonal factors and obviously a variety of social, psychological and physical factors are likely to be involved.

Following childbirth reduced sexual interest and activity may persist for several months and there is a widespread clinical impression that this is a common time for the onset of sexual problems. In a prospective study of 119 primiparous women, Robson et al (1981) found that sexual intercourse had been resumed in nearly all women by the 12th week after delivery, with a third restarting by the sixth week. The frequency of intercourse, however, remained subdued for some time in many of the women and a year post-natally about 20% were having intercourse less than once weekly compared with 6% in the few months prior to conception (Fig. 2.42).

Whereas hormonal changes during pregnancy are invariably massive (see p. 30), during the post-partum period we have the specific effect of lactation to consider. The breastfeeding woman, whose prolactin levels remain high and whose ovaries are largely suppressed, has a very different hormonal profile to the artificially feeding mother in whom normal cyclicity may have returned within 6 weeks of childbirth (Howie et al 1982; Fig. 2.8). Comparison of the sexuality of lactating and non-lactating mothers is therefore of particular interest. Surprisingly, very little attention has been paid to this variable. Whilst Robson et al (1981) reported no association between breastfeeding and changes in the frequency or enjoyment of sexual intercourse, they did not take into account the complexity of breastfeeding, which is not an all-or-nothing phenomenon. Not only is the duration of breastfeeding important, so too is the timing of the introduction of supplementary feeds and the associated reduction in suckling frequency, determining when ovarian cyclicity returns (Howie et al 1981). There is however more to breastfeeding which we must consider than its effects on the ovary. Suckling induces release of oxytocin from the posterior pituitary, which then provokes the release of milk. Oxytocin may also produce contraction of the uterus and in this way contribute to the uterine changes accompanying orgasm. The reverse has also been demonstrated; not only in animals but also in lactating women, sexual stimulation commonly leads to milk ejection, presumably also because of oxytocin release.

Newton (1973) has also emphasised the sensual aspects of breastfeeding. The breasts are sensual organs for most women and nipples are erect during both suckling and sexual arousal. The consequences may be varied and difficult to predict. Some women may enjoy breastfeeding more because of these erotic effects; others may feel guilty about them and be reluctant to continue with breastfeeding. The effect on the male partner is also likely to vary; some men may be sexually stimulated by their partners' breastfeeding, while others are put off by it.

Masters & Johnson (1966) interviewed 101 women during pregnancy and 3 months post-partum. They found the highest level of sexual interest postpartum in the breastfeeding women. This is surprising, but their results are difficult to interpret. They give no details of how their subjects were selected or of such crucial variables as social class. Only 24 women 'were successful in nursing their babies for at least 2 months after delivery.' This is a low incidence and a short duration of breastfeeding and it is possible that at the time of the study attitudes to breastfeeding were different, with those women electing to breastfeeding tending to have a different and more positive attitude to sexuality.

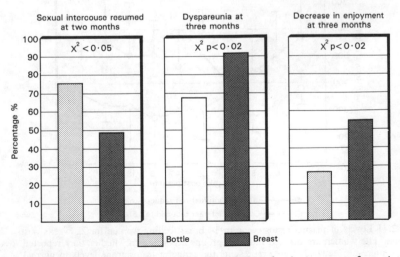

Fig. 2.43 Comparison of breast and bottle-feeding mothers for three aspects of sexual activity at 3 months post-partum. (from Alder & Bancroft 1988)

In a more recent prospective study (Alder & Bancroft 1988) 90 primiparous women were assessed early in pregnancy for their sexual attitudes and prepregnancy sexual activity. They were then followed-up at 3 and 6 months post-partum. A total of 42% were still fully and 21% partially breastfeeding at 3 months and 52% partially at 6 months. There were no differences between those who persisted with breastfeeding and those who did not (or did not start) in terms of their prepregnancy sexual attitudes or activity. The persistent breastfeeders were however significantly more likely to experience loss of sexual interest and enjoyment and pain or discomfort during intercourse (Fig. 2.43). A number of factors must be considered in interpreting these results. Greater interruption of sleep and resulting fatigue associated with breastfeeding may have been important. But hormonal factors are also likely to be relevant. Pain during intercourse, though initially it is often the result of episiotomies or other forms of birth trauma, may well be aggravated and kept going by the effects of lactation-induced oestrogen deprivation on the vagina. Masters & Johnson (1966) described the vaginae of the post-partum lactating women they investigated in their laboratory as 'almost senile to direct observation' and other aspects of these women's pelvic and genital responses were also subdued. In another study (Alder et al 1986) we found an association between loss of sexual interest and low androgen levels in lactating women (Fig. 2.44), though no association with circulating oestradiol. This finding requires replication, but it remains possible that, at least in some breastfeeding women, androgens may be relevant to sexual interest and oestrogens to impaired genital response and vaginal soreness.

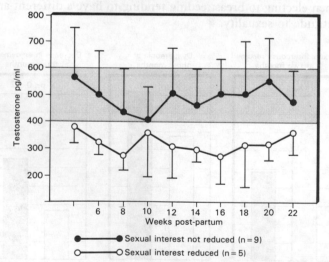

Fig. 2.44 Levels of plasma testosterone in 14 breastfeeding women for 22 weeks post-partum. The women are divided into two groups according to whether they reported loss of sexual interest. The shaded area represents the range of testosterone levels in normal women. (Analysis of variance $P < 0.05$). (Alder et al 1986)

Oral contraceptives

The sexual effects of oral contraceptives remain obscure. Obviously many women, perhaps the majority, have no obvious sexual problems whilst using them though there may be a tendency for normal cyclical variation in interest to be 'flattened out' (Udry et al 1973), or for an increase in sexual interest to occur towards the end of the pill-free week (Bancroft et al 1980). There is also evidence that a substantial number of women do have sexual difficulties on the pill (Royal College of General Practitioners 1974) and we know very little about the number of women who start on oral contraceptives and give them up for this reason. The available evidence will be considered in more detail in Chapter 12.

Effects of oophorectomy and oestrogen replacement

Oophorectomy (i.e. surgical castration) is a common operation. Whilst it is often carried out as part of the management of hormone-dependent malignancies of breast or uterus, it is still widely recommended as a prophylactic procedure in women close to the age of menopause who are undergoing hysterectomy for non-malignant indications. The reasoning is that soon their ovaries will be of little use to them, and by removing them they will avoid the possibility of ovarian carcinoma, a particularly unpleasant malignancy. This is a controversial issue; many believe the post-menopausal ovary has a worthwhile endocrine function (see Chapter 5) and hormone replacement, which is usually required after oophorectomy in premenopausal women, is not without its problems.

Kinsey and his colleagues (1953) concluded that bilateral oophorectomy had negligible sexual effect. Utian (1975), in a partially controlled study of hormone replacement after oophorectomy, found that oestrogen benefited vaginal dryness but not loss of libido. Dennerstein & Burrows (1982), in a further controlled study, found that both vaginal dryness *and* sexual interest and orgasmic capacity were improved by oestrogen, an effect which was reduced if progestagens were added to the hormone replacement. Sherwin et al (1985), in what is probably the best controlled study to date, found that oestrogens had no effect whereas androgens increased sexual interest. Dow et al (1983) compared oestrogen and oestrogen–androgen combination in oophorectomised women with loss of sexual interest and found that both regimes helped to a similar extent. Similar confusion prevails in the studies of hormone replacement in women following natural menopause and this evidence will be considered in Chapter 5.

Thus, whilst there is general agreement that oestrogens are necessary for normal vaginal response and oestrogen deficiency will lead to vaginal dryness and painful intercourse, the role of oestrogens in the maintenance of sexual interest is uncertain. Androgens will be considered further in a later section.

Primary hypogonadism and hyperprolactinaemia

Primary hypogonadism in women, whilst not rare, has received very little attention from the sexual point of view. Hyperprolactinaemia in women has an uncertain relationship to sexuality (Buvat et al 1978) in contrast to its predictable effect in men. Prolactin levels are high during lactation, but we found no correlation between prolactin levels and sexual function in breast-feeding women (Alder et al 1986). Lundberg et al (1985) reported a series of 109 women with hypothalamo–pituitary disorders of various kinds. More than 60% reported absent or markedly diminished sexual interest. This was not correlated with levels of either oestrogen or androgen, but there was an association with hyperprolactinaemia. However this was not straightforward; reduction in prolactin levels with dopaminergic drugs did not produce a predictable return sexual interest, as one would expect in men.

Androgens and the sexuality of women

For some time androgens have been regarded as the libido hormones for women (Money 1961). This has been based mainly on anecdotal observations following the administration of androgens for various gynaecological conditions (Shorr et al 1938; Greenblatt 1942; Salmon & Geist 1943) or following oophorectomy and adrenalectomy for malignancy (Waxenburg et al 1959). We now have rather more and better evidence but the picture is far from clear.

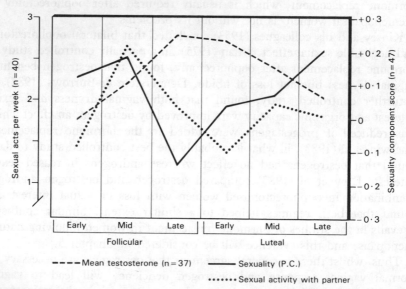

Fig. 2.45 Changes in sexual activity, sexual feelings and plasma testosterone during the six phases of menstrual cycle. The sexuality component score is based on a principal components (P.C.) analysis of daily subjective ratings (Sanders et al 1983); details of testosterone levels are given in Bancroft et al (1983).

Testosterone varies predictably through the menstrual cycle with levels highest in the middle third. According to our study of 55 women, this peak of androgens coincides with the phase when sexual interest and activity is relatively low (Fig. 2.45; Bancroft et al 1983). However we should not assume that the behavioural effects of this mid-cycle rise in testosterone will be rapid; effects of androgen replacement in hypogonadal men are not apparent for several days. If a similar temporal relationship exists in women we might expect mid-cycle rises in testosterone to have behavioural effects later in the cycle. Schreiner-Engel and her colleagues (1982) also found evidence that testosterone was related to cyclical responsiveness. They divided their female subjects into high and low testosterone groups on the basis of their average levels. The high testosterone group showed significantly higher levels of sexual response during the luteal phase of their cycles than the low testosterone group.

Apart from cyclical changes, are androgens related to women's sexuality in any more persistent fashion? Paradoxically, whereas correlations between circulating testosterone levels and measures of sexuality are seldom significant in men (see above) we might expect to find such correlations in women. The reason for this is shown diagramatically in Fig. 2.37. Normal males are overdetermined in their behavioural dependence on androgens, i.e. they produce more than they need for behavioural purposes. Thus when androgens vary in that part of the range that is behaviourally irrelevant, any correlation with behaviour will be obscured. It is only when androgens vary *below* this threshold level, as in hypogonadal men, or in boys around puberty (Fig. 2.39) that we find positive correlations. In women, on the other hand, the behaviourally relevant range of circulating androgen may extend well beyond the laboratory normal range. Hence if androgen–behaviour relationships do exist they are likely to be demonstrable as correlations.

Oestrogens, by contrast, show enormous increases at certain stages of the ovarian cycle which are unlikely to be behaviourally relevant and we may only expect to find correlations between oestrogen levels and behaviour when levels are low, as in post-menopausal women. The evidence is consistent with this view. Oestrogen levels do not correlate with sexual behaviour in ovulating women (Persky et al 1978a), though in post-menopausal women they correlate with vaginal lubrication and response (Chakravarti et al 1979).

With androgens the story is different. Persky and his colleagues (1978b) studied 11 married couples and found a significant correlation between mid-cycle testosterone and frequency of sexual intercourse through the cycle. A comparable relationship was reported by Morris et al (1987) in a larger group of women. Other evidence, however, has not been so straightforward. In our previous study (Bancroft et al 1983) there was a high correlation (0.79) between mid-cycle testosterone and frequency of masturbation in those women who masturbated. Correlations with aspects of the sexual relationship with the partner, however, were absent or in the opposite direction. A similar contrast was found by Schreiner-Engel et al (1981); subjects with high testosterone levels produced greater vaginal responses to erotic stimuli in the laboratory, but reported less satisfactory relationships with their male partners than the low testosterone group. Thus in these two studies we find positive correlations between androgens and aspects of autoeroticism, but negative associations with sexual interaction. We will consider this paradox later.

Udry et al (1986) in their developmental study of boys and girls around the age of puberty found that in girls, whereas androgen levels were correlated with measures of sexual interest, coital experience was more dependent on other social factors, such as peer group relationships. This contrasts with the findings in the boys (see p. 98) and illustrates how the greater importance of social factors in determining female sexual behaviour is already more evident at this stage of development.

Androgen levels in women are affected by oral contraceptives. In a previous study we explored the possibility that oral contraceptives may impair sexual interest and enjoyment by lowering androgens. We compared two groups of women who were matched for type of oral contraceptive. One group had sexual problems which they attributed to the pill; the other group had no sexual difficulties. Both groups showed low levels of testosterone and androstenedione and were indistinguishable in this respect. The problem-free group, however, showed a significant correlation between their testosterone levels and measures of sexual interest; the problem group did not (Bancroft et al 1980).

Effects of exogenous androgens or anti-androgens on women

Whereas for many years there has been anecdotal evidence that androgens enhance the sexuality of women, controlled evidence has become available only recently (and only in women with sexual problems). In the first such study (Carney et al 1978) we did find apparent evidence of an enhancing effect of androgens in women with loss of sexual interest or enjoyment. Two subsequent studies have, however, failed to replicate this finding (Mathews et al 1983; Dow 1985). In contrast, uncontrolled clinical reports continue to appear, showing beneficial effects of testosterone injections or implants. In all of the three controlled studies cited above, testosterone has been administered in the pure form sublingually in doses of 10 or 20 mg daily. It has been suggested that this would be less effective in increasing circulating levels than the parenteral methods of administration. Until recently there was no evidence of the absorption of sublingual testosterone in women. We have now found that very high levels of plasma testosterone occur for several hours after sublingual administration (Fig. 2.46) making it unlikely that the ineffectiveness of testosterone in the above studies was due to insufficient absorption.

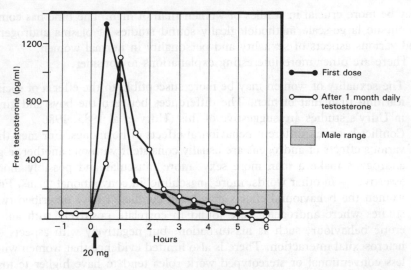

Fig. 2.46 Absorption of sublingual testosterone in women. Mean plasma levels of free testosterone at 30 minute intervals after a 20 mg sublingual dose of pure testosterone (Testoral, Organon) on two occasions, the first dose and after one month of daily dosage, in two women. (Unpublished observations)

As mentioned earlier, androgens have been shown to benefit sexuality when given to women after oophorectomy (Sherwin et al 1985) or the menopause (Studd et al 1986; Hailes et al 1986) though in a further study androgens were no more effective than oestrogens (Dow et al 1983). In each of these studies testosterone was administered by implant or injection. Further controlled evidence is required of the effects of these methods of administration in premenopausal women.

Anti-androgens, such as cyproterone acetate, are being widely used for the treatment of hirsutism or acne in women. Evaluation of their sexual effects in such cases is complicated by the psychological impact of the original condition on the woman's sexual development. As yet adequate controlled evidence is lacking, though early results from Hamburg (Appelt 1983) suggest that, when there is an existing active sexual relationship, a substantial proportion of women receiving this treatment experience a reduction of sexual interest or enjoyment.

Hormones and the sexuality of women — an interpretation

There is little consistency in the above data for women. With the possible exception of oestrogens and vaginal function, there is as much evidence against as for the role of hormones in female sexuality. How can we account for this seeming confusion? Perhaps the simplest and least interesting explanation is that in too many of the studies there have been important methodological deficiencies. Measurement of free testosterone, for example, may be more crucial in studies of women than of men. The time has come to pursue large-scale methodologically sound studies of plasma androgens and various aspects of sexuality and personality in normal women.

There are other more interesting explanations to consider.

1. The sexuality of women may be more susceptible to the effects of social learning than that of men. The differences between the boys and girls in Udry's studies are suggestive of this (Udry et al 1985, 1986).
2. Conflict between different behavioural effects of hormones. For men the various effects of androgens are usually consistent with one another; e.g. androgens make a man more sexy, more muscular and possibly more assertive — in other words, more 'masculine' in conventional terms. For women the behavioural effects may be in conflict. I have described two studies where androgens were found to correlate positively with auto-erotic behaviour, such as masturbation, but negatively with aspects of heterosexual interaction. There is also limited evidence that women with less conventional or stereotyped work roles tend to have higher testosterone levels* (Purifoy & Koopmans 1980; Bancroft et al 1983). It is therefore possible that some women may be made more sexy by andro-gens, but also more career-orientated or assertive and less prepared to conform with the expectations of their traditional husbands and society. If such conflicts do occur it would not be surprising to find some women with higher testosterone levels adopting a homosexual lifestyle where the combination of sexiness and 'non-conformity' would cause no conflict. We find some evidence of that kind; a proportion of lesbian women do have higher than normal testosterone levels (Meyer-Bahlburg 1979).
3. Confounding effect of psychological factors. It is possible that once sexual problems become established, whatever their original cause, the hormone–behaviour relationship may be obscured by psychological repercussions. Thus we found a significant correlation between testos-terone and sexual interest in problem-free women but not in those with established sexual difficulties (Bancroft et al 1980). The association between low testosterone and loss of sexual interest in breastfeeding women (Alder et al 1986) may have been observable because we were studying these women right at the start of their behavioural change, before psychological repercussions had become established. The positive findings for androgens and sexuality in the post-oophorectomy studies (e.g. Sherwin et al 1985) were in groups of women who were being studied soon after surgery and who were not initially complaining of sexual problems. In the study by Dow et al (1983), on the other hand, when no difference was found between androgens and oestrogens, the

---

* Further evidence reported by Baucom et al (1985) that women students with high levels of 'masculinity' had higher testosterone levels than did feminine sex-typed women must be treated with considerable caution as the testosterone levels were based on single saliva samples with no regard to time of day collected and no indication whether the subjects were taking oral contraceptives.

women were selected for the study on the basis of established sexual difficulties. Thus it may be important to distinguish between studies of normal subjects and those involving people with established sexual problems.

4. Greater individual variability in hormone–behaviour relationships. In comparison with men, women may be much more variable in their behavioural susceptibility to hormones. There are two reasons why this might be so.

    a. Early hormonal organisation. I have already postulated that men are 'overdetermined' by androgens, whereas women are exposed to levels of androgens of which the variability may be much more crucial to their organisational effects. Such early variation may be reflected in adulthood as greater variability of target organ sensitivity.

    b. Genetic variability. We know that for most mammals behavioural sensitivity to hormones is in part genetically determined, though in rodent research this fact is often obscured by the use of genetically pure strains of animal. But we also know that in subprimates the period of sexual receptivity of the female is usually restricted to a relatively brief period around ovulation. We have already seen that with primates, the extent to which sexual activity is restricted to this brief fertile phase varies considerably from one species to another. Where it is so restricted, as in the gorilla, it is then crucially important for the female to show a behavioural dependence on her hormones comparable to that seen in rodents. Any female who does not do so is unlikely to reproduce herself. Consequently we can expect that species to breed relatively true for this particular genetic characteristic.

In a species such as the human, where sexual activity is far in excess of that required for optimum fertility, the woman's degree of behavioural responsiveness to her reproductive hormones will have little bearing on whether she reproduces herself optimally through her fertile life span. The human male, on the other hand, who tends to initiate sexual pairings, has both his sexual appetite and his fertility dependent on the same hormone. Men who are behaviourally unresponsive to that hormone may be *less* likely to reproduce themselves. The result, I am postulating, is greater genetic variability of hormone–behaviour responsiveness in women than in men, leading, together with the other factors I have discussed, to the complexity and confusion of our female evidence to date.

The subject of hormone–behaviour relationships in women is a sensitive one. The notion that 'biology is destiny' is inflammatory for many in the women's movement. I have been told that I should not do research in this area — that, as with research into racial differences in intelligence, the scientist is simply colluding with undesirable social or political influences. I am not totally resistant to this view, and have some sympathy with it in relation to intelligence and race. But each case should be judged rationally on its merits. What I am postulating is that, first, as far as sexual destiny is concerned, men are biologically determined in a more predictable way than women. Secondly, I have emphasised the interaction that may occur between biological and social influences and the importance of avoiding an 'either–or' approach. Some women may experience more difficulty because their particular biological natures conflict with what is expected of them by conventional society. That may be a reason for modifying the social influences but not for denying the biological ones.

Thirdly I am proposing that instead of looking for the hormone that 'turns women on', we should be looking for different types of women with different hormonal sensitivities and needs — some apparently immune to hormonal influence, others unduly sensitive. This seemingly obvious concept will, if taken seriously, fundamentally change our approach to hormone–behaviour research, not just in relation to sexual behaviour, but also to other possible consequences of women's reproductive systems, such as premenstrual syndrome, post-natal depression and the menopause.

THE NEUROPHARMACOLOGY OF SEXUAL BEHAVIOUR

The inter-relationship of steroid hormones, cerebral amines and sexual behaviour

If we accept that steroid hormones influence sexual behaviour by their effects on the brain, how are those effects mediated and to what extent are cerebral amines involved?

Cerebral amines

There are two main types of cerebral amine: the *indoleamines*, of which serotonin or 5-hydroxytryptamine (5-HT) is the principal form and *catecholamines*, of which dopamine, noradrenaline and adrenaline are the principal examples. Their chemical origins and inter-relationships are shown in Fig. 2.47.

There is increasing evidence that the hypothalamus of both primates and subprimates is sensitive to sex steroids. Receptors for androgens, oestradiol and progesterone are found in large numbers of neurones in the medial preoptic area (MPOA) and ventromedial nucleus (VMN) of the hypothalamus. In castrated male rats the MPOA is particularly sensitive to testosterone implants for the restoration of sexual behaviour. In the female rat the VMN is uniquely sensitive to the receptivity-inducing effects of oestradiol implants (Everitt & Hansen 1983). However, the situation is not straightforward. The effects of MPOA lesions, discussed on p. 68, are not the same as the effects of castration (Hart & Leedy 1985). Everitt (personal communication) has recently evolved an ingenious procedure for differentiating between motivation for sexual contact and the process of

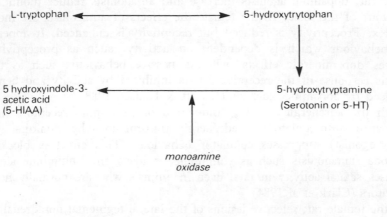

INDOLEAMINES

L-tryptophan ⟷ 5-hydroxytrytophan

5 hydroxyindole-3-
acetic acid
(5-HIAA) ⟵ 5-hydroxytryptamine
(Serotonin or 5-HT)

monoamine
oxidase

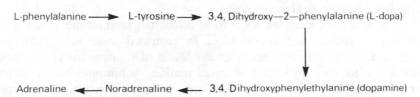

CATECHOLAMINES

L-phenylalanine ⟶ L-tyrosine ⟶ 3,4, Dihydroxy—2—phenylalanine (L-dopa)

Adrenaline ⟵ Noradrenaline ⟵ 3,4, Dihydroxyphenylethylanine (dopamine)

Fig. 2.47

sexual interaction itself. He uses an operant paradigm which enables him to measure the amount of work a male will do to gain access to a female. The MPOA-lesioned male rat does not show any less motivation than the intact animal; it is when he gains access to the female and attempts to mount her that he runs into difficulties. (Is this a rodent model of erectile dysfunction?) The testosterone-deficient male rat, on the other hand, shows reduced motivation to gain access, reinforcing the basic thesis that androgens are more related to sexual appetite than to sexual function per se. The role of testosterone-dependent mechanisms in the function of the MPOA is not therefore clear and is certainly not simple. To what extent may these testosterone-sensitive pathways interact with the aminergic systems in the hypothalamus?

The catecholamine systems of the hypothalamus are involved in most appetitive behaviours, including sex. Is it possible that the hormone-sensitive neurones of the MPOA modulate the activity of ascending dopaminergic and noradrenergic fibre tracts that run in the lateral hypothalamus and medial forebrain bundle in serving goal-directed behaviour. We cannot yet answer that question, but we can look at the results of manipulating the aminergic systems pharmacologically.

Pharmacological studies in animals

In the rat, dopamine agonists increase and antagonists reduce mounting behaviour of the male. In the female the effects of antagonists are more complex. Proceptivity is reduced but receptivity is enhanced. It appears that behaviour which is dependent on activity, such as proceptivity, requires dopaminergic effects, whereas passive behaviour, such as the lordosis response of the receptive rat, is inhibited by activity and hence enhanced by dopamine blockade (Everitt & Hansen 1983).

With the adrenergic system, stimulation of the alpha$_2$ receptors (i.e. presynaptic autoregulators of adrenergic transmission) by clonidine (an alpha$_2$ agonist) suppresses copulator behaviour. This effect is blocked by alpha$_2$ antagonists such as yohimbine or idazoxan. Yohimbine alone increases sexual activity in rats, even in animals who are normally non-copulators (Clark et al 1984).

In the female rat, selective lesions of the lateral tegmental noradrenaline neurones also result in dissociation of proceptive and receptive behaviours. Proceptivity continues, but the capacity to display lordosis is severely impaired (Everitt & Hansen 1983).

Clark and his colleagues went on to assess the relationship between the adrenergic system and testosterone. In castrated male rats, yohimbine increased sexual activity, and after low levels of testosterone replacement, which on its own produced sluggish mating, yohimbine had a further enhancing effect. This suggests that the adrenergic mechanisms are operating later in the sequence than testosterone receptor mechanisms (Clark et al 1985).

With the indoleamine system 5-HT re-uptake blockers and post-synaptic 5-HT agonists stimulated seminal emission whilst suppressing erectile reflexes in the male rat (Mas et al 1985). In the female rhesus monkey the decrease in proceptivity following adrenalectomy can be restored not only with androgens (testosterone or androstenedione) but also with P-chloro-phenylalanine (PCPA) a drug which reduces 5-HT levels in the brain.

Thus various pharmacological ways of manipulating the cerebral amine systems produce effects on sexual behaviour. It is not clear from these various experiments how specific the effects are. With dopamine agonists in female rats, for example, is the separation of proceptivity and receptivity a result of some generalised alteration in activity which would also be evident in other behavioural systems? Is the impairment of receptivity of the female rat produced by lateral tegmental noradrenaline lesions the result of some non-specific impairment of the capacity to respond to tactile cues? Obviously the hormone-sensitive mechanisms in the hypothalamus make use of these aminergic pathways to express their sexual effects. But the mechanisms mediating between the systems are not understood, and crude, unselective manipulation of aminergic function pharmacologically is likely to produce a wide variety of behavioural effects which will not be recognised unless the experimental procedures measure them. This is obviously relevant when considering the clinical use of such pharmacological agents.

Human studies

Prolactin, as we have seen is related to male sexuality in some way, although the effects of hyperprolactinaemia may be pharmacological or pathological rather than physiological. But prolactin is mainly under the control of the dopaminergic system; prolactin rises when dopaminergic activity in the pituitary is inadequate. One of the few non-hormonal drugs which appears to have specific negative effects on male sexuality in humans is a butyrophenone, benperidol. In a controlled study, similar in design to that evaluating cyproterone acetate and ethinyloestradiol, referred to earlier (Bancroft et al 1974), benperidol (1.25 mg daily) was found to be more effective than placebo in reducing sexual interest, but had no effects on erections to erotic stimuli in the laboratory (Tennent et al 1974). The effects were strikingly similar to those of the anti-androgen and oestrogen, although there was no change in either gonadotrophin or testosterone during benperidol administration (human prolactin assays were not yet available at that time) and there were side-effects of the kind one would expect with such drugs. Also evaluated in this study was chlorpromazine (125 mg daily) which did not differ from placebo in its sexual effects. Both benperidol and chlorpromazine have dopamine antagonistic properties, though the latter has a much wider variety of pharmacological effects in addition. It is possible that, in the doses being used, benperidol was having a more selective dopamine-blocking effect than the chlorpromazine, although in view of the side-effects, the drug action was not specifically sexual.

Apomorphine is a dopamine agonist which, as we have seen, enhances mounting in rodents in appropriate dosage. In an interesting placebo-controlled human study, involving normal male volunteers, apomorphine induced spontaneous erections (i.e. not in response to erotic stimuli) during a 75-min period after subcutaneous injection (Lal et al 1984). Some erectile response was also produced in an uncontrolled study of a few men with erectile dysfunction of varied aetiology (Lal et al 1987)

Alpha$_2$ adrenergic antagonists have been shown to enhance male sexual response in rats (Clark et al 1984). Morales et al (1982) have claimed some success in treating erectile failure in men with yohimbine, a specific alpha$_2$ antagonist. This was not a placebo-controlled study, however, and the results are more difficult to evaluate because of their decision to select men with organic erectile failure, many of whom may be unlikely to respond to a centrally acting drug because of peripheral damage. In a more recent placebo-controlled study, this group reported some benefit in the treatment of psychogenic erectile problems (Morales et al 1987) but the study was confounded by design problems and the results are difficult to interpret.

In an interesting study of normal volunteers, Charney & Heninger (1986) assessed the effects of yohimbine, naloxone (an opiate antagonist) and a combination of the two. Yohimbine on its own produced no observable effects, whereas naloxone produced partial erection in three of the six men studied. The combination of the two drugs produced a full erection, lasting at least 60 min, in all six men, though it also produced a substantial anxiety response. These authors suggested that an interaction between adrenergic and opiate mechanisms may be important in erectile response as well as anxiety.

So far the only attempt to look at the interaction between androgens and amines was reported by Benkert (1973) who found that PCPA, P-chloro-methamphetamine (PCMA) and methysergide (which all reduce 5-HT effects) had sexually enhancing effects in men when combined with a synthetic androgen, mesterolone. This evidence should be interpreted with caution for methodological reasons.

Thus it remains possible that the sexual effects of androgens depend on catecholaminergic mechanisms and the field is open for investigating the role of catecholamines in restoring the sexuality of hypogonadal men. The possible role of neuropeptides will also have to be taken into consideration when attempting to clarify this complex neuroendocrine picture, though as yet the relevant evidence is confined to subprimates (see p. 100).

We have already learnt the importance of distinguishing between different components of sexual behaviour in investigating both hormonal and amine effects. The distinction which emerged between spontaneous erections (e.g. during sleep) and those in response to erotic stimuli may be of particular value in this respect. In Figure 2.48 I have presented a theoretical schema which attempts to account for this differential response and which leads to a number of interesting possibilities for future research. Erection is seen as a response at a late stage of a sequence of events in the system. Interference with erection can occur at various points in this sequence. Within the brain (and possibly spinal cord) I am postulating an androgen-dependent neurophysiological substrate for both sexual interest or desire and spontaneous erections, such as occur during sleep. I have called this the central arousability system. In addition, external stimuli mediated by specific sensory systems in the brain may lead to erections by means of pathways which are not androgen-dependent and hence are inde-pendent of this central arousability system. The part that internal stimuli, such as fantasies, play in this scheme is not yet clear.

If this scheme has any heuristic value it follows that the *systematic* assess-ment of erectile responses firstly, during sleep and secondly, in response to erotic stimuli (external and internal) offers a method for differentiating between the effects of hormones or drugs on the various components of this system, with measurement of sleep erections providing a *quantitative* evalu-ation of the central arousability component, providing that the peripheral mechanisms are intact. The use of intracavernosal injections adds to this

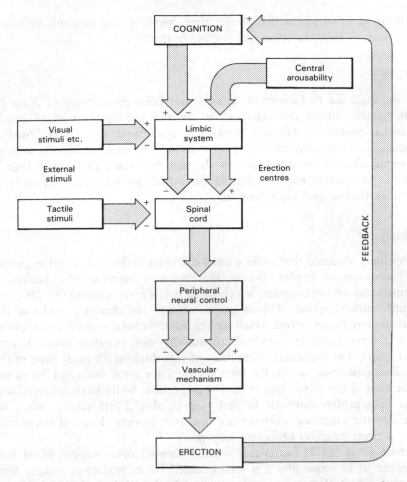

Fig. 2.48 Psychosomatic circle of sex. Two possible inputs leading to erection are shown: from central arousability, the androgen-dependent system linked with sexual desire, and from external stimuli (visual and/or tactile). The effects of visual stimuli are not androgen-dependent; it is not yet known whether the erotic effects of tactile stimulation depend on androgens.

scheme the ability to test *local* mechanisms serving erection. As yet it is more difficult to propose such an experimental model for investigating human female sexuality.

PSYCHOLOGICAL PROCESSES

In the psychosomatic circle of sex (Fig. 2.1; 2.48) psychological processes were shown to play an important part, both as cognitions mediating the influence of attitudes and expectations, and also as awareness or perception of the genital and somatic changes which are occurring. Sexual desire is best understood as an interaction of affective, cognitive and neurophysiological components. How do affect and cognition operate?

AFFECT

As we shall see in Chapter 8, anxiety has been given pride of place by both psychoanalysts and behaviourists in their explanations of the causes of sexual problems. Anger, hostility and resentment are also regarded as crucial. Less attention has been paid to mood. We will consider these three types of affect in more detail. In the last few years there have been a number of relevant experimental studies which we will consider, many of them by Barlow and his colleagues.

Anxiety

It is widely assumed that anxiety has a disruptive effect on sexual response. A long-favoured explanation is that anxiety activates the peripheral sympathetic nervous system, which in turn has a vasoconstrictive effect on genital vasocongestion. This is an example of the dualistic model of the autonomic nervous system which sees parasympathetic activity as associated with positive states and sympathetic activity with negative ones (Wenger et al 1968). The misleading simplicity of this dualism for most parts of the autonomic nervous system has been apparent for some time, and the earlier discussion of the physiology of genital responses should have indicated that it is unhelpfully simplistic in that respect also. Furthermore, when we consider the empirical evidence we find that anxiety does not necessarily have a negative effect on sexual response.

Hoon et al (1977) found that women showed more vaginal blood flow response to an erotic film if it was preceded by an anxiety-provoking film. A comparable effect in men was reported by Wolchik et al (1980). Whilst this suggested that in some way the anxiety was facilitating the sexual arousal, it was also possible that some contrast effect, due to switching from negative to positive stimuli, or some anxiety relief effect was operating (Beck & Barlow 1984). Barlow et al (1983) therefore tested the effect of anxiety in parallel with sexual stimulation. Subjects were told that they were likely to receive electric shocks whilst watching an erotic film. In one group shock would depend on their showing a sexual response; in the other group it would be random. The two groups did not differ in their response and in fact the threat of shock seemed to enhance their sexual arousal. Lange et al (1981) simulated the physiological experience of anxiety with subcutaneous injections of adrenalin. These injections were compared with placebo. Erections to erotic stimuli were no different in the two conditions, except that after adrenalin injections the erections subsided more quickly once the stimuli were withdrawn.

In a series of studies using non-physiological measures of sexual response, such as sexual imagery when reacting to thematic apperception test (TAT) cards, genuinely anxiety-provoking situations have apparently increased sexual response (e.g. Dutton & Aron 1974).

In his classical study of prepubertal boys, Ramsey (1943) found many boys between the ages of 10 and 12 years who reported experiencing erections during a variety of non-sexual but arousing situations, many of which were frightening (e.g. being chased by a policeman). It seemed that at that stage of development there was relatively non-discriminated genital response to any form of arousing stimulus (see p. 179). I have previously reported relevant evidence from studies of aversion therapy in which a proportion of men under threat of shock if they produced an erection found their erectile responses enhanced. Thus in 10 men who gave subjective ratings of anxiety during such procedures, eight showed no correlation between level of anxiety and latency, whereas two showed a significant *negative* correlation, i.e. the more anxious they were the more rapidly their erections developed. One of these men described how since his early teens he would get slight erections whenever he was feeling anxious (Bancroft 1980a). In a study of systematic desensitisation in homosexual men it was apparent that whether anxiety accompanied erection or not depended on whether the erotic stimulus was anxiety-provoking. Thus one subject produced erections to both hetero- and homosexual stimuli but only reported anxiety with the first. As treatment proceeded this pattern was reversed and subsequently he only experienced anxiety when homosexual responses (i.e. which he recognised as an indicator of treatment failure) occurred (Bancroft 1978).

We can therefore conclude from the available evidence that anxiety per se does not necessarily impair sexual response and may in certain circumstances enhance it. If anxiety is sufficiently marked it may interfere with the attention to erotic stimuli, resulting in a reduced sexual response. Perhaps most important for understanding the origins of sexual problems is that anxiety may be a signal that the sexual situation is threatening in some way, though the individual may respond to that threat in a variety of ways, including the direct inhibition of genital responses. We will consider this further in relation to cognitive processes.

We can therefore define a number of different relationships between anxiety and sexual response.

1. Anxiety produces peripheral autonomic effects which interfere with sexual response. (As yet the evidence for this is most convincing in relation to speed of ejaculation.)
2. Anxiety disrupts cognitive processes which would otherwise facilitate sexual response to erotic stimuli.
3. Anxiety and neurophysiological inhibition of genital response coexist, both being reactions to some perceived threat.
4. Sexual responses are inhibited in order to avoid anxiety.

5. Anxiety occurs as a reaction to failure of sexual response.
6. Anxiety may facilitate sexual response.

We will consider some of these relationships more closely in Chapter 8.

Anger

The relationship between anger and sexual response needs to be approached in a similar way as anxiety. There is some experimental evidence to suggest that sexual response and anger may facilitate each other. Clark (1953) found that men who had looked at sexually stimulating pictures showed more evidence of aggressive fantasies in response to TAT cards. Jaffe et al (1974) instructed their subjects to punish with electric shocks confederates who had made incorrect responses to some task. After reading erotic literature they gave stronger shocks. Two studies (Barclay & Haber 1965; Barclay 1969) have shown that inducing anger leads to greater sexual imagery in response to TAT cards. The relationship between anger and sexuality is profoundly important and will be discussed further in relation both to sexual violence (Chapter 13) and interpersonal sexual problems (Chapter 8). But again we need to postulate a variety of possible relationships.

1. Anger may facilitate sexual response.
2. Anger may reduce sexual response. Some individuals appear to find it difficult to be angry and sexually aroused at the same time.
3. Avoidance or rejection of sexual activity may be a way of expressing anger.
4. Sexual response may facilitate anger.
5. Sexual response may reduce anger (i.e. sexual interaction may be used to defuse an angry situation).
6. Failure to respond sexually may cause anger (either in the subject or the partner).

Mood

Although it would not be surprising if a person were less likely to feel sexual when depressed, or more likely when elated, remarkably little attention has been paid to the relationship between mood and sexuality.

I have already commented how women's experience of sexual feelings vary with their general well-being through the menstrual cycle (p. 108). Sanders et al (1983) found that one-third of the variability in women's self-ratings of sexual interest could be accounted for by changes in their well-being.

There has been little attempt to manipulate mood in experimental studies of sexual response. One exception was reported by Wolchik et al (1980), who found that by first showing a film inducing a depressed mood, the sexual response to a later erotic film was reduced, in contrast to anxiety-provoking films, which, as already mentioned, have an enhancing effect.

Recently, detailed investigations of men and women with loss of sexual desire have found an association with depressive illness, at least at the time of onset of the low sexual desire (Schreiner-Engel & Schiavi 1986). Clearly mood is likely to influence sexuality by its effect on cognition — we will think more negative thoughts if depressed. But the possibility must also be considered that underlying biochemical changes may be relevant to both mood and sexuality. It is of interest that impaired sleep erections, which, as already discussed, are found in cases of low sexual desire and androgen deficiency states, are also found during depressive illnesses (Roose et al 1982; Thase et al 1987).

COGNITION

Voluntary control and feedback

Masters & Johnson (1966) asserted that erection 'cannot be "willed"; it can only happen'. This assertion is not generally true. Experimental studies have shown that many men and women can produce genital responses at will, usually by concentrating on sexual thoughts or fantasies (Laws & Rubin 1969; Henson & Rubin 1971; Heiman 1977; Stock & Geer 1982).

Many individuals are also capable of responding in the laboratory setting to non-tactile external erotic stimuli (e.g. visual or auditory) with erections or vaginal responses (Bancroft & Mathews 1971; Heiman 1977; Bancroft & Bell 1985). Many men can also voluntarily inhibit erections in response to such stimuli (Laws & Rubin 1969; Henson & Rubin 1971; Rosen et al 1975). One condition which predictably interferes with such responding is distraction by non-erotic cognitive tasks. Geer & Fuhr (1976), using a dichotic listening paradigm, showed that the more difficult the task, involving listening in one ear, the lower the sexual response to an auditory erotic stimulus in the other ear. Przybyla & Byrne (1984) extended this experiment by looking at the effect of such distraction on visual (erotic film) as well as auditory erotic stimuli. They found that in the case of men such distraction was relatively ineffective in reducing the response to visual stimuli, whereas women were distracted with both auditory and visual stimuli — an interesting and potentially important sex difference.

Generally, erotic films are more powerful in eliciting sexual responses in men than are fantasies or non-moving visual stimuli (e.g. slides; Bancroft 1978; Bancroft & Bell 1985) and these results from distraction experiments support my earlier suggestion that at least in men moving visual erotic stimuli are effective without any intervening cognitive mediation, whereas non-moving visual stimuli (and presumably auditory stimuli also) require such mediation to bring the stimulus to life (Bancroft & Mathews 1971; Bancroft 1978). Whether internal imagery or fantasy is more effective in eliciting a sexual response if it involves vivid *visual* imagery is not clear.

Dekker et al (1984) conjectured whether the cognitive mediation was effective simply by focusing on the external stimulus or whether it was necessary in some way to focus on or imagine the sexual response. Their male and female subjects listened to an erotic tape. In one condition they were asked not only to attend to the scene being described on the tape but also to concentrate on their own feelings and responses; in another condition they were asked simply to attend to what was being described in the tape. Their reported sexual arousal was greater in the first condition, and these workers concluded that cognitive mediation needs to focus on response if it is to lead to sexual arousal. A weakness of this study was that no objective measure of sexual response was involved and the higher levels of sexual arousal reported during the first condition may have been simply because by focusing on their reactions they were more aware of them. This raises another key issue. Are our sexual responses enhanced by our paying attention to them? Masters & Johnson (1966) have blamed the spectator role as a crucial factor in causing or maintaining sexual dysfunction. What is the available evidence?

Price (1973) and Rosen et al (1975) found that in men the provision of feedback of their erectile response had if anything a slightly beneficial effect on their voluntary production of erection. A comparable effect was found in women (Hoon et al 1977). It is of course possible that people who develop sexual dysfunction are different in this respect or at least become so. In general terms, however, dysfunctional men have not differed from normal men in their response to laboratory-based feedback. Csillag (1976) compared six normal volunteers with six men with erectile dysfunction. In neither group did feedback apparently impair their erectile response, but whereas the normal men reached their peak response in the second testing session and thereafter declined somewhat, the dysfunctional men steadily improved with repeated testing. Perhaps something else was happening; perhaps they were becoming increasingly reassured by their responses, a form of deconditioning of performance anxiety. But clearly feedback was not having a negative effect on this process.

Other studies have demonstrated that various aspects of feedback and self-awareness must be taken into consideration. Beck et al (1983) and Abrahamson et al (1985) investigated the possible effect of the partner's response. They compared two groups of sexually functional and dysfunctional men. If the partner was showing low sexual arousal both groups of men responded better by concentrating on their own responses rather than the partner's. If however the partner was showing high arousal, the functional men responded better by focusing their attention on the partner, whereas with dysfunctional men the reverse applied. Here we see the meaning of the impact of a particular situation. High arousal in the partner of a dysfunctional man might be more threatening than low arousal.

Sakheim et al (1984) considered the effect of visual feedback, i.e. what happens if you can see how your penis is responding? With normal volunteers, being able to see their penis had an enhancing effect if they were responding to a strong erotic stimulus but had the opposite effect in the case of a relatively weak stimulus. In other words, perceiving a good sexual response is in itself sexually arousing; perceiving a poor response is sexually inhibiting. Heiman & Rowland (1983) found that normal men were not adversely affected by demand for a response in the experimental situation, whereas dysfunctional men were.

Thus the most sensible conclusion we can draw at this stage is that the effect of awareness, feedback, being a spectator and performance demand depend on the circumstances and how they are interpreted by the individual. Awareness of our genital responses and those of our partner can in some circumstances lead to a positive feedback loop, resulting in escalating sexual arousal, and in other circumstances may have a negative feedback effect with inhibition of sexual response.

Fantasy

The final question to consider is whether the individual's capacity for internal imagery or fantasy influences his or her capacity for sexual response. We have raised the possibility earlier that hormones might influence the effectiveness of erotic fantasy in producing arousal, though at this stage this is a very speculative suggestion. What other evidence do we have?

Zimmer et al (1983) found a significant relationship between frequency of fantasy and sexual activity in both men and women. According to Harris et al (1980), subjects of either sex reporting greater ability to form clear vivid images also reported higher arousability. Stock & Geer (1982) found that the more frequently a woman used fantasy during masturbation the greater the genital response she showed in the laboratory.

Dekker et al (1984) found to their surprise that whereas the ability to respond to fantasy with arousal in the laboratory correlated positively with frequency of masturbation, there was a negative correlation with frequency of sexual interaction with the partner. Schreiner-Engel (personal communication) found that the women in her study (Schreiner-Engel et al 1981) who responded the most strongly to fantasy in the laboratory reported the worst sexual relationships with their partners. This raises the interesting question of whether in some instances fantasy may provide a form of controllable sexuality which real sexual interaction does not. Nutter & Condron (1985), on the other hand, found that women with low sexual desire reported a lower frequency of sexual fantasies than normal controls, though the types of fantasy were not apparently different. It may be that 'switching off' sexual desire is one way of coping with interpersonal problems, whilst actively using certain types of sexual fantasy is another. Hariton & Singer (1974) in their study of women's fantasies concluded that the use of fantasies during sexual intercourse was in general quite normal, but they did identify certain types of women whose use of fantasy reflected dissatisfaction with their relationship. We will be considering the role of sexual fantasy in more detail in Chapter 4.

To summarise the role of psychological processes, we must again restate the complex interaction that occurs between cognitive processes, mood and the physiological arousability of the brain. It does not help to be simplistic or to generalise about the effects of anxiety, anger, feedback or performance demands. Awareness of the response of us or our partner can be either sexually exciting or inhibiting depending on the circumstances and various aspects of our personal histories. We will be considering the sources of negative thinking and the role of learning more closely in Chapter 8 in a discussion of the causes of sexual problems. The only predictable effect is that of distraction. We should always aim to formulate the individual's experience taking into account his or her idiosyncrasies.

There may be certain types of external erotic stimuli, e.g. moving visual stimuli, which have predictable sexual effects — at least in men — without cognitive mediation. But in most cases external stimuli require internal processing with all the complexity and scope for individual reactions this entails.

As for sexual fantasy, whether this is a stimulus or response or both at the same time remains a tantalising question which is as yet unanswered.

REFERENCES

Abrahamson D J, Barlow D H, Beck J G, Sakheim D K, Kelly J P 1985 The effects of attentional focus and partner responsiveness on sexual responding: replication and extension. Archives of Sexual Behavior 14: 361–372

Adams D B, Gold A R, Burt A P 1978 Rise in female initiated sexual activity at ovulation and its suppression by oral contraceptives. New England Journal of Medicine 299: 1145–1150

Alder E, Bancroft J 1983 Sexual behaviour of lactating women: a preliminary communication. Journal of Reproductive and Infant Psychology 1: 47–52

Alder E, Bancroft J 1988 The relationship between breast feeding persistence, sexuality and mood in post-partum women. Psychological Medicine 18: 389–396

Alder E, Cook A, Davidson D, West C, Bancroft J 1986 Hormones, mood and sexuality in lactating women. British Journal of Psychiatry 148: 74–79

Andrew R J 1978 Increased persistence of attention produced by testosterone and its implications for the study of sexual behaviour. In: Hutchison J (ed) Biological determinants of sexual behaviour. Wiley, Chichester, pp 255–276

Appelt H 1983 The effects of anti-androgen treatment on the sexuality of hirsute women. Proceedings of 7th World Congress of Psychosomatic Medicine, Hamburg

Bancroft J 1970 Disorders of sexual potency. In: Hill O W (ed) Modern trends in psychosomatic medicine. Butterworths, London pp 246–261

Bancroft J 1978 Psychological and physiological responses to sexual stimuli in men and women. In: Levi L (ed) Society, stress and disease, vol 3. The productive and reproductive age. Oxford University Press, Oxford, pp 154–163

Bancroft J 1980a Psychophysiology of sexual dysfunction. In: Van Praag H M, Lader M H, Rafaelsen O J, Sachar E J (eds) Handbook of biological psychiatry. Dekker, New York, pp 359–392

Bancroft J 1980b Endocrinology of sexual function. Clinics in Obstetrics and Gynaecology 7: 253–281

Bancroft J 1987 Hormones, sexuality and fertility in humans. Journal of Zoology
213: 445–454
Bancroft J, Bell C 1985 Simultaneous recording of penile diameter and penile arterial pulse
during laboratory-based erotic stimulation in normal subjects. Journal of Psychosomatic
Research 29: 303–313
Bancroft J, Wu F C W 1983 Changes in erectile responsiveness during androgen therapy.
Archives of Sexual Behavior 12: 59–66
Bancroft J, Tennent G, Loucas K, Cass J 1974 The control of deviant sexual behaviour by
drugs: behavioural changes with oestrogens and antiandrogens. British Journal of
Psychiatry 125: 310–315
Bancroft J, Mathews A 1971 Autonomic correlates of penile erection. Journal of
Psychosomatic Research 15: 159–167
Bancroft J, Davidson D W, Warner P, Tyrer G 1980 Androgens and sexual behaviour in
women using oral contraceptives. Clinical Endocrinology 12: 327–340
Bancroft J, Sanders D, Davidson D W, Warner P 1983 Mood, sexuality, hormones and the
menstrual cycle. III Sexuality and the role of androgens. Psychosomatic Medicine
45: 509–516
Bancroft J, O'Carroll R, McNeilly A, Shaw R W 1984 The effects of bromocriptine on the
sexual behaviour of hyperprolactinaemic man: a controlled case study. Clinical
Endocrinology 21: 131–137
Barclay A M 1969 The effect of hostility on physiological and fantasy responses. Journal of
Personality 37: 651–667
Barclay A M, Haber R N 1965 The relation of aggressive to sexual motivation. Journal of
Personality 33: 462–475
Barlow D H, Sakheim D K, Beck J G 1983 Anxiety increases sexual arousal. Journal of
Abnormal Psychology 92: 49–54
Baucom D H, Besch P K, Callahan S 1985 Relation between testosterone concentration, sex
role identity, and personality among females. Journal of Personality and Social
Psychology 48: 1218–1226
Baum M J, Everitt B J, Herbert J L, Keverne E B 1977 Hormonal basis of proceptivity
and receptivity in female primates. Archives of Sexual Behavior 6: 173–191
Beach F A 1976 Sexual attractivity, proceptivity and receptivity in female mammals.
Hormones and Behavior 7: 105–138
Beach F A, Westbrook W H, Clemens L G 1966 Comparison of the ejaculatory response in
men and animals. Psychosomatic Medicine 28: 749–763
Beck J G, Barlow D H 1984 Current conceptualisations of sexual dysfunction: a review and
an alternative perspective. Clinical Psychology Review 4: 363–378
Beck J G, Barlow D H, Sakheim D K 1983 The effects of attentional focus and partner
arousal on sexual responding in functional and dysfunctional men. Behaviour Research
and Therapy 21: 1–8
Benkert O 1973 Pharmacological experiments to stimulate human sexual behaviour. In: Ban
T A et al (eds) Psychopharmacology of sexual disorders and drug abuse. North Holland,
Amsterdam, pp 489–495
Benkert O, Jordan R, Dahlen H G, Schneider H P G, Gammel G 1975 Sexual impotence: a
double blind study of LHRH nasal spray versus placebo. Neuropsychobiology 1: 203–210
Benkert O, Witt W, Adam W, Leitz A 1979 Effects of testosterone undecanoate on sexual
potency and the hypothalamic–pituitary–gonadal axis of impotent males. Archives of
Sexual Behavior 8: 471–480
Benson G S 1983 Penile erection: in search of a neurotransmitter. World Journal of
Urology 1: 209–212
Benson G S, McConnell J A, Lipshultz L I, Corriere J N Jr, Wood J 1980
Neuromorphology and neuropharmacology of the human penis. Journal of Clinical
Investigation 65: 506
Bentler P M, Peeler W H 1979 Models of female orgasm. Archives of Sexual Behavior
8: 405–424
Black S L, Biron C 1982 Androstenol as a human pheromone: no effect on perceived
physical attractiveness. Behavioural and Neurological Biology 34: 326–330
Bohlen J G, Held J P, Sanderson M O, Ahlgren A 1982 The female orgasm: pelvic
contractions. Archives of Sexual Behavior 11: 367–386

Bonnar J, Franklin M, Nott P N, McNeilly A S 1975 Effect of breast freeding on pituitary–ovarian function after childbirth. British Medical Journal 4: 82–84

Bors E, Comarr A E 1960 Neurological disturbances of sexual function with special reference to 529 patients with spinal cord injuries. Urological Survey 10: 191–222

Brindley G S 1982 Sexual function and fertility in paraplegic men. In: Hargreave T (ed) Male infertility. Springer Verlag, Berlin, pp 261–279

Brindley G S 1983 Cavernosal alpha-blockade: a new treatment for investigating and treating erectile impotence. British Journal of Psychiatry 143: 332–337

Brindley G S 1984 Pharmacology of erection. Paper presented at 10th annual meeting of International Academy of Sex Research, Cambridge, England

Brown J B, Harrisson P, Smith M A 1978a Oestrogen and pregnanediol excretion through childhood, menarche and first ovulation. Journal of Biosocial Science (suppl 5): 43–62

Brown W A, Monti P M, Corriveau D P 1978b Serum testosterone and sexual activity and interest in men. Archives of Sexual Behavior 7: 97–103

Bruhl E E, Leslie C H 1963 Afrodex, a double blind test in impotence. Medical Records and Annals 56: 22

Burnstock G 1986 The changing face of autonomic neurotransmission. Acta Physiologica Scandinavica 126: 67–91

Buvat J, Asfour M, Buvat-Herbaut M, Fossati P 1978 Prolactin and human sexual behaviour. In: Robyn C, Harter M (eds) Progress in prolactin physiology and pathology. Elsevier, Amsterdam

Buvat J, Lemaire A, Buvat-Herbaut M, Fourlinnie J C, Racadot A, Fossati P 1985 Hyperprolactinaemia and sexual function in men. Hormone Research 22: 196–203

Cameron J 1989 Factors controlling the onset of puberty in primates. In: Bancroft J, Reinisch J (eds) Adolescence and puberty. The third Kinsey symposium. Oxford University Press, New York (in press)

Carney A, Bancroft J, Mathews A 1978 Combination of hormonal and psychological treatments for female sexual unresponsiveness: a comparative study. British Journal of Psychiatry 133: 339–346

Carter J N, Tyson J E, Tolis G, Van Vliet S, Faiman C, Friesen H G 1978 Prolactin-secreting tumours and hypogonadism in 22 men. New England Journal of Medicine 299: 847–852

Chakravarti S, Collins W P, Thom M H et al 1979 Relation between plasma hormone profiles, symptoms and response to oestrogen treatment in women approaching the menopause. British Medical Journal ii: 983–985

Chambless D L, Stern T, Sultan F F et al 1982 The pubococcygeus and female orgasm: a correlational study in normal subjects. Archives of Sexual Behavior 11: 479–490

Charney D S, Heninger G R 1986 Alpha$_2$ adrenergic and opiate receptor blockade. Archives of General Psychiatry 43: 1037–1041

Christensen E, Hertoft P 1980 Sexual activity and attitude during pregnancy and the post-partum period. In: Forleo R, Pasini W (eds) Medical sexology. Elsevier/North Holland, Amsterdam, pp 357–364

Clark R A 1953 The effects of sexual motivation on fantasy. Journal of Experimental Psychology 44: 3–11

Clark J T, Smith E R, Davidson J M 1984 Enhancement of sexual motivation in rats by yohimbine. Science 225: 847–849

Clark J T, Smith E R, Davidson J M 1985 Testosterone is not required for the enhancement of sexual motivation by yohimbine. Physiology and Behavior 35: 517–521

Cochran C A, Perachio A A 1977 Dihydrotestosterone propionate effects on dominance and sexual behaviors in gonadectomised male and female rhesus monkeys. Hormones and Behavior 8: 175–187

Cohen H D, Rosen R C, Goldstein L 1976 Electro-encephalographic laterality changes during human sexual orgasm. Archives of Sexual Behavior 5: 189–199

Cooper A J, Ismail A A A, Smith C G, Loraine J A 1973 A controlled trial of Potensan forte in impotence. Irish Journal of Medical Science 142: 155–167

Costell R, Lunde D, Kopell B, Wittner N 1972 The contingent negative variation as an indicator of sexual object preference. Science 177: 718–720

Csillag E R 1976 Modification of penile erectile response. Journal of Behavioral Therapy and Experimental Psychiatry 7: 27–29

Cunningham G R, Karacan I, Ware J C, Lantz C D, Thornby J I 1982 The relationship between serum testosterone and prolactin levels and nocturnal penile tumescence (NPT) in impotent men. Journal of Andrology 3: 241–247

Cutler W B, Preti G, Krieger A M, Huggins G R, Garcia C R, Lawley H J 1986 Human axillary secretion influences women's menstrual cycles. The role of donor extract from men. Hormones and Behavior 20: 463–473

Davies T F, Mountjoy C W, Gomez-Pan A et al 1976 A double-blind cross-over trial of gonadotrophin releasing hormone (LH-RH) in sexually impotent men. Clinical Endocrinology 5: 601–608

Davidson J M 1984 Response to 'Hormones and human sexual behavior' by John Bancroft. Journal of Sexual and Marital Therapy 10: 23–27

Davidson J M, Camargo C A, Smith E R 1979 Effects of androgens on sexual behavior of hypogonadal men. Journal of Clinical Endocrinology and Metabolism 48: 955–958

Daw S F 1970 Age of boys' puberty in Liepzig, 1729–49 as indicated by voice breaking in J. S. Bach's choir members. Human Biology 42: 87–89

Deakin J F W, Crow T J 1986 Monoamines, rewards and punishments — the anatomy and physiology of the affective disorders. In: Deakin J F W (ed) The biology of depression. Gaskell, London, pp 1–25

DeAloysio D, Codispoti O, Bottiglioni F 1980 Gynecologic aspects of sexuality during pregnancy. In: Forleo R, Pasini W (eds) Medical sexology. Elsevier/North Holland, Amsterdam, pp 332–348

de Groat W C, Booth A M 1984 Peripheral neuropathy, vol I Saunders, Philadelphia

Dekker J, Everaerd W, Verhelst N 1984 Attending to stimuli or to images of sexual feelings: effects on sexual arousal. Behaviour Research and Therapy 22: 139–149

Delitala G, Masala A, Alagna S, Lotti G 1977 Luteinizing hormone, follicle stimulating hormone and testosterone in normal and impotent men following LH-RH and HCG stimulation. Clinical Endocrinology 6: 11–15

Dennerstein L, Burrows G D 1982 Hormone replacement therapy and sexuality in women. Clinics in Endocrinology and Metabolism 11: 661–679

Deslypere J P, Vermeulen A 1984 Influence of age and sex on steroid concentration in different tissues in humans. Excerpta Medica International Congress Series 652, Amsterdam (abstract 572)

Deysach L J 1939 The comparative morphology of the erectile tissue of the penis with special emphasis on the probable mechanisms of erection. American Journal of Anatomy 64: 111–132

Dickinson R L 1949 Human sex anatomy, 2nd edn. Williams & Wilkins, Baltimore

Dieckmann G, Hassler R 1976 Unilateral hypothalamotomy in sexual delinquents. Confinia Neurologia 37: 177–186

Dixson A F 1983 The hormonal control of sexual behaviour in primates. Oxford Reviews of Reproductive Biology 5: 131–218

Dixson A F 1987 Neuroendocrine control of sexual initiating behaviour in the female common marmoset (Callithrix jacchus). Primate Report 16: 3–19

Dixson A F, Lunn S F 1987 Post-partum changes in hormones and sexual behaviour in captive groups of marmosets (Callothrix jacchus). Physiology and Behaviour 41: 577–583

Dixson A F, Kendrick K M, Blank M A, Bloom S R 1984 Effects of tactile and electrical stimuli upon release of vasoactive intestinal polypeptide in the mammalian penis. Journal of Endocrinology 100: 249–252

Dow M G T 1985 Unpublished Ph D, University of Glasgow

Dow M G T, Hart D M, Forrest C A 1983 Hormonal treatment of sexual unresponsiveness in postmenopausal women: a comparative study. British Journal of Obstetrics and Gynaecology 90: 361–366

Dufy B, Vincent J D 1980 Effects of sex steroids on cell membrane excitability: a new concept for the action of steroids on the brain. In: de Wied D, van Keep P A (eds) Hormones and the brain. MTP, Lancaster

Dutton D G, Aron A P 1974 Some evidence for heightened sexual attraction under conditions of high anxiety. Journal of Personality and Social Psychology 30: 510–517

Edwards A E, Husted J R 1976 Penile sensitivity, age and sexual behavior. Journal of Clinical Psychology 32: 697–700

Evans I M, Distiller L A 1979 Effects of luteinising hormone releasing hormone on sexual arousal in normal men. Archives of Sexual Behavior 8: 385–395

Everitt B J, Hansen S 1983 Catecholamines and hypothalamic mechanisms. In: Wheatley

D, (ed) Psychopharmacology and sexual disorders. Oxford University Press, Oxford, pp 3–14

Fenwick P B C, Mercer S, Grant R et al 1986 Nocturnal penile tumescence and serum testosterone levels. Archives of Sexual Behavior 15: 13–22

Fisher S 1973 The female orgasm. Basic Books, New York

Fisher C, Cohen H D, Schiavi R C et al 1983 Patterns of female sexual arousal during sleep and waking: vaginal thermo-conductance studies. Archives of Sexual Behavior 12: 97–122

Forest H G, Deperetti E, Bertrand J 1976 Hypothalamic–pituitary–gonadal relationships from birth to puberty. Clinical Endocrinology 5: 551–569

Fournier G R, Juenemann K-P, Lue T F, Tanagho E A 1987 Mechanism of venous occlusion during canine penile erection: or anatomic demonstration. Journal of Urology 137

Fox C A, Fox B 1969 Blood pressure and respiratory patterns during human coitus. Journal of Reproduction and Fertility 19: 405–415

Fox C A, Ismail A A A, Love D N, Kirkham K E, Loraine J A 1972 Studies on the relationship between plasma testosterone levels and human sexual activity. Journal of Endocrinology 52: 51–58

Franks S, Jacobs H S, Martin N, Nabarro J D N 1978 Hyperprolactinaemia and impotence. Clinical Endocrinology 8: 277–287

Gebhard P H, Johnson A B 1979 The Kinsey data: marginal tabulations of the 1935–1965 interviews conducted by the Institute for Sex Research. Saunders, Philadelphia

Geer J H, Fuhr R 1976 Cognitive factors in sexual arousal: the role of distraction. Journal of Consulting and Clinical Psychology 44: 238–243

Ginestie J-F, Romieu A 1978 Radiologic exploration of impotence. Martinas Nijghof, The Hague

Gold A R, Adams D B 1978 Measuring the cycles of female sexuality. Contemporary Obstetrics and Gynecology 12: 147

Gooren L J G 1985 Human male sexual functions do not require aromatisation of testosterone: a study using tamoxifen, testolactone and dihydrotestosterone. Archives of Sexual Behavior 14: 530–548

Gooren L J G 1988 Hypogonadotropic hypogonadal men respond less well to androgen substitution treatment than hypergonadotropic hypogonadal men. Archives of Sexual Behavior 17: 265–270

Gorski R A, Gordon J H, Shryne J E, Southam A M 1978 Evidence for a morphological sex difference within the medical preoptic area of the rat brain. Brain Research 148: 333–346

Graber B, Kline-Graber G 1979 Female orgasm — role of pubococcygeus. Journal of Clinical Psychiatry 40: 34–39

Graber B, Rohrbaugh J W, Newlin D B, Varner J L, Ellingson R J 1985 EEG during masturbation and ejaculation. Archives of Sexual Behavior 14: 491–504

Grafenburg E 1950 The role of the urethra in female orgasm. International Journal of Sexology 111: 145–148

Graham C A, McGrew W C 1980 Menstrual synchrony in female undergraduates living on a co-educational campus. Psychoneuroendocrinology 5: 245–252

Greenblatt R B 1942 Androgenic therapy in women. Journal of Clinical Endocrinology and Metabolism 2: 665–666

Hailes J, Nelson J, Menelaus M, Burger H 1986 The treatment of loss of libido in post-menopausal women with implants of oestradiol alone or in combination with testosterone: clinical results. In: Dennerstein L, Fraser I (eds) Hormones and behaviour. Elsevier, Amsterdam

Hamilton J B 1943 Demonstrated ability of penile erection in castrated men with markedly low titers of urinary androgens. Proceedings of Society for Experimental Biology and Medicine 54: 309–312

Hariton E B, Singer J L 1974 Women's fantasies during sexual intercourse: normative and theoretical implications. Journal of Consulting and Clinical Psychology 42: 313–322

Harris et al 1980

Hart B L, Leedy M G 1985 Neurological bases of male sexual behavior: a comparative analysis. In: Adler N, Goy R W, Pfaff D W (eds) Handbook of behavioral neurobiology, vol 7. Plenum, New York, pp. 373–422

Heap R B, Flint A P E 1984 Pregnancy. In: Austin C R, Short R V (eds) Hormonal control of reproduction. Reproduction in mammals, vol 3, 2nd edn. Cambridge University Press, Cambridge, pp 153–194

Heath R G 1972 Pleasure and brain activity in man. Journal of Nervous and Mental Diseases 154: 3–18

Heiman J 1977 A psychophysiological exploration of sexual arousal patterns in females and males. Psychophysiology 14: 266–273

Heiman J R, Hatch J P 1981 Conceptual and therapeutic contributions of psychophysiology to sexual dysfunction. In: Hayner S, Gannon L (eds) Psychosomatic disorders: a psychophysiological approach to etiology and treatment. Gardner, New York

Heiman J R, Rowland D L 1983 Affective and physiological sexual response patterns: the effects of instructions on sexually functional and dysfunctional men. Journal of Psychosomatic Research 27: 105–116

Henson D E, Rubin H B 1971 Voluntary control of eroticism. Journal of Applied Behavioral Analysis 4: 37–47

Herbert J 1977 The neuroendocrine basis of sexual behavior in primates. In: Money J, Musaph H (eds) Handbook of sexology. Excerpta Medica, Amsterdam, pp 449–459

Herms V, Gabelmann J, Müller M, Schmid A, Kubli F 1980 Sexual behaviour during pregnancy. In: Forleo R, Pasini W (eds) Medical sexology. Elsevier/North Holland, Amsterdam

Hirshkowitz M, Karacan I, Thornby J, Ware J 1984 Nocturnal penile tumescence and EEG asymmetry. Research Communications in Psychology, Psychiatry and Behavior 9: 87–94

Hite S 1976 The Hite report. Talmy Franklin, London

Hoch Z 1980 The sensory arm of the female orgasmic reflex. Journal of Sex Education and Therapy 6: 4–7

Höckfelt T, Everitt B, Meister B et al 1986 Neurons with multiple messengers, with special reference to neuroendocrine systems. Recent Progress in Hormone Research 42: 1–70

Hoon P W, Wincze J P, Hoon E F 1977 The effects of biofeedback and cognitive mediation upon vaginal blood volume. Behaviour Research and Therapy 8: 694–702

Hopwood N J, Kelch R P, Hale P M, Mendes T M, Foster C M, Bertius I Z 1989 The onset of human puberty — biological and environmental factors. In: Bancroft J, Reinisch J (eds) Adolescence and puberty, the third Kinsey symposium. Oxford University Press, New York (in press)

Howie P W, McNeilly A S 1982 Effects of breast feeding patterns on human birth intervals. Journal of Reproduction and Fertility 65: 545–557

Howie P W, McNeilly A S, Houston M J, Cook A, Boyle H 1981 Effect of supplementary food on suckling patterns and ovarian activity during lactation. British Medical Journal 283: 757–759

Howie P W, McNeilly A S, Houston M J, Cook A, Boyle H 1982 Fertility after childbirth: post partum ovulation and menstruation in bottle and breast feeding mothers. Clinical Endocrinology 17: 323–332

Huffman J W 1948 The detailed anatomy of the periurethral ducts in the adult human female. American Journal of Obstetrics and Gynecology 55: 86–100

Imperato-McGinley J, Guerrero L, Gautier T, Peterson R E 1974 Steroid 5-alpha-reductase deficiency in man; an inherited form of male pseudo-hermaphroditism. Science 186: 1213–1215

Ismail A A A, Davidson D W, Loraine J A 1970 Assessment of gonadal function in impotent men. In: Irvine W J (ed) Reproductive endocrinology. Livingstone, Edinburgh, pp 138–147

Jaffe Y, Malamuth N, Feingold J, Feshback I 1974 Sexual arousal and behavioural aggression. Journal of Personality and Social Psychology 30: 759–764

Jakobovitz T 1970 The treatment of impotence with methyl testosterone thyroid. Fertility and Sterility 21: 32–35

Johnson D F, Phoenix C H 1976 Hormonal control of sexual attractiveness, proceptivity and receptivity in rhesus monkeys. Journal of Comparative and Physiological Psychology 90: 473–483

Kaplan H S 1979 Disorders of sexual desire. Brunner/Mazel, New York

Karacan I, Salis P J, Thornby J I, Williams R L 1976 The ontogeny of nocturnal penile tumescence. Waking and Sleeping 1: 27–44

Kendrick K M, Dixson A F 1985 Luteinizing hormone releasing hormone enhances proceptivity in a primate. Neuroendocrinology 41: 449–453

Kendrick K M, Dixson A F 1986 Anteromedial hypothalamic lesions block proceptivity but not receptivity in the female common marmoset (*Callithrix jacchus*). Brain Research 375: 221–229

Keverne E B 1978 Olfactory cues in mammalian sexual behaviour. In: Hutchison J B (ed) Biological determinants of sexual behaviour. Wiley, Chichester, pp 727–763

Kinsey A C, Pomeroy W B, Martin C F 1948 Sexual behavior in the human male. Saunders, Philadelphia

Kinsey A C, Pomeroy W B, Martin C F, Gebhard P H 1953 Sexual behavior in the human female. Saunders, Philadelphia, pp 759–761

Korenchevsky V 1937 The female prostatic gland and its reaction to male sexual compounds. Journal of Physiology 90: 371–376

Kraemer H C, Becker H B, Brodie H T H, Doering C H, Moos R H, Hamburg D A 1976 Orgasmic frequency and plasma testosterone levels in normal human males. Archives of Sexual Behavior 5: 125–132

Krall J F 1986 Smooth muscle tension; the biochemistry of regulation in the vasculature. Paper presented at Scientific Basis of Sexual Dysfunction, NIH, Baltimore, June 1986

Krantz K E 1958 Innervation of the human vulva and vagina. Obstetrics and Gynecology 12: 382

Kuhn R A 1950 Functional capacity of the isolated human spinal cord. Brain 73: 1

Kwan M, Greenleaf W J, Mann J, Crapo L, Davidson J M 1983 The nature of androgen action on male sexuality a combine laboratory and self report study in hypogonadal men. Journal of Clinical Endocrinology and Metabolism 57: 557–562

LaFerla J J, Anderson D L, Schalch D S 1978 Psychoendocrine response to sexual arousal in human males. Psychosomatic Medicine 40: 166–172

Lal S, Ackman D, Thavundayil J X, Kiely M E, Etienne P 1984 Effect of apomorphine, a dopamine receptor agonist, on penile tumescence in normal subjects. Progress in Neuro-Psychopharmacology and Biological Psychiatry 8: 695–699

Lal S, Laryea E, Tharundayil J X et al 1987 Apomorphine-induced penile tumescence in impotent patients — preliminary findings. Progress in Neuro-Psychopharmacology and Biological Psychiatry 11: 235–242

Landis J, Thomas P, Peffenberger S 1950 The effects of first pregnancy upon the sexual adjustment of 212 couples. American Sociological Review 15: 766

Lange J D, Brown W A, Wincze J P, Zwick W 1980 Serum testosterone concentration and penile tumescence changes in men. Hormones and Behavior 14: 267–270

Lange J D, Wincze J P, Zwick W, Feldman S, Hughes K 1981 Effects of demand for performance, self-monitoring of arousal, and increased sympathetic nervous system activity on male erectile response. Archives of Sexual Behavior 10: 443–464

Lawrence D H, Swyer G I M 1974 Plasma testosterone and testosterone binding affinities in men with impotence, oligospermia, azoospermia and hypogonadism. British Medical Journal i: 349–351

Laws D R, Rubin H B 1969 Instructional control of an autonomic sexual response. Journal of Applied Behavioral Analysis 2: 93–99

Lee P A, Jaffe R B, Midgley A R 1974 Lack of alteration of serum gonadotrophins in men and women following sexual intercourse. American Journal of Obstetrics and Gynecology 120: 985–987

Levi L 1969 Sympatho-adreno-medullary activity, diuresis and emotional reactions during visual sexual stimulation in human males and females. Psychosomatic Medicine 31: 251–268

Levin R J 1980 Physiology of sexual function in women. Clinics in Obstetrics and Gynaecology 7: 213–252

Levin R J, Wagner G 1985 Orgasm in women in the laboratory — quantitative studies on duration, intensity, latency and vaginal blood flow. Archives of Sexual Behavior 14: 439–450

Levin R M, Wein A J 1980 Adrenergic alpha receptors outnumber beta receptors in human penile corpus cavernosum. Investigative Urology 18: 225

Lifshitz K 1966 The averaged evoked cortical response to complex visual stimuli. Psychophysiology 3: 55–68

Lincoln G A 1974 Luteinising hormone and testosterone in man. Nature 252: 232–233

Littler W A, Honour A J, Sleight P 1974 Direct arterial pressure, heart rate and electrocardiogram during human coitus. Journal of Reproduction and Fertility 40: 321–331

Lue T F 1986 The erectile mechanism. Paper presented at Conference on Scientific Basis of Sexual Dysfunction. NIH Baltimore, Maryland

Luisi M, Franchi F 1980 Double-blind group comparative study of testosterone undecanoate and mesterolone in hypogonadal male patients. Journal of Endocrinological Investigation 3: 305–308

Lundberg P O, Muhr C, Hutler B, Brattberg A, Wide L 1985 Sexual libido in patients with hypothalamo–pituitary disorders. Proceedings of 7th World Congress Sexology, New Delhi, November

McClintock M 1971 Menstrual synchrony and suppression. Nature 229: 244–245

McEwen B S 1976 Interactions between hormones and nerve tissue. Hormones and reproductive behavior. Readings from Scientific American. W H Freeman, San Francisco, pp 106–116

Maclean P D 1976 Brain mechanisms of elemental sexual functions. In: Sadock B T, Kaplan H I, Freeman A M (eds) The sexual experience. Williams & Wilkins, Baltimore, pp 119–127

Maclean P D, Ploog D W 1962 Cerebral representation of penile erection. Journal of Neurophysiology 25: 29–55

MacMahon B 1973 Age at menarche. Vital and health statistics, series 11, no 133. Rockville, National Center for Health Statistics, USA

Manni A, Pardridge W M, Cefalu W et al 1985 Bioavailability of albumin bound testosterone. Journal of Clinical Endocrinology and Metabolism 61: 705–710

Marrama P, Carani C, Montamini V et al 1984 Gonadal function: sexual behavior in bromocriptine treated men with prolactinoma. In: Segraves T, Haeberle E (eds) Emerging dimensions of sexology. Praeger, New York

Marshall E A, Tanner J M 1969 Variations in patterns of pubertal changes in girls. Archives of Diseases of Childhood 44: 291–303

Marshall E A, Tanner J M 1970 Variations in patterns of pubertal changes in boys. Archives of Diseases of Childhood 45: 13–23

Mas M, Zahradnik M A, Martino V, Davidson J M 1985 Stimulation of spinal serotonergic receptors facilitates seminal emission and suppresses penile erectile reflexes. Brain Research 342: 128–134

Masters W H, Johnson V E 1966 Human sexual response. Churchill Livingstone, London

Masters W H, Johnson V E 1970 Human sexual inadequacy. Churchill Livingstone, London

Mathews A, Whitehead A, Kellett J 1983 Psychological and hormonal factors in the treatment of female sexual dysfunction. Psychological Medicine 13: 83–92

Matteo S, Rissman E F 1984 Increased sexual activity during the midcycle portion of the human menstrual cycle. Hormones and Behavior 18: 249–255

Meyer-Bahlburg H F L 1979 Sex hormones and female homosexuality: a critical examination. Archives of Sexual Behavior 8: 101–119

Meyers R 1961 Evidence of a locus of the neural mechanisms of libido and penile potency in the septo-fornico-hypothalamic region of the human brain. Transactions of the American Neurological Association 86: 81–85

Meyers R 1962 Three cases of myoclonus alleviated by bilateral ansotomy, with a note on post-operative alibido and impotence. Journal of Neurosurgery 19: 71–81

Michael R P, Bonsall R W, Warner P 1974 Human vaginal secretions: volatile fatty acid content. Science 186: 1217–1219

Michael R P, Richter M C, Cain J A, Zumpe D, Bonsall R W 1978 Artificial menstrual cycle behaviour and the role of androgens in female rhesus monkeys. Nature 275: 439–440

Money J 1961 Components of eroticism in man I. The hormones in relation to sexual morphology and sexual desire. Journal of Nervous and Mental Disease 132: 239–248

Money J, Alexander D 1969 Psychosexual development and absence of homosexuality in males with precocious puberty: a review of 18 cases. Journal of Nervous and Mental Diseases 148: 111–123

Money J, Yankowitz R 1967 The sympathetic inhibiting effects of the drug Ismelin on human male eroticism, with a note on Melleril. Journal of Sex Research 3: 69–82

Morales A, Surridge D H C, Marshall P G, Fenemore J 1982 Nonhormonal pharmacological treatment of organic impotence. Journal of Urology 128: 45

Morris N M, Udry J R 1978 Pheromonal influences on human sexual behavior: an experimental search. Journal of Biosocial Science 10: 147–157

Morris N M, Udry J R, Khan-Dawood F, Dawood M Y 1987 Marital sex frequency and midcycle female testosterone. Archives of Sexual Behavior 16: 27–38

Mortimer C H, McNeilly A S, Fisher R A, Murray M A F, Besser G F 1974 Gonadotrophin releasing hormone therapy in hypogonadal males with hypothalamic or pituitary dysfunction. British Medical Journal 4: 617–621

Mosovich A, Tallafero A 1954 Studies on EEG and sex function orgasm. Diseases of the Nervous System 15: 218–220

Moss R L, Dudley C A 1982 Hypothalamic peptides and sexual behavior. In: Freeman R (ed) Behavior and the menstrual cycle. Dekker, New York, pp 65–76

Muller D, Roeder R, Orthner H 1973 Further results of stereotaxis in the human hypothalamus in sexual deviation. First use of the operation in addiction to drugs. Neurochirurgia 16: 113–126

Nadelhaft I, de Groat W C, Morgan C 1980 Location and morphology of parasympathetic preganglionic neurons in the sacral spinal cord of the cat revealed by retrograde axonal transport of horse-radish peroxidase. Journal of Comparative Neurology 193: 265–281

Nadler R D 1977 Sexual behaviour of captive orang-utans. Archives of Sexual Behavior 6: 457–476

Nadler R D 1980 Determination of sexuality in the great apes. In: Forleo R, Pasini W (eds) Medical sexology. Elsevier/North Holland, Amsterdam, pp 215–222

Naftolin F, Ryan K J, Davies I J et al 1975 The formation of estrogens by central neuroendocrine tissues. Recent Progress in Hormone Research 31: 295–320

Newman H F 1970 Vibratory sensitivity of the penis. Fertility and Sterility 21: 791–793

Newman H F, Northup J D 1981 The mechanism of human penile erection — an overview. Urology 17: 399–408

Newton N 1973 Interrelationships between sexual responsiveness, birth and breast feeding behavior. In: Zubin J, Money J (eds) Critical issues in contemporary sexual behavior. Johns Hopkins Press, Baltimore, pp 77–98

Nutter D, Condron M R 1985 Sexual fantasy and activity patterns of males with inhibited sexual desire and males with erectile dysfunction versus normal controls. Journal of Sexual and Marital Therapy 11: 91–98

O'Carroll R E 1984 Androgen administration to hypogonadal and eugonadal men — effects on measures of sensation seeking, personality and spatial ability. Personality and Individual Differences 5: 595–598

O'Carroll R, Bancroft J 1984 Testosterone therapy for low sexual interest and erectile dysfunction in men: a controlled study. British Journal of Psychiatry 145: 146–151

O'Carroll R, Shapiro C, Bancroft J 1985 Androgens, behaviour and nocturnal erections in hypogonadal men: the effect of varying the replacement dose. Clinical Endocrinology 23: 527–538

Ottesen B, Wagner G, Virag R, Fahrenkrug J 1984 Penile erection: a possible role for vasoactive intestinal polypeptide as a neurotransmitter. British Medical Journal 288: 9–11

Parkes A S 1976 Patterns of sexuality and reproduction. Oxford University Press, London

Penfield W, Jasper H 1954 Epilepsy and the functional anatomy of the human brain. Little, Brown, Boston

Perachio A A, Marr L D, Alexander M 1979 Sexual behavior in male rhesus monkeys elicited by electrical stimulation of preoptic and hypothalamic areas. Brain Research 177: 127–144

Persky H, Charney N, Lief H I, O'Brien C P, Miller W R, Strauss D 1978a The relationship of plasma estradiol levels to sexual behavior in young women. Psychosomatic Medicine 40: 523–535

Persky H, Lief A I, Strauss D, Miller W R, O'Brien C P 1978b Plasma testosterone levels and sexual behavior of couples. Archives of Sexual Behavior 7: 157–173

Persky H, Driesbach L, Miller W R et al 1982 The relation of plasma androgen levels to sexual behaviors and attitudes of women. Psychosomatic Medicine 44: 305–319

Peters R S 1960 The concept of motivation, 2nd edn. Routledge & Kegan Paul, London

Pfaff D, Modianos D 1985 Neural mechanisms of female reproductive behavior. In: Adler N, Goy R W, Pfaff D W (eds) Handbook of behavioral neurobiology vol 7. Plenum, New York, pp 423–493

Pirke K H, Kockott G, Dittmar F 1974 Psychosexual stimulation and plasma testosterone in man. Archives of Sexual Behavior 3: 577–584

Pirke K M, Kockott G, Aldenhoff J, Besinger U, Feil W 1979 Pituitary gonadal system function in patients with erectile impotence and premature ejaculation. Archives of Sexual Behavior 8: 41–48

Pollen J J, Dreilinger A 1984 Immunohistochemical identification of prostatic acid phosphatase and prostate specific antigens in female periurethral glands. Urology 23: 303–304

Price K P 1973 Feedback effects of penile tumescence. Paper presented at Eastern Psychological Association, Washington D C, May 1973

Przybyla D P J, Byrne D 1984 The mediating role of cognitive processes in self-reported sexual arousal. Journal of Research in Personality 18: 54–63

Purifoy F E, Koopmans L H 1980 Androstenedione, T and free T concentrations in women of various occupations. Social Biology 26: 179–188

Purvis K, Landgren B M, Cekan Z, Diszfalusy E 1976 Endocrine effects of masturbation in men. Journal of Endocrinology 70: 439–444

Raboch J, Starka L 1973 Reported coital activity of men and levels of plasma testosterone. Archives of Sexual Behavior 2: 309–315

Raboch J, Mellan J, Starka L 1975 Plasma testosterone in male patients with sexual dysfunction. Archives of Sexual Behavior 4: 541–545

Racey P A, Ansari M A, Rowe P H, Glover T D 1973 Testosterone in impotent men. Journal of Endocrinology 59: xxiii

Ramsey G V 1943 The sexual development of boys. American Journal of Psychology 56: 217–234

Reid K, Surridge D H C, Morales A et al 1987 Double-blind trial of yohimbine in the treatment of psychogenic impotence. Lancet iii 421–423

Reinberg A, Lagoguey M 1978 Circadian and circannual rhythms in sexual activity and plasma hormones (FSH, LH and testosterone) of five human males. Archives of Sexual Behavior 7: 13–30

Robbins M B, Jensen G D 1978 Multiple orgasm in males. In: Gemme R, Wheeler C C (eds) Progress in sexology. Plenum, New York

Robinson B W, Mishkin M 1968 Penile erection evoked from the forebrain structures in *Macaca mulatta*. Archives of Neurology 119: 184

Robson K M, Brant H A, Kumar R 1981 Maternal sexuality during first pregnancy and after childbirth. British Journal of Obstetrics and Gynaecology 88: 882–889

Roose S P, Glassman A H, Walsh B T, Cullen K 1982 Reversible loss of nocturnal penile tumescence during depression: a preliminary report. Neuropsychobiology 8: 284–288

Root W S, Bard P 1947 The mediation of feline erections through sympathetic pathways with some remarks on sexual behavior after deafferentiation of the genitalia. American Journal of Physiology 151: 80–89

Rosen R C, Shapiro D, Schwartz G E 1975 Voluntary control of penile tumescence. Psychosomatic Medicine 37: 479–483

Rosen R C, Goldstein L, Scoles V, Lazarus C 1986 Psychophysiological correlates of nocturnal penile tumescence in normal males. Psychosomatic Medicine 48: 423–429

Rowell T E 1972 Female reproduction cycles and social behavior in primates. Advances in the Study of Behavior 4: 69–105

Royal College of General Practitioners 1974 Oral contraceptives and health. Pitman, London

Sakheim D K, Barlow D H, Gayle Beck J, Abrahamson D J 1984 The effect of an increased awareness of erectile cues on sexual arousal. Behaviour Research and Therapy 22: 151–158

Salmimies P, Kockott G, Pirke K M, Vogt J J, Schill W B 1982 Effects of testosterone replacement on sexual behaviour in hypogonadal men. Archives of Sexual Behavior 11: 345–353

Salmon U J, Geist S H 1943 The effects of androgen upon libido in women. Journal of Clinical Endocrinology 3: 235–238

Sanders D, Warner P, Backström T, Bancroft J 1983 Mood, sexuality, hormones and the menstrual cycle. I. Changes in mood and physical state: description of subjects and method. Psychosomatic Medicine 45: 487–501

Sarrel P M 1976 Biological aspects of sexual function. In: Gemme R, Wheeler C C (eds) Progress in sexology. Plenum, New York, pp 227–244

Schreiner-Engel P 1980 Female sexual arousability: its relation to gonadal hormones and the menstrual cycle. Dissertations Abstracts International 41.02: 80–17, 527

Schreiner-Engel P, Schiavi R C 1986 Lifetime psychopathology in individuals with low sexual desire. Journal of Nervous and Mental Disease 174: 646–651

Schreiner-Engel P, Schiavi R C, Smith H, White D 1981 Sexual arousability and the menstrual cycle. Psychosomatic Medicine 43: 199–214

Schreiner-Engel P, Schiavi R C, Smith H, White D 1982 Plasma testosterone and female sexual behavior. In: Hoch Z, Lief H I (eds) Proceedings of Fifth world congress of sexology. Excerpta Medica, Amsterdam

Schwartz M F, Kolodny R C, Masters W H 1980 Plasma testosterone levels of sexually functional and dysfunctional men. Archives of Sexual Behavior 9: 335–366

Schwartz M F, Banman J E, Masters W H 1982 Hyperprolactinaemia and sexual dysfunction in men. Biological Psychiatry 17: 861–876

Semans J H, Langworthy O R 1938 Observations on the neurophysiology of sexual function in the male cat. Journal of Urology 40: 836–846

Sherfey M J 1966 The evolution and nature of female sexuality in relation to psychoanalytic theory. Journal of American Psychoanalytic Association 14: 28–128

Sherwin B B, Gelfand M M, Brender W 1985 Androgen enhances sexual motivation in females: a prospective, crossover study of sex steroid administration in the surgical menopause. Psychosomatic Medicine 47: 339–351

Shorr E, Papanicolou G N, Stimmel B J 1938 Neutralisation of ovarian follicular hormones in women by simultaneous administration of male sex hormones. Proceedings of the Society for Experimental Biology and Medicine 38: 759–762

Short R V 1979 Sexual behaviour in red deer. Animal reproduction. In: Hawk H (ed) BARC symposium no 3. Allanheld, Osmun, Montclair, pp 365–372

Short R V 1980a Hormonal control of growth at puberty. In: Lawrence T L J (ed) Growth in animals. Butterworth, London, pp 25–45

Short R V 1980b The origins of human sexuality. In: Austin C R, Short R V (eds) Human sexuality. Cambridge University Press, Cambridge, pp 1–33

Singer I 1973 The goals of human sexuality. Wildwood House, London

Skakkebaek N E, Bancroft J, Davidson D W, Warner P 1981 Androgen replacement with oral testosterone undecanoate in hypogonadal men: a double-blind controlled study. Clinical Endocrinology 14: 49–67

Smals A G H, Kloppenborg P W C, Benraad T J 1976 Circannual cycle in plasma testosterone levels in man. Journal of Clinical Endocrinology and Metabolism 42: 979–983

Spitz C J, Gold A R, Adams D B 1975 Cognitive and hormonal factors affecting coital frequency. Archives of Sexual Behavior 4: 249–263

Stearn E L, Winter J S D, Faiman C 1973 Effects of coitus on gonadotrophin, prolactin and sex steroid levels in man. Journal of Clinical Endocrinology and Metabolism 37: 687–691

Steinman D L, Wincze J P, Sakheim D K, Barlow D H, Mavissakalian M 1981 A comparison of male and female patterns of sexual arousal. Archives of Sexual Behavior 10: 529–548

Stock W E, Geer J H 1982 A study of fantasy-based sexual arousal in women. Archives of Sexual Behavior 11: 33–47

Studd J, Montgomery J, Appleby L, Versi E, Tapp A 1986 Prospective randomised study of oestradiol and testosterone implants in the treatment of psychiatric and psychosexual problems at the menopause. In: Dennerstein L, Fraser I (eds) Hormones and Behaviour. Elsevier, Amsterdam

Swaab D F, Fliers E 1985 A sexually dimorphic nucleus in the human brain. Science 228: 1112–1115

Tauber E S 1940 Effects of castration upon the sexuality of the adult male. Psychosomatic Medicine 11: 74–87

Tennent G, Bancroft J, Cass J 1974 The control of deviant sexual behavior by drugs: a double-blind controlled study of benperidol, chlorpromazine and placebo. Archives of Sexual Behavior 3: 261–271

Thase M E, Reynolds C F, Glanz L M et al 1987 Nocturnal penile tumescence in depressed men. American Journal of Psychiatry 144: 89–92

Toone B K, Wheeler M, Nanjee N, Fenwick P, Grant R 1983 Sex hormones, sexual activity and plasma anticonvulsant levels in male epileptics. Journal of Neurology, Neurosurgery and Psychiatry 46: 824–826

Tutin C E G 1980 Reproductive behaviour of wild chimpanzees in the Gombe National Park, Tanzania. Journal of Reproduction and Fertility (suppl 28): 43–57

Udry J R, Morris N M 1967 Seasonality of coitus and seasonality of birth. Demography 4: 673–680

Udry J R, Morris N M 1968 Distribution of coitus in the menstrual cycle. Nature 220: 593–596

Udry J R, Morris N M 1977 The distribution of events in the human menstrual cycle. Journal of Reproduction and Fertility 51: 419–425

Udry J R, Billy J O G, Morris N M, Groff T R, Raj M H 1985 Serum androgenic hormones motivate sexual behavior in adolescent boys. Fertility and Sterility 43: 90–94

Udry J R, Talbert L M, Morris N M 1986 Biosocial foundations for adolescent female sexuality. Demography 23: 217–229

Utian W H 1975 Effect of hysterectomy oophorectomy and estrogen therapy on libido. International Journal of Obstetrics and Gynaecology 84: 4314–315

Vance E B, Wagner N N 1976 Written descriptions of orgasms — a study of sex differences. Archives of Sexual Behavior 5: 87–89

van Wieringen J C, Wafelbakker F, Verbrugge H P, De Haas J H 1971 Growth diagrams 1965, Netherlands. Wolters-Noordhoff, Groningen

Veith J, Buck M, Getzlaf S, Van Dalfsen P, Slade A 1983 Exposure to men influences the occurrence of ovulation in women. Physiology and Behavior 31: 313–315

Virag R, Ottesen B, Fahrenkrug J, Levy C, Wagner G 1982 Vasoactive intestinal polypeptide release during penile erection in man. Lancet 4: 1166

Wagner G, Brindley G 1980 The effect of atropine and beta blockers upon human penile erection — a controlled pilot study. In: Zorgniotti A (ed) First international conference on vascular impotence. Charles C Thomas, New York

Wagner G, Levin R J 1980 Effect of atropine and methyl atropine on human vaginal blood flow, sexual arousal and climax. Acta Pharmacologica et Toxicologica 46: 321–325

Wagner G, Bro-Rasmussen F, Willis E A, Nielsen M H 1982 New theory on the mechanism of erection involving hitherto undescribed vessels. Lancet ii: 416–418

Ward I L 1977 Regulation of sexual behavior by hormones in male non-primates. In: Money J, Musaph H (eds) Handbook of sexology. Excerpta Medica, Amsterdam, pp 377–392

Warner P, Bancroft J 1988 Mood, sexuality, oral contraceptives and the menstrual cycle. Journal of Psychosomatic Research (in press)

Waxenburg S E, Drellich M G, Sutherland A M 1959 The role of hormones in human behaviour. 1. Changes in female sexuality after adrenalectomy. Journal of Clinical Endocrinology and Metabolism 19: 193–202

Wenger M A, Averill J R, Smith D D B 1968 Autonomic activity during sexual arousal. Psychophysiology 4: 468–478

Whalen R E, Yahr P, Luttge W G 1985 The role of metabolism in hormonal control of sexual behavior. In: Adler N, Pfaff D, Goy R W (eds) Handbook of behavioral neurobiology, vol 7. Plenum, New York, pp 609–649

Whitelaw G P, Smithwick R H 1951 Some secondary effects of sympathectomy: with particular reference to disturbance of sexual function. New England Journal of Medicine 245: 121–130

WHO Task Force on Psychosocial Research in Family Planning 1982 Hormonal contraception for men: acceptability and effects on sexuality. Studies in Family Planning 13: 328–342

Wolchik S A, Beggs V, Wincze J P, Sakheim D K, Barlow D H, Mavissakalian M 1980 The effects of emotional arousal on subsequent sexual arousal in men. Journal of Abnormal Psychology 89: 595–598

Wu F C, Bancroft J, Davidson D W, Nicol K 1981 The behavioural effects of testosterone undecanoate in adult Klinefelter men: a controlled study. Clinical Endocrinology 16: 489–497

Yerkes R M 1939 Sexual behavior in the chimpanzee. Human Biology 11: 78–111

Zimmer D, Borchardt E, Fischle C 1983 Sexual fantasies of sexually distressed and non-distressed men and women: an empirical comparison. Journal of Sexual and Marital Therapy 9: 38–50

Zuckerman M 1971 Physiological measures of sexual arousal in the human. Psychological Bulletin 75: 297–329

3

Sexual development

People may differ in what they regard as mature sexual behaviour; such judgement inevitably involves values. But few would disagree that their route to sexual maturity is complicated, with many points of possible and untoward departure. When we look at this developmental process a number of points strike us. First, that even before birth important stages may go wrong. Second, through childhood and early adolescence various strands of development eventually combine to produce the sexual adult. Third, the adult continues to develop sexually well into the latter part of his or her life.

THE DEVELOPMENTAL PROCESS

When considering an individual's development from the early embryonic stage to the mature sexual adult we are faced with a dynamic process shaped by a multitude of influences. Various theoretical models have been offered to explain this process. None, it is probably true to say, claims the ability to predict how an individual's development will proceed, but rather explains in retrospect what has gone before. Certain limited stages of development, e.g. prenatal sexual differentiation, may be looked at separately, allowing the generation of testable hypotheses. But when we attempt to fit the whole developmental story into one explanatory system our powers of prediction are soon overwhelmed. And yet we must not lose sight of these many influences if we are to avoid being misled.

Although argument has raged as to whether sexual development depends on inborn determinants (nature) or environmental influences (nurture), few scientists now enter such debate as it is evident that both are involved. The challenge is rather to formulate in a useful way the continuing interaction between these two sources of influence.

RELEVANT MODELS OF DEVELOPMENT

There are now well described models of sexual differentiation based on biological mechanisms, including the mediation of genetic effects and the

146

organising action of reproductive hormones. These mechanisms are most clearly relevant prenatally, but they are possibly important during post-natal development as well. We will consider these biological mechanisms later.

We must also consider appropriate models of learning as they apply to sexual development, in particular the social learning (Mischel 1966) and cognitive learning (Kohlberg 1966) paradigms.

Social learning is the process by which behaviour is shaped by its consequences; encouraged and discouraged by reward and punishment, its modification is facilitated by modelling or the example of others. This type of learning has equal relevance to animal and human development. Awareness of what is taking place during such learning is no more than an epiphenomenon of the human experience. We will be drawing parallels between sexual learning of this kind in primates and humans.

Cognitive learning is perhaps uniquely human. In this case the stimuli which impinge upon the individual and the responses elicited are cognitively organised according to categories. This has an added and often crucial effect on the basic social learning process. Consequences become rewarding or punishing according to the category they are assigned.

Kohlberg (1966) drew the distinction between these two paradigms with the following illustration. 'In social learning "I want reward, I am rewarded for doing boy's things, therefore I want to be a boy". In cognitive learning "I am a boy, therefore I want to do boy's things, therefore the opportunity to do boy's things is rewarding".' To take this illustration further, any reward given for behaving like a boy will, through cognitive processes, strengthen the concept 'I am a boy'. Failure to be rewarded, or to be punished for such behaviour will challenge and possibly weaken the concept 'I am a boy'.

Thus these two types of learning process interact, raising learning to a much more complex plane than that of social learning alone. We assume that cognitive learning is unique to humans because it depends on the use of language, which animals do not have, except perhaps in a most rudimentary form.

How we conceptualise and categorise our environment and experiences must also develop. Piaget has elegantly shown how this ability goes through crucial stages of development in a stepwise rather than continuous fashion, analogous to the development of the motor nervous system. Curiously, the Piagetian school has almost totally ignored the development of thinking as it applies to sexuality and reproduction. We will return to this later. But cognitive learning is of particular significance for the gender development of the child, who at some time between the ages of 18 months and 3 years becomes able to categorise people in simple ways and assigns itself to the category of boy or girl. It is also possible that this same process of 'either—or' categorisation or labelling plays an important part much later in development when the young adolescent is responding to socially prescribed categories such as homosexual or heterosexual.

The best known and most influential model of sexual development has been the psychoanalytic model. As indicated earlier (p. 4), I have not found psychoanalytic theory or concepts helpful in this respect, though undoubtedly psychoanalysts have drawn our attention to some crucially important aspects of development. I have found some of the major modifications of psychoanalytic theory to be more useful, in particular those of the ego-analysts such as Erikson (1950). This may be because the ego-analysts have concerned themselves with explaining the normal rather than extrapolating from the abnormal, which is more characteristic of orthodox psychoanalysis.

Miller & Simon (1980) have usefully compared various models of sexual development. They point out that, in the Freudian view, the child enters adolescence with 'an articulated set of erotic meanings that seek appropriate objects and behaviour', whereas Erikson (1950) sees the child making this entry with a number of skills which are relevant to the sexual encounters of adolescence but not confined to them, e.g. the capacity for intimacy and trust. Erikson also proposes useful ways of recognising and describing different stages of identity development which allow us to see childhood experiences as crucially important to later sexual development without requiring the assumption of the degree of early sexual organisation which is central to the Freudian view.

Sociologists such as Gagnon and Simon have also contributed to our thinking. Using concepts entirely consistent with the cognitive learning model, they talk of scripts, or ways people can or should behave in certain situations; this plays a fundamental part in the unfolding of our sexuality. Such scripts, which we acquire from our social group — in particular the peer group of the adolescent — help us to attribute meaning to internal states, organise sequences of specific sexual acts, decode novel situations, set the limits for sexual response and link meanings from non-sexual aspects of life to specifically sexual experience (Gagnon & Simon 1973). Such a view attaches major importance to social and cultural factors in determining our sexuality, and Gagnon and Simon may perhaps be criticised for emphasising such mechanisms at the expense of other more biological factors.

AN ECLECTIC INTERACTIONAL MODEL OF SEXUAL DEVELOPMENT

Despite this wealth of theoretical models relevant to sexual development, there have been few attempts to integrate them in a way which gives balanced consideration to both biological and psychosocial influences (Serbin & Sprafkin 1987). Borrowing from these various approaches, let me therefore present the model I have found most useful in tackling the complexity of sexual development.

First, there are two dimensions: strands and stages. There are three main strands:

1. sexual differentiation into male or female and the development of gender identity.
2. sexual responsiveness.
3. the capacity for close dyadic relationships.

Stages can be defined in varying degrees of detail, but, to be brief, there are six basic stages:

1. prenatal stage;
2. childhood;
3. adolescence and early adulthood;
4. marriage (or the establishment of a stable sexual relationship);
5. early parenthood, late parenthood;
6. mid-life.

At the prenatal stage, sexual differentiation is taking place most obviously in anatomical terms, but also, to some extent, in the organisation of brain function along male or female lines. We will consider the evidence for this shortly. Little can be said, at the present time, about the other two strands at this prenatal stage. During most of childhood, the three strands are developing in relative independence of one another. During late childhood and early adolescence the strands begin to be woven together or integrated to form the young sexual adult. Further periods of integration or reorganisation, though less fundamental than that during adolescence, do occur at a number of important transitional phases during adult life, and account for many of the crises we see in marriage and families. This varying

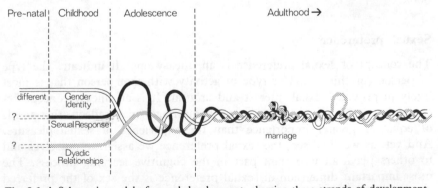

Fig. 3.1 A Schematic model of sexual development, showing three strands of development, gender identity, sexual response and the capacity for close, dyadic relationships, at different stages of the life cycle. During childhood these three strands are relatively independent of each other. During adolescence they start to integrate to form the sexual adult.

interaction of strands of sexual development over time is shown schematically in Figure 3.1.

There are two other aspects of the interactional model to consider — the variety of *functions* or consequences of sexual behaviour which determine the interactional process at each stage, and *sexual preferences* for certain types of sexual partner or activity which first result from these interactions, and then influence our subsequent sexual behaviour as labels or parts of sexual scripts.

The functions of sexual behaviour

In addition to the basic function of reproduction, many other functions or purposes of sexual behaviour can be recognised:
1. Assertion of masculinity or femininity.
2. Bolstering or maintenance of self-esteem.
3. Exertion of power or dominance.
4. Bonding dyadic relationships and fostering intimacy.
5. Source of pleasure.
6. Reduction of tension.
7. Expression of hostility.
8. Risk-taking as a source of excitement.
9. Material gain.

Many of these functions are not peculiarly human and many can be recognised in the behaviour of non-human primates. They provide the variety of rewards that affect sexual learning, with some functions being more in evidence than others at certain stages of development. Many of the problems of human sexual relationships stem from the participants using sex for different purposes at the same time. We will consider these functions and the problems they may generate at various stages in this book.

Sexual preference

The concept of sexual preference is an uneasy one. It indicates the type of person (or thing) and/or type of activity with that person that is most likely to provoke sexual interest and arousal. It is an uneasy concept because the choice of partner (e.g. as in marriage) may reflect other needs of equal or greater importance than the experience of sexual pleasure. And yet, as we shall see, the sexual preference we assign to ourselves and to others plays an important part in the cognitive learning process. The most important dimension of sexual preference is the sex of the preferred partner: whether the preference is heterosexual or homosexual. This development will be considered in more detail later in this chapter. The possible origins of other variations of preference (e.g. fetishism or sadomasochism) will be considered in Chapter 7.

The prevailing controversy is between those who see sexual preference as a manifestation of early organisation or learning and those who regard it as the product of an on-going development process, not necessarily fixed and immutable. Most psychoanalytic theorists have emphasised the importance of early experience in determining later sexual preference. Some, more biologically oriented, such as Money (1980) and more recently Perper (1985), talk of templates. For Perper this is a 'pre-figured gestalt' of an ideal (woman) sexual partner. 'It is not', he suggests, '"encoded" in the genes, but is created by a slow developmental process involving genetic regulation of neural development and later neurophysiological construction of an increasingly detailed and recognisably female image of a woman'. Money calls his templates 'lovemaps' and talks of 'schemas implanted in the brain'. Like a native language, a lovemap is not completed on the day of birth. It requires input from the social environment. The critical period for its development is not puberty, as is often assumed, but before the age of 8.' The implication of the template concept is that, whilst it is influenced by environmental factors, it is formed fairly early and thereafter is relatively fixed. It is not clear on what evidence such ideas are based or, as theoretical models, how they could be tested. The models are reminiscent of psychoanalytic concepts reformulated with modern biological terminology. Ironically, the template or lovemap is a good example of what Perper himself disparagingly describes as ethnobiology or folk beliefs about biology rather than scientifically useful concepts. It may be helpful to think in terms of a gestalt of a sexually attractive person, which is relatively unique for each individual. But we should keep open minds about how that gestalt evolves and how fixed it becomes.

Sources of evidence

Before putting 'the meat on the bones' of this interactional model let us briefly consider the available sources of evidence of early sexual development. There has been considerable reliance on animal experiments. Whilst undoubtedly important, we must be cautious in our extrapolation, as much of the evidence, especially that requiring the sacrifice of the experimental animal, comes from lower mammals, mainly rodents.

At the prenatal stage we can make use of clinical studies of developmental abnormalities. During childhood certain types of behaviour and functioning, such as intelligence, play behaviour and peer group relationships are relatively accessible and there is a considerable body of evidence from which to draw. Explicitly sexual behaviour of children is much less accessible. Parents' and nursery staff's observations of small children's behaviour have been reported by a number of workers. A few studies of children's sexual thinking and knowledge have been carried out (e.g. Goldman & Goldman 1982; see Serbin & Sprafkin 1987 for a review). Kinsey also made use of the documented observations of a few paedophiles who recounted the sexual responses of young children with whom they had been sexually involved.

Kinsey was prepared to accept any information which was likely to throw light on otherwise inaccessible aspects of human sexuality, and in doing so he carefully avoided passing or implying moral judgement. Not everyone would agree that he was right to do so, though until recently his use of such evidence, clearly and openly described in his first volume (Kinsey et al 1948), has not attracted criticism or moral censure. In the last few years, with mounting concern about sexual abuse of children, attempts have been made to denigrate Kinsey's reputation by accusing him and some of his early colleagues of being paedophiles themselves, though on no more evidence than the observations and comments in the first Kinsey volume, which has been open to public scrutiny for 40 years. There is no justification for these accusations and no evidence that Kinsey in any way encouraged or condoned sexual abuse of children. But these reactions serve to remind us that childhood sexuality is an extremely emotive subject, so much so that any adult wanting to study it must be prepared for accusations of this kind. Bornemann (1984), an Austrian psychiatrist who has been studying childhood sexuality for 40 years, describes the various stages his methods of investigation went through in order to avoid this problem. He has relied mainly on eliciting from children comments about children's songs, rhymes or games which may have sexual connotations, using an older child with a tape recorder as his experimenter. Langfeldt (1981) from Norway has reported observations through a one-way screen of preschool children attending a nursery school; these children were allowed to play without any clothes on, circumstances which would not be allowed in most communities in the western world, particularly in the present climate of opinion. We will discuss some of his interesting observations later. Public concern about child sexual abuse is reaching such a level that it is conceivable that a need for better understanding of childhood sexuality will be more widely recognised and research into this aspect of childhood may become easier to carry out in the future.

Many workers have recorded retrospective accounts by adults of their own childhood, but there is good reason to be cautious in accepting these accounts as valid. Not only do most of us need to deny the sexuality of children, we also tend to deny its existence in our own childhood. Freud described the latent period of sexual development: after the stage of infancy, when sexual inhibitions are not apparent and children may show masturbatory behaviour apparently without guilt, the child enters the latent period when it is assumed the child is sexually inactive. It is now generally agreed that during this phase the child's sexuality is not so much latent as actively concealed from adult view. This reflects the onset of sexual shame which our society fosters and which results in the child restricting his or her sexual expression to a 'child's world' where adults are not in evidence. Fortunately children, at least those who are not sexually abused, do not usually get sex out of proportion — it is one of the many aspects of the adult world about which they feel curious. It is when they approach puberty, and their physiology as well as the sexual scripts provided for them give sexuality greater emphasis, that the so-called latent period is over.

These sources of evidence are insufficient as yet to give us a complete picture of childhood sexual development and for the present time we must rely on informed speculation.

SEXUAL DIFFERENTIATION AND THE DEVELOPMENT OF GENDER IDENTITY

We tend to take our gender for granted: 'Of course you are male if you have a penis'. Usually we can afford to do so, but the processes leading to the ascription of gender identity are so complex it is little wonder they occasionally go wrong.

Gender can be manifested in at least seven different ways:

1. chromosomes;
2. gonads;
3. hormones;
4. internal sexual organs;
5. external genitalia and secondary sexual characteristics;
6. the gender assigned at birth ('It's a boy');
7. Gender identity ('I am a girl').

Each of these levels leads on to the next during this fascinating developmental process. An eighth stage, sexual differentiation of the brain, develops in parallel with the other later stages.

Problems are fortunately rare, but can occur at any of these stages. We will look at the normal process as far as we understand it and then consider some of the anomalies.

CHROMOSOMAL GENDER

The most basic manifestation of gender lies in our sex chromosomes, which are present in every cell of the body. The normal female has two X chromosomes; the male has one X and one Y. The Y chromosome determines maleness (in some animals, e.g. birds, it is the other way round — the female is XY). How this process of determination operates is not known. At one time, the male-determining factor on the Y chromosome was believed to be related to an antigen on the chromosome called the HY antigen, so-called because it was discovered to be a cause of tissue incompatibility between very closely inbred male and female mice (hence histocompatibility (H) antigen on the Y chromosome). However, this now seems unlikely, although it is possible that different mechanisms are involved in the differentiation of somatic and germ cells.

THE GONADS

The primitive gonad has a medulla and a cortex. In the presence of the somatic male-determining factor the medulla develops into a testis, and the cortex regresses. This process starts in about the sixth week of fetal life. In the absence of the male factor the cortex develops into an ovary, though this happens a little later, starting at the 12th week. The full development of the gonad and its functioning does however depend on both somatic and germ cells, which need to be sexually consistent with one another. Thus in Turner's syndrome, where one X chromosome is missing (i.e. 45X) the remaining X chromosome is sufficient for female somatic development and a primitive ovary forms. However, the absence of the second X chromosome results in no oocyte formation and without these the ovary does not develop as a hormonally secreting organ and eventually atrophies.

HORMONES

In the male fetus the Leydig cells in the testis start to produce steroids, in particular testosterone, from about the eighth week, reaching a maximum between the 10th and 18th weeks. Following this, steroidogenesis is much reduced, though the testis continues to grow in size. This phase of maximal fetal steroid production is a crucial time for differentiation of the male internal and external genitalia. The fetal testis is stimulated by the placental human chorionic gonadotrophin, but also by fetal gonadotrophins which predominate during the second half of pregnancy. (For a detailed review of reproductive hormones and their actions see Chapter 2.)

In the female fetus, differentiation of the reproductive tract does not depend on steroids and in fact ovarian steroidogenesis is minimal. Oestrogens circulating in the fetus are largely derived from the placenta.

THE INTERNAL SEXUAL ORGANS

The early fetus has the potential for developing both male and female internal sexual organs (Fig. 3.2). The Wolffian duct can develop into the vas deferens, seminal vesicles and ejaculatory ducts of the male. The Müllerian duct can develop into a uterus, fallopian tube and upper vagina. The fetal testis secretes two types of hormone: testosterone, which stimulates male development of the Wolffian duct, and a large molecular weight protein, probably produced by the Sertoli cells of the testis, which causes regres-

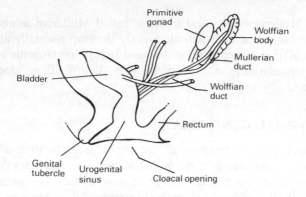

Primitive gonad · Wolffian body · Mullerian duct · Wolffian duct · Bladder · Rectum · Genital tubercle · Urogenital sinus · Cloacal opening

Undifferentiated 8-10 weeks

♀ Ovary · Fallopian tube · Uterus · Wolffian remnants · Bladder · Genital tubercle (clitoris)

♂ Testis · Vas · Mullerian remnants · Bladder · Genital tubercle (penis)

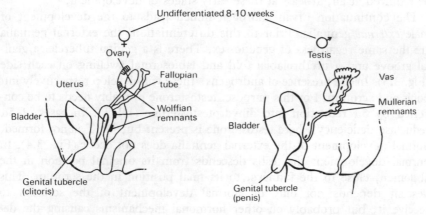

12-16 weeks

Wolffian remnants · Fallopian tube · Ovary · Uterus · Vagina · Clitoris · Urethra · Labia

Epididymis · Mullerian remnant · Testis · Vas deferens · Bladder · Prostate · Penis · Urethra · Scrotum · Site of testis after descent

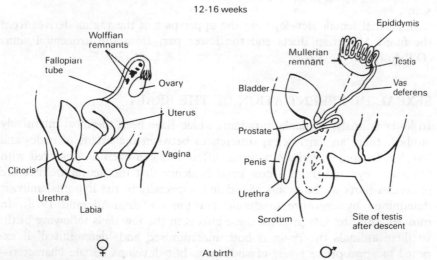

♀   At birth   ♂

Fig. 3.2 Differentiation of the genitalia. The existence of a primitive gonad capable of developing into either a testis or ovary and both Wolffian (male) and Müllerian (female) systems gives the potential for either male or female differentiation. The presence of androgens and Müllerian-Inhibiting Factor leads to male development. The absence of both leads to female development.

sion of the Müllerian duct, and hence is called Müllerian-inhibiting factor (MIF). The Müllerian duct will apparently develop normally along female lines unless MIF is present, and it does not require oestrogenic or any other hormonal stimulation, in the way that the Wolffian duct requires testosterone.

THE EXTERNAL GENITALIA

Thus, between the development of the gonads and the internal sexual organs we have a characteristic hormonal status. For male development the right hormones are required; for female development hormones may not be required at all, at least at these early stages of development.

The continuation of an androgen milieu leads to the development of male *external* genitalia. Prior to this differentiation, the external genitalia are the same regardless of genetic sex. There is a genital tubercle, a genital groove and a urethrolabial fold and labioscrotal swelling on each side (Fig. 3.3). In the presence of androgens, these will develop respectively into penis and scrotum. For this purpose, testosterone probably needs to be converted by 5α reduction into dihydrotestosterone (DHT). In cases of 5α reductase deficiency where testosterone is present but DHT is not formed, normal development of the external genitalia does not occur (Fig. 3.4). In normal development the testis descends from its original position in the abdomen, close to the kidneys, to its final position in the scrotum. This descent depends not only on normal development of the scrotum to receive it, but probably on other hormonal mechanisms causing the descent.

In normal female development the upper part of the vagina derives from the fused Müllerian ducts and the lower part from the urogenital sinus (O'Rahilly 1977).

SEXUAL DIFFERENTIATION OF THE BRAIN

In lower animals, particularly rodents which have been the most intensively studied, there are fairly clear differences between the brains of males and females. In some species structural differences can even be observed with the naked eye and there is now good evidence that the neural architecture of certain parts of the brains of rodents, especially in the hypothalamus, is determined by exposure to steroid hormones (Toran-Allerand 1978). In most rodents steroids produce these effects in the few days following birth. In these animals the brain is both masculinised and 'defeminised' if exposed to appropriate levels of androgens but develops female characteristics if no such androgenic influence occurs. In other words, as with the genitalia, the genetic sex may be male or female, but the development is along female lines unless androgens are involved. (Structural differences are present in the human hypothalamus, with the so-called 'sexually

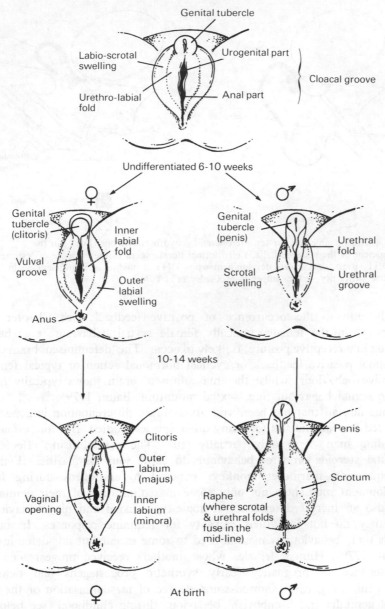

Fig. 3.3 Differentiation of the external genitalia. The undifferentiated structures at 6–10 weeks develop along female (left) or male (right) lines, depending on whether androgens are present or absent.

dimorphic nucleus' 2.5 times bigger in the male. But the function of this nucleus is not known; see p. 69).

This sexual differentiation of the brain is manifested in two ways. First, the female hypothalamus and pituitary show typical endocrine function

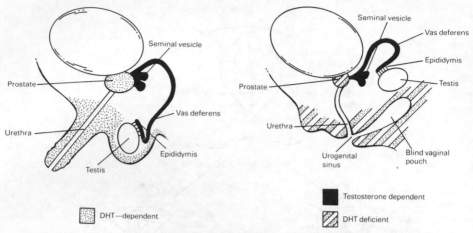

Fig. 3.4 The possible role for testosterone and dihydrotestosterone (DHT) in the development of the male genitalia. Left: normal development in the presence of testosterone and DHT. Right: incomplete development when DHT is missing or insufficient, as in 5α reductase deficiency. (From Imperato-McGinley et al 1974)

mainly due to the occurrence of positive feedback (see Chapter 2). Secondly, in the female, typically female sexual behaviour (e.g. back-arching in a receptive posture) is likely to occur. The 'defeminised' brain does not show positive feedback or cyclical hormonal action or typical female receptive behaviour, whilst the 'masculinised' brain shows typically masculine sexual behaviour (e.g. sexual mounting; Baum 1979).

Thus far, all that has been said about brain differentiation is generally accepted for rodents and for many other species studied. But for primates, including man, it is only partially true. The masculinising effects of prenatal steroids on later behaviour do show some similarities. Female macaque and marmoset monkeys exposed to androgens during fetal development may show not only some masculinisation of their genitalia, but also an increased tendency to male-type sexual and play behaviour. But they do not lose their capacity for feminine responses. In other words their behaviour is masculinised to some extent but not defeminised (Baum 1979). Human females whose mothers received progestagens for maintenance of pregnancy (early synthetic progestagens had definite androgenic properties) showed some degree of masculinisation of the external genitalia and 'tomboyish' behaviour during childhood (see below). The anatomical effect would depend on androgenic stimulation relatively early in fetal development; the behavioural effects on exposure at a later stage in pregnancy (Money & Ehrhardt 1972). Similarly, women with the adrenogenital syndrome (see below) exposed to high androgen levels during fetal development and childhood show a similar picture. It is not known in which part of the primate or human brain androgens exert these behavioural influences.

In all these cases, however, normal menstruation usually occurs, though probably with somewhat delayed onset. This emphasises the fact that the similarity with rodents is much less striking as far as the hormonal function of the hypothalamus is concerned. The androgenised female rhesus monkey continues to show evidence of positive feedback. Conversely, humans with the androgen-insensitivity syndrome (see below), who because of a metabolic defect are insensitive to androgenic steroids in all their cells, show a male pattern of hypothalamic function (Van Look et al 1977). In other words, in primates and humans, something other than or in addition to the fetal hormonal status determines the later sex-specific hormonal characteristics of the hypothalamus.

GENDER OF ASSIGNMENT

How a child, once born, develops in terms of psychological gender depends to a large extent on how he or she is brought up. That in turn depends on the initial observation of anatomical gender — 'it's a boy'. This seemingly obvious remark in the delivery room is therefore of crucial importance. If anatomical development has proceeded normally, there will be no problem. But if not, there may be varying degrees of ambiguity of the external genitalia. The gender of assignment is then based on a decision which is somewhat arbitrary but with far-reaching consequences. Some of the causes of such ambiguity will be considered later. What would happen if, quite arbitrarily, an anatomical female was brought up as a male or vice versa? Would the effects of rearing determine the psychological gender of that child? A few such attempts have been described (Diamond 1965); each apparently failed.

Clinical experience with cases of pseudohermaphrodism and ambiguous external genitalia has pointed to a critical stage in psychological development when the belief 'I am a male' or 'I am a female' becomes fixed. Stoller (1968) has called this the core gender identity. This occurs between the ages of about 2 and 4 years, presumably related to the appropriate stage of cognitive development when gender begins to have meaning. There is uncertainty about how fixed the core gender identity remains after this critical phase, and whether reassignment can succeed at a later stage. Diamond (1965) cites evidence of an incorrect assignment being successfully reversed as late as 13 or 14 years of age. Whilst this issue remains controversial, it probably depends on the degree of uncertainty about the child's identity in the first place. If, at the age of 4 or later, the child feels unequivocally male (or female) then later attempts to change identity will probably fail. If however gender identity remains equivocal, with the individual feeling uncomfortable with the assigned gender, then reassignment may be quite successful even at a relatively late stage.

SEX DIFFERENCES IN BEHAVIOUR

Apart from the core gender identity, the child also develops a sense of masculinity or femininity and will express this in typically masculine or feminine behaviour. It is this issue that generates the fiercest arguments. In our society there are clear differences between the behaviour of boys and girls (Serbin & Sprafkin 1982). Boys not only show more physical activity, rough and tumble play and exploration, they also have different interests preferring, for example, war games in contrast to girls' preferences for domestic roles. Obviously, whilst these generalisations apply to the majority, there is considerable overlap between the sexes. Also these sex role stereotypes vary from culture to culture. In some societies, women typically adopt roles which have masculine connotations for us and vice versa. The controversy surrounds the extent to which these roles are socially or innately determined. Do boys become typical boys because they are taught to be so? Are women in these contrasting societies genetically prone to develop in the way they do? The more primitive the society, and hence the less interbreeding with other social groups that has occurred, the more likely it is that genetic factors would be expressed in relatively pure culture. There is therefore a limit to how much one can use cultural differences of that kind as evidence of environmental rather than innate determinants. This issue is at the heart of the political campaign to liberate women. Much of the control of women by men in our society depends upon these stereotyped roles. Women are expected to stay at home, look after the children and the house and do the cooking. This effectively ties the woman, making it more difficult to develop her own career or even separate identity.

Those who defend the status quo often justify it on the basis of innate determinance of these sex roles. Those who reject it tend to rely on the argument that sex role stereotypes are simply the products of a culture that has a vested (male) interest in fostering such roles. The result is that what appears to be a scientific argument is often a political one with a consequent loss of scientific objectivity. I am uneasy about prevailing social values relating to sex roles and have no doubt that alteration of the balance of power and opportunities between men and women is one of the most fundamental needs for human societies at the present time. But this need for change exists whether sex roles are constitutionally or socially determined and arguing about the relative importance of nature or nurture seems politically irrelevant. The constitutional origins of a disadvantage do not justify its exploitation. But, on the other hand, it may be foolish to ignore or even inhibit constitutionally determined advantages on the grounds that everybody ought to have the same opportunities.

The nature–nurture polemic is also futile on scientific grounds except when considering the relative importance of different determinants at specific stages of development. It seems inescapable that genetic factors as well as intrauterine experiences all determine how we interact later with our environment (see p. 271-5 for further discussion).

It is nevertheless an intriguing question to what extent typical boy or girl behaviour is learnt. Unfortunately, interesting and potentially important findings in certain studies are cancelled out by contrary findings in others. Maccoby & Jacklin (1974), both avowed feminists, have presented the most comprehensive and probably the most balanced review of these various studies and their main conclusions will be summarised.

Girls have greater verbal ability than boys, though this is not obvious until about the age of 11. Boys, on the other hand, are superior in visual—spatial tasks, though again this is not apparent until adolescence. At a similar age, boys' mathematical skills grow faster than those of girls. Males, from an early age, are more aggressive than girls, both verbally and physically. However, Maccoby & Jacklin could find no support for the following commonly held views: that girls are more social, or more suggestible than boys; that girls have lower self-esteem; that boys are better at tasks requiring higher level cognitive processing and the inhibition of previously learned responses, whereas girls are better at rote learning of simple repetitive tasks; that girls lack achievement motivation; that girls are 'auditory', boys 'visual'. They did find weak but unconvincing support for the following: that girls are more sensitive to touch; girls are more timid or anxious; boys are more active and more competitive; that boys are more concerned with dominance in their relationships; girls are more compliant and show more nurturant behaviour. For most of these, Maccoby & Jacklin found some studies reporting such differences but a greater number finding no difference.

Perhaps the only convincing difference which could contribute to sex role differentiation rather than be a result of it is greater male aggression. The other more equivocal differences may be relevant in subtle and variable ways. We considered earlier the possible sexual implications of the male superiority in visuospatial skills that becomes apparent from puberty onwards (see Chapter 2). It seems unlikely that this nature–nurture issue will ever be finally resolved and perhaps this is just as well. There would seem to be an inherent advantage in assuming that nature and nurture are both fundamental and that we cannot shape our children's destinies completely by controlling their environments. The importance of social and cognitive learning is nevertheless crucial and a matter of concern, and it is undoubtedly desirable to reappraise continually the influences to which our children are subjected.

Society influences the learning of the child in three principal ways: in the family, in the child's peer group and in relation to adults at school. The effects of television together with other external influences such as books or comics are a fourth factor in industrial societies, the importance of which is now being recognised. As far as gender identity development is concerned, it is easiest to investigate the role of the family. Several studies have shown that the absence of the father or the dominance of the mother in the family is associated with increased femininity or less masculinity in boys. Once again, it is difficult to interpret this association. It does not follow that absence of a father necessarily leads to impaired masculinity in boys. In some instances, the father's absence may be linked with an attitude in the mother that actively fosters masculine development. Conversely, an overtly dominant father may sometimes undermine his son's masculinity. The unmasculine son of a subordinate father may be expressing a genetic tendency to low masculinity, and so on.

The social class and educational level of parents are also relevant. Kagan & Moss (1962) in their longitudinal study of American children found that boys and girls with well educated parents were more likely to develop interests more typical of the opposite sex and in less educated families conventional sex roles were more likely to become established. These associations may be sensitive to cultural factors, however, and we should not assume that they would be the same now or in other cultures.

Goldman & Goldman (1982) investigated children's knowledge and styles of thinking about sexual- and gender-related issues in four countries — Australia, England, the USA and Sweden. They interviewed children in the age range 5 to 15 years. Their conclusions from this study include the following:

1. Piaget's cognitive developmental stages are evident in sexual thinking in terms of pre-operations, concrete operations and formal operations. There are non-sexual, transitional sexual and fully sexual stages of cognition which closely parallel the Piagetian stages.
2. There was some evidence of Kohlberg's (1969) three levels of pre-conventional, conventional and post-conventional moral thinking in relation to some aspects of sexuality in children's thinking.
3. Freud's cloacal theory of children's conceptualisation of pregnancy and childbirth was supported for children aged 5—7 years, but they found no support for the Oedipal phase as a part of normal child development.
4. The evidence against the latency period was so strong that they referred to the 'myth of latency'.
5. There were cultural differences as to when children evolved sexual thinking, with the Swedish children being ahead of the English-speaking groups.

The peer group world of the prepubertal schoolchild is undoubtedly a powerful source of learning, though not an easy one to study. The fascinating work of the Opies (1959) shows how ritualised and adult-free this world is, with rules, games and songs handed down through generations of children. The rules or scripts for successful boyhood and girlhood are probably clear in this world, and it is difficult to know how much they are determined by adult influences. They do nevertheless reflect adult sex role stereotypes with physical assertiveness, risk-taking and warlike interest characterising the boy, and childlike domesticity or home-making, characterising the girl. Boys' games are perhaps more competitive and girls' more tied to the home base.

CHILDHOOD TO ADOLESCENCE

One of the most fascinating stages of development as far as gender identity is concerned is the transition from childhood to adolescence. There are important hormonal changes during this stage which underlie the development and maturation of secondary sexual characteristics and which are considered in detail in Chapter 2.

The prepubertal child may have become extremely competent and confident in the childhood gender role, and yet be thrown into gender confusion by the events accompanying puberty. Changes in body shape — sometimes dramatic — produce a phase of uncertainty about the future: 'What shape am I going to end up?' Some of the emotional instability at this stage may well stem from the endocrine changes which are occurring (Nottelman et al 1988). Changes in the sexual response system are also occurring, as will be discussed later. But the rules for succeeding as a male or female are also changing. Sexuality now becomes a very important aspect of gender: 'Am I sexual in a masculine or feminine way?' Success in sexual encounters may be used to bolster self-esteem or exert control or dominance.

Some adolescents, for one reason or another, postpone entry into this sexual phase, and rely on non-sexual supports for both their gender identity and self-esteem. For example, a boy may concentrate on sport, justifying avoidance of sexual contact as a necessary part of his dedication. Whilst this may be effective in some respects, it may also alienate him from his peer group or at least delay learning how to manage relationships with the opposite sex. For many, on the other hand, early attempts at forming sexual relationships are largely aimed at proving their newly re-established gender identity. In some subcultures this process is almost institutionalised within the same sex peer group, when sexual activity with the opposite sex is manifestly a way of scoring points in competition with one's peers. This is what Gagnon & Simon (1973) call 'homosocial sexual behaviour'. In primitive societies ritual forms of transition into adulthood are common; these are discussed in Chapter 4.

Kagan & Moss (1962) in their cohort study assessed the degree of heterosexual interaction (i.e. interaction with children of the opposite sex) and opposite sex activity (i.e. interest in and practice of activities traditionally associated with the opposite sex) at different stages of childhood and adolescence. Between the ages of 6 and 10 years boys and girls played predominantly in same-sex groups. Children, especially boys, who did not conform in this respect were often rejected by their same-sex peers. With opposite sex activity they again found greater predictability in boys than girls. Even as young as 3 to 6 years, the extent of opposite sex behaviour was highly correlated with opposite sex behaviour of adults. Competitiveness and involvement in mechanical, gross motor and aggressive games during the pre-school years were prognostic of sex role activities 20 years later (Kagan & Moss 1962). Fagot (1977), in another study of preschool children, found that boys who engaged in stereotypical feminine behaviour received a considerable amount of negative reinforcement from their peers, and to a lesser extent from their teachers. This pattern was not observed in girls. Fagot asked the interesting question why this behaviour persisted in the face of such unremitting discouragement, and suggested that either opposite influences in the child's home were operating or that possibly some biological factor, unresponsive to social learning, was involved.

Kagan & Moss also assessed anxiety about sexual behaviour at the late adolescent and early adult stages. For the boys, but once again not for the girls, the absence or lack of clearly masculine behaviour between the ages of 3 and 10 years was associated with greater anxiety about sex in early adulthood. In addition early masculine behaviour was predictive of earlier dating and involvement in erotic heterosexual activity during adolescence. We will need to reconsider these associations when discussing the development of sexual preferences later in this chapter.

The timing of puberty, the determinants of which are still obscure, also has a bearing on gender identity and personality development. Boys who are late in reaching puberty tend to be less popular and less assertive McCandless 1960) though once again such factors are likely to vary across cultures. As Rutter (1983) puts it: 'Manliness and sexual vigour are highly regarded attributes among adolescent males, and boys who have still not reached puberty by 16 years or so may well begin to doubt their masculinity and become anxious and introspective about their development.' Girls' reactions to early or late puberty are more complex and there are less clearcut advantages to early maturation (McCandless 1960).

This is the age, therefore, when gender identity, sexual responsiveness and sexual preferences are becoming integrated and we will need to consider these two other aspects. But before doing so, it is worth mentioning that our gender identity experiences further periods of development and change as we age. In early adulthood the work role becomes an important aspect of gender identity. Ironically, its effects tend to reflect the prevailing sex role stereotypes and whilst an effective work role will tend to bolster the male's sense of masculinity, for the woman it frequently produces conflicts with her femininity — fearing that if she is effective in a career, she will be less attractive as a woman or less successful as a mother. Clearly, with changing values about women's roles, this issue is in a state of flux but it is still commonplace to find women suffering from this conflict.

As other factors, such as work or parenthood, reinforce gender identity, it becomes less necessary to use sexuality for this purpose. This makes it easier to establish mutually rewarding and mature sexual relationships. The two participants are not pursuing incompatible goals for their sexuality and can concentrate on the process of establishing intimacy and the dyad. Conversely, if there is any crisis in the work role or in other non-sexual areas which undermines gender identity and self-esteem, this may reverberate in the individual's sexuality, leading to renewed attempts to exploit sexual relationships for these purposes.

Whilst the first part of our developmental history involves the progressive recruitment of maturing abilities into our pattern of sexual behaviour, there comes a time when our continuing development requires adaptation to declining function — the effects of ageing. This is sufficiently important to require a separate chapter (Chapter 5).

THE SEXUAL RESPONSE SYSTEM AND SEXUAL BEHAVIOUR

The capacity for genital response is present from early infancy. In the male infant this is obvious, as erections are commonplace. In the female infant we are less certain of the presence of vaginal vasocongestive responses, though they seem equally likely.

MASTURBATION AND SEX PLAY

Although erections in little boys can occur spontaneously, they commonly result from genital handling and it is clear from observations of both boys and girls that genital stimulation is a source of pleasure. One of the first to describe this was Moll who in 1912 wrote: 'When we see a child lying with moist, widely opened eyes, and exhibiting all the other signs of sexual excitement as we are accustomed to observe in adults, we are justified in assuming that the child is experiencing a voluptuous sensation'. Freud regarded various types of non-genital self-stimulation such as thumbsucking as forms of sexual activity. Moll preferred to restrict sexual significance to genital stimulation.

Galenson & Roiphe (1974), observing infants and small children in a nursery, reported that boys usually begin genital play at about 6–7 months of age, whereas girls start a little later at 10 or 11 months. They found boys continued with this form of stimulation until more obvious masturbation became established at 15–16 months of age. The girls showed more intermittent genital play. There is also a tendency for girls to transfer to less direct methods of stimulation, such as thigh pressure or rocking. Both boys and girls may use direct genital contact with an inanimate object such as a doll or toy, as if mounting it.

Masturbation to the point of obvious orgasm has been observed in children of both sexes as young as 6 months. (Bakwin 1973). Behaviour of this kind in the young child, unassociated with any embarrassment or self-consciousness, can be observed and is occasionally reported by parents and others in contact with small children. As the child gets older, he or she learns that such behaviour is frowned upon, or at least regarded as private and the behaviour becomes more concealed, and its incidence uncertain.

Elias & Gebhard (1969) have reported evidence from interviews with prepubescent boys and girls. Table 3.1 gives the proportion reporting masturbation and sex play with other children. They commented that these percentages were close to those reported retrospectively by adults. The average age for onset of masturbation and sex play was about 8–9 years for boys, being somewhat younger for the girls.

Table 3.1 Percentage of children reporting masturbation and sex play

	n	Mean age	% having masturbated	% sex play with boys	% sex play with girls
Boys	305	10.3 years	56	52	34
Girls	127	8.1 years	30	37	35

From Elias & Gebhard (1969); Kinsey et al (1948); Kinsey et al (1953).

Genital exhibition was almost invariably involved in sex play, both hetero- and homosexual, for both boys and girls. The reported frequencies of other types of activity are shown in Table 3.2.

Whereas masturbation starting during childhood is likely to carry on into adolescence without interruption in both boys and girls, the prepubertal play with other children is usually discontinued in girls and often in middle-class boys. This probably reflects the parental and social constraints imposed on such sociosexual behaviour, whilst masturbation continues as a solitary and private activity. There were some striking associations between this prepubertal sexual activity and social class. Working-class children were almost twice as likely to masturbate as middle-class children. They were three times as likely to have attempted coitus during sex play. By comparison, the middle-class children were better

Table 3.2 Percentage of children experiencing sex play

	Genital manipulation	Genital union	Oral–genital	Vaginal insertion	Femoral/anal intercourse	
Boys	81	55	9	—	—	(hetero)
	67	—	16	—	17	(homo)
Girls	52	17	2	3	—	(hetero)
	62	—	3	18	—	(homo)

From Kinsey et al (1948, 1953).

informed about sexual matters (except for coitus). For working-class children, their peer group was the most important source of sexual information.

ORGASM

The incidence of orgasm or the capacity for it at different prepubertal ages is difficult to judge. Questions about age at first prepubertal orgasm were not asked systematically in Kinsey's male study (Kinsey et al 1948). Neither a boy, who does not ejaculate until puberty nor a girl may understand what orgasm is. But clearly a substantial proportion of both sexes is capable of orgasm before puberty.

For boys, as for adult males, the speed of response varies considerably. Some are able to reach orgasm after only 10 sec of stimulation, while others require 20 min or more. An interesting observation in Kinsey's studies is that a majority of prepubertal boys who experience orgasm are capable of going on to a second orgasm within a short time (ranging from 10 sec to 30 min, but with a mean of 6 min). Nearly a third of the orgasmic boys documented by Kinsey were able to experience five or more orgasms in rapid succession. Although there are some adult males capable of this performance, the proportion of pre-adolescent boys with this capacity is probably much higher. The typical refractory period of the adult is less in evidence before puberty. The reasons for this are not yet clear.

Kinsey and his colleagues held the view that, whereas orgasmic potential seemed to increase with age during the prepubertal period, its realisation depended on the occurrence of appropriate stimulation. If a child is discouraged or inhibited, or simply not aware that orgasm is a possible end point, then orgasm is unlikely to happen. They concluded, perhaps a little speculatively, that in an uninhibited society more than half of boys would experience orgasm by the age of 3 or 4 years and nearly all within the 3 or 4 years prior to puberty. It would indeed be interesting to know whether this is so. If there were important constitutional or biological differences in the orgasmic potential before puberty these may play an important part in influencing subsequent sexual development.

A similar picture emerges for girls. In Kinsey's sample (Kinsey et al 1953), 0.3% recalled experiencing orgasm by 3 years of age, and the proportion rose gradually to 14% by 13 years of age. In the large majority, the orgasm occurred during masturbation.

Boys commonly learn about masturbation and hence orgasm from their peer group or from adults. Girls, on the other hand, usually discover masturbation during self-exploration or by accident (e.g. sliding down a rope). The occurrence of prepubertal orgasm in girls is probably less than it might be for that reason.

The anatomical sexual differences between boys and girls contribute in a variety of ways to the differences in their sexual development. The obviousness of the boy's external genitalia results in a definite vocabulary for their description. Interest and curiosity about genitalia amongst boys is common and facilitates peer group learning as well as homosexual play. Girls, by contrast, are strikingly unaware of their genitalia, a fact reflected in the almost complete absence of a suitable vocabulary for these parts. Not surprisingly, the clitoris, vagina and urethral opening remain, for many girls, uncharted territory and not a matter for mutual discussion or exploration. Indeed girls are much more likely to show an awareness and interest in boys' penises, a fact which frequently encourages psychoanalysts to regard girls as suffering from penis envy. In addition, the boy has a clear indication of genital response (the erection) which the girl lacks, at least until she is able to label more subtle and concealed physiological changes. Not only does the erect penis feature as important in the play and communication of young boys (and to some extent in their interaction with girls) it also presumably facilitates the learning of genital responsiveness to sexual signals. The implications of this in the development of sexual preferences will be considered later.

CHANGES AT PUBERTY

The onset of dating behaviour appears to be more related to age than to pubertal development (Dornbusch et al 1981). Kagan & Moss (1962) found that dating behaviour of boys between the ages of 10 and 14 was a strong predictor of later heterosexual activity. Such early dating is highly likely to be influenced by social factors — the normal scripts established in the young boys social group. But such young dating does not necessarily involve more intimate or erotic behaviour. At what stage are these initiated and under what influence?

In an extensive study of young West German adolescents, Schoof-Tams et al (1976) found that sexual behaviour proceeded in a sequential pattern from social dating to kissing, petting and coitus. By age 11, 69% of boys and 55% of girls had had at least one date; 56% of boys and 47% of girls had kissed a member of the opposite sex. By that age 25% of boys and 12% of girls had experienced heavy petting, and whereas none of them reported experience with sexual intercourse, by the age of 13 31% of the boys and 21% of the girls had done so. These findings may reflect different attitudes and patterns of teenage sexuality in West Germany compared with Britain or the USA, and these issues will be considered further in Chapter 4.

Whereas sociologists such as Gagnon & Simon (1973) assume that social factors are responsible for these patterns of emerging sexuality, biological commentators have assumed that hormonal changes are also involved — though until recently their only evidence was the temporal association of the increases of sexual activity and hormonal changes

(Kinsey et al 1953). The direct effects of the hormones may have been on the stage of pubertal development which in turn affected the social influences.

Udry et al (1985) reported a remarkable study in which 102 boys of eighth, ninth and 10th grades completed questionnaires about their recent past and intended sexual behaviour and also gave blood samples for hormone assay. Of all variables studied, the free testosterone index (FTI) was found to be the most important correlate of sexual activity, such as number of sexual outlets in the past month (masturbation to orgasm, wet dreams and coitus) and frequency of thoughts about sex. In a multiple regression analysis neither age nor level of pubertal development added to the predictive value of the FTI. The main weakness of this study is its reliance on self-rating of stages of pubertal development. But the authors nevertheless present persuasive evidence that, in boys at this stage of sexual development, increases in biologically active (i.e. free) testosterone are more important in initiating erotic behaviour than socially mediated factors.

If we accept this evidence there are still some unanswered questions. What aspect of sexuality is primarily affected by these hormonal changes? We know from studies of androgen-deficient men that androgen replacement has a primary effect on sexual appetite, ejaculation and sleep erections (See Chapter 2). This may also be the case at this stage of pubertal development. In boys whose patterns of masturbation and orgasm are established well before puberty the principal change may be the onset of ejaculation and perhaps an increase in masturbatory frequency, reflecting an enhanced sexual appetite. In other boys masturbation and orgasm may occur for the first time in association with ejaculation, as if the hormonal surge had activated a latent interest or at least lowered the stimulus threshold for sexual arousal. But there may also be effects on erectile responsiveness. In Chapter 2 we considered evidence suggesting that erections during sleep are sensitive to changing levels of androgens, whereas erections in response to erotic stimuli in the waking state are not. Sleep erections increase during childhood, reaching a peak in adolescence and thereafter undergoing a gradual decline (Karacan et al 1976). Thus it is unlikely that sleep erections are entirely dependent on androgens, as their increase probably precedes the hormonal increase, but they may well be enhanced by androgens. There is also an undoubted stimulation of penile growth accompanying the prepubertal androgen surge. Later in this chapter we will consider Ramsey's (1943) evidence of a phase of enhanced erectile responsiveness during the waking state in prepubertal boys. It is a distinct possibility that androgens contribute to this phenomenon, though the direct effects may be on central arousability rather than erectile responsiveness per se (see Chapter 2 for a fuller discussion).

For girls the evidence presents a different picture. According to Kinsey, there is a much less dramatic upsurge in sexual responsiveness in the pubertal girl. Whereas the large majority of boys reach their maximum responsiveness within a year or two of puberty, girls reach their peak over a much longer time scale. The sexual learning of girls may be much more susceptible to social influences. In Udry et al's (1986) study of girls around the age of puberty, carried out in parallel with their study of boys, they found that, whereas self-rated sexual interest was correlated with androgen levels, the best predictors of whether a girl engaged in sexual activity with a partner were not hormonal but social, such as the type of peer group she was involved with. It is not clear why there should be this sex difference in the relative importance of biological and social influences at this stage of development, but it is likely to be of considerable relevance in understanding sex differences in adulthood. The relevance of the fact that the girl does not have the clear sexual signalling system the boy has with his erections is considered further below.

SEXUAL LEARNING AND THE ROLE OF EDUCATION

Given the central role that learning has been allotted in sexual development it is appropriate to consider the part education plays in the process. Obviously the effects of modelling by parents, siblings and peers are important. Parents may have powerful effects on a child's beliefs and attitudes about appropriate sex role behaviour, his or her own body, emotional expression and responsibility in relationships simply by the example they set. But how important is their role in providing factual information? To what extent should this form of education be provided by schools or responsible adults other than the parents?

Roberts et al (1978) carried out a survey of parents of 3- to 11-year-old children in a large industrial city in the USA. A total of 856 mothers and 605 fathers were interviewed at length and asked about the sex education they had given their children. Topics for sex education were categorised by these authors as 'easy' (e.g. pregnancy and birth, male–female differences), 'control' (e.g. nudity, child molestation, atypical gender behaviour, sex play) and 'erotic' topics (e.g. masturbation, intercourse, premarital sex and homosexuality). In general mothers discussed all of these topics more than fathers. A majority had discussed at least some of the easy topics, whereas two-thirds of mothers and four-fifths of fathers had never discussed any of the erotic topics with either son or daughter. Control topics tended to be discussed only as a reaction to undesirable or threatened behaviour on the part of the child. No more than one-quarter of parents had discussed sex play with their children, and most had expressed strong disapproval.

The child was the most likely person to initiate such discussions; with younger children this was usually following some incident in the home or neighbourhood, while with older children it was most often a reaction to something seen on television, usually when the mother was also watching. In general, the older the child and the more sexual the question the less likely was the parent to discuss it. This and other studies indicate that parents find it difficult to provide their children with the factual information about sex which they consider should be given.

Sex education in schools has been and probably always will be a controversial topic. There will inevitably be disagreement about the content of such teaching. In spite of this there has been a considerable increase in the amount of such teaching in the UK. Between 1964, when Schofield (1965) assessed sex education in British schools, and 1974, when the 16-year-olds in the National Child Development Study (Fogelman 1983) completed a related questionnaire, there had apparently been considerable improvement in terms of the children's satisfaction. Certainly many innovations have been tried in recent years, in particular using television programmes as stimuli for group discussion. Rogers (1974) has gathered reports on a number of these TV series. Evaluation of such methods is not easy; immediate gains in factual knowledge may be demonstrated, but long-term effects on behaviour and attitudes are much more difficult to assess. Two American studies have however suggested that such formal education has little effect on the sexual behaviour of teenagers, and probably less than informal methods (e.g. family, friends and the media; (Weichman & Ellis 1969; Spanier 1976).

At the time of writing the role of parents in sex education is of particular topical interest, for a variety of reasons. There have been fears in some sections of society that sex education in schools has too often promulgated undesirable sexual values. Attempts have also been made to curb the provision of contraceptives to girls under the age of 16 without the permission of their parents, on the grounds that the parents are the best people to judge whether they should have them. The assumption underlying these reactions is that values about sexuality should properly come from within the family. The USA is a striking example of how confused messages about sexual morality within a society cause confusion amongst teenagers which is manifested most dramatically in high rates of teenage pregnancy and abortion. In Chapter 4 we consider further the results of a cross-cultural study which shows that in societies other than the USA where different attitudes to sex education and the availability of contraceptives prevail, the results are substantially lower levels of teenage pregnancies and abortions with no evidence of greater promiscuity amongst teenagers.

Ironically, whilst this reaction develops in favour of the family as the main source of influence on sexual morality, we are faced with growing evidence of sexual abuse of children within the family. All of this requires us to reappraise the proper role of parents and family in sex education, and in particular the assumption that the parents are both the best and the proper people to take responsibility for this role. But we have already seen that the large majority of parents find this role difficult. Why is that so? There are two possibilities. For the parental couple, the adolescent's curiosity and questions about sex pose a threat to the intimacy of their own sexual relationship. It is difficult for parents to discuss the more erotic aspects of sex without in some way revealing something about their own sexual life. Many parents feel inhibited sexually with adolescent children in the house, fearing that they will be overheard or spied upon. It is therefore not surprising that within the intimacy of the family group the special intimacy of the parental pair is protected by a conspiracy of silence. Secondly, as a child approaches puberty his or her emerging sexuality leads to awkwardness in the relationship with the opposite-sex parent. The sexuality of this parent–child relationship, whilst normally contained by the strong incest taboo, is nevertheless a potentially important part of the child's sexual development. For a young girl, her father is the first important man in her life and the sexuality of this relationship endows it with a special tenderness as well as awkwardness. This is why abuse of this special relationship has such a traumatic effect on the girl's sexual development (see p. 705).

We should therefore question the assumption that the parents are the best people to be advisers and educators at this particularly sensitive stage of the parent–child relationship. Perhaps the large majority of parents who avoid these issues may be doing the right thing, at least during this short but important phase of adolescence. There is little doubt that parents have a crucial and probably the most important role in educating the prepubertal child, both in terms of factual knowledge and attitudes. After the first painful stages of adolescent separation have passed, most young people will need and benefit from parents in whom they can confide their sexual anxieties. But in between these two phases of parenthood is a sensitive and important time when the role of educator may conflict with the role of parent. If so, then the young person will need to turn to another responsible adult. In Chapter 4, when considering cross-cultural evidence from non-industrial societies, we find that in general the guidance of sexual development of the adolescent is not something that is left to the parents or even the immediate family.

SEXUAL PREFERENCES

One of the sexual characteristics of humans is our tendency to prefer certain kinds of partner or sexual activity. Although there are themes which we share with each other, each individual is probably unique in his or her pattern of preferences. Fundamental to our sexual lives is the type of person we are attracted to, because this plays a large part in determining our important relationships. Perhaps most fundamental to our choice of person is the gender of that person — are we attracted to someone of the same or opposite sex, are our preferences predominantly homo- or heterosexual?

But there are many other qualities which enter the composition of the sexually attractive person: body shape, face, age, certain types of body movement or behaviour. We still know little about the determinants of sexual attraction. There is reason to believe that current fashion influences our preferences. At certain times, large-breasted women hold a wide appeal; at other times, women with more modest-sized breasts may be generally preferred. But apart from these vicissitudes of fashion we still have our personal idiosyncrasies — there will always be some men who prefer large breasts or big bottoms.

It may be that whereas for men visual appearance is important, for women a wider range of qualities contribute to the attractive man: indicators of social class, wealth or power, for example. These issues are discussed more fully in Chapter 4.

For most of us, these relatively superficial cues are part of the initial attraction and other more subtle and interpersonal factors determine whether that attraction leads to any kind of bond or relationship. For many of us, once such a bond is established, the existence all around us of other examples of such erotic stimuli produces conflict or at least threatens the stability of our current dyadic relationship. For some, the attraction of the alternative stimuli has a destructive effect on their relationship; for others, their value when set against the rewards of a stable relationship is seen to be trivial, even if tantalising.

But for some people the erotic stimulus remains outside any interpersonal relationship because the attractive person is characteristically unattainable, or because the erotic stimulus is of a kind which precludes any interpersonal relationship, or because the individual for other reasons has difficulties in establishing close relationships.

Thus in some cases the erotic stimulus is part of the body, e.g. the top of the thigh or foot, sometimes called 'partialism'. The preoccupation with the part precludes a satisfactory relationship with the whole person. Or the erotic stimulus may be an extension of a person, e.g. an article of clothing. Such fetishes may be compatible with a sexual relationship but often they are so powerful that they prevent or destroy relationships rather than bind them. It is not easy to maintain a sexual relationship with a person who is far more interested in your suspender belt than in you.

Our preferences for particular types of sexual activity also vary and may contribute to or detract from our interpersonal relationships. We may prefer certain positions during intercourse, oral–genital or anal stimulation, being tied down or chastised. If our preferences in such matters complement those of our partner then they may strengthen or at least enhance the relationship. If they are unacceptable or threatening to our partner they may weaken the relationship. Some types of sexual activity, such as voyeurism or exhibitionism, preclude their incorporation into any form of relationship other than the most fleeting.

How are these preferences established? To what extent are they learnt rather than innately determined? Once established, how fixed or immutable are they? Even with the most fundamental aspect of our preferences — the sex of our preferred partner — these questions are surprisingly difficult to answer. Let us look at the evidence from the animal world of the possible determinants of homo- and heterosexual behaviour and see whether this gives us any clues.

HETEROSEXUAL, HOMOSEXUAL OR BISEXUAL?

Sexual preferences in animals

The clearest examples of sexual preferences in animals are in birds. Some species show sexual imprinting at an early stage; this is a form of learning during a critical period of development. For example, the polymorphous snowgoose tends to mate with geese the same colour as those it was exposed to early in its life (usually its parents). The mechanism of such imprinting is not understood and its relevance to mammals or man is very uncertain (Bateson 1978).

Evidence of preferences in mammals requires some test of choice of mate and there is little evidence of that kind. Beagle bitches, when in heat, show a preference for male dogs even when they have had no previous mating experience (Beach & Le Boeuf 1967). Similar evidence has been reported in some female rodents (Larsson 1978). It may be relevant that this limited evidence appears to be confined to female animals.

Most of the evidence we have from mammals concerns sexual behaviour rather than sexual preferences per se, i.e. how an animal responds to mounting or being mounted rather than the type of animal it prefers to mount or be mounted by. Beach (1979) has emphasised the importance of complementarity of sexual behaviour. This is the tendency for an animal to adopt a receptive posture when being mounted or to mount an animal presenting in a receptive posture. It so happens that males are more likely to show mounting and females to be receptive, and this tendency can be influenced by hormones during development. However, the fact that a male animal mounts another male does not mean that either animal has a homosexual preference. Beach (1979) made a pungent critique of studies that used such animal interaction as a model for human homosexuality.

The extent of same-sex behaviour, or at least that which is observed, varies considerably across species (Tyler 1984). Goy & Goldfoot (1975) have pointed out that for mammals the main variable is the extent of bisexuality. Not only do species vary in this respect, but within species the sexes usually differ, i.e. in species where the male shows a lot of bisexual behaviour the female tends to show little and vice versa. In most species it is the female which shows more bisexual behaviour (i.e. mounting other females as well as adopting the characteristic posture for being mounted — lordosis in rodents, presenting in primates).

In the case of primates the early organisational effects of hormones are more related to the degree of later bisexuality than whether sexual behaviour is *either* heterosexual *or* homosexual. Thus a female given large amounts of testosterone may show increased mounting behaviour as a result, but not a decrease in her presenting behaviour.

When animals are living in their natural habitat it is unusual to observe sexual behaviour, whether hetero- or homosexual, either because it is infrequent or because it is usually concealed. Most of our evidence comes from animals in captivity and we must be cautious in our extrapolations. There are of course degrees of captivity — a colony of animals living in a substantial compound may be much closer to nature than a pair of animals put together in a small cage for 30 minutes for the purpose of a mating test. In extrapolating from animals to humans we must also consider what we mean by a natural human habitat. Is a commuter living in a small house in a dense suburb, trapped within a nine-to-five repetitive job demonstrating 'natural' behaviour? Or should we restrict our attention to the !Kung of the Kalahari desert?

The primate for which we have the most evidence is the rhesus monkey. According to Goy & Goldfoot (1975) the male rhesus shows much more bisexual behaviour than the female, particularly during the prepubertal years. During its first year of life the male rhesus mounts other males and females in its peer group with more or less equal frequency. Mounting of the mother is also common. If separated from the mother but left with its peer group, the male initially shows more mounting of females, though this appears to be part of the assertion of dominance in the motherless group. After a while there is a return to a more equal ratio of male:female mounts. When the male reaches adolescence any mount of a female which results in intromission is usually followed by more exclusively heterosexual mounting behaviour (Goy 1979). This pattern suggests that early mounting by males is more an expression of dominance or masculinity than an erotic response. Once puberty is reached, however, and erotic responses become enhanced by hormonal effects, the dominance function is superseded by the sexual.

Akers & Conoway (1979), somewhat in contrast to Goy, reported relatively frequent homosexual interactions between adult female rhesus monkeys living in a heterosexual group. The mounter was usually in the follicular phase of her oestrous cycle, while the female being mounted was in her periovulatory phase. Little activity of this kind occurred during the luteal phase. These authors did not see this behaviour as a substitute for heterosexual activity. These homosexual pairs tended to spend much more time soliciting than in actual physical contact and affectional ties may have been important. They suggested that 'sexual gratification may be a fringe benefit of a relationship that develops for a variety of reasons'; this is a possibility that crops up frequently in our attempts to understand many human relationships.

Field studies of troops of rhesus monkeys have identified a predictable pattern with a group of leader or alpha males in the centre surrounded by the females. The subordinate males are not admitted to the central group and are progressively forced to the periphery of the troop where they show a considerable amount of homosexual behaviour (Goy & Goldfoot 1975).

Goldfoot et al (1984) have also demonstrated that the extent of bisexual behaviour can be influenced by manipulating environmental factors. At the age of 3 months, infant rhesus monkeys were assigned either to heterosexual groups (i.e. with both male and female infants) or to isosexual groups (i.e. all infants of the same sex). The isosexual condition increased the likelihood of homosexual behaviour (i.e. presenting by males and mounting by females), though this effect was more marked in the males than the females. The authors concluded from this evidence that 'presenting behaviour is extremely responsive to social conditions, mounting behaviour is intermediate in this regard and rough and tumble play seems to be only mildly influenced by the social environment'.

Early experience in same-sex peer groups is one form of environmental manipulation. There is also a considerable amount of evidence of the effects of more extreme forms of social deprivation on later adult sexual behaviour. In all species of mammals studied so far, including the rat, guinea-pig, cat, dog and rhesus monkey, being deprived of tactile contact with either the mother or peer group during infancy and early childhood results in abnormal or disrupted adult sexual behaviour in male animals. The same disruptive effect has not been demonstrated in females. In the rat such disruption can be easily treated by subsequent sexual experience, i.e. the rat readily learns to overcome this disability. In the rhesus monkey, on the other hand, the disability is relatively intractable, suggesting that there may be a critical period during the first 6 or so months for this crucial learning to take place (Larsson 1978). Such disruption results in a failure of normal copulation in the older animal, but the precise reason for this failure is not entirely clear. It is unlikely to be due to an impaired sexual appetite as such animals show fairly frequent masturbation. Some workers have suggested that the primary deficit is a problem of motor co-ordination, making successful mounting (a fairly acrobatic performance in many species) and intromission impossible. Others, such as Harlow (1971) and Goy (1979), see this as a failure in the formation of affectional bonds, both homophilic and heterophilic. Mounting behaviour, in their view, is a way of establishing such bonds, which in the heterophilic case become more obviously erotic with the onset of puberty. The female's development in this respect seems obscure or at least passive.

How relevant are these observations, particulary of primates, to the establishment of sexual preferences in humans? We have seen sexual behaviour serving more than one function (i.e. mounting being used to establish and maintain dominance); early relationships with both parents and peers affecting later sexual behaviour (though not sexual preference per se); facultative homosexuality occurring among males denied access to females. In general we have seen how innate factors (e.g. hormonally mediated mechanisms) and social learning interact during the course of childhood development to determine the pattern of post-pubertal sexual behaviour. What we have *not* seen is any primate equivalent of exclusive homosexuality. Examples of a primate choosing a same-sex partner in preference to an available and receptive heterosexual partner have been so rare as to warrant one or two special reports (Erwin & Maple 1976). We should therefore give serious consideration to the possibility that exclusive homosexual preference is a uniquely human phenomenon — and one that may not necessarily occur with equal frequency in different social systems. Before discussing this possibility further let us consider the different types of experience and mechanisms which may contribute to the development of human sexual preferences, some of which may be similar to those factors we have related to primate sexual development.

POSSIBLE DEVELOPMENTAL MECHANISMS IN BOYS

Sexual mounting in children

Lewis (1965) described movements of infants in contact with their mothers which involved pelvic thrusting similar to coital movements. According to his observations, these movements occur for a short period around the age of 8 to 10 months. 'In a moment of apparent delight the child clasps the mother . . . throwing his arms about her neck, nuzzling her chin, he begins rapid rotatory pelvic thrusts at about two per second'. Lewis regarded this behaviour as 'clearly directed at the loved one'. He is unable to tell us how common this is, though he considered it unlikely to occur except in conditions of 'maximum security'. He also does not make clear whether it is confined to male infants.

Various kinds of sexual play are common amongst children, as we have already indicated, and are perhaps comparable to the mounting of young rhesus monkeys. In many sexually permissive societies sexual play, including simulated coitus, is commonly observed by adults and accepted as normal (Ford & Beach 1952). In western societies such behaviour is likely to be actively discouraged by adults. Langfeldt (1981) has nevertheless offered some interesting observations of such play in Norwegian children. He describes such mounting in playgroup settings with children of 4 to 5 years old. Whilst both boys and girls may mount or be mounted, he noticed that boys were more likely to have erections if they were actively mounting. There is a tendency, he says, for children to prefer their own gender pattern (i.e. males to mount, females to be mounted) and if they exhibit a cross-gender pattern, they are likely to show their own gender pattern in the same play session — as if to reassert their gender. He describes agreement to mutual role exchange as a condition often preceding such behaviour when it occurs in same-sex pairs. Age plays a part in this respect;

younger boys will often accept mounting by older boys as if accepting their dominance.

As with monkeys, sexual play amongst children may therefore be an assertion of both gender and dominance without necessarily being motivated by any obviously sexual reward. It may also facilitate the development of friendships with both the same and opposite sex.

Erotic identification

The interest boys show in each other's penises has already been mentioned as a factor facilitating homosexual play. But sexual interest in one's peers may influence the development of our preferences in another subtle way. It is commonplace for early-adolescent children to hero-worship other adolescents slightly older than themselves. They admire them, want to emulate them and to be with them and they envy them their sexual success (real or imagined). In some instances this process becomes sexualised, i.e. thoughts of the admired person or of being with him, or of his sexual exploits become associated with sexual arousal. Such a response may be of no more significance than the arousal younger boys experience when observing each other's erections, but it often causes confusion and uncertainty about the individual's sexual identity and it is not uncommonly described as an early experience by teenage boys who regard themselves as homosexual. It may thus interact with the cognitive learning to reinforce a homosexual identity.

Langfeldt (1981) believes that boys are sexually activated by seeing other boys' erections. As they get older this leads to group activity which is more secretive and exclusive whilst at the same time various methods are used for denying possible homosexual implications of such behaviour. They say they are thinking of girls at the time, or that they have no access to girls. In a comparable way, if delinquent teenage boys become involved in homosexual activity with adults, they may protect their heterosexual identity by taking money or by avoiding any affection or by insulting or bullying their adult partner (Reiss, 1967). Here we see the effect that the social meaning of a particular behaviour may have on its subsequent development. The behaviour will either be modified to avoid the label of homosexual or else it will be regarded as homosexual and hence in some way incompatible with heterosexuality. The assumption 'if you are one thing you can't be the other' reflects particular values and beliefs about homosexuality which are presumably socially determined and certainly are not present in all cultures. We will consider this process of social polarisation later in relation to cognitive learning and the establishment of exclusive homosexual preferences.

Homosocial behaviour

A further social influence on sexual development has been mentioned earlier. Gagnon & Simon (1973) describe as homosocial the tendency for adolescent boys to engage in heterosexual activity as a way of improving their status in their male group. This is in contrast to heterosocial behaviour where it is the relationship with the *girl* that is important rather than with one's male friends. Gagnon & Simon believe that homosocial sexual behaviour is more prevalent in working-class groups, as reflected in the greater incidence of coitus in young working-class males. Such homosocial factors illustrate the functions of sex in asserting gender identity and bolstering self-esteem, and are likely to have a significant effect on the development of sexual preferences. The animal counterpart is seen when dominance in a male hierarchy is reflected in access to available females. The relevance of this behaviour to the sexual double-standard will be considered further in Chapter 4.

Non-specific responsiveness and peer group learning

Ramsey (1943) found that a majority of boys just prior to puberty (aged 12–14) described the occurrence of erections in a variety of arousing but not necessarily sexual situations. These ranged from going for a ride in an aeroplane to being chased by a policeman; in other words the associated affect could be pleasant or frightening. They also included physical contact such as wrestling or other high-contact sports. Within 2 or 3 years this type of experience apparently largely disappears, and erections become more specifically linked to sexual stimuli.

These interesting reports suggest that although the younger male child is capable of erections, there is a transient phase just prior to puberty when the threshold for erections is lowered and they occur to a variety of non-specific stimuli. During the next few years penile erection becomes more clearly linked to sexual stimuli. Some process of discrimination is presumably taking place and there is good reason to believe that peer group learning may influence that process. How boys interpret these responses will influence their subsequent development. If you regard a stimulus as sexual you will react to it as sexual and hence reinforce its sexual effect. Here we see cognitive learning at work as behaviour becomes labelled. The peer group is likely to be the main source of such labels leading to a normalisation of meaning. It is a common clinical observation that boys who develop abnormal sexual preferences (i.e. erectile responses to abnormal stimuli) are often isolated from an appropriate peer group (Langfeldt 1981). The occurrence of non-specific responses in such a boy may result in a non-sexual stimulus being self-labelled as sexual, thus leading to an abnormal pattern of response.

This type of mislabelling may interact with other factors to influence sexual learning. For example, it is not unusual to find that masochistic preferences arise in a boy who is inhibited and guilty about sex and has experienced a non-specific erection during some occasion of corporal punishment.

The guilt about sex and the need for punishment may in some way reinforce the sexualisation of this non-specific response and lead to the masochistic pattern. When one considers the minimal communication between adult and child about the meaning of the child's emerging sexual responses, it is little wonder that the child relies on his peer group for sorting out appropriate meaning and no surprise that the isolated child is prone to inappropriate labelling.

The effects of anxiety

Much of the theorising about sexual development has stressed the importance of anxiety or fear. Anxiety associated with certain types of sexual activity or partner may push us away from such a preference — the so-called 'push factor' in our sexual learning. Two types of threat may be involved, leading to fear of failure and fear of success. Fear of sexual failure or rejection by a sexual partner is usually associated with lack of self-confidence or low self-esteem, or uncertainty about one's gender identity, sexual attractiveness or sexual competence. For such an individual, rejection or failure may be less likely with certain kinds of partner. For example, a man unsure of his masculinity or his attractiveness to women may feel safer in a sexual involvement with another male, or with a child of either sex.

Fear of success is the fear of the actual sexual encounter and may stem from guilt about sexual enjoyment or fear of its consequences, learnt during childhood and perhaps reinforced by a sexually repressive environment. More specifically, guilt or anxiety about the sexuality of one's relationship with the opposite-sex parent may be involved — the Oedipus complex, which plays such a central part in psychoanalytic theory. If for some reason the boy learnt to be threatened by the sexual implications of his relationship with his mother, he may avoid sexual relationships which bear any similarity — e.g. with a similar type of woman, or relationships involving love. He may even avoid heterosexual relationships altogether.

Little will be said in this book about psychoanalytic theory, even though a very large proportion of writing on the subject of human sexual development has been of that genre. In my view, the psychoanalytic tradition has done us a service in drawing attention to certain key issues, such as the sexuality of the parent–child relationship. But it is of limited value because of its unsatisfactory and unscientific conceptual basis. Readers will have no difficulty in finding good summaries of the psychoanalytic viewpoint; examples are found in Kaplan (1974) and Rosen (1978).

Paradoxically, anxiety may in some circumstances act as a 'pull factor' towards homosexual preferences, when sex becomes a method of dealing with a threatening relationship. It has been commonly observed amongst monkeys that one male may appease another aggressive dominant male by presenting himself in a sexually receptive posture. There is little evidence that this situation is exploited sexually by the dominant male, though the presentation obviously has an appeasement function. A comparable mechanism has been suggested in human males. Bieber (1965), a psychoanalyst, believes that males cope with other threatening males by sexual techniques of a comparable kind. He relates this to his observed association between development of homosexual preferences in the presence of a detached or hostile father. The possible relevance of the pattern of parent–child interaction on sexual development will be considered shortly. An example of threat stemming from a sibling relationship and sexualised in this way is given by Hoffman (1968). But if sexual interaction is used to deal with threat between males, then its significance may become confounded by the social polarisation mechanism (see below) and homosexual preferences may be reinforced. The monkey, in contrast, can probably exploit such appeasement behaviour without affecting his sexual preferences or identity.

The relevance of the parent–child relationship to sexual development

For some years, particular types of parent–child relationship have been implicated in the causation of homosexuality. Studies have varied, some showing particular types of mother–son relationships (in particular, the so-called 'closed binding intimate' mother); others the father–son relationship (in particular, detached, absent or hostile father). Most of these observations have involved psychiatric patient populations. More recently it has become clear that such relationships are more obviously related to personality characteristics rather than homosexual preferences per se. In a series of studies of non-clinical populations, Siegelman (1974, 1978) found that homosexual men did report more disturbed relationships with their parents than did the heterosexual controls. However, the homosexual group were also more neurotic and when low-neuroticism groups were compared, then these differences in parental relationships disappeared. Siegelman also found that high femininity, in both homosexual and heterosexual males, was associated with neuroticism. Gender identity problems, as already mentioned, could well influence sexual preferences but we have to allow for the possibility that disturbed parent–child relationships could be as much a consequence as a cause of such disturbed gender identity.

Preparedness for learning and possible innate determinants

So far we have considered the determinants of sexual preference which rely on learning for their effects. It is inconceivable that learning does not play a major role. But to what extent are we programmed to learn certain things more than others? This is what Seligman & Hager (1942) call preparedness for learning — something in our constitution which makes us particularly susceptible to certain types of environmental influence or perhaps the effects of earlier learning on later learning. Such a possibility suggests itself particularly when we consider the development of heterosexual and homosexual preferences. Whilst it seems sensible to allow for such innate factors, their importance remains to be demonstrated. Perhaps the most convincing evidence is genetic. There is greater concordance for homosexuality amongst monozygotic than dizygotic twins. This concordance is not 100%, however, but probably somewhere between 40–60% (Heston & Shields 1968). Genetic factors must therefore be playing a part. But that may mean no more than a genetically determined likelihood to react to environmental influences in a similar way, rather than a specific predisposition to learn either hetero- or homosexual preferences.

In the early part of this century, Hirschfeld (1913) put forward the view that homosexuality was a form of hormonal intersex. Evidence obtained during the 1940s countered this view. But more recently, with the development of modern hormone assay techniques, interest in this possibility has been revived. Quite a number of studies have looked for endocrine differences between adult homosexuals and heterosexuals. Most of these studies have been notable for their naivety and for the almost total lack of control of the many variables that can influence isolated hormone levels. Not surprisingly, they present a totally contradictory set of findings. We can conclude that as yet no endocrine pattern distinguishes male homosexuals from heterosexuals (Meyer-Bahlburg 1977; Bancroft 1983). There are two possible exceptions to this general conclusion. One particular difference was found in two studies. The ratio of androsterone and etiocholanolone, two metabolites of testosterone excreted in the urine, was found to differentiate between homosexual and heterosexual men (Evans 1972; Margolese & Janiger 1973). The relevance of this obscure finding to the sexual preferences in these men is another matter.

Of rather greater interest is a study by Dörner et al (1975). These authors compared groups of exclusively homosexual and heterosexual men in their responses to oestrogen provocation. The homosexual group showed a pattern of luteinising hormone response which was closer to the normal female positive feedback response than that found in the heterosexual group. Dörner's conclusion was that the brains of the homosexual men had been inadequately defemininised and this was evidence of the biological basis of their homosexuality. These findings have always been controversial and the homologous nature of this so-called positive feedback response has been seriously questioned. More recently this study was replicated by Gladue et al (1984) with the crucial difference that, in addition to including a heterosexual female comparison group, the authors also assessed the effects of the oestrogen provocation on the testes of the male subjects. They found a luteinising hormone response to the oestrogen provocation which in the male homosexual group was midway between the heterosexual women and men — in other words, they replicated Dörner's findings. However Gladue et al found that the testicular response also differed, with the homosexual group showing a more prolonged suppression of testosterone. The greater reduction in negative feedback of testosterone on the pituitary which would result in the homosexual men is therefore the most likely explanation for the more pronounced rise in luteinising hormone in that group. In other words, the difference in hypothalamic response was really a difference in testicular response, and as such was probably unrelated to defemininisation of the brain. For some reason Gladue and his colleagues rejected this interpretation of their findings, which they took to reinforce Dörner's conclusions. But there is little doubt that the testicular explanation is the more likely.

Perhaps the final nail in the coffin of Dörner's model is provided by Gooren (1986) who showed in both male and female transsexuals that the hypothalamic response to oestrogen provocation was consistent with the prevailing hormonal milieu at the time. Thus before sex reassignment surgery the hypothalamic response was consistent with the genetic sex. After surgery (and castration) it was in the opposite direction. The response was not a fixed product of early organisation of the brain but a function of the dynamic organising effects of the prevailing hormonal milieu (see Bancroft 1988 for fuller discussion).

Earlier claims that homosexuals differed from heterosexuals in their body build were also shown to be due to faulty sampling. The relatively feminine physique reported in male homosexuals has been observed in psychiatric patient populations. Coppen (1959) showed that homosexual psychiatric patients had similar physical androgyny scores to other neurotic psychiatric patients; this is a further example of the pitfalls of generalising from the psychiatric population to people in general.

Although no evidence has been put forward linking homosexual preferences to abnormalities in the central nervous system, this link has been made with some abnormal types of sexual preference. Temporal lobe epilepsy is occasionally associated with abnormal sexual preferences (Taylor 1969). Most striking is the high incidence of electroencephalogram abnormalities in transsexuals (though this involves a disturbance of gender identity rather than of sexual preference), but the significance of this intriguing finding awaits explanation (Hoenig & Kenna 1979). Without specifying any direct link between central nervous system function and the development of sexual preference, it is nevertheless sensible to assume that any factor which disturbs normal sexuality during childhood or adolescence, whether by neurological or hormonal means, may facilitate the development of abnormal preferences simply by interfering with normal learning.

One crucial question about sexual learning which remains unanswered is its relative fixity. To what extent do we learn sexual preferences that become immutable and resistant to any further learning? Or to what extent can we go on learning new ways of responding and new preferences? It is a common clinical experience to find some men with interests so fixed and specific that they must resort to specific fantasies and activities to get any sexual pleasure. For the majority preferences are much more adaptable but to what extent can they change, say from heterosexual to homosexual? This aspect of learning may well prove to be crucial to our understanding of sexual development.

DEVELOPMENT OF SEXUAL PREFERENCES IN GIRLS

Although it is reasonable to assume that many of the mechanisms we have postulated to be relevant to the male may also be relevant to the female, we should nevertheless keep an open mind. We have less evidence concerning the human female, and the animal evidence alerts us to the possibility that there may be important sex differences in development.

One striking and interesting sex difference is that the more bizarre and fetishistic types of male preference rarely if ever arise in women. Women do develop homosexual preferences, though probably less commonly than men (see Chapter 6). They may have a greater facility for enjoying both homo- and heterosexual relationships (i.e. bisexuality). They do show sadomasochistic tendencies, though to a limited extent (see Chapter 7), but they do not develop fetishes and are seldom involved in anti-social sexual behaviour such as voyeurism or exhibitionism. Sexual abuse of children by women, though probably more common than has previously been realised, is undoubtedly much less common than such abuse by men (see Chapter 13).

We can only speculate why these differences exist. It may be that males have more learning to do in establishing their preferences, giving more scope for variety and error. We have already learnt that the disruptive effects of early experiences on adult sexuality of animals is observed in males but not females, and that the limited evidence of innate sexual preference in mammals has been confined to females. Perhaps the overlap of dominance and erotic functions of sexual behaviour is greater for the male. A further interesting possibility is that the female lacks the clear genital signal which the male gets from erection of his penis and which may facilitate learning of sexual responses to both normal and abnormal stimuli. Perhaps for this reason the developing sexuality of the adolescent female is less genitally oriented.

Where possible constitutional factors are concerned, there is relatively little evidence. Hormonal studies of homosexual women have been few, but more consistent in their findings than those involving males. It has been found that about one-third of lesbians studied have testosterone levels which are higher than those in heterosexual controls, while the remaining two-thirds show normal levels (Meyer-Bahlburg 1979). The possible relevance of this fact to sexual development in women is discussed further on p. 120. Also of interest is the evidence from endocrine abnormalities, such as the adrenogenital syndrome and prenatal exposure to steroid hormones. This will be considered later in this chapter.

Interestingly, whereas attempts to find endocrine abnormalities in male-to-female transsexuals have consistently failed, there is evidence that some female-to-male transsexuals may be hormonally unusual. Some have been found to have raiséd testosterone levels and others show responses to oestrogen provocation which are more characteristic of males than females (Seyler et al 1978; Meyer-Bahlburg 1979; Futterweit et al 1986).

HOMOSEXUAL IDENTITY AND THE EXCLUSIVE HOMOSEXUAL

The various mechanisms and formative experiences discussed above can be seen to combine to increase or decrease the probability that an individual will participate or feel interested in homosexual activity. This is consistent with the social learning paradigm and we can draw close parallels with non-human primates. Such a view is also compatible with the well-known Kinsey scale (see Chapter 6) on which individuals are placed according to the relative predominance of homosexuality or heterosexuality in their lives. Kinsey's concept allowed him to emphasise the large number of people who have been involved in homosexual activity at some stage of their lives. But although Kinsey, for good reasons, wanted to counter the idea that people are *either* heterosexual *or* homosexual, he nevertheless found a substantial number of people whose preferences were exclusively homosexual. This is an aspect of human sexuality which does not appear to have any counterpart in the animal world. Animals, as we have seen, are frequently involved in same-sex sexual activity, some more than others. But the animal which has an exclusive preference for the same sex, even in the presence of available opposite-sex partners, is hard to find (Tyler 1984).

Thus there seems to be something uniquely human about exclusive homosexuality. Paradoxically it is the exclusive form of homosexuality that is often attributed to biological causes (e.g. Feldman & McCulloch 1971). Yet if that were so it is unlikely that such a pattern should be confined to humans. Why shouldn't such biological determinants operate in some primates also? My suggested solution to this paradox is that the uniquely human phenomenon of exclusive homosexuality is a product of the uniquely human process described earlier — cognitive learning (Bancroft 1983).

The principal weakness of the Kinsey scale, in my view, is that it pays no attention to the crucial cognitive variable — sexual identity. Just as children are encouraged to see themselves as *either* male *or* female, so adolescents and young adults are required to categorise or label themselves as *either* heterosexual *or* homosexual. It is important to stress that this is not invariably so, but depends on the social system involved. It applies in most western societies, but there are other cultures where this polarisation does not seem to apply. Herdt (1981) has vividly described one society in which homosexual activity between adult men and adolescent boys is an accepted or assumed stage in the boy's sexual development, whilst at the same time provides an alternative source of sexual pleasure for the adult men. This pattern in no way undermines or threatens the normality of their sexual identities or their heterosexual lifestyles, though their tendency to conceal this behaviour from their women folk suggests that they may feel a little corporate guilt at such indulgence.

There are other societies where homosexual behaviour has different meanings and where the polarising binary distinction between the homosexual and the heterosexual is less evident or absent (Hotvedt 1983). What may be more universal is the clear binary distinction between the reproductive roles of men and women, and most societies recognise that some anatomical males are feminine in important ways — the shaman or berdache of some societies, the transvestite or transsexual of the western world. But whereas such 'female' men are often involved in sexual activity with other men, their 'femaleness' results in such activity being seen as an extension of heterosexuality.

Anthropological evidence of sexual behaviour in primitive societies is seldom substantial enough to draw firm conclusions, but there are reasons to believe that apart from the 'female male', the exclusive homosexual is unusual in those societies which accept homosexual expression as compatible with normal sexuality. This lends weight to the conclusion that the heterosexual–homosexual dichotomy, so evident in western societies, is a social construct which, through the mechanisms of cognitive learning, leads in some cases to the establishment of an exclusive homosexual identity. (These issues are discussed further in Chapter 6.)

Such sexual identity development is obviously a complex process which can be simplified into three stages:

1. The pre-labelling stage, when childhood and early adolescent sexual experiences occur without the need to categorise them as either homo- or heterosexual.
2. The self-labelling stage: at some stage the individual asks the question 'Am I straight or gay?' and begins to interpret experiences as evidence for or against.
3. Social labelling: at some later stage, the social world asks the same question about the individual, influencing the cognitive learning process and reinforcing labels as well as providing the underlying assumption: 'You are either one thing or the other'.

The complexity of such a multifactorial developmental process has been well illustrated in two case histories described by Richardson & Hart (1981), showing the wide variety of of influences which impinge on the developmental process — the 'push' and 'pull' factors away from or towards a hetero- or homosexual identity. Obviously we cannot exclude the possibility that in some sense an individual is more prepared to follow the homosexual rather than the heterosexual option (or vice versa) at various crucial points in the developmental sequence. Certainly many homosexuals, in describing their own early development, emphasise the strong unequivocal attraction they felt to people of the same sex at a relatively early age. But such accounts must be interpreted with caution. How many individuals have similar experiences but follow a different course, and how much do we all, heterosexual and homosexual, need to recall our past in ways which serve our current needs?

THE RELATIONSHIP BETWEEN GENDER IDENTITY AND SEXUAL IDENTITY

We have considered a variety of factors which might contribute to both social and cognitive learning. But from the few substantial studies of the childhood of homosexuals only two factors occur with sufficient frequency to be regarded as key influences. Adults who develop homosexual preferences are more likely to report gender non-conformity or relative isolation from their peer group during childhood. Such evidence comes from prospective studies of effeminate boys (see Chapter 7 for further details) as well as from the retrospective accounts of adults (Siegelman 1974, 1978; Bell et al 1981).

This raises a crucial issue. Does this gender non-conformity lead to homosexuality by its contribution to the social and cognitive learning processes (since uncertainty about one's masculinity may lower self-confidence and reduce one's attractiveness in the eyes of a potential heterosexual mate, so that heterosexual interaction poses a threat of failure or rejection)? Or is it a manifestation of some central nervous system state which also determines sexual preference, i.e. a marker of biological determination? This is the explanation that Dörner would favour. No firm conclusion on this point is possible at the present time, but it is important to realise that gender non-conformity is only evident in the histories of a proportion of adult homosexuals and is therefore not *necessary* for homosexual development. I therefore favour the view that such personality characteristics are important but not sufficient factors in the multifactorial learning process. Biological factors may therefore influence the development of sexual preference indirectly by their effects on these mediating personality characteristics. We will consider homosexual identity further in Chapter 6.

BIOLOGICAL ABNORMALITIES IN DEVELOPMENT

What can we learn about normal sexual development from studying biological abnormalities? Most such conditions are rare and thus can be considered appropriately here rather than in the clinical section of the book. There are three main types of condition:

1. Sex chromosome abnormalities.
2. Inborn errors of metabolism affecting the reproductive hormones.
3. Exposure to exogenous steroids during fetal development.

SEX CHROMOSOME ABNORMALITIES

Variations from the normal sex chromosome karyotype (i.e. 46 XY or 46 XX) are complex, with mosaicism adding to the complexity. We will confine our attention to the simplest and most common: 45XO, 47 XXY, 47 XYY and 47 XXX. Although chromosomal status may influence development in a variety of ways, some of the most obvious effects are mediated through the gonads and sex endocrine system.

46 XO: gonadal dysgenesis or Turner's syndrome

Although this is the commonest sex chromosome anomaly to arise, the large majority of fetuses so affected are aborted and consequently this karyotype occurs in less than 1 in 5000 live births.

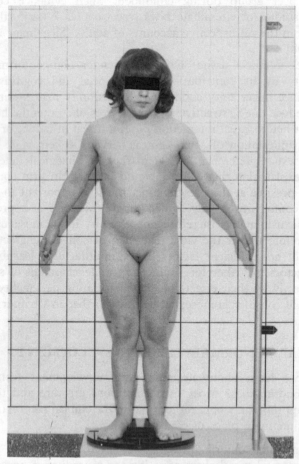

Fig. 3.5 Twelve-year-old girl with Turner's syndrome. (photograph courtesy of Dr Shirley Ratcliffe)

Ovarian development starts normally, but presumably because of the absence of normal oocytes (which require two X-chromosomes, see p. 154) the ovaries soon regress and by birth are no more than streaks of connective tissue. There is thus a marked deficiency of sex steroids, resulting in absence of breast development and secondary sexual characteristics, and amenorrhoea. The genitalia are otherwise normally female. Growth is stunted (presumably due to the steroid lack) and there may be a variety of somatic anomalies, the best known being webbing of the neck. (see Fig. 3.5)

Intelligence is usually normal, though spatial aptitude may be impaired. Gender identity is unequivocally female (Money & Ehrhardt 1972). Menstruation can be initiated and maintained with long-term oestrogen substitution therapy. The available evidence does not provide information about the development of sexual preferences, sexual appetite or response in these girls, though Money & Ehrhardt (1972) stress that without hormone substitution therapy it is difficult for them to establish psychosocial maturity.

This syndrome tells us little about the role of hormones and sexual development except that female prepubertal genitalia and gender identity develop in the absence of any ovarian steroid production.

47 XXX or triple-x anomaly

This has a frequency of about 1 in 1250 live female births. Sexual development appears to be normal in most cases although a proportion do not menstruate normally. At least some of these women are fertile (producing normal children). There is an increased likelihood of intellectual impairment.

47 XXY or Klinefelter's syndrome

About 1 in 700 newborn males has this karyotype. Development is invariably along male lines. The full picture of Klinefelter's syndrome includes small testes (about 2–6 ml) with tubular dysgenesis, hypogonadism, infertility, tall stature and gynaecomastia. There may be intellectual impairment, personality problems and abnormal sexual preferences. Considering the frequency of this condition at birth, the full syndrome is rare. This presumably means that the majority of such men must be relatively free from such stigmata. This is borne out by their relative frequency amongst otherwise normal men attending infertility clinics (approximately 5% of male clinic attenders).

The endocrine pattern of this condition shows a somewhat low plasma testosterone concentration (though overlapping the normal range) and raised gonadotrophins (both luteinising hormone (LH) and follicle-stimulating hormone (FSH)). Although the raised FSH is to be expected in

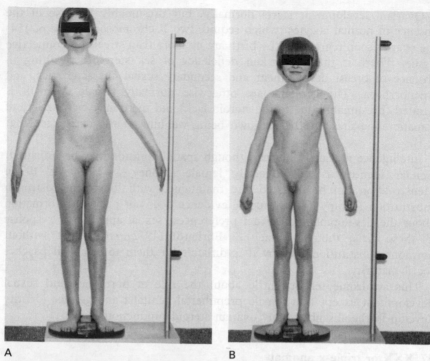

A   B

Fig. 3.6 Ten-year-old twins. The taller one (A) has an XXY chromosome constitution; his penis is proportionally smaller and he has increased fat deposition on the hips and more marked increase in leg length. (photograph courtesy of Dr Shirley Ratcliffe)

view of the tubular dysgenesis, the high LH is probably not simply due to impaired Leydig cell function, as it is difficult to suppress the LH level to the normal range with exogenous androgens. These men usually have a relatively high oestrogen:testosterone ratio which may account for their tendency to gynaecomastia.

The tall stature, which is by no means invariable, is not fully understood. It is detectable throughout childhood before epiphyseal closure normally occurs, and is therefore not simply a result of delayed closure (see Fig. 3.6).

Tubular degeneration in the testes proceeds throughout childhood and it is only in late childhood that the testis size and consistency is noticeably different from normal.

Raboch et al (1979) found evidence of delayed development of heterosexual interest and sociosexual behaviour in XXY males attending clinics. A recent study of adolescent boys with 47 XXY karyotypes identified at birth found them to have slightly lower intelligence than a group of normal matched controls (Ratcliffe et al 1981). Most developed normally except for being behind their peer group in the onset of adolescent sexual interest, relatively impaired in peer group relationships and more tender-minded than the controls (Bancroft et al 1982).

A recent study has found evidence of a positive feedback response in XXY adult males, suggesting that their abnormal chromosome constitution may influence hypothalamic development in spite of relatively normal male androgen levels (Barbarino et al 1979).

There is no evidence that XXY males are more likely to develop homosexual preferences.

A rarer and possibly related conditions is that of the 46 XX male. It is thought possible that a Y chromosome, or at least Hy antigenic material, is hidden in such cases, perhaps by translocation to an autosome. These men are similar in many ways to the 47 XXY male, though not showing a tall stature to the same extent.

47 XYY

This condition has approximately the same incidence as 47 XXY, i.e. 1 in 700 to 1000 live male births. There are no obvious sexual consequences except that testicular abnormalities with impaired spermatogenesis and tubular atrophy may occur (Polani 1972). They are often fertile, fathering chromosomally normal children, though their fertility is apparently reduced by a low incidence of marriage. Hormonally, they have slightly raised gonadotrophins (both LH and FSH). The FSH may well reflect the tubular atrophy. The raised LH is more difficult to explain. Most studies have reported normal testosterone levels, though one study found raised testosterone compared with matched controls (Schiavi et al 1978).

These men show tall stature, similar to the XXY male, though their body shape is somewhat different. They first attracted attention because of their apparently high incidence amongst patients of special hospitals (i.e. for mentally disturbed offenders). It was suggested at one time that they had a tendency to high aggression, presumably a naive extrapolation from their extra Y chromosome. In fact the XYY men found in the special hospital populations are characterised by offences against property rather than people. They show inadequacy rather than aggression. It may be that they have an increased incidence of behavioural problems of various kinds, though the risk of an XYY male becoming convicted, although increased, is very small. As with XXY males, the majority live their lives without obvious problems or stigmata. There is no evidence of an increased likelihood of homosexual development.

INBORN ERRORS OF METABOLISM

Of the various types of innate metabolic deficiencies, there are some which directly affect the production of sex hormones. They are all rare and we will consider only the most important. (For a description of the full range of metabolic defects, see Lev Ran 1977.)

Androgen insensitivity syndrome (or testicular feminisation syndrome)

The basic defect in this condition is a reduced affinity of cellular receptors for androgens. This results in a more or less complete failure of androgenic effects at cellular level and probably in all cells of the body. The syndrome is transmitted either as an X-linked recessive trait or a male-limited dominant trait, so only genetic males are affected.

During embryonic development, the Mullerian-inhibiting factor is produced normally so that no fallopian tubes, uterus or upper vagina develop. In other respects the body develops along female lines, with external genitalia indistinguishable by their outward appearances from those of a normal female. Such children are therefore reared as girls.

Testes are found in the abdominal cavity or more commonly in the groin or labia. They have a tendency to neoplastic change and are usually removed during adulthood. They secrete normal male amounts of androgens and also relatively large quantities of oestrogen, which is responsible for the feminisation (hence the original term 'testicular feminisation', used before the actual mechanism was understood). At puberty good breast development and feminine contours arise, though there is a deficiency of body and pubic hair even by female standards (see Fig. 3.7). As mentioned earlier, women with androgen insensitivity syndrome do not show positive feedback as genetic females normally do.

The first sign of something wrong may be failure to menstruate. Psychologically, development is along almost stereotyped female lines. Money & Ehrhardt (1972) have reported 10 such women, whose sexual lives appeared to be unexceptional. Six of them reported average libido, were usually orgasmic but were reserved and passive during coitus. Two reported above-average libido, were always orgasmic and usually initiated sexual activity. Two were sexually inexperienced. Erotic arousal was predominantly dependent on touch.

In this interesting condition we have striking evidence that, in the presence of apparently normal male chromosomal structure, female development occurs simply because of the absence of androgenic effects and the presence of oestrogens. Although the evidence is limited, such individuals apparently show fairly normal sexual interest and preferences. Further evidence is required before we can be sure that they do not differ sexually from normal women.

In some cases the androgen insensitivity is incomplete, and partial masculinisation occurs. These children are more likely to be assigned to the male gender and their psychosexual development tends to conform to this.

Adrenogenital syndrome (congenital adrenal hyperplasia)

This is the result of an autosomal recessive gene defect in cortisol synthesis, usually due to a deficiency of the 21-hydroxylase enzyme. If severe, serious electrolytic disturbance and Addisonian crises occur. Usually the defect is

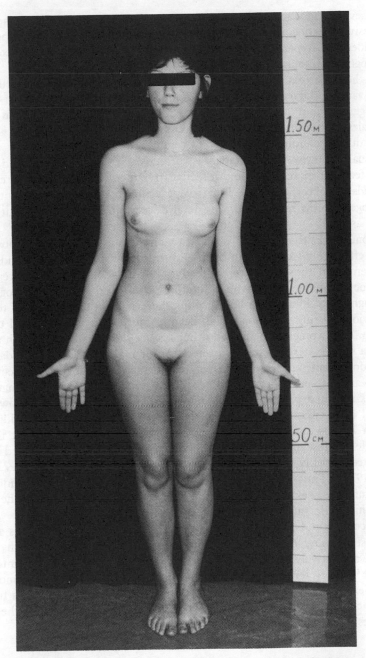

Fig. 3.7 Woman with androgen insensitivity syndrome. Notice the normal breast development and absence of sexual hair. (photograph courtesy of Professor David Baird)

less severe, and adequate cortisol production is maintained by means of excessive adrenocorticotrophic hormone stimulation, but at the expense of considerable hyperplasia of the adrenal cortex and a resulting excess of androgenic steroids.

In the male this causes precocious puberty. In girls it leads to virilisation with varying degrees of masculinisation of the external genitalia (i.e. clitoral enlargement and labioscrotal fusion). Some such children have been reared as males, and have apparently adapted successfully, though needing surgery both during childhood and later to remove the uterus.

Usually, however, the anomaly is correctly diagnosed and the child reared as a female. In recent years, effective treatment, in the form of cortico-steroids, has been available. Previously, lack of appropriate treatment led to androgen excess not only during fetal development but throughout child-hood as well.

Money & Ehrhardt (1972) studied two groups of such women: those who were effectively treated from birth and thus only suffered excess androgens in utero, and those who were already adult or adolescent when treatment became available and who therefore continued to be androgenised throughout childhood. In both groups there is definite evidence of tomboy behaviour during childhood, significantly more than in a matched control group. The women also showed other features more consistent with a male than a female stereotype, e.g. preference for male clothes and avoidance of self-adornment, and putting career before marriage. In these respects, the early- and late-onset groups did not differ, presumably indicating that these effects reflected prenatal androgenisation. The two groups did show some sexual differences, however. The late-treated group were more likely to report homosexual or bisexual fantasies than those treated early, though definite homosexual orientation did not occur. Also the late-treated group reported possibly greater sexual arousability (Money & Ehrhardt 1972; Lev Ran 1977). Thus we have some evidence from this source that androgens may influence sexual appetite and sexual preference, although in the latter case this could once again be via effects on gender identity.

Precocious puberty in boys due to the adrenogenital syndrome is also of interest. Money & Alexander (1969), describing a series of such cases, found a relatively early onset of sexual interest, although the content of sexual imagery tended to be consistent with the boys' social and emotional age. Sexual behaviour problems did not arise in these boys. This is further evidence that androgens 'energise' the sexual experience, whilst the form it takes is more determined by social learning.

5α reductase deficiency

5α reductase is necessary for the conversion of testosterone to DHT. DHT is necessary for the male development of the urogenital sinus into normal external genitalia (see Fig. 3.4).

Imperato-McGinley et al (1974) studied a small community in the Dominican Republic in which there were 24 genetic males all related to one another and with 5α reductase enzyme deficiency. They were all born with ambiguous genitalia. The vas deferens, epididymis and seminal vesicles developed normally, being dependent on testosterone. The urogenital sinus, however, remained as a blind vaginal pouch, with a clitoral-like phallus, labia-like scrotum and inguinal or labial testes. Most of these individuals were reared as girls, but at puberty not only did growth of the penile stump and scrotum occur but there was also a change to a masculine gender identity with sexual feelings directed at females. Why testosterone should show this effect at puberty and not cause normal development earlier has not yet been adequately explained. The change of gender identity at this age is also surprising, though it seems possible that those children born more recently were not reared as normal girls, but as something unusual. If so, their earlier gender identity may have been relatively ambiguous. Unfortunately it is difficult to be certain on this theoretically crucial point because of lack of more definite evidence. If they were reared unequivocally as girls and their childhood gender identity was clearly female, then the change at puberty suggests that exposure to testosterone during early development effectively counteracts subsequent environmental influences. If, on the other hand, the gender identity was ambiguous until puberty, then we can draw no conclusions on that particular point.

THE EFFECTS OF EXOGENOUS STEROIDS DURING PREGNANCY

The administration of steroid hormones to the mother during pregnancy, and hence to the fetus, provides us with evidence of the effects of steroids on physical and behavioural development. Of particular interest, therefore, are those female children born to mothers given synthetic steroids during pregnancy in order to prevent spontaneous abortion. The early progestagens used for this purpose had androgenic properties. The effects observed depended on the stage of pregnancy when the steroids were administered. If early enough, ambiguity of the genitalia sometimes resulted; if later, behavioural characteristics of tomboy type have been reported, though sexual preferences have usually been heterosexual (Ehrhardt & Meyer-Bahlburg 1979).

The effects of steroids with androgenic properties are therefore consistent with the animal data; some degree of masculinisation is to be expected. With oestrogenic steroids and progestagens which are not androgenic the effects are much less clearcut. This is not surprising, as in subprimates the effects of such steroids on development are varied and unpredictable (Baum 1979). The fetus is normally exposed to high levels of oestrogen and progesterone from the placenta. In some animals there is good evidence that the organisational effects of androgens depend on aromatisation of testosterone to oestradiol within the brain cells. The brain is presumably protected from the circulating oestrogens, and it has been postulated that some protective binding mechanism, perhaps involving α-fetoprotein, stops the extracellular oestrogen from entering the cell; only the testosterone can get in (McEwan 1976). It is not clear how relevant this is to the human, but the human fetus is exposed to oestradiol and progesterone so it is difficult to see how giving additional steroids will make any difference. Synthetic steroids, however, may act differently; there is evidence that diethylstilboestrol (DES) enters the fetal brain cells and is not blocked by a protective mechanism. Of considerable interest, therefore, is recent evidence that women exposed prenatally to DES have an increased likelihood of developing homosexual preferences (Ehrhardt et al 1985). These results should be regarded as preliminary however. These workers have not yet reported the gender identity development of these DES-exposed women and it is conceivable that the primary hormonal effect was on that aspect of development rather than directly on sexual preference per se.

In one study *boys* were assessed whose diabetic mothers had received oestrogens or oestrogen/progestagen combinations during pregnancy. There was some inconclusive evidence that the boys were less aggressive and less masculine than the normal controls. The possibility that this was related to having diabetic mothers rather than steroid effects was not excluded (Yalom et al 1973). Green (1979) and colleagues have followed up people in adulthood whose mothers received various other steroids during pregnancy and compared them with matched controls. The results are confusing and inconclusive; this is not surprising considering there is no clear basis on which to predict effects.

CONCLUSIONS

Whilst we remain basically ignorant about the determinants of sexual preference, both normal and abnormal, learning probably plays a major part. Certain types of preference are more likely to be reinforced and established if they conform with our developing gender identity, and avoid threatening or anxiety-provoking consequences. In particular, our ability to incorporate our sexuality into relationships which are otherwise loving and emotionally rewarding plays a fundamental part. Social learning tells us what is normal and abnormal, hence acceptable or unacceptable. This process also has its effects. Through childhood we are exposed to a complex set of 'push' and 'pull' factors, learning to avoid certain types of sexual activity and to be in some way rewarded by others. Underlying this learning we must nevertheless allow for some biologically determined predisposition, particularly in relation to our preference for male or female partners. This may be determined by genetic or hormonal mechanisms. At the same time, we should not assume that these determinants are the same in both male and female development.

REFERENCES

Akers J S, Conoway C H 1979 Female homosexual behavior in *Macacca mulatta*. Archives of Sexual Behavior 8: 63–80

Bakwin H 1973 Erotic feelings in infants and young children. American Journal of Diseases of Childhood 126: 52–54

Bancroft J 1983 Problematic gender identity and sexual orientation; a psychiatrist's view. In: Schwartz M F, Moraczwewski A S, Monteleone J A (eds) Sex and Gender; a theological and scientific inquiry. The Pope John Center, St Louis, Missouri, pp 102–124

Bancroft J 1988 Biological factors in development of sexual preferences. In: McWhirter D, Reinisch J (eds) Homosexuality, heterosexuality. The second Kinsey symposium. Oxford University Press, New York (in press)

Bancroft J, Axworthy D, Ratcliffe S G 1982 The personality and psychosexual development of boys with 47 XXY chromosome constitution. Journal of Child Psychology and Psychiatry 23: 169–180

Barbarino A, DeMarinis L, Lafuente G, Muscatello P, Matterici B R 1979 Presence of positive feedback between estrogen and LH in patients with Klinefelter's syndrome and Sertoli-cell-only syndrome. Clinical Endocrinology 10: 235–242

Bateson P P G 1978 Early experience and sexual preferences. In: Hutchison J (ed) The biological determinants of sexual behaviour. Wiley, Chichester

Baum M J 1979 Differentiation of coital behaviour in mammals: a comparative analysis. Neuroscience and Behavioural Reviews 3: 265–284

Beach F A 1979 Animal models for human sexuality. In: Sex, hormones and behaviour. Ciba Foundation Symposium 62. Excerpta Medica, Amsterdam

Beach F A, LeBoeuf B J 1967 Coital behavior in dogs I. Preferential mating in the bitch. Animal Behavior 15: 546–558

Bell A P, Weinberg M S, Hammersmith S N 1981 Sexual preferences: their development in men and women. Indiana University Press, Bloomington

Bieber I 1965 Chapter 1 In: Marmor J (ed) Clinical aspects of homosexuality in sexual inversion. Basic Books, New York

Bornemann E 1984 Progress in empirical research on children's sexuality. In: Segraves T, Haeberle E (eds) Emerging dimensions of sexology. Praeger, New York

Coppen A J 1959 Body build of male homosexuals. British Medical Journal 2: 1443

Diamond M 1965 A critical evaluation of the ontogeny of human sexual behaviour. Quarterly Review of Biology 40: 147–175

Dornbusch S, Carlsmith M, Gross R et al 1981 Sexual development, age and dating: a comparison of biological and social influences upon one set of behaviour. Child Development 52: 178

Dörner G, Rohde W, Stahl F, Krell L, Masius W G 1975 A neuroendocrine predisposition for homosexuality in men. Archives of Sexual Behavior 4: 1–8

Ehrhardt A A, Meyer-Bahlburg H F L 1979 Psychosexual development: an examination of the role of prenatal hormones. In: Sex hormones and behaviour. Ciba Foundation Symposium 62. Excerpta Medica, Amsterdam, pp 41–50

Ehrhardt A A, Meyer-Bahlburg H F L, Rosen L R et al 1985 Sexual orientation after prenatal exposure to exogenous estrogen. Archives of Sexual Behavior 14: 57–77

Elias J, Gebhard P 1969 Sexuality and sexual learning in childhood. Reprinted in: Rogers R S (ed) Sex education — rationale and reaction. Cambridge University Press, London, pp 143–154

Erikson E H 1950 Childhood and society. Norton, New York

Erwin J, Maple T 1976 Ambisexual behavior with male–male anal penetration in male rhesus monkeys. Archives of Sexual Behavior 5: 9–14

Evans R B 1972 Physical and biochemical characteristics of homosexual men. Journal of Consulting Clinical Psychology 39: 140–147

Fagot B I 1977 Consequences of moderate cross-gender behavior in preschool children. Child Development 48: 902–907

Feldman M P, McCulloch M J 1971 Homosexual behaviour: therapy and assessment. Pergamon, Oxford

Fogelman 1983 Growing up in Great Britain. Papers from the National Child Development Study. Macmillan, London, pp 287–298

Ford C S, Beach F A 1952 Patterns of sexual behaviur. Eyre & Spottiswoode, London

Futterweit W, Weiss R A, Fagerstrom R M 1986 Endocrine evaluation of 40 female-to-male transsexuals: increased frequency of polycystic ovarian disease in female transsexualism. Archives of Sexual Behavior 15: 69–78

Gagnon J, Simon W 1973 Sexual conduct: the social sources of human sexuality. Aldine, Chicago

Galenson E, Roiphe H 1974 The emergence of genital awareness during the second year of life. In: Friedman R C, Richart R M, Van de Wiele R L (eds) Sex differences in behavior. Wiley, New York, pp 233–258

Gladue B A, Green R, Hellman R E 1984 Neuroendocrine response to estrogen and sexual orientation. Science 225: 1496–1499

Goldfoot D A, Wallen K, Neff D A, McBrair M C, Goy R W 1984 Social influences on the display of sexually dimorphic behavior in rhesus monkeys: isosexual rearing. Archives of Sexual Behavior 13: 395–412

Goldman R, Goldman J 1982 Children's sexual thinking. Routledge & Kegan Paul, London

Gooren L 1986 The neuroendocrine response of luteinizing hormone to estrogen administration in the human is not sex specific but dependent on the hormonal environment. Journal of Clinical Endocrinology and Metabolism 63: 589–593

Goy R W 1979 Discussion. In: sex, hormones and behaviour. Ciba Foundation Symposium 62. Excerpta Medica, Amsterdam, pp 141–142, 264–265

Goy R W, Goldfoot D 1975 Neuroendocrinology: animal models and problems of human sexuality. Archives of Sexual Behavior 4: 405–420

Green R 1979 Sex-dimorphic behaviour in the human: prenatal hormone administration and post-natal socialisation. In: Sex, hormones and behaviour. Ciba Foundation Symposium 62. Excerpta Medica, Amsterdam, pp 59–68

Harlow H F 1971 Learning to love. Albion, San Francisco

Herdt G H 1981 Guardians of the flutes. Idioms of masculinity. McGraw-Hill, New York

Heston L L, Shields J 1968 Homosexuality in twins: a family study and a register study. Archives of General Psychiatry 18: 149–160

Hirschfeld 1913 Die Homosexualität des Mannes und des Weibes. In: Bloch I (ed) Handbuch der Sexualwissenschaft in Einzeldarstellungen, vol. III. Marcus, Berlin

Hoenig J, Kenna J C 1979 EEG abnormalities and transsexualism. British Journal of Psychiatry 134: 293–300

Hoffman M 1968 The gay world. Basic Books, New York

Hotvedt M 1983 Gender identity and sexual orientation: the anthropological perspective. In: Schwartz M F, Moraczewski A S, Monteleone J A (eds) Sex and gender: a theological and scientific inquiry. The Pope John Center, St Louis, Missouri

Imperato-McGinley J, Guerrero L, Gautier T, Peterson R E 1974 Steyeroid 5α-reductase deficiency in man; an inherited form of male pseudo-hermaphroditism. Science 186: 1213–1215

Kagan J, Moss H A 1962 Birth to maturity. A study in psychological development. Wiley, New York

Kaplan H S 1974 The new sex therapy. Brunner Mazel, New York

Karacan I, Salis P J, Thornby J I, Williams R L 1976 The ontogeny of nocturnal penile tumescence. Waking and Sleeping 1: 27–44

Kinsey A S, Pomeroy W B, Martin C F 1948 Sexual behaviour in the human male. Saunders, Philadelphia

Kinsey A C, Pomeroy W B, Martin C F, Gebhard P H 1953 Sexual behaviour in the human female. Saunders, Philadelphia

Kohlberg L 1966 A cognitive–developmental analysis of children's sex role concepts and attitudes. In: Maccoby E E (ed) The development of sex differences. Stanford University Press, Stanford

Kohlberg L 1969 Stages in the development of moral thought and action. Holt, Rinehart & Winston, New York

Langfeldt T 1981 Sexual development in children. In: Cook M, Howells K (eds) Adult sexual interest in children. Academic Press, London

Larsson K 1978 Experimental factors in the development of sexual behaviour. In: Hutchison J (ed) Biological determinants of sexual behaviour. Wiley, Chichester

Lev Ran A 1977 Sex reversal as related to clinical syndromes in human beings. In: Money J, Musaph H (eds) Handbook of Sexology. Excerpta Medica, Amsterdam

Lewis W C 1965 Coital movements in the first year of life. International Journal of Psychoanalysis 46: 372–374

McCandless B R 1960 Rate of development, bodybuild and personality. Child development and Child Psychiatry 88: 42–57

Maccoby E E, Jacklin C N 1974 The psychology of sex differences. Stanford University Press, Stanford

McEwan B S 1976 Interaction between hormones and nerve tissues. Reprinted in: Silver R, Feder H H (eds) Hormones and reproductive behaviour. Readings from Scientific American. Freeman, San Francisco

Margolese M S, Janiger O 1973 Androsterone/etiocholanolone ratios in male homosexuals. British Medical Journal 3: 207–210

Meyer-Bahlburg H F L 1977 Sex hormones and male homosexuality in comparative perspective. Archives of Sexual Behavior 6: 297–235

Meyer-Bahlburg H F L 1979 Sex hormones and female homosexuality. A critical examination. Archives of Sexual Behavior 8: 101–119

Miller P Y, Simon W 1980 The development of sexuality in adolescence. In: Adelson J (ed) Handbook of adolescent psychology. Wiley, Chichester

Mischel W 1966 A social-learning view of sex differences in behavior. In: Maccoby E E (ed) The development of sex differences. Stanford University Press, Stanford

Moll A 1912 The sexual life of the child. Translated by Paul E. McMillan, New York

Money J 1980 Love and love sickness: the science, gender difference, and pair bonding. Johns Hopkins University Press, Baltimore

Money J, Alexander D 1969 Psychosexual development and absence of homosexuality in males with precocious puberty: a review of 18 cases. Journal of Nervous and Mental Diseases 148: 111–123

Money J, Ehrhardt A A 1972 Man and woman, boy and girl. Differentiation and dimorphism of gender identity from conception to maturity. Johns Hopkins University Press, Baltimore

Nottelman E D, Inoff-Germain G, Susman E J, Chrousos G P 1988 Hormones and behavior at puberty. In: Bancroft J, Reinisch J (eds) Adolescence and puberty. The third Kinsey symposium. Oxford University Press, New York

Opie I, Opie P 1959 The lore and language of schoolchildren. Clarendon Press, Oxford

O'Rahilly R 1977 The development of the vagina in the human. In: Blandau R J, Bergsma D (eds) Morphogenesis and malformation of the genital system. The National Foundation — March of Dimes. Birth defects: original article series, vol 13, no 2. Alan Liss, New York

Perper T 1985 Sex signals. The biology of love. ISI Press, Philadelphia

Polani P E 1972 Sex chromosome anomalies. In: Ounsted C, Taylor D C (eds) Gender differences: their ontogeny and significance. Churchill Livingstone, Edinburgh

Raboch J, Mellan I, Starka L 1979 Klinefelter's syndrome: sexual development and activity. Archives of Sexual Behavior 8: 333–339

Ramsey G V 1943 The sexual development of boys. American Journal of Psychology 56: 217–234

Ratcliffe S G, Bancroft J, Axworthy D, McLaren W 1982 Klinefelter's syndrome in adolescence. Archives of Diseases of Childhood 57: 6–12

Reiss A J 1967 The social integration of queers and peers. In: Gagnon J, Simon W (eds) Sexual deviance. Harper Row, New York

Richardson D, Hart J 1981 The development and maintenance of a homosexual identity. In: Hart J, Richardson D (eds) Theory and practice of homosexuality. Routledge & Kegan Paul, London, pp 73–92

Roberts E, Kline D, Gagnon J 1978 Family life and sexual learning: a study of the role of parents in the sexual learning of children, vols 1–3. A report of the project on human sexual development. Cambridge, Massachusetts

Rogers R 1974 Sex education. Rationale and reaction. Cambridge University Press, Cambridge

Rosen I (ed) 1978 Sexual deviation, 2nd edn. Oxford University Press, Oxford

Rutter M 1983 Psychosexual development. In: Rutter M (ed) Scientific foundations of developmental psychiatry. Heinemann, London, pp 322–338

Schiavi R C, Owen D, Fogel M, White D, Szechter R 1978 Pituitary–gonadal function in XXY and XYY men identified in a population survey. Clinical Endocrinology 9: 233–239

Schofield M 1965 The sexual behaviour of young people. Longman, London

Schoof-Tams K, Schlaegel J, Walczak L 1976 Differentiation of sexual morality between 11 and 16 years. Archives of Sexual Behavior 5: 353–370

Seligman M E P, Hager J L 1972 Biological boundaries of learning. Appleton-Century-Crofts, New York, pp 1–6

Serbin L A, Sprafkin C H 1987 A developmental approach: Sexuality from infancy through adolescence. In: Geer J H, O'Donohue W T (eds) Theories of human sexuality. Plenum, New York, pp 163–196

Seyler L E, Canalis E, Spare S, Reichlin S 1978 Abnormal gonadotrophin secretory responses to LRH in transsexual women after diethylstilboestrol priming. Journal of Clinical Endocrinology and Metabolism 47: 176–183

Siegelman M 1974 Parental background of male homosexuals and heterosexuals. Archives of Sexual Behavior 3: 3–18

Siegelman M 1978 Psychological adjustment of homosexual and heterosexual men: a cross-national replication. Archives of Sexual Behavior 7: 1–12

Siegelman M 1981 Parental backgrounds of homosexual and heterosexual men: a cross-national replication. Archives of Sexual Behavior 10: 505–514

Spanier G B 1976 Formal and informal sex education on determinants of premarital sexual behavior. Archives of Sexual Behavior 5: 39–68

Stoller R 1968 Sex and gender. On the development of masculinity and femininity. Hogarth, London

Taylor D C 1969 Sexual behaviour and temporal lobe epilepsy. Archives of Neurology 21: 510–516

Toran-Allerand C D 1978 Gonadal hormones and brain development: cellular aspects of sexual differentiation. American Zoologist 18 (3): 553–566

Tyler P A 1984 Homosexual behaviour in animals. In: Howells K (ed) The psychology of sexual diversity. Blackwell, Oxford

Udry J R, Billy J O G, Morris N M, Groff T R, Raj M H 1985 Serum androgenic hormones motivate sexual behavior in adolescent boys. Fertility and Sterility 43: 90–94

Udry J R, Talbert L, Morris N M 1986 Biosocial foundations for adolescent female sexuality. Demography 23: 217–229

Van Look P F A, Hunter W M, Corker C S, Baird D T 1977 Failure of positive feedback in normal men and subjects with testicular feminisation. Clinical Endocrinology 7: 353–366

Weichman G H, Ellis A L 1969 A study of the effects of 'sex education' on premarital petting and coital behaviour. Reprinted in: Rogers R (ed) Sex education. Cambridge University Press, Cambridge

Yalom I, Green R, Fisk N 1973 Prenatal exposure to female hormones; effects on psychosexual development in boys. Archives of General Psychiatry 28: 554–561

4

Patterns of sexual behaviour — heterosexuality

THE SOURCE OF OUR INFORMATION

Interest in human sexual behaviour and the factors influencing it has probably never been greater than it is today as, threatened with a new and uniquely dangerous epidemic of sexually transmitted disease (AIDS), we speculate about how our sexual behaviour will need to change to lessen this formidable threat.

There are three important sources of information: historical evidence of changing patterns of sexual behaviour; cross-cultural anthropological studies of mainly primitive societies and surveys of sexual behaviour and attitudes in modern societies.

Social history, particularly as it applies to sexuality and marriage, is a relatively new discipline. In the last few years some important studies have been published (e.g. Shorter 1975; Stone 1979; Boswell 1981; Gillis 1985). They make compelling reading and seductively offer interpretations of the past which have considerable potential relevance to our situation today. We must undoubtedly treat them seriously, whilst at the same time recognising that they are as susceptible to bias as any other source of evidence, and in some respects more so. As we shall see they do not always reach the same conclusions.

Anthropological data are also a rich, appealing and intrinsically important source. As yet relatively few anthropological studies have focused specifically on sexuality (Malinowski 1929; Mead 1929, 1931; Herdt 1981; Marshall & Suggs 1971) and the scope for biased interpretation in such studies is obviously considerable. Much of the writing on cross-cultural comparisons has relied on the Human Relations Area File (e.g. Ford & Beach 1952; Barry & Schlegel 1980), a collection of information about 186 cultures which varies considerably in the amount of attention paid to sexual behaviour, and which has been gathered by a motley collection of observers whose sexual values and prejudices were probably highly influential (Broude & Greene 1980).

Our main sources of information are the various surveys of modern western societies. In 1965 Schofield was able to list 33 such surveys carried out in the previous 50 years. There have been quite a few more since and again their value is very variable.

Standing out from the others in terms of size and importance are the Kinsey reports on the male (Kinsey et al 1948) and the female (Kinsey et al 1953). These monumental studies, involving interviews with 5300 males and 5900 females, are not only the most comprehensive source of information available even to this day, but also provide a yardstick against which later studies may be compared. In the male volume, Kinsey did not report on attitudes to or satisfaction with sex. He believed that overt behaviour was the best indicator of a person's attitudes (Gebhard & Johnson 1979). Fortunately, in the female volume he did include some interesting information about attitudes and emotional reactions. Most later studies have assessed attitudes in addition to or instead of behaviour.

How valuable are these various surveys? What can we learn from them? In attempting to answer these questions, two principal issues arise: how representative are the samples (i.e. to what extent can we generalise from the findings?) and how valid is the information obtained? Before we look at the reported evidence, it is therefore relevant to consider a number of methodological issues which underlie its validity. (The reader less interested in this aspect may wish to omit the next section and turn to p. 211.)

METHODOLOGICAL ISSUES

The sample

Probability sampling has now become a sophisticated technique which allows generalisations to be drawn about a population from a small but appropriately selected sample. Such inferences are based on statistical principles rather than judgement. One starts with a defined population, e.g. an electoral register or general practitioner's list, and takes a random sample. In order to obtain geographical representation a small sample of localised areas may be randomly selected first, providing a number of limited populations for further sampling. Such sampling techniques are used with considerable precision for opinion polls and market research. In surveying sexual behaviour the task is not so easy. Defining the individuals in a probability sample is not the same thing as obtaining information from them. With such a sensitive topic as sex, a substantial refusal rate is to be expected. The higher it is, the less one is able to make statistically based inferences.

Kinsey started his work in the late 1930s at a time when probability sampling was in its infancy. He was in any case suspicious of random sampling methods and believed that the solution to sampling problems was to increase the size and diversity of the sample. Kinsey regarded himself as a taxonomist. Gebhard & Johnson (1979) describe him as a collector. He obtained his subjects by making contact with a wide variety of groups, e.g.

student groups, trade unions, religious groups, inmates of penal institutions etc. An attempt was then made to recruit as many of each group as possible. About one-quarter of his subjects came from '100% groups' (i.e. groups where every member was interviewed). This sampling method has been much criticised, although usually with accompanying praise for the overall importance of the work. The American Statistical Association set up a committee in 1950 to assess the first Kinsey volume (Cochran et al 1953), and various other thoughtful and authoritative critiques have been published (e.g., Hobbs & Lambert 1948; Terman 1948; Wallin 1949; Hyman & Barmack 1954). The main criticisms of the sampling, on which there was general agreement, were as follows:

1. A substantial proportion of the population, i.e. those not affiliated to organised groups, had no chance of being represented.
2. Nothing can be said about those who were not interviewed and it is a distinct possibility that in general they differed from the volunteers in their sexual attitudes or behaviour. Kinsey compared data from the '100% samples' and partially sampled groups and found little difference in a number of behavioural variables. However, we cannot conclude with confidence that groups in which 100% sampling was achieved were similar in the distribution of such responder variables to those where only partial recruitment was possible.
3. A substantial majority of the subjects came from Indiana, hence we should be cautious in generalising to the US population elsewhere, let alone to populations outside the USA.
4. Social class and educational attainment were represented disproportionately, e.g. three-quarters of the women came from the 13% of American women who had gone to college, while the 40% of American women who never went beyond eighth grade were represented by 3% of the study population. There were similar problems with age.

Gebhard & Johnson (1979) published a re-analysis of the Kinsey data with the addition of data collected since publication of the last report. It provides an interesting and previously inaccessible breakdown of the data as well as insights into the original method used. An attempt has also been made to 'clean' the data, by removing individuals who were derived from sources with known sexual biases. Most important is the exclusion of the substantial proportion of less-educated individuals who had been recruited from penal institutions or who had criminal records. It is now clear that as a group they differ in terms of sexual attitudes and behaviour from those never convicted. Although Gebhard & Johnson conclude that the major findings of the early work regarding age, gender, marital status and socio-economic class remain intact, these new figures are substantially different in many respects, particularly where the non-college educated subjects are concerned (see sections on masturbation, premarital intercourse and Chapter 6 on homosexuality, this volume). Throughout this book, wherever possible, this more recent report has been used in preference to the original Kinsey reports. In spite of the extensive and largely constructive criticism of the Kinsey sampling method, only limited progress has been made in improving sampling in subsequent studies. To some extent this reflects the substantial difficulties facing the researcher in this area. A number of studies have made serious attempts at probability sampling, however. The first, a study of English adolescents by Schofield (1965), used a variety of methods to identify local populations of teenagers, including GP lists, school attendance registers and use of a market research agency to locate teenagers in selective areas. Schofield then took random samples and contacted those who were selected. The non-response rate was 34%, but much of this was due to inadequacies in the original sample, with the teenagers having moved. A total of 15% clearly refused.

In 1971, Gorer reported a survey which used the English electoral register to draw a probability sample of 2000 men and women under 45 years of age. There was a 35% non-response rate, including 18% refusal, the remainder being unobtainable. Kantner & Zelnik (1972) obtained a national probability sample of the 15–19-year-old female population living in US households. In all, 92% were unmarried; there were 2839 white and 1400 black. The authors obtained another sample, differing in some sampling respects, in 1976 (Zelnik & Kantner 1977) which involved 1232 white and 654 black unmarried women in the same age group. In both samples there was a wide representation of social class. The refusal or non-response rates were not reported.

Sorensen (1973) reported a study of American adolescents in which a representative sample of 2042 households yielded a total of 839 adolescents. But by the time the consent of both the parents and the adolescent were obtained, only 393 could be interviewed (53% non-response rate). Frenken (1976), using the Dutch census, obtained a response from 500 married men and women with only a 15% non-response rate. Their sample was however predominantly broad middle-class.

In 1978, Farrell reported a British survey which obtained a sample of 16–19 year-olds from the electoral register. They identified 2100 teenagers, and were able to interview 74% of them — 16% refused and 10% were not available for interview. Garde & Lunde (1980) interviewed a small but representative sample of Danish women who were all aged 40. This was part of a larger study of general health in which 88% of women contacted through the Central Person Register participated. A subsample of these were invited to undergo the sexual interview, and 94% agreed, giving a total of 227 interviews.

Hagstad & Janson (1984) sent questionnaires to a random sample of 579 Swedish women in the 37–46 year-old age group and obtained a 77% response. Wyatt (1987) interviewed a stratified probability sample of Afroamerican & white American women (aged 18 to 36) with 126 and 122 in each group. Russell (1983) interviewed a probability sample of 930 married women in San Francisco: 19% of her selected cases refused to participate, and 17% of households would not give details of the occupants of the household. This gave a refusal rate of 36%. Add to those the women who were not at home or unavailable to be interviewed and the failure rate becomes 50%. This was a rigorous study and emphasises the difficulty of obtaining satisfactory samples.

Whilst the non-response in the Sorensen study makes it of uncertain value, the other studies have certainly achieved worthwhile samples.

Chesser (1956) asked English GPs to hand out questionnaires to their female patients. Approximately 6000 were completed, representing a response rate of between 30 and 40%. Chesser concluded, rather unconvincingly, that the biases affecting the GPs' choice of women were sufficiently varied to represent a random sample, but one must remain sceptical on this point. There was an obvious bias to the higher social classes.

Hunt (1974) started with some undefined random sample of names in 24 cities in the USA. These individuals were then contacted by telephone and asked to participate anonymously in small, private panel discussions of present trends in American sexual behaviour, for the benefit of a group of behavioural researchers. They achieved about 20% success. Having attended the group, the volunteers were asked to complete anonymous questionnaires. 'Motivated by the discussion and unwilling to walk out on the group, virtually 100% of the discussants completed usable questionnaires'. The powerful selection involved in such a recruitment method makes this sample of very dubious value in terms of representativeness. Pietropinto & Simenauer (1977) in their study of the American male used agents placed at booths in public places such as shopping precincts, airport lounges etc. They approached men and asked them to complete the questionnaire there and then. The criteria for selecting the men were not specified and it was estimated that approximately 50% of those approached cooperated. They obtained about 4000 participants.

Starr & Weiner (1981) handed out questionnaires to older people after talking to groups on the subject of love, intimacy and sex in the later years. They had 800 questionnaires returned — a 14% response. Blumstein & Schwartz (1983) in their survey of American couples appealed for participants through television, radio and the press. They responded to 22 000 requests for questionnaires. After selecting those with responses from both partners they ended up with 3574 married couples, 642 cohabiting couples, 957 gay male and 772 lesbian couples. They did not indicate what the response rate was. They selected 300 couples for indepth interviews.

A method gaining in popularity is to enclose questionnaires in magazines, asking the readers to return them anonymously. Such magazines include Psychology Today (Athanasiou et al 1970), Woman's Own (Chester & Walker 1979), Woman (Sanders 1985, 1987) and Nineteen (April 1980). The Hite Report (Hite 1976) comes into this category; early distribution was done through national mailings to women's groups of various kinds;

later distribution used magazines such as Oui, The Village Voice, Mada-memoiselle, Brides and Ms. Most of these surveys have produced very large numbers of respondents — Psychology Today more than 20 000; Woman's Own and Nineteen around 10 000 each. This usually means that a random sample of say 2000 of the respondents is used for the analysis. However, one is usually not told what proportion of the questionnaire distributed was returned. It is likely to be low. In Hite's survey, the return rate was only 3%. Furthermore, there is the additional selection factor resulting from the particular appeal of the magazine involved. Hite countered this to some extent by using a variety of magazines, but the population must still be seen as selected and excluding important sections of American women. Brecher (1984) used a slightly different approach in his survey of love, sex and ageing. He included an announcement in the monthly magazine Consumer Reports, inviting readers born before 1928 to apply for a questionnaire. More than 5000 requested 9800 questionnaires, of which 4246 were returned in usable form.

In only a few surveys can we therefore speak of representative samples; for the remainder, we will appraise their possible usefulness later. Let us first consider the validity of the information obtained in such surveys, irrespective of the representativeness of that sample.

The method

The most basic question about surveys into sexual behaviour is whether the information obtained has any validity. It would not be surprising if, with information as sensitive and confidential as this, people gave false accounts or strove for social desirability in their answers. Although this is difficult to prove, most researchers who are experienced in talking to people about their sex lives have the impression that they are prepared to be frank and honest, providing that they see a good reason for revealing such intimate information, and that they can trust the recipient to treat information revealed with respect and confidentiality. The main methodological question in trying to achieve these criteria is whether to use an interviewing method or a self-completed questionnaire. This issue is of course central to much of social and psychological research, and there is a substantial body of evidence of a general kind available. But sexual surveys do present special problems. Let us briefly consider the pros and cons of each approach.

The interview

The obvious *advantages* of obtaining information in a face-to-face interview are as follows:

1. It is possible to ensure that the questions are comprehended — the question can be phrased in more than one way, the subject's interpretation

can be checked and inconsistencies in answers given can be cross-checked. As a consequence, a wide range of information can be investigated by this means. As the interviewer can respond appropriately to the level of comprehension of the subject, a wide range of intelligence can be tackled and satisfactory answers are not so dependent on verbal ability or a facility for filling in forms.
2. It is possible to establish a good rapport with a subject and engender trust so that the subject feels that the information will be treated with respect. Obviously this can work both ways — a poor relationship between interviewer and subject may seriously impair the information obtained. A good relationship often means that the subject gains from having someone to talk to and confide in. As Gebhard & Johnson (1979) wrote of the Kinsey interviews: 'we did not distance ourselves from the respondent by assuming a coldly objective impersonal role . . . we presented ourselves as interested and sympathetic researchers'. The fact that not infrequently subjects gain emotionally from being able to discuss their feelings increases the likelihood that they will give honest answers whilst at the same time increasing the ethical justification for the research.

The main *disadvantages* of the interview method are:

1. It is extremely time-consuming for the researcher, particularly if the interviewer allows time to listen to what the subject wants to say rather than just concentrating on research items. Such allowance is necessary to ensure the good relationship needed.
2. The interviewer is obviously very susceptible to bias in the way questions are asked or answers interpreted. The Kinsey interview method has been criticised for the policy of 'placing the burden of denial (for sexual activity) on the respondent'. Whilst it may be easier for some people to admit to behaviour they regard as socially unacceptable when asked in this way, it may also be that some will feel the need to admit to behaviour in order to avoid sounding abnormal.
3. Anonymity is not possible, hence confidentiality of records becomes a major concern. Kinsey and his colleagues went to great lengths in dealing with this, memorising an extensive code and storing information which was incomprehensible to all but a handful of researchers.

The questionnaire

The main *advantages* are that:

1. Questions can be standardised, hence avoiding interviewer bias.
2. Information can be collected relatively cheaply with highly economical use of the researcher's time.
3. Anonymity is possible, rendering safeguards for confidentiality unnecessary.

The *disadvantages* are:

1. The impossibility of checking whether the proper meaning of the questions has been grasped. Although much can be done by careful design and piloting of questionnaires, there are nevertheless serious limits to the questions which can be asked about sex without ambiguity or misinterpretation. Some aspects of sexual response and behaviour are difficult to define in simple terms. Orgasm, for example, may require some explanation. Interest in sex is a concept sometimes taken to mean a spontaneous desire for sex and sometimes as enjoyment of sexual activity (see p. 416). In order to establish unambiguous response categories, there is also a tendency for questionnaires to become stark, insensitive or somewhat absurd in their wording (e.g. a question from the Sorensen (1973) questionnaire: 'number of different boys whose sex organs I have felt in the past month').
2. The method of answering often requires a level of sophistication in form-filling that is beyond large sections of the population.

For these various reasons, questionnaires tend to be more successful with the better educated.

It is of course possible to combine the advantages of both approaches. Thus Frenken (1976) ensured that a researcher introduced his questionnaire to the subjects, stayed with them until it was completed and answered any queries about meaning of questions or alternative responses. In our current research we rely on an interview during which we introduce questionnaires and self-rating items for those aspects which are more suited to that approach. It is nevertheless inevitable that any method that requires a researcher to be present, whether for interviewing or not, will be much more time-consuming and expensive to execute.

Kinsey and his colleagues had no doubts about the need for a lengthy face-to-face interview. The same conclusion was reached by Schofield (1965), Gorer (1971) and Farrell (1978). Zelnik & Kantner (1977) used a self-administered questionnaire to deal with the more sensitive questions during the interview of their first 1971 sample. For the 1976 study they relied on interviews throughout and concluded that the questionnaire had no obvious advantage. Clearly there are some aspects which are better dealt with by questionnaire, in particular questions about attitude which in view of the subjectivity need standard questions and answers (e.g. Frenken 1976). More research is needed to establish what information can effectively be obtained by questionnaire and which aspects need a sensitive, trained interviewer. For most of the studies cited, questionnaires appear to have been used for simple expediency, with little attempt to establish that this method was the most appropriate. When combined with the highly dubious sampling involved, this makes much of the evidence of very limited value.

HOW USEFUL ARE SURVEYS OF SEXUAL BEHAVIOUR?

Bearing in mind the methodological problems and short-comings we have just discussed, it is pertinent to ask how useful such surveys are. It is difficult to carry out a survey of any extent, even when methodologically unsatisfactory, without considerable expenditure of time and money. When is the cost justified? It is worth pointing out that financial reward must have figured as the main objective in many of these studies. When it was realised that the Kinsey reports, particularly the first volume on the male, provided some of the most indigestible reading material ever published but nevertheless became bestsellers, the sex survey was launched as a way of making money. Not all have been so successful (although The Hite Report was a bestseller) and there must be a point when the market becomes saturated, but obviously popular magazines see the cost of carrying out questionnaire surveys is commercially justified when they can present reports that have scientific respectability, albeit of a rather spurious kind. Presentation of data from such surveys to the scientifically unsophisticated population poses some ethical questions which we will discuss further below. Financial considerations apart, what other benefits can we look for?

1. Establishing norms for comparative purposes. Unless we have evidence of the prevalence of particular behaviours or attitudes in the population in general, it is difficult and often misleading to assess the significance of such prevalence figures in specific groups, such as those attending clinics of various kinds. This issue is discussed in relation to sexual problems in Chapter 8. We do lack good epidemiological evidence of the prevalence of sexual difficulties and there may be a tendency to assume that relatively high prevalence rates in specific groups are of more relevance than they really are.
2. Policy-making in education and health care. It is important in making policy decisions about sex education and the provision of contraceptive services to have some idea of the extent of sexual behaviour amongst young people. Obviously there is a need for good representative samples for this purpose, but precise figures may be less important than evidence of change or trends. A number of studies have used similar methods repeated after intervals of time, allowing some conclusions to be drawn about changing patterns of sexual behaviour in specific types of population. We will consider some of this evidence below.
3. Challenging false myths. The widely held view that 'normal' women experience orgasm during intercourse without additional physical stimulation is difficult to sustain with the evidence from various studies such as The Hite Report (Hite 1976) and Woman's Own survey (Chester & Walker 1979). Although the precise figures from these surveys mean very little, it is justifiable to conclude that large numbers, possibly the majority of women, normally require such additional stimulation. Information of this kind is therefore useful in reassuring patients.

4. Changing social attitudes. It is an ironic fact that public opinion is affected less by the scientific validity of the evidence put before it than by the political skill with which the evidence is used. Attitudes to human sexuality were almost certainly affected by the Kinsey reports, perhaps more readily because of their apparent dispassionate, non-judgmental objectivity. And yet as Robinson (1976) has pointed out, 'throughout the reports the reader was treated to an array of bleak moral posturings', mainly reflecting Kinsey's ethic of tolerance for the variety of sexual behaviour. Whatever scientific merit the Kinsey reports have, they were undoubtedly used by Kinsey, unwittingly or not, as propaganda devices. Gagnon & Simon (1973) have commented that sheer numbers are important in the decriminalisation of deviant behaviour. They cite the example of marijuana use; although the precise incidence of such use is not known, there is evidence that it is sufficiently large to make the anti-marijuana laws unenforceable. So, with homosexuality, it matters not whether the incidence is 5 or 10% but rather that very large numbers of people are involved.

The use of figures in this way is nevertheless a double-edged weapon. They can be used to support dubious causes or indiscriminately with little concern for ensuing effects. Thus the recent rash of surveys in popular magazines, selling copies as they obviously do but with very limited scientific validity, may have effects on public opinion which are difficult to foresee and not necessarily advantageous. There is reason to believe that such influence may have increased many people's dissatis-faction with their sex lives, without offering them any solutions.

5. Testing hypotheses about relationships between sexuality and other vari-ables. Eysenck (1976) emphasises the value of unrepresentative samples in his defence of his study Sex and Personality. Although he somewhat overstates his case, he has a valid point. In his questionnaire sample, which is about as unrepresentative as any, his prime purpose is to study the relationship between aspects of sexuality reflected in his question-naire and his own measures of personality, in particular neuroticism, extroversion and psychoticism. He asserts that his sample is sufficiently varied both in terms of sexuality and personality to allow these relation-ships to be investigated. The validity of associations observed in this way then needs to be established with replication using further samples. He studiously avoids drawing any inferences about the population incidence of these aspects of his data. It is noticeable how few of these surveys have built-in hypothesis-testing of this kind, when they could easily have done so. Nonetheless, the same principle can be used in drawing conclusions about the relationship between sexual behaviour and social class, educational attainment, religion, etc, as was done by Kinsey. As we shall see later in this chapter, however, the importance of replication of such conclusions is paramount. Much of the strength of Kinsey's assertions about the effects of social class has been weakened by the

'cleaning' of the data because of the marked distortion on the figures produced by his 'delinquent population'.

Thus, in spite of the difficulties in obtaining representative population samples, there is much to be gained by surveying sexual behaviour. Let us look at some of the available evidence. The evidence is largely confined to western countries, but we will consider some cross-cultural data if only to remind ourselves that the so-called civilised countries of the western world are very different in many respects to the second and third worlds.

The evidence will be considered under four headings:

1 masturbation;
2 premarital sex;
3 marriage;
4 sexual fantasy.

MASTURBATION

Self-stimulation to achieve sexual pleasure and orgasm is so effective and so widespread that one is tempted to ask why we bother with sexual partners. At least part of the answer lies in the negative attitudes to masturbation and other forms of non-procreative sex which have prevailed universally. Since the time of the Old Testament, people have argued as to whether the sin of Onan, for which he was severely punished, was masturbation or coitus interruptus (Genesis 38, 8–10). The attitudes to masturbation in different cultures and at different periods have usually reflected the general attitudes to sex at the time. Thus in ancient China, with its poetic mysticism, life was seen as a balancing act between the active and passive forces of yin and yang. Sex was an important example of this harmonious balance. The essence of sexual yang in the male was the man's semen, and that of yin was the woman's vaginal fluids. Whereas the latter were thought to be inexhaustible, the former was by contrast precious, needing to be maintained by a regular supply of yin (Tannahill 1980). Thus coitus reservatus was widespread and masturbation regarded as a waste of vital yang essence. Female masturbation was more or less ignored (Bullough 1976). In the Middle Ages, when venereal pleasure was only tolerated when associated with procreation, lust was regarded as a vice because, according to St Thomas Aquinas, 'it exceeded the order and mode of reason'. In Aquinas's league of sins against nature (i.e. non-procreative and hence sins against God), masturbation was the least serious, but it nevertheless carried heavier penalties than sexual sins against the person, such as adultery or even rape.

These two examples illustrate the two themes that have recurred in social attitudes to masturbation; first as a threat to health and secondly as a form of immorality. As religion gave way to medical science as the main influence on sexual standards in the late 18th and 19th century, these two themes became combined. Tissot's Onanism, or a Treatise upon the Disorder of Masturbation, used medical authority to declare that masturbation was a serious danger to be avoided. The threat to health appeared to be used to reinforce the traditional moral message. The idea of immorality in non-procreative sex has obvious biological implications on a social group struggling to maintain population size, as was undoubtedly the case during the Middle Ages. But it is impossible to judge the extent to which such basic biological advantages determine such social attitudes in the first place. More apparent has been the moral threat stemming from lack of sexual control. Procreative sex is tolerated because it would be difficult to do otherwise without offending God's plan, but perhaps it is the dignity and civilised status of man that is being primarily protected by such moral strictures, rather than the population size. Bullough (1976) has made the interesting suggestion that the reinforcement of repressive sexual attitudes which occurred in the late 18th century was a reaction not only to the period of sexual permissiveness that had preceded it, but also the anxieties engendered by the French Revolution: 'the emerging middle-classes of the 19th century seized upon sexual purity as a way of distinguishing themselves from the sexual promiscuity of the noble and the lower-classes'. Sex, he suggests, is a manifestation of the beast in man that appeared to surface in the bloodier aspects of the French Revolution. We will return to this theme later when considering changing attitudes to premarital sexuality.

The social significance of this fear of sexual excess and the uncontrolled aspect of human nature underlying it remains an issue of some importance. Now, when the biological advantages of discouraging non-procreative sex have not only disappeared but have been put into reverse, the conventional sexual taboos remain resistant to change in most cultures.

When considering the 'naturalness' of human behaviour, attention is often paid to the incidence of such behaviour amongst lower animals as well as more primitive cultures. Ford & Beach (1952) summarised much of the evidence for both. Masturbation occurs in many subhuman mammals, and male primates have been observed to induce ejaculation by such means, even in circumstances when coitus would have been possible. There is general agreement, however, that masturbation by female mammals is much less common and has rarely been observed to lead to orgasm.

In several primitive societies studied, there is evidence that masturbation occurs but in almost all cases the practice is frowned upon, usually on the grounds that it is an inferior form of sexual activity, only used by those who are unable to obtain a sexual partner. In one society, the Lesu Islanders, masturbation was apparently expected of women who became sexually excited but had no male partner available. What evidence do we have for the western world?

Our rather limited evidence concerning childhood and the role of masturbation in sexual development is considered in Chapter 3. Kinsey and his colleagues provide the most substantial data for adults. In the re-analysis

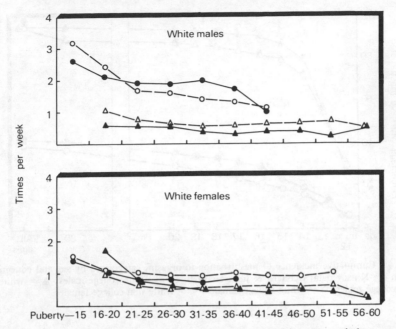

Fig. 4.1 Mean frequency of masturbation per week, categorised by age, marital status and education (for those who masturbate). From the Kinsey data; Gebhard & Johnson 1979. ○ = never married, college-educated; ● = never married, non-college educated; △ = married, college-educated; ▲ = married, non-college educated.

of the Kinsey data (Gebhard & Johnson 1979), 94% of men and 40% of women had masturbated to orgasm at some time in their lives. This is a somewhat lower proportion for women than had been originally reported (58%), presumably due to the 'cleaning' of the data described above. In the original report about 4% of women had masturbated without experiencing orgasm, whereas less than 1% of men came into this category.

The frequency of masturbation depends on the availability of alternative sexual outlets, particularly in men, as the difference between married and unmarried subjects shows in Figure 4.1. In the unmarried, for whom masturbation frequency is some measure of their level of sexual interest unconfounded by the sexual needs of a spouse, the frequency is highest (in those who masturbate at all) in the early teens for both males and females. Figure 4.2 gives the cumulative incidence (the percentage who had ever masturbated by a particular age), showing that by the age of 20 about 30% of women and 87% of men had already masturbated. The different pattern for men and women is apparent not only in the overall incidence but also the age of onset.

How do Kinsey's figures compare with other studies? The high percentage in men has been fairly consistent. Landis et al (1940) questioned 295 American women and found that 54% had masturbated at some time; the majority started during adolescence and ceased when heterosexual

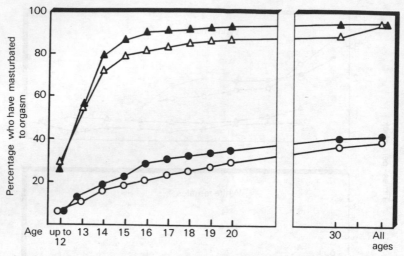

Fig. 4.2 Cumulative incidence of masturbation to orgasm, categorised by sex and education. From the Kinsey data; Gebhard & Johnson 1979. △ = White college males; ▲ = white non-college males; ○ = white college females; ● = white non-college females.

interest became predominant. In an earlier study, Davis (1929) reported that two-thirds of 1180 unmarried women with college education had masturbated at some stage in their lives, but many had never induced orgasm by this means. Hunt (1974), comparing his results with those of Kinsey, reported an increased incidence in frequency of masturbation, particularly amongst women. Whereas between 25 and 30% of the 16–25-year-old age group in Kinsey's study were masturbating, 60% of a similar age group in Hunt's study were doing so. There was also some evidence of increased frequency. Hunt also reported a greater frequency of masturbation amongst married men compared with Kinsey. However, as he did not give details of educational level or social class, and these proved to be powerful factors in Kinsey's data, this comparison is of dubious value. Garde & Lunde (1980) in their survey of 40-year-old Danish women found that 47% had masturbated at some time in their lives. The average age of onset was 18 years, ranging from 6 to 38 years.

In Hagstad & Janson's (1984) questionnaire survey of Swedish women of similar age, 64% had masturbated at some time, but for the majority this was infrequent. Only 8% masturbated once a week or more often. Masturbation was more common in single women, and women having infrequent intercourse tended to masturbate more frequently.

Sorensen (1973) in his study of American adolescents reported 43% of boys and 30% of girls masturbating between the ages of 13 and 15, and 70 and 42% respectively between 16 and 19 years. By comparison, Kinsey's figures (see Fig. 4.1) show incidences lower than Sorensen's for the boys and higher for the girls. Clement et al (1984) reported a comparison of West

German students in 1966 and 1981. In the earlier survey 89% of males had masturbated by the age of 20, in contrast to 46% of females. In 1981 the percentages were 92 and 73%. The age of onset of masturbation fell during this 15-year interval and the difference between males and females lessened considerably. Sex differences in the frequency of masturbation did not change however; although overall the frequency had increased over the 15 years, it remained twice as high for men as for women. Masturbation remains the form of sexual behaviour showing the greatest difference between the sexes, at least as far as West German students are concerned. Another change over time was an increase in masturbation as the first sexual experience for girls, and for masturbation to continue in the presence of regular sexual intercourse for both sexes. These authors concluded that greater heterosexual permissiveness is accompanied by more interest in masturbation.

In the Woman's Own survey (Chester & Walker 1979), 56% of women said they masturbated (14% often) and there was no obvious association with age. In the Nineteen survey (April 1980), the majority of respondents were in the 16–24-year age range (i.e. 77%) and mostly unmarried. In all, 52% said they masturbated to orgasm (15% quite often). In the Woman survey (Sanders 1985) two-thirds of unmarried and 56% of married woman said they masturbated, but frequency was not given. Many of them felt guilty about it. Thus these various figures, with all their limitations, do suggest that the proportion of women who masturbate at some stage of their lives has increased slightly, and that women are trying masturbation for the first time at an earlier age than they used to.

When one considers the negative attitudes to masturbation that prevail, it is not surprising to find that the frequency of masturbation in men is related to religious affiliation (Kinsey et al 1948) and is definitely less common among more devout women (Kinsey et al 1953). This association has been found in other studies and was still evident in West Germany students in 1981 (Clement et al 1984). More interesting is the effect of social class and educational level. This is most striking when one considers the incidence of masturbation in married men (see Fig. 4.1). The lesser educated show a much lower incidence, a difference which is apparent but less marked in women. Masturbation during marriage appears to be less acceptable to the lower socioeconomic groups. We have already mentioned the increased frequency of early masturbation by females in the higher educated group. Education level of the parents, however, had no relation to masturbation in the study of Clement et al (1984) of West German students. Also of interest are the reasons people give for worrying about masturbation. According to the Kinsey data, the college-educated are more likely to give moral reasons, while the non-college-educated report fear of mental or physical debility (Gebhard & Johnson 1979). This is relevant to our earlier discussion of the hypochondriacal and moralistic themes in attitudes against masturbation.

Techniques of masturbation

For the male by far the commonest method is manual stimulation. Other methods are used occasionally by many men and predominantly by a few. These include lying face down, making pelvic thrusts against a bed or pillow; use of a vibrator; holes in objects or water jets. A few men insert objects into their urethra and there are three or four men in Kinsey's sample who relied on self-fellatio, a technique which many men try to use but find anatomically impossible (Gebhard & Johnson 1979). For women, the principal method is direct stimulation of the clitoris, sometimes associated with the insertion of something into the vagina; 73% of Hite's women came into this category (Hite 1976). Other techniques, such as squeezing the thighs together, are used predominantly by a small proportion of women, although only 1–3% rely on inserting objects into their vaginas (Hite, 1976; Gebhard & Johnson 1979).

Orgasms which occur during masturbation do not appear to differ physiologically from those during sexual activity with a partner (Masters & Johnson 1966). The controversy over the possible subjective difference between clitoral and vaginal orgasms is discussed on p. 82. Any such difference, if real, is not related to masturbation per se, but rather the method of stimulation. Whether masturbation is as enjoyable as sexual activity with a partner is an even more complex question. According to Hite, many women enjoy masturbation physically but usually not psychologically. Her subjects described the experience as 'lonely, guilty, unwanted, selfish, silly and generally bad'. This, Hite believes, reflects the negative attitudes to masturbation; 'sex with a partner legitimises the activity, whatever it is, to call it masturbation demeans it'.

THE SIGNIFICANCE OF MASTURBATION

We must conclude that whereas masturbation is a common if not universal form of behaviour, it is usually regarded as undesirable and is an aspect of sexuality that causes embarrassment, particularly to the young. We have already discussed the possible origins of these various attitudes. It remains to be considered whether there are any rational grounds for regarding masturbation as undesirable as a private form of sexual activity. For the male it would be difficult to dispute that masturbation is perfectly compatible with normal sexual adjustment, and no convincing evidence has been presented to the contrary. There may be occasional cases where the habitual pattern of masturbation works against a good sexual relationship. A man seen by the author first learnt to masturbate with his adolescent peer group in a 'circle jerk'. He was extremely tense on the first occasion and thereafter would feel tense throughout masturbation. Presumably as a consequence he found ejaculation and orgasm unrewarding. In spite of this he masturbated at least once a day up to the age of 30. He found that his habitual tension and unrewarding orgasm also occurred during sexual intercourse with a partner. By cutting down his masturbation to once a week or less and practising relaxation in association with it, he obtained considerable improvement, both during masturbation and intercourse. Sometimes negative feelings concerning ejaculation are reinforced by masturbation — as in the man who ever since he started masturbating always ejaculated into the lavatory pan. It is not surprising that he found ejaculating into the vagina difficult. Such cases are the exception.

For women, claims that masturbation interferes with the capacity for orgasm during intercourse have been much more widespread. Kinsey, however, presented evidence that women who had experienced orgasm before marriage, usually by means of masturbation, were less likely to have orgasmic difficulty once married than those who had not experienced it previously. Once again, there are instances when the pattern of masturbation seems to have been a disadvantage. Women who have habitually used thigh adduction as a method of achieving orgasm may find the abduction during intercourse to be incompatible with orgasm. However, there is now an increasing tendency to encourage men and women with sexual problems to masturbate in order to overcome their difficulties and learn to let themselves go (see Chapter 10). Also, faced with the AIDS threat, greater attention is being paid to safe sex, both homosexual and heterosexual. Masturbation is likely to receive a boost from this campaign. How much such influences will reverse the predominantly negative attitudes to masturbation remains to be seen.

PREMARITAL SEX

Marriage in one form or another is a universal human institution. Forms of marriage vary considerably, as we shall see later, but in all cases some control over sexual behaviour is imposed. The term 'premarital' refers to the period of a person's life before marriage, including childhood and adolescence. We have already considered sexual behaviour during childhood in Chapter 3. Let us now consider the adolescent and young adult not yet married. It is this phase of the sexual lifespan that most clearly reflects the influence of social and religious factors.

CROSS-CULTURAL AND HISTORICAL ASPECTS

In their review of sexual behaviour in primitive societies, Ford & Beach (1952) divided their societies into three types:

1. restrictive societies in which sexuality outside marriage was generally discouraged;
2. semi-restrictive societies in which there were formal prohibitions which were not enforced with any vigour. Sexual behaviour amongst the unmarried was accepted provided it was in secret, but if pregnancy ensued marriage was expected;

3. permissive societies; in some cases the permissiveness applied to early childhood only, but often continued at least until marriage. Sexual activity between young people was expected, but once again, the occurrence of pregnancy was seen as an indication for marriage.

In a more recent anthropological analysis of the Human Relations Area File (HRAF), Broude & Greene (1980) examined 141 societies for which adequate information on premarital sexuality was available. They reported attitudes to premarital *female* sexuality (Table 4.1). Premarital sexual activity was regarded as uncommon for females in 43%, and for males in 31% of societies. According to Whyte (1980) a double standard for premarital sexuality was evident in 44% of cultures.

Table 4.1 Attitudes to premarital female sexuality (from Broude & Greene 1980)

Attitude to premarital sex	Percentage
Expected and approved; virginity has no value	24
Accepted if discreet	21
Mildly or moderately disapproved; virginity is valued	26
Disallowed except with bridegroom	4
Strongly disapproved; virginity is required (virginity tests, severe reprisals for non-virginity)	26

Societies also vary in their view of adolescence. In some cultures, such as our own, adolescence is a long period involving different expectations and responsibilities from both childhood and full adulthood. In other societies this period may be very short or only recognised as the occurrence of puberty, often marked by some puberty ritual, so that the child passes suddenly into adulthood.

Schlegel & Barry (1980) reviewed the HRAF data from 183 societies for cross-cultural evidence of adolescent initiation ceremonies. These occurred in a minority of the societies, at ages usually close to puberty, though ranging from 8 to 18 years. In 25% there were ceremonies for both sexes, in 21% only for girls and in 9% only for boys. For both sexes the major themes were fertility–sexuality and responsibility, but for boys responsibility was more important, and for girls fertility–sexuality clearly predominated. Same-sex bonding was a characteristic of 37% of boys' ceremonies, but of only 8% of girls' ceremonies, supporting the widely held assumption that men form same-sex bonds outside the kin circle much more than women do. Genital operations (e.g. circumcision, clitoridectomy) were involved in 32% of boys' and only 8% of girls' ceremonies, although other unpleasant or painful experiences were involved in 32% and 25% respectively.

In general, adolescent initiation ceremonies are more likely in societies which attach greater social significance to gender identity.

Another form of institution for regulating and influencing adolescent sexuality in some pre-industrial societies is the dormitory, where older children and teenagers are segregated as a group from their nuclear families.

The form and influence of such dormitories vary considerably however. Hotvedt (1988) contrasts the Sambian model (described by Herdt 1981) with that of the Munda of north-east India (described by Elwin 1968). The Sambian dormitory represents sexual segregation in an extreme form, with homosexual initiation of younger boys by older youths as a method of re-inforcing masculinity and male bonding, in a society in which heterosexual relationships are somewhat antagonistic (see p. 301). The Munda, on the other hand, have mixed-sex dormitories; they are similar in the respect that it is the older adolescents who are the sex educators, but in this case the education is in heterosexual behaviour and relationships. (The author's recollection of his own childhood in an English single-sex boarding school suggests to him that the dormitory model is not confined to pre-industrial societies, and that the traditional English version is closer to the Sambian than the Munda model!).

So we find a rich variety of patterns of attitudes and behaviour in relation to premarital sexuality. Hotvedt (1988) has reviewed the more recent attempts to account for these cultural variations. The important dimensions include the importance of wealth and inheritance, the degree of differen-tiation of sexual roles, sexual segregation and sexual stratification (i.e. when one gender group has greater access to rewards, prestige and power), and the complexity of social structure. Drawing from cultural materialism, Hotvedt explains how much of this variability can be accounted for by the level of social development. The contrast is between the hunter–gatherer society, now largely extinct (the !Kung of the Kalahari desert remain as one of the few surviving examples, much researched by anthropologists), and the pre-industrial agricultural society (i.e. with mechanised food production), with pastoral and horticultural societies falling in between. The hunter–gatherer society is characterised by nuclear families combining and co-operating as small residential groups. These are classless societies with egalitarian decision-making and restrictions on personal wealth and power. Horticultural and pastoral systems introduce the important compo-nent of wealth (either land or domestic animals). This dimension becomes of much greater importance in the agricultural societies, where because of relatively efficient food production by a minority, other productive roles can be developed, resulting in the elaboration of more complex social systems; this process was greatly amplified by the industrial revolution.

Thus we find that the hunter–gatherer society is the one most likely to be permissive towards premarital sexuality and the class-ridden agricultural society to be restrictive, as the need to protect lineage and the inheritance of wealth becomes more relevant.

This analysis combines an overview of relatively recent and existing pre-industrial societies with a historical perspective of human societies in general. It therefore provides us with a bridge to the ever-growing social history of western European society, as well as a relevant model for inter-preting some of the changes and variations we see there.

When considering the social history of sexual behaviour and marriage in Europe we have two dimensions to consider: one geographical, the other temporal. We find repeated indications that north (or perhaps more correctly north-western) and south (or south-eastern) Europe have different early sources of influence on this aspect of behaviour, perhaps exemplified by the Viking culture in the north and the Christian and Islamic cultures in the Mediterranean south. This divide becomes compounded by the religious divide after the Reformation, which in itself probably reflects this basic difference.

Temporally, there is a turning point, which by general agreement appears to be the latter part of the 18th century, in the early stages of the Industrial Revolution. Figure 4.3 shows the demographic evidence of a dramatic rise in both prenuptial pregnancy and illegitimacy *and* an associated fall in the age at marriage; this combination led to the extraordinary increase in birth rate which continued until the 1930s. Both Stone (1979) and Gillis (1985) have documented the associated changes in behaviour in Britain over this period. Gillis's account commends itself because of its greater attention to

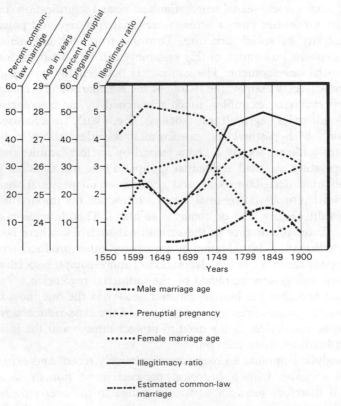

Fig. 4.3 Age of marriage, pre-nuptial pregnancy, illegitimacy, and common-law marriage in Britain 1550–1900. (Collected by Gillis (1985) from various sources)

the poorer classes, and the contrasts between the social classes. In pre-industrial Britain there was not only late marriage but predominant chastity amongst the unmarried. This was facilitated by the tendency for young people to live in with the families of their rural employers. Early hetero-sexual experience was dominated by what Gillis calls polygamous play: the innocent sexuality of the group that protects the young person from premature pairing. Courtship, once started, was highly ritualised, with betrothal the most important event. Sexual licence was given once betrothal was established, on the understanding that pregnancy would lead to marriage. This was a time of relatively high prenuptial pregnancy. Courting in rural Britain was of the 'bundling' or night-visiting variety, where it was assumed that the courting couple would spend time together at night, often in the girl's sleeping quarters. But sexual activity would usually be limited, epecially in the early stages of courtship. Hertoft (1977) has described this courtship pattern as typical of peasant communities in Scandinavia and northern Europe, also spreading to New England colonies in North America. According to his description, girls invited boys of their choice to spend the night with them. A traditional set of rules required them to keep all their clothes on initially but if the relationship flourished in other ways and familiarity increased, sexual activity would progress until full inter-course occurred. At this stage (it is not clear whether it was usually before or after first intercourse) the couple would announce their betrothal, often marrying once pregnancy resulted. This custom was still widespread in Nordic countries in the mid 19th century and may still be found occasionally in remote rural areas. Although there may have been variations on this theme, the important element was the graduated process of mate selection which preceded coitus and pregnancy, and the commitment associ-ated with coitus. There was a single standard of premarital sexuality (i.e. equal for boys and girls), applied within a clear set of rules and linked to betrothal and marriage. Such a society would be regarded as permissive according to our definition.

Then came the 'sexual revolution' with its dramatic changes between 1750 and 1850 which were apparent in almost every region of Europe and the USA. Shorter (1973) considered various possible explanations for this change, rejected an increase in fertility on the grounds that no such increase in birth rate applied to women over the age of 30, and concluded that there had been a dramatic increase in premarital sexual behaviour, a trend which in his view was predominantly amongst the urban working class. Gillis (1985) attributed a large part of this increase in illegitimacy in Britain to a simultaneous increase in the number of common-law unions, whose offspring would be recorded as illegitimate, rather than to desertion of the pregnant woman. These were times of important changes in attitudes to marriage in Britain, which can be seen as part of the complex evolution of values about both the individual and religion. Stone (1979) summarises this evolutionary process as follows. In the 16th century and earlier, the purpose of life was to assure continuity of the family, the class, the village or the state. Personal preference should always be subordinated to the common good. In the 16th and 17th centuries there was an increasing tendency to recognise the uniqueness of the individual, leading to competition, which required control by the power of the stern patriarchal family or the state. In the late 17th and 18th centuries the sense of individual uniqueness and pursuit of personal happiness was tempered by respect for the rights of others. Stone discusses the socioeconomic changes associated with this evolution of the human spirit. One crucial aspect was the growth of the wealthy bourgeoisie or middle class, who shared some of the political and social as well as economic power that had previously been in the hands of the landed gentry. It was this emerging class that espoused the new religious attitude, starting with Puritanism, that led to greater emphasis on *Holy* matrimony and hence the importance of personal choice in selecting one's spouse. This resulted in conflict with the continuing importance of patriarchal authority over marriage and a state of relative confusion over attitudes to mate selection, which we will consider in more detail later in the chapter.

Thus the Hardwicke Marriage Act of 1753, provoked by a steady increase in clandestine marriages in which young couples were evading the control of their parents over their choice of marriage partner, reflected a reactionary establishment attempting to stem the tide of change. The basis of marriage as a continuation of the family line and property was being undermined, as the rights of the individual took precedence. The Hardwicke Act required residential qualifications, including banns, and strict parental consent for anyone aged under 21. At the same time it brought to an end the binding effect of the betrothal, and paved the way for a flourishing business in cross-border weddings in Scotland where the law was different.

Around that time there were other factors encouraging early marriage, particularly amongst the poor. Poor relief discriminated against single men and women and employment was easier to obtain for the married or co-habiting couple who were seen more or less as two for the price of one. The agricultural workers, who previously had 'lived in' at the employers' household in circumstances favouring celibacy, were now expected to fend for themselves in the community with various encouragements to sexual activity.

The married couple, whilst benefiting from the work input of younger teenage children, would nevertheless need to encourage them to leave the home once they were of marriageable age. A pregnancy became a means of securing a marriage or parish maintenance. From Gillis's (1985) account we see clearly the separation of sexual values of the poor working class, who had no property to protect or pass on to their children, and for whom fertility was important for several reasons, from those of the propertied classes who were still intent on protecting lineage and appropriate inheritance of wealth, and eventually the bourgeoisie who strove to establish a foundation for the family based on the work ethic and Puritan values. Thus we see the origins of the profound influence of social class on sexual behaviour which was still very much in evidence when Kinsey carried out his surveys. Furthermore, from the mid 18th century we see the affluent classes attempting to impose their standards on the rest of society with varying degrees of success. Gillis, somewhat contrary to Shorter (1975), saw the vanguard of this changing sexual morality in the countryside rather than the city. In his view the more traditional objectives of marriage, with the couple waiting until they had accumulated enough material possessions and income to provide a secure basis for family life, prevailed for longer in the city where perhaps the opportunities for such self-improvement were greater. Prostitution, on the other hand, flourished in the cities.

By the early Victorian era the cities had changed places with rural areas in terms of early marriage. By then the full impact of the Industrial Revolution and of the new middle class could be seen. Somehow during this period the double standard of sexual morality became established not only across Europe but also across the social classes.

Schmidt (1977) drew an interesting comparison between the views of Shorter, an American, and van Ussell, a Belgian historian of Marxist persuasion. Industrialisation, according to van Ussell, resulted in small social groups becoming less self-sufficient and more dependent on each other, an extension of the process described earlier as societies developed from the hunter–gatherer to the agricultural model. Discipline as a guarantee for complicated social interaction became the value of the emerging bourgeoisie. 'The body was transformed from an organ of pleasure to an organ of achievement'. Body function, including sex, became something to be concealed. Nudity became unacceptable. Expressions of feelings became inhibited, and keeping oneself under control was regarded as a moral virtue. A parallel with these changes was the breakdown of large family groups, with people becoming more private in their habits, particularly when affluent. Premarital sex became forbidden, a taboo that was almost certainly effective amongst bourgeois girls. However, the more people struggled against sexuality, the more the environment became sexualised. The combination of sexual preoccupation and taboo led to a dissociation between love and sexuality that previously had been combined so effectively in the 'bundling' scene. Men started to exploit female partners from a lower social class or increasingly through prostitution. The double standard and all the negative consequences of human sexuality for the role of women had arrived — or at least returned. Schmidt concluded that whereas the bourgeois girl was protected by strict parental control, the working-class girl was, as a result of industrialisation and urbanisation and the relative collapse of the family as a close community, deprived of the security of the 'bundling' system. At the same time, she fell victim to the uncaring, exploitative sexuality of the dominant double standard male.

This analysis has however assumed that prior to industrialisation and urbanisation the relatively permissive Nordic system was the norm. Schmidt, based in West Germany, is perhaps more familiar with the northern Europe pattern, and as we shall see later, the double standard receded first in north Europe. But Mediterranean societies probably had a repressive system of much longer standing; the tradition of the virgin bride (enforced by strict chaperonage) and the dowry dates back to ancient Chaldean, Jewish and other codes (Kinsey et al 1953) and is still very much in evidence in rural Italy today (Littlewood 1978). In such systems, the importance of virginity and the associated dowry places the woman as a form of property, handed over from one man (i.e. the father) to another. Such a double standard, which is also evident in many modern machismo cultures in the Latin American world, is less easily attributable to industrialisation and more to the deep-rooted dominance of the male. We are therefore left with an important gap in our understanding of this aspect of European history. Did the virginity ethic spread to northern Europe, at least as far as the propertied classes were concerned, becoming more socially spread as industrialisation took its toll? Or have such values always been present when wealth and property are involved, as our earlier anthropological summary had hinted? As far as Britain is concerned we must take into account its peculiarly deep class divisions. And in the USA we are now seeing the results of a mixture of very different cultural backgrounds in which the Nordic, Mediterranean and Afroamerican all play a part.

When we consider modernisation in other parts of the world an even more varied historical background influences the situation. In Africa, many of the old traditional values prevail but migration and urbanisation are leading to a weakening of their effects (Sai 1978). Muslim countries typically maintain powerful restrictions on premarital sexuality. To a large extent this has been possible because of early marriage for girls. The disadvantages of such early marriage, both in terms of overpopulation and reduction in women's status, are considerable. Many countries are combating this by raising the minimum legal age for marriage (Farman-Farmaian 1978) but the taboos on premarital sex remain strong. The severity of penalties for breaking such taboos are being demonstrated with depressing frequency since the Islamic revolution of 1978 in Iran. The adaptation of migrant Iraqi Muslims to the sexual mores of Israel was reported by Klausner (1964), though this acculturation was more noticeable for the Iraqi male than female. Evidence of what is happening to sexual norms in Russia is hard to come by and since the Revolution, the picture to the outsider has been somewhat confused (Murstein 1974). Visitors to China are usually impressed by the apparent desexualisation of young people in spite of a relatively late age of marriage (Money 1977). Certainly strong social discouragement of unplanned or excessive fertility appears to have had striking effects, but what has happened to the sexual feelings and experience of the premarital Chinese between puberty and the late 20s remains a mystery to the westerner, though it may not be so different to the picture that Gillis (1985) painted for Britain in the 16th century.

We must therefore avoid any tendency to oversimplify the historical and sociological antecedents of the present situation. But we have no difficulty in recognising the historical precedents for the association between premarital (and marital) sexuality and social class.

THE INCIDENCE OF PREMARITAL INTERCOURSE IN THE 20TH CENTURY

Several writers (e.g Bell 1966; Reiss 1969) have concluded from the available evidence that after a significant increase in premarital sexuality in the

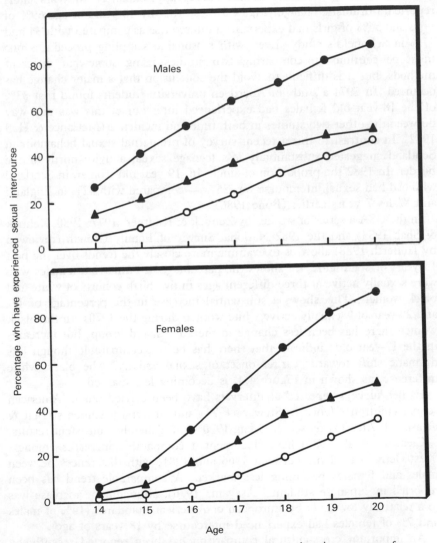

Fig. 4.4 Cumulative incidence of sexual intercourse amongst American teenagers from 1938–1963. From the Kinsey data; Gebhard & Johnson 1979.
○ = White college youths; ● = black college youths; ▲ = white non-college youths.

1920s the picture remained relatively stable until the 1960s. Since then, as we shall see, there have been further major changes.

The Kinsey data in its re-analysed form covers the period from 1938–1963 (Gebhard & Johnson 1979). The incidence of premarital intercourse amongst teenagers is given in Figure 4.4, showing the striking difference between blacks and whites and between educational groups. We will return to these sociological aspects later.

Schofield's (1965) survey of British teenagers of the early 1960s found an incidence comparable to that of the whites in Kinsey's study (Fig. 4.5A). Farrell (1978), in a further British survey approximately 10 years later, reported a dramatic change (Fig. 4.5B), so that by 18 years of age 69% of boys and 55% of girls had experienced intercourse as compared with 34 and 17% in Schofield's study. Even with reasonable sampling procedures one must be cautious in comparing two studies using somewhat different methods, but it is difficult to avoid the conclusion that a major change has occurred. In 1971 a study of Aberdeen university students found that 33% of the 18-year-old females had experienced intercourse; this was mid-way between the other two studies in both time and incidence (McCance & Hall 1972). In contrast to this a recent survey of premarital sexual behaviour in Scotland suggested substantially less teenage sexual activity north of the border. In 1982 the proportion of single 16–19 year-old women in Scotland who had had sexual intercourse was 26% — compared with 42% in England and Wales 7 years earlier (Bone 1986).

In the USA a series of studies by Zelnick & Kantner (1977; 1980; Zelnick & Shah 1983) and the 1982 National Survey of Family Growth (reviewed by Hofferth 1988) allow us to examine more closely the trends over the past 15 years or so. Figure 4.6 shows the percentage of unmarried females who were sexually active at three different ages in five birth cohorts of white and black women. This shows a substantial increase in the percentage of 17- and 20-year-old sexually active white women during the 1970s. In the black women there has been less change in the 20 year-old group, but increases in the 17-year-olds indicate that there has been a comparable though less dramatic shift towards earlier onset of sexual activity. The black–white difference, as shown in Figure 4.4, is becoming less marked.

Earlier surveys repeated at intervals have been carried out in American school children (Vener & Stewart 1974) and university students (Bell & Chaskes 1970; Christensen & Gregg 1970) with generally consistent results.

Clement et al (1984) have documented comparable increases amongst West German students between 1966 and 1981, with differences between males and females becoming less marked. A comparable trend has been reported in Japanese students (Asayama 1976), although the increase was to a relatively low level by European or American standards (14% of males and 7% of females had experienced intercourse by 18 years of age).

An important cross-cultural comparison has been reported recently by Jones et al (1985), and we will be considering this study in more detail later in the chapter. The comparable figures for premarital sexual experience in six countries is shown in Figure 4.7. This universal trend has been noticeable since the mid 1960s; it accelerated most rapidly during the 1970s and has probably levelled off during the 1980s.

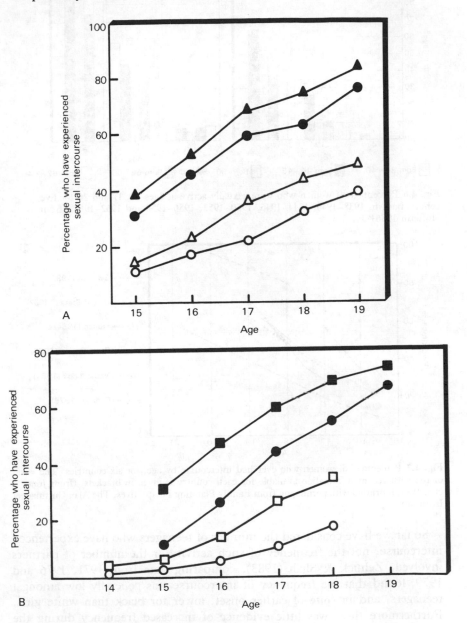

Fig. 4.5 Cumulative incidence of sexual intercourse, by age, amongst UK teenagers for A. 1964 and B. 1974. (from Schofield 1965 (A) and Farrell 1978 (B))

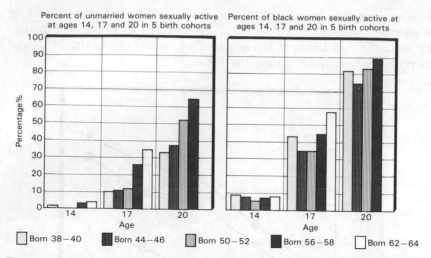

Fig. 4.6 Percentage of women who were sexually active at ages 14, 17 and 20 for five cohorts born in 1938–1940, 1944–1946, 1950–1952, 1956–1958 and 1962–1964. (from Hofferth 1986)

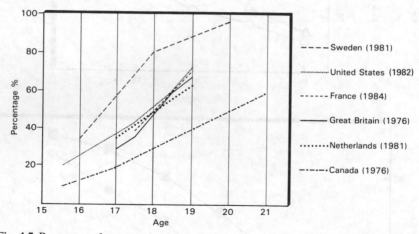

Fig. 4.7 Percentage of women who ever had intercourse by age, for six countries. The year of the most recent information available for each country is given in brackets. (from Jones et al 1985, reprinted with permission from Family Planning Perspectives, The Alan Guttmacher Institute)

So far we have considered the number of teenagers who have experienced intercourse, not the frequency of such activity or the number of partners involved. Zelnick & Shah (1983), comparing data from 1971, 1976 and 1979, found that the frequency of intercourse was generally low amongst teenagers, and in spite of earlier onset, lower for black than white girls. Furthermore there was little evidence of increased frequency during the period under study. Frequency of sexual activity during the previous 3 months was assessed in the 1982 National Survey of Family Growth (Hofferth 1987), as shown in Table 4.2.

Table 4.2 Frequency of sexual activity in the previous 3 months in unmarried white and black women (from the 1982 National Survey of Family Growth; Hofferth 1987)

	White		Black	
	Age 15–19	Age 20–24	Age 15–19	Age 20–24
No sexual intercourse in past 3 months	20.7	27.8	9.5	15.0
Once a month	12.4	14.5	30.8	12.6
Two to three times a month	24.1	20.5	27.2	29.8
Once a week	21.6	17.0	17.4	21.3
More than twice a week	17.6	19.3	12.3	18.8
Daily	3.6	0.9	2.7	2.5

Clement et al (1984) found a modest increase in frequency in their German students. The mean monthly frequency for males was 6.6 in 1966 and 9.4 in 1981; for females it was 2.4 and 3.5 respectively.

As far as number of partners in concerned, Zelnick & Shah (1983) found that of 15–19-year-old sexually experienced women in 1979, half of the white and two-fifths of the black women had only had one partner, whilst 9% of the white and 5% of the black women had had six or more partners. This represents a fall in the number with only one partner, an increase in the number with two or three partners, and no real change in the proportion with many partners. The West German students reported more partners. In 1981 42% of both men and women had had more than six partners, compared with 27% for men and 14% for women in 1966. There was also an increased tendency to engage at least occasionally in sexual relations outside the steady relationship — with women in 1981 showing as much if not more infidelity than men — a further example of the disappearing sex differences in the sexuality of West German students. Clement et al (1984) have interpreted this trend as a reduction in the double standard and in the importance of virginity. Whether the double standard has receded to the same extent in Britain or the USA is not so clear. Schofield (1965) found that although fewer girls than boys were sexually experienced, those who were had intercourse more frequently but with fewer partners than boys. In other words, the pattern of female teenage sexuality was more linked to stable relationships than it was for boys. In the USA Bell & Chaskes (1970) found that engagement (i.e. betrothal) was becoming less of a prerequisite of premarital intercourse in their female subjects. But in a later study in the USA half of women were going steady with or engaged to their first sexual partner, compared with only two-fifths of white and one-fifth of black men. But there are some reasons to believe that we are moving in the same direction as West Germany, and away from the double standard which reinforces so much that is bad about male–female relationships and sexuality in our society. Although we are seeing a shift from premarital monogamy to serial premarital monogamy there is no evidence of any major increase in promiscuity (i.e. of having a number of casual sexual relationships) amongst teenage girls.

Other forms of premarital sexual activity

Most teenagers engage in 'necking' (i.e. kissing and caressing of breasts and above) and 'petting' (i.e. including genital caressing with or without orgasm) before they first experience intercourse. In Kinsey's sample 46% of the women first experienced orgasm in a heterosexual relationship whilst petting (Kinsey et al 1953). As we shall see later, there have been striking social class differences in the extent to which teenagers engage in non-coital sexual behaviour. Kinsey discussed the moral and religious objections to petting as a form of non-procreative sex, whilst stressing the universal occurrence of non-coital genital stimulation amongst mammalian species (Kinsey et al 1953).

It is possible, though not as yet demonstrated, that as recognition and concern about the level of teenage coital activity grows, so a more positive and accepting public attitude to non-coital forms of premarital sexual activity may emerge. This is a likely consequence of the fear of AIDS.

Of particular interest are the changing trends amongst the unmarried in oral sexual activity (i.e. fellatio — oral stimulation of the penis — and cunnilingus — oral stimulation of the vulva). In the Kinsey surveys oral sex was more or less confined to males and females who were already coitally active — and the more active, the more likely they were to engage in oral sex. In 1967, some 20 years later, Gagnon & Simon (1987) found a doubling in the proportion of coitally active unmarried males and females who had experienced oral sex (from 45 to 80% for females), but still it remained a behaviour that occurred *after* regular coitus had been established. More recently, in a 1982 survey of schoolchildren (Newcomer & Udry 1985), there was an appreciable minority of virgin boys (25%) and girls (15%) who had given or received oral–genital stimulation, though in this study cunnilingus was more frequently reported than fellatio. We can thus conclude that not only has oral sex become more accepted as a form of premarital sexual interaction, it is also beginning to occur as a precursor of coital sex.

Social class

Kinsey's data indicate a striking social class difference for teenage sexuality which was also apparent in the sexual play of children (see Chapter 3). Working-class adolescents were more likely to experience sexual intercourse and at an earlier age than those from the middle classes. Conversely, middle-class adolescents were more likely to participate in sexual activity other than coitus (e.g. heavy petting, mutual masturbation and oral sex).

Schofield (1965) found broadly similar associations, particularly for the boys. His middle-class girls were much more likely to have experienced genital stimulation short of intercourse than the working-class girls, though the proportions with experience of intercourse were similar.

Schmidt and his colleagues have paid particular attention to social class differences by comparing young workers with students in West Germany. In their first study of 20-year-olds carried out between 1966 and 1968, they found a striking social class difference in sexual experience (Schmidt & Sigusch 1971). Whereas 81% of the male workers had experienced coitus by the age of 20, only 44% of the male students had done so. This difference had been evident from the age of 13 onwards, the workers showing two to four times higher incidence at each age. Similarly, for the females, 83% of the workers and 33% of the students had experienced coitus, a difference also maintained throughout adolescence. On average, the workers, both male and female, started their sexual careers about 4 years earlier than the students (though it should be remembered that they also married earlier so that the duration of the premarital sexual activity was not so different). There was also a social class effect on the sex difference in number of sexual partners. The male workers had experienced sex with more partners than the female workers. This difference was not marked for the students. We will return to this point when further discussing the double standard. The pattern of sexual activity other than coitus also showed class differences similar to those reported by Kinsey. The students were more likely to report manual–genital and oral–genital contact as well as nudity during love-making than were the workers, who were more likely to limit their activities to coitus proper.

Schmidt & Sigusch (1972) went on to reveal striking changes in this pattern between 1962 and 1970. This was mainly in the higher education group. By the age of 17, male and female schoolchildren in the Gymnasium stream (i.e. pre-university) had had as much sexual experience as students born 8 years earlier had had by the age of 20. Thus the striking social class difference in age of onset of sexual activity had largely disappeared. Conversely, the lower educational group were now experiencing more non-coital forms of sexual activity. In general, Schmidt & Sigusch found that girls were starting their sexual careers with much more positive attitudes, more enjoyment, less guilt and less under pressure from their partners than had previously been the case.

This lessening of social class differences may also be happening elsewhere (see review by Fisher & Byrne 1981). Kantner & Zelnick (1972) found little social class differences in their American teenager females except for the blacks, where poverty was associated with earlier sexual experience. Unfortunately, they did not comment on these associations for their 1976 sample. Farrell (1978) still found differences between working-class and middle-class boys in the UK, however, suggesting that the change noticed in West Germany may not be general in Europe. More recently, McCabe & Collins (1983) found no effect of social class on the dating behaviour of Australian adolescents.

In spite of the almost universal nature of the trends reported above, we should not expect the speed or pattern of change to be uniform and it is probable that the determinants of change will vary according to the culture involved. Schmidt considers that West Germany is becoming more like the Scandinavian countries in losing the double standard for premarital sexuality, in reinforcing permissiveness with affection (the romantic love ideology) and in allowing teenage girls to approach sex with the same positive attitude as their boyfriends. Scandinavian countries probably made this change somewhat earlier (Linner 1967). Changes in the USA are perhaps slower and more complex, reflecting the rich cultural mix that makes up American society. The Mediterranean virginity ethic is probably much more deeply rooted in large sections of the US population than was ever the case in northern Europe. The UK is probably different again, though one might expect it to have more in common with other north European countries than with the USA as a whole.

A serious attempt to analyse the various factors contributing to these widespread trends would be a major sociological exercise of great complexity and well beyond the scope of this book. Bury (1983) has pointed to a variety of cultural factors, including changing attitudes to premarital sexuality, changes in parenting behaviour, rising incidence of marital breakdown, lessening influence of religion, influences of the media and product advertising and peer group pressures, as well as biological factors in the form of earlier sexual maturity and fertility. Also to be taken into account are socioeconomic factors and the availability of modern methods of fertility control.

Let us briefly consider a few of these issues under three headings:

1. The virginity ethic.
2. The role of fertility — both these dimensions were related earlier to the differing historical cultural backgrounds of northern and southern Europe.
3. The influence of the family.

THE VIRGINITY ETHIC

The importance of virginity of the woman at marriage has, as was previously mentioned, been linked with the property rights of men over women, a pattern which has a long tradition in Mediterranean countries in particular (Kinsey et al 1953). The sociobiological view is that men prefer chaste women in order to ensure their paternity (Daly & Wilson 1978). (We will need to consider this point further when discussing extramarital sex.) Whereas the basic economic implications of the bride price and dowry may have largely disappeared except in ritualistic form, the importance of 'owning' the woman for the self-esteem of many men has not lessened. By the same token, 'scoring' with women represents a method of asserting dominance over other men, the so-called 'homosocial' form of sexuality discussed in Chapter 3. It has been suggested that such supports for the self-esteem of men will be used less frequently as alternative sources of self-esteem gain in importance. Thus in modern urban societies both the virginity ethic and the homosocial exploitation of women have been somewhat more marked amongst the lower socioeconomic groups (Gagnon & Simon 1973). Although, according to Schmidt (1977) the social class distinction is disappearing, this form of exploitation is now most noticeable amongst the more deprived unstable working class. Whyte (1943) provided a vivid picture of this in his description of adolescence in an Italian slum of an American city. Whereas promiscuity carried high prestige for the boys, promiscuous girls were generally scorned. Girls sought either to be virgins who were highly respected, or 'one-man girls' going steady. If the latter got pregnant, she would marry. For the promiscuous girl, marriage was most unlikely within that community. Thus according to this analysis, the machismo attitude to adolescent sexuality is more likely to survive in conditions of socioeconomic deprivation when the male may have little else to boost his morale. Schmidt's view of change away from this amongst the stable working class is therefore an encouraging one, although he has perhaps played down the extent to which traditional working-class attitudes to male/female roles may still take their toll once the couple enter marriage.

Another product of the double standard is female prostitution. Available evidence indicates that young men are much less likely to resort to prostitutes than they used to, and prostitution is increasingly serving the needs of those with abnormal sexual interests. The apparent increase in the popularity of massage parlours is an interesting development. The system would appear to provide both the customer and the proprietor with an alternative to prostitution in which, if the circumstances seem right, sexual gratification can be paid for and obtained. This may be one way of avoiding some of the stigma currently associated with prostitution (Armstrong 1978). Fear of AIDS is also likely to have a major impact on prostitution.

The black American

The black American requires special consideration. The figures already given show a striking difference between blacks and whites which has persisted. The gap in terms of adolescent sexuality may be narrowing simply because the black population has more limited scope for increase. If the double standard is fostered by social deprivation, then black Americans should have more than their fair share. Kantner & Zelnick (1972) found by controlling the socioeconomic variables, such as educational level of parents and poverty, that the black–white difference persisted, making a simple socioeconomic explanation unlikely. Wyatt (1987) has suggested that the ethnic differences in the earlier studies may have been exaggerated by inadequate control of relevant demographic characteristics. In her well controlled study of black and white Californian women reporting retrospectively on their adolescence she found a difference, though less marked than in earlier studies.

Obviously the ethnic or cultural differences towards sexual permissiveness should also be considered. Reiss (1964) found that whereas church attendance was a good indicator of sexually non-permissive attitudes amongst American whites (especially women), this was not the case with blacks. A comparable though less marked ethnic difference in relation to church attendance was reported by Kantner & Zelnick (1972). The origins of such ethnic differences have been the cause of bitter controversy in the USA and it is clearly desirable to avoid over-simplification. Nevertheless, there is no reason to assume that the black American is any less subject to cultural tradition than, say, American Italians, and there is likely to be interaction between such factors and current socioeconomic forces. Homosocial determinants of black adolescent sexuality need not be any different to those affecting whites, but there appears to be a different attitude to virginity which may reflect the earlier impact of slavery on the black American and the resulting systematic weakening of the family structure. Visotsky (1969) described the attitudes to adolescent sexuality amongst blacks in a deprived area of Chicago. It was assumed that every girl would have sexual relations, whether married or not, and if this did not happen by the age of 18 or 19, then there was something wrong with her. Boys not only gained in status by demonstrating their potency, but also by fathering children. 'Girls seek to please boys by having babies' was the attitude, even though the girl was expected to take responsibility for the offspring. Although lip service was paid to the undesirability of pregnancies out of wedlock, illegitimate children were usually accepted by the girls' mothers.

THE ROLE OF FERTILITY

In the early northern European pattern of premarital sexuality, the so-called 'bundling' system, pregnancy was expected to lead to marriage and in many respects was required in order to demonstrate the young woman's fertility. To what extent does fertility, or the need to demonstrate it, influence modern premarital sexual behaviour?

The first issue to be considered is the relevance of adolescent *infertility*. Humans and some of the higher primates are typically infertile for a period of time following puberty. Ford & Beach (1952) mentioned several permissive societies where premarital intercourse was usual for periods of 2 to 3 years, but pregnancy unusual. A more recent study of the !Kung, hunter–gatherers of the Kalahari desert, found that menarche and marriage occur at the age of $15\frac{1}{2}$ years, whereas the average age for bearing the first child is $19\frac{1}{2}$ years (Kolata 1974). Short (1976) suggested that in man and other primates who rely on pair-bonding a period of adolescent sterility may be important for allowing proper sexual learning and mate selection to occur, free from the complications of early pregnancy. Short also comments that the human female is the only primate in which full breast development occurs at puberty, rather than at the time of first pregnancy. This, he suggests, is to allow sexual attractiveness to develop in advance of fertility. Thus one way of looking at adolescent sexuality is that it is a biologically important stage of sexual development protected by adolescent sterility. The converse is that it may be particularly important to prove fertility after a period of infertile sexual activity. It must be also taken into account that over the past 100 years or so age at menarche has declined in most developed countries. In 1900 the average age was probably around 14 years, and it has declined steadily since, levelling off in the past decade and will probably stabilise around 12.5 years (Tanner 1962). This has been associated with a reduction in the age of first fertility, though it is important to remember that there is, and always has been, considerable individual variability in the interval between menarche and fertility. In 1970 it was calculated that 94% of girls were fully fertile by 17.5 years. By contrast, it has been estimated that in 1870 only 13% would have been fully fertile at that age (Bury 1983). Earlier menarche may also mean earlier onset of sexual responsiveness, although according to Kantner & Zelnick (1972) the association between age at menarche and onset of sexual activity was only evident in their black teenagers. And Udry et al (1986) have shown that the onset of coital activity in white girls is determined more by social than biological influences, whereas puberty was the main determinant with the black girls (see p. 170). Nevertheless if we give any credence to the sociobiological importance of adolescent infertility, it is clear that adolescents of today will need to exploit it at an earlier age.

Teenage pregnancies

In Britain, since 1938, when statistics of the age of mother at birth started to be recorded, the birth rate amongst teenagers has risen, reaching a peak in the early 1970s and then showing an unsteady decline since. Trends in abortion have been substantially altered by the legal availability of the procedure, and meaningful statistics have only been vailable since 1968, when the Abortion Act was implemented.

The incidence of teenage pregnancies is impossible to establish precisely because of the unknown number of spontaneous abortions, which are probably more frequent in this age group. However, a combination of births and abortions gives us a fairly close estimate. In England and Wales there has been a decline in teenage pregnancies over the past 15 years.

An important cross-cultural study of teenage pregnancy has been carried out by the Alan Guttmacher Institute in the USA (Jones et al 1985), prompted by evidence of disturbingly high levels of teenage pregnancy (Dryfoos 1978). The authors first considered a number of socioeconomic indices and their relationship to adolescent fertility in 37 developed countries. They found that teenage child-bearing was *positively* associated with a measure of low socioeconomic status (i.e. the proportion of the workforce employed in agriculture) and with the level of maternity benefit. On the other hand, birth rates were lower in countries with more liberal attitudes to sex, and with more equitable distribution of income. The USA, with its high levels of teenage pregnancy, partially fitted this pattern, being less open about sex and having less equitable income distribution than most countries. But it did not fit the pattern by having much higher socioeconomic status than other countries with comparable teenage birth rates.

This contrast was studied further in a more detailed comparison of six

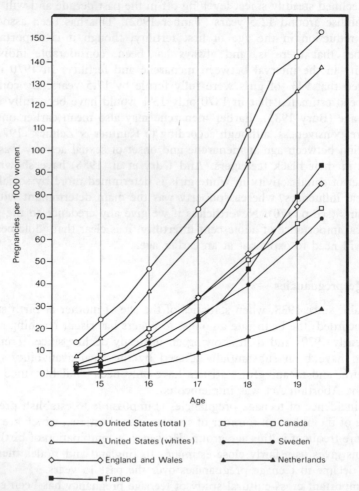

Fig. 4.8 Teenage pregnancies in seven countries. (from Jones et al 1985, reprinted with permission from Family Planning Perspectives, The Alan Guttmacher Institute)

countries, all highly developed socioeconomically; the countries were the USA, Canada, England and Wales, France, Sweden and the Netherlands. A comparison of the level of teenage sexual activity is shown in Figure 4.7, though this must be treated with caution because of the different times and methods of collecting the data. Nevertheless the median age at first inter-course appears to be similar for the USA, the UK, France and the Netherlands — just under 18 years — whereas for Sweden it is about 1 year younger, and Canada 1 year older. Teenage pregnancy rates (births plus abortions) in 1981 for the six countries are shown in Figure 4.8; the USA rates are dramatically higher, especially for the younger teenagers, while the Netherlands show noticeably lower rates for all ages. Dutch women aged 19 have the same likelihood of getting pregnant as 15–16 year-old Ameri-cans. It is therefore clear that these differences in teenage pregnancies cannot be attributed to differences in the level of teenage sexual activity. Sweden has higher teenage abortion rates than the other countries, with the notable exception of the USA, where the teenage abortion rate alone is as high or higher than the overall teenage pregnancy rate in any of the other countries.

Evidence was also collected from each country about sex education and the availability of contraceptives to teenagers. The USA stands out as being different in both respects, with more restrictions on sex education and with contraception less accessible, particularly at low cost. Although Sweden is unusual because of its long-standing commitment to sex education, the Netherlands is of interest in that information about contraception is dissemi-nated in a variety of ways, encouraged by the government, and results in a high level of knowledge amongst young people about avoiding pregnancy. It is therefore particularly noteworthy not only that the pregnancy rates were so low in the Netherlands, but that the level of sexual activity was no higher than any of the other countries except Canada. The authors of this report drew attention to the unusual degree of religiosity in the USA which they believe contributes to the American problem.

> American teenagers seem to have inherited the worst of all possible worlds regarding their exposure to messages about sex: movies, music, radio and TV tell them that sex is romantic, exciting, titillating; premarital sex and coha-bitation are visible ways of life among the adults they see and hear about; their own parents or their parents' friends are likely to be divorced or separated but involved in sexual relationships. Yet at the same time young people get the message 'good girls should say no'. Almost nothing that they see or hear about sex informs them about contraception or the importance of avoiding pregnancy (Jones et al 1985).

This cross-cultural evidence also undermines the view that the provision of contraception or access to abortion increases the likelihood of teenage sexual behaviour. The changes over time show that the important increase in teenage sexuality preceded the availability of contraception (in particular oral contraception). Initially this trend in behaviour resulted in an increase in teenage pregnancies. Since teenagers have begun to use contraception, teenage pregnancies and abortions have started to decline (Bury 1983). Teenage pregnancies are declining in the USA as well and this can also be attributed to increased contraceptive use. The worrying aspect of the American figures is that the improvement is mainly in the 18–19-year-old group; the situation for the 15–17 age group has worsened (Dryfoos 1978).

The link between adolescent sexuality and fertility is particularly striking for the black girl in the USA. In spite of the relatively low *frequency* of sexual intercourse amongst black teenagers reported by Kantner & Zelnick, the birth rate for unmarried 15–17 year-old black girls was about eight times that for white girls of the same age during the late 1970s.

This reminds us that whereas sexual success may be an important source of self-esteem for the young male, fertility has comparable importance for the young female. In societies where falling population is a problem and pronatalism is the general view, fertility as a source of status is likely to have widespread importance amongst women. In most modern western societies where not only is there a problem with overpopulation but also substantial changes in women's role, there are many more alternative ways for the young girl to gain status and bolster her self-esteem. Nevertheless, for the underprivileged, socially deprived girl of today, confronted with appallingly high levels of youth unemployment, fertility may be one of the very few options open to her. It should therefore not be surprising that such girls get themselves pregnant in spite of the many major long-term disadvantages that often follow. In the case of the black teenager, it is not clear how much the especially high illegitimacy rate can be attributed to such socioeconomic factors and how much to culturally different attitudes to fertility. Bury (1983) has considered the balance of advantages and disadvantages of motherhood for the British teenager and how this might influence the decision to proceed with a pregnancy once conceived. She doubts that teenagers *choose* to get pregnant for such reasons. But on the other hand, in a social climate where alternative roles and opportunities are so palpably lacking, awareness of such deficiencies may well influence the level of contraceptive risk-taking.

Obviously it is important to avoid over-simplification. Modern contraception may well have had a major influence on the changing status of women and thus indirectly on the sexual attitudes of young people. But it is probably wise to assume that the determinants of adolescent behaviour differ in many ways from those affecting adults and that the common sense of the adult world has only limited relevance to the teenager. There is evidence from many studies that much adolescent sexual intercourse is unprotected by contraception. It is difficult to know how much this is due to restricted availability for this age group, and there is a tendency to assume that greater availability would solve the problem. This is no more reasonable than the contrary view that the provision of contraceptives will encourage adolescent sexuality. We need greater empathy with the emerging sexuality of the adolescent before we can improve our policies in this important area of health care and education (see Chapter 12). Changes in availability of contraception probably need to be combined with changing attitudes to teenage sexuality.

With the statistics available, it is difficult to keep a check on the relevance of social class to these variations of teenage fertility during the past two decades. But there is some evidence that it is easier for middle-class married women to use contraception and postpone their fertility (Cartwright 1970) and this may be relevant to the teenagers also.

We are entitled to have mixed feelings about these apparent trends in adolescent sexuality. The weakening of the double standard is to be strongly welcomed as so many of the problems of our society are fostered by it. The emergency of a more positive attitude to sexuality amongst young females is also encouraging, although the lifting of constraints on the young is not without its problems. Our traditional and often deep-seated attitudes to fertility need to adjust to suit the pressing problems of the modern world. Also these more positive trends in adolescent sexuality are occurring whilst society is still prone to exploit sexuality. One hopes that the positive values of today's young will carry through into the adult world as they get older, but there will inevitably be casualties on the way.

THE INFLUENCE OF THE FAMILY

Social historians have described vividly how changes in the family have influenced premarital sexual behaviour over the last few centuries (Shorter 1975; Stone 1979; Gillis 1985). To what extent have changes in the family contributed to the more recent changes in teenage sexuality over the past 20 years? According to Shorter (1975), 'In the 1960s and 1970s the entire structure of the family has begun to shift'. Certainly increasing numbers of families are being affected by marital breakdown. But in spite of the considerable amount of attention paid to the modern family, our knowledge of its impact on teenage sexuality remains limited and fragmentary. The most striking evidence involves the effects on the age of onset of female sexual activity of the number and consistency of parents in the home. Kantner & Zelnick (1972) found that the lowest incidence of premarital sexuality occurred in girls living in families headed by their natural fathers. Whereas 70% of the white teenagers came into this category, only 41% of the black girls did so. However, whereas the incidence of sexual activity was 60% higher if the white girl's family was headed by her mother rather than her father, the effect was less marked with the black girls (i.e. 15% higher). It is therefore difficult to know to what extent this factor could account for the ethnic differences. Wyatt (1987) found that the presence of both biological parents *and* a more consistent pattern of parenting (i.e. without change of parental figures) were associated with later onset of sexual activity in both black and white Californian women.

Schofield (1968) found that sexual experience was more likely in teenagers subjected to less parental discipline. Single parents offer more information about sex whilst tending to be more permissive (Fox 1981). Teenagers whose parents are more open about sex are more likely to use contraception (Bury 1983). Fox & Inazu (1980) assessed a large group of mothers and daughters and found that daughters who discussed birth control with their mothers had more knowledgeable and responsible attitudes and were more likely to use contraceptives.

The extent to which adolescents are influenced predominantly by their parents rather than their peer group is very variable and there is an important need for better understanding of the factors accounting for this variability.

MARRIAGE

Human beings are unusual amongst mammals in maintaining an alliance between a sexual pair that persists through gestation and lactation. Although the form of this alliance varies enormously, it is in the general sense a 'universal' amongst human societies which formalise it as marriage. Furthermore, the marital state is adopted by the large majority of people, both male and female. In its various forms, it involves a mutual obligation between the married partners, social sanctions, sexual access and the legitimisation of the status of any offspring (Daly & Wilson 1978). A further common characteristic, which is of considerable relevance in the understanding of the place of marriage in modern society, is the accompanying institutionalisation of the social dominance of the male over the female. Marriage can be seen as a contract between men involving a formalised exchange of women as commodities (Levi-Strauss 1969). Whatever the needs are for a revision of this state of affairs, we must acknowledge its long heritage and if we are effectively to revise it, we will need to understand its universal nature.

In Murdock's (1967) survey of more than 800 human societies, 83% were polygamous, 16% monogamous and 0.5% polyandrous. In most polygamous societies however, the majority of men are monogamously married because they cannot afford more than one wife.

In Whyte's (1980) analysis of 93 societies, 57 were polygamous but in 35 (38%) polygamous unions formed less than 20% of all marriages. The relative status of women in these societies varied considerably. Whyte concluded that cross-culturally there appeared to be no such thing as the status of women, e.g. women in one society may have important property rights whilst being excluded from key religious posts; they may have important roles in political life whilst suffering from a severe sexual double standard. However there is little doubt that for more or less all the variables Whyte examined, if there was a preference for one sex in terms of power, privilege or opportunity it would be in favour of men. In 70% of societies there was an explicit view that men should and did dominate their wives, although in only 29% was there a clearly stated belief that women were generally inferior to men.

The relative weakness of the position of women is to some extent amplified by the age difference between husband and wife. In only 13% of societies were women likely to be of the same age or older than their husbands, whereas in 44% the men were usually more than 4 years older than their wives (Whyte 1980). The marriage of girls soon after puberty, or even before, maximises their reproductive potential whilst at the same time reducing, if not eliminating, their opportunities for alternative forms of status. We have already commented on the recent attempts by some Muslim countries to raise the legal age of marriage to counter this effect (and to reduce the birth rate). Unfortunately, we find little encouragement for women in the four societies that Murdock regarded as polyandrous. The two most convincing examples are in the Indian subcontinent. The Tibetan system has been practised amongst a particular group of prosperous land-holding serfs. Families of brothers would take a common wife in order to avoid partitioning the family holdings. The importance of land as the determinant is shown by the occasional family in which all the children were daughters, who would then take a common husband. Amongst the Pahari of North India, wives are very expensive to buy. Consequently brothers club together to buy one and invest in another later when they can afford it. This leads eventually to group marriage rather than polyandry.

The emphasis on monogamy in the western world has been strongly reinforced by the Christian Church. Until relatively recently, divorce and re-marriage was difficult, if not impossible. The major increase in both during the 20th century which we shall consider shortly indicates that when the social constraints are lessened, lifelong monogamy gives way to serial monogamy in an increasing number of people.

The 19th century saw many novel experiments in marriage and sexual alliances, most of them taking place in the USA where some degree of isolation suitable for experimentation was possible. Many were attempts at Utopia, which were usually short-lived. In some cases, e.g. the Owenites, the principles were sound but before their time. In others, the ideas were bizarre. Some, such as the Mormons, had a strong religious quality and it is of interest that it was the polygamous aspect of Mormonism that provoked such hostility from others in the USA (and it is said from many of the female Mormons also). Since forgoing polygamy the Mormons have prospered, and they are the only one of these experimental groups really to have done so (Murstein 1974).

Of the more modern experiments in marriage, in particular group and commune living, we have little evidence of their success or failure, though it would seem that relatively few such communes achieve any stability (Murstein 1974). Of unmarried cohabitation, Trost (1978) made some interesting observations about trends in Sweden. The falling marriage rate was to some extent compensated by an increase in the number of unmarried couples cohabiting. In 1974, 12% of couples came into this category, with the proportion rising. They tended to be younger than the average married couple and showed a dissolution rate seven to eight times that of married couples. In England and Wales, in marriage occurring between 1978 and 1981, approximately one-third of the couples had been cohabiting before marriage. In couples in which neither of the partners had been married previously, this applied to one-fifth of the total (Haskey & Coleman 1986). Trost (1978) points out that, given the established legal procedures for divorce, it is now becoming easier for a married couple to separate than for an unmarried couple, who may have considerable complications relating to division of property. Although this pattern can be seen as serial monogamy before settling into a more permanent marriage, there is also evidence that more couples are prepared to rear children outside marriage. In the UK there has been an increase in the number of illegitimate births registered jointly by both parents (50% of such births in 1974; Rothman & Capell 1978).

SEXUAL ATTRACTION, FALLING IN LOVE AND PARTNER CHOICE

What are the characteristics of a sexually attractive person? Which factors lead from sexual attraction to the establishment of a sexual relationship and possibly marriage? And what part does falling in love play in this process?

Sexual attraction, as we considered in Chapter 2, involves the visual signals of how a person looks and how he or she behaves. Smell may also be important, at least for some people; this factor could operate without their knowledge. Once two people begin to interact, personality factors will also operate. It is nevertheless difficult to go much beyond this rather obvious statement in our attempts to explain what is often referred to as the 'chemistry' of sexual attraction.

Physical attractiveness does not necessarily imply sexual attractiveness. The face is of particular importance. Certain types of face are generally regarded as attractive. Galton (1883) produced an 'average' face by photographically combining the face of a number of individuals, eliminating the irregularities and peculiarities in the process. The result was regarded as beautiful, though obviously there was a different average face for a woman and for a man. This type of attractiveness is important; even preschool children see such attractiveness as desirable in a potential friend, tending to see unattractive children as unfriendly or more likely to be aggressive. And a similar stereotyping of attributes has been demonstrated in young adults (Dion 1981).

It is therefore likely that such attractiveness plays an important part in personality development, enhancing self-esteem and hence adding further benefits in the establishment and maintenance of relationships. It has been suggested that such an asset is not always an unqualified advantage in the long term. If an individual comes to rely too much on physical attractiveness then he or she may find it more difficult to cope if and when that attractiveness declines, either with age or illness, whereas those who are less well endowed physically may have developed other more resilient resources for maintaining self-esteem (Wilson & Nias 1976).

However, a generally attractive looking person is not necessarily *sexually* attractive — particularly in the case of men. Dion (1981) has reviewed the evidence that women are more dependent on their appearance both for their self-esteem and their attractiveness. The distinction between ascribed and achieved roles means that the male can achieve attractiveness by what he *does*, but the female has to rely much more on what she *is*.

Eysenck & Wilson (1979) have suggested that the essence of sexual attractiveness is the difference between male and female features. In other words, an attractive woman is one who is clearly non-male and vice versa, hence the importance of breasts, hips, body hair, physique etc. This is probably an oversimplification. Whilst it is possible to distil the characteristics of a more or less universally attractive woman, there are not only cultural differences but also many individual differences — this is just as well or we would either evolve with monotonous homogeneity or a lot of individuals would remain disappointed! Mathews et al (1972), using photographs of women and asking men to rate them for sexual attractiveness, found an attractiveness factor relevant to all the male respondents. A further factor, however, which appeared to relate to the sexiness or sexual availability of the woman, showed much more variation of ratings amongst the men. Wiggins et al (1968) investigated the importance of size and shape of breast, buttock and leg by varying these three characteristics separately in an otherwise unchanging silhouette. The authors found an association between preferences for large breasts, buttocks etc. and certain personality types. As far as women are concerned there is no convincing evidence that the size of a man's penis is particularly important as a visual clue of sexual attractiveness; women usually deny its importance though it is noticeable that the issue often features in women's humour. According to a study by Beck (1978), it is the sight of a man's buttocks, preferably small, firm and suitably clad, which is most appealing. Bulging muscles are not particularly popular amongst women.

A study, parallel to that of Mathews et al (1972), which involved showing photographs of men to women from various occupational groups did reveal a general factor of attractiveness, but the women's ratings of sexual attractiveness were generally lower than the men's in the earlier study, and social class differences were much more evident; women preferred men who appeared to belong to the same social class (Bancroft 1978).

In their cross-cultural analysis, Ford & Beach (1952) concluded that whereas the characteristics of a sexually attractive woman were predominantly physical, though varying in particular features from one culture to another, a man's sexual attractiveness was most often attributable to his skills and prowess.

Blumstein & Schwartz (1983), in their study of American couples, made the interesting observation that whereas good looks were important in their heterosexual and gay male couples, this did not apply to their lesbian couples. The male is influenced by the physical appearance of his partner, whether he is straight or gay; the heterosexual woman is concerned about being physically attractive to her mate, but the lesbian woman rejects male standards of female attractiveness as indicators of a woman's worth. If there are physical attributes which are important to lesbian attraction they have not been identified.

Sexual attraction, it would seem, is not a passive process — the response of the individual to the subject may influence how attractive that individual appears. Perhaps the most interesting evidence of this involves the eyes. Eye contact is an important part of the courting process. Our pupils dilate when we look at something which interests us and women with dilated pupils are judged more attractive by male observers (Hess 1965).

Perper (1985) has described the typical behaviour of two people meeting and establishing a sexual contact in a singles bar in the USA. He calls this the 'courtship sequence'. When two people are strangers courtship begins when one approaches or moves next to the other. After initial conversation, the next step is when the two people turn to face each other (a step which can take from 10 minutes to 2 hours or more!) The next step involves touching — one person touches the other. As the sequence develops further, eye contact becomes prolonged. Then the couple start to move or gesture in a synchronised manner. By then the courtship sequence is well on its way. Turning to face or touching the other person are examples of what Perper calls 'escalation points' — what happens next depends on how the other person responds; if he or she responds positively the sequence 'escalates'.

Perhaps the most interesting conclusion drawn by Perper is that it is women who tend to control these sequences, showing proceptive behaviour in a variety of subtle ways. Although it could be said that Perper goes beyond his data, he develops the interesting idea that selection of a mate is a process that is principally under the woman's control. She decides when to let the sequence develop; she feels entitled to stop it at any stage.

Being sexually attracted to someone, and 'escalating' in a singles bar is one thing; choosing that person as a partner in a more permanent relationship, possibly leading to marriage, is another. Here cultural differences are fundamental. We have already considered how control of choice of spouse by parents has changed in Europe over the last few centuries. We find a comparable variation and a tendency to progress from arranged marriages to free choice across cultures. We are familiar with arranged marriages in Asian and Jewish communities; the pattern in rural Ireland, reflecting the economic constraints on marriage, is probably less well known (Mullan

1984). Arranged marriages are also common in some African countries and other parts of the world. There is a tendency for such arrangements to move gradually towards free choice. In 1950 the People's Republic of China legislated against the previous tradition of arranged marriages. The general tendency is for parental control to remain strongest where parental affluence and hence the importance of inheritance is greater, or where ethnic communities are alienated within a culture and therefore need to intermarry to maintain their ethnic identity, as in the Jewish example. According to Rosenblatt & Anderson (1981), movement towards freedom of choice is fraught with difficulties. Given the rate of marital breakdown in societies where such free choice is well established, the arranged marriage has quite a good record.

Mullan (1984) has suggested that, as we have moved away from parental influence on choice of spouse, we have seen the growth of dating agencies and marriage bureaux which, whilst often run in a dubious fashion, nevertheless appeal to a need for sensible rather than emotional influences on partner choice.

What happens when there is freedom of choice? The available evidence presents rather a dull picture. People tend to choose partners with a similar degree of physical attractiveness (Dion 1981). They tend to marry within the same ethnic or religious group, though this tendency is lessening. And they tend to marry within the same social class and level of education (Udry 1974). When these boundaries are crossed there is a higher rate of marital breakdown. People tend to marry those living near them (Ineichen 1979). All of these tendencies underline the importance of accessibility rather than suitability. There are some interesting variations on this theme. The tendency to marry someone from the same social group is greatest in the highest status group (not surprising, when there is property or wealth at stake), but second highest in the lowest status group. For men, those in social class I are most likely to marry, whereas for women the reverse applies; those in social class V are most likely to be married in any age group (Haskey 1983).

In general, therefore, there is a tendency for like to marry like. Although it would seem intrinsically likely that choice of partner will also reflect the matching of needs, this concept of complementarity, as proposed by Winch (1958), has proved difficult to demonstrate. It may be that similarity is easier to demonstrate than complementarity. Either model is simplistic — what Murstein (1981) calls 'monolithic'. He reviews a number of more complex theories of partner selection which take into account the *process* of establishing a relationship. Mate selection is not a 'one-off' process, like choosing a commodity off the shelf, but one of an evolving relationship. Having considered a number of such theoretical models somewhat critically, Murstein (1981) favours his own stimulus–value–role theory, which is an example of an exchange theory, i.e. it stems from the assumption that attraction and interaction in a relationship are based on the exchange value of the assets and liabilities each person brings into the relationship. The kinds of variable involved in this 'trade-off' are considered under three headings; stimulus, value and role. Stimulus variables are most important in the initial stages, reflecting in particular physical attractiveness. As indicated earlier, equality of attractiveness is believed to be important. The value comparison stage follows and involves the matching of attitudes and values which results when the couple are getting to know each other. The role stage involves working out the respective role of each person in the relationship, a process which sometimes only really begins after the couple has married. Whilst there is experimental evidence supporting Murstein's theory, it is mainly relevant to the exchange aspect of the model, i.e. the characteristics brought into the relationship, and less to the developmental aspects, such as the role stage, which are more difficult to study.

Sitting awkwardly in the midst of this is the concept of love. Whilst those in the artistic world have grappled persistently and often effectively with this topic, scientists have been somewhat half-hearted, perhaps revealing an ambivalence. Falling in love therefore remains an enigma, possibly the last defended stronghold against the analytical prying of scientific man. Tennov (1979), who coined the word 'limerence' to describe the state of being in love, had problems when tackling the subject with traditional methods of scientific enquiry. Eventually she turned to 'searching discussions in which informant and investigator jointly sought clarification'. Limerence, she decided, was not an emotion, a perception, a form of learning, a cognitive process or a behaviour, although it included components of all of them. 'Linguistically invisible under ordinary circumstances, limerence was clearly present when present and fully absent when absent' (Tennov 1980).

The term 'love' has a variety of meanings. Katchadourian (1985) has summarised various attempts to define these different meanings, including that of C. S. Lewis who distinguished between affection (storge), friendship (philia), sexual love (eros) and charity (agape), differentiating also between 'need-love' and 'gift-love'.

Sexual love, or limerance, has certain features which most writers have recognised: a preoccupation with the loved one, with intrusive thoughts; a dominant yearning for a return of feelings from the loved one, who tends to be idealised and his or her good points are emphasised and bad points played down. The distinction is often made between romantic love and conjugal love — the less passionate, possibly more durable variety that develops in long-standing and mutually rewarding relationships (Udry 1974).

Boswell (1980) believes that in Ancient Greece and Rome there were fewer boundaries between friendship and romantic love than we see today. Love between men was often presented by Greek writers as 'the only form of eroticism which could be lasting, pure and truly spiritual'. The concept of platonic love stems from Plato's conviction that only love between persons of the same gender could transcend sex. A recurring theme of Boswell's book, usually only implied, is that love between men is regarded by men as of greater value than love between men and women. He is not restricting his attention to men of homosexual orientation, though it is possible that he is biased by his own gay viewpoint. Nevertheless, his somewhat disturbing implication is less surprising when one considers societies in which women are substantially devalued by men, and allowed much lower status.

It is often assumed that women are more 'romantic' than men. The evidence, such as it is, suggests that men more readily fall in love. Women show more caution before becoming involved and are more likely to decide when an affair ends, while men take longer to get over a love affair (Hatfield & Walster 1978).

Various attempts have been made to measure love with questionnaires. Thus Rubin (1970) distinguished loving from liking. Lee (1976) had a more ambitious objective. His questionnaire measured different types of love — eros (characterised by physical attraction, sensuality, close intimacy and rapport); ludus (love that is playful, hedonistic and uncommitted); storge (affectionate, compassionate). These three types, together with two dimensions, mania (feverish, obsessive and jealous love), and pragma (practical, realistic and compatibility-seeking) could combine in various ways.

Other workers have looked for behavioural characteristics of people who are in love. Probably the most convincing is the tendency to engage in prolonged eye contact and also to stand close to one another (Hatfield & Walster 1978). In general, one is left with a sense of incompleteness in these attempts to capture the essence of romantic love.

How important is romantic love when choosing a partner for marriage? It is often assumed that romantic love as the basis for marriage is a relatively new phenomenon, leading to expectations of marriage which are difficult to realise. Margaret Mead (1950), considering the modern American style of marriage, said: 'It is one of the most difficult marriage forms that the human race has ever attempted and the casualties are surprisingly few, considering the complexities of the task'.

Stone (1979), in his social history of marriage in England, reached firm conclusions. He describes:

> . . . the imposition on the sexual drive of an ideological gloss known as romantic love, which thanks to nature imitating art, at times has taken on a life of its own. Beginning as purely extramarital emotions in the troubadour literature of the 12th century, it was transformed by the invention of the printing press and the spread of literacy in the 16th and 17th century. Among the upper classes the demand for romantic love and sexual fulfillment was stimulated, especially among women, by the reading of romances and love stories, which created exaggerated expectations of marital felicity which were very often frustrated.

Prior to the 19th century it was, according to Stone, the accepted wisdom that marriage based on romantic love or sexual attraction was less likely to lead to lasting happiness than one based on common sense considerations. 'Almost everyone agreed that both physical desire and romantic love were unsafe bases for an enduring marriage since both were violent mental disturbances which would inevitably be of only short duration'.

Gillis (1985) paints a rather different and to me more attractive historical picture. 'As we turn to the 16th and 17th century it is not the capacity for love but the *form* of affection that separates their world from ours' 'Direct and personal expressions of love were inhibited and in their place we find highly ritualised forms of courtship, whose actions and symbols seem to us strangely impersonal'. In other words, we should be not be surprised to find that romantic love has been expressed in different ways at different times in history and in different cultures. Gillis saw romantic love and its associated passion as an important part of the courtship process which was 'exorcised at the time of the wedding' as 'too much affection was perceived as unnatural and a threat to the broader social obligations that come with the establishment of a household'. This exorcism was sometimes ritualised by the bride removing her garter at the wedding celebration and ceremoniously passing it on to other single people who would require it to make their own marriages. As mentioned earlier, Gillis, in his account, dealt more with ordinary working people than Stone. Such people, as described on p. 222, had negligible property or possessions and hence were generally freer to make their own choice of partner. They nevertheless saw marriage as a long-term serious business of coping and rearing a family — the adult phase of life. Romantic love, whilst important for the bonding process, was perhaps too couple-centred, too light-hearted for the serious business of living. In the more affluent families, who provided much more of the evidence reported by Stone, the need for arranged marriages was stronger. It is not difficult to see how in such circumstances romantic love would seem to the parents of the aspiring bride or groom a threat to the orderly choice of suitable partner, whilst for the young person the inevitability of major parental influence would discourage the development of emotional attachments which could so easily be thwarted.

The cross-cultural evidence indicates that societies differ markedly in the importance attached to love as a basis for marriage; it tends to be greater in those societies with freedom of choice of spouse (Rosenblatt & Anderson 1981). A variety of factors could result in the restriction or inhibition of the expression of romantic love, for example, jealousy amongst one's family members if a couple are seen to be too close. The availability of private sleeping quarters may also be important. Without such privacy too much expression of passion could be disturbing for relatives (Rosenblatt & Anderson 1981).

In all societies rules determine who it is acceptable to mate with and it is striking to what extent romantic associations are kept within such rules.

The most striking set of rules involves kinship — the taboos on incest, which will be considered in more detail in Chapter 13. At the end of the 19th century Westermark, an anthropologist, proposed that incest avoidance amongst siblings occurs as a result of childhood familiarity (see p. 698). Support for this view has come from studies of children brought up in Israeli kibbutzim. They are most unlikely to have sexual relationships with or marry anyone brought up on the same kibbutz. According to Shepher (1971) this effect probably depends on their living together during the first 6 years of life. In the Sim-Pua marriages of Taiwan, the couple are wed as young children, usually less than 3 years old. They grow up together intimately throughout childhood. These couples have more difficulty in establishing a sexual relationship, have fewer children and are more likely to resort to extramarital sex or divorce than other types of marriage (Wolf 1970). Thus there is some evidence of a negative factor in mate selection operating during childhood.

These various sources of evidence point to the power of social controls over this aspect of mate selection. Udry (1974), having reviewed the evidence, concludes that 'the emotion of love has probably existed as a natural social phenomenon wherever young people were allowed to associate with the opposite sex. Wherever it has existed it has had as much influence on mate selection as the society would let it'. He was also unable to find any evidence that marriages based on romantic love have a worse outcome — which might reassure the romantics amongst us.

INCIDENCE OF MARRIAGE

The proportion of the adult population married in the UK and its change over time is shown in Figure 4.9. Marriage rates (i.e. per 1000 of marriageable age) rose from the early years of the century, reaching a peak in the

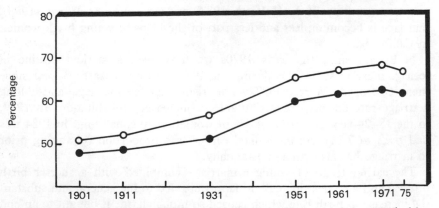

Fig. 4.9 Percentage of UK population, aged 15 and over, who are married, categorised by sex. (from Thompson 1977)
o = males; ● = females.

late 1960s and early 1970s. Since then they have declined steadily to levels below those of the 1920s, with a steep decline in rates of first marriages in the last few years, partly compensated by some increase in remarriage. The substantially higher rates of remarriage for widowers and divorced men than for widows and divorced women is due to the much higher number of the women, particularly in older age groups. The major increase in remarriages in the early 1970s followed the Divorce Reform Act of 1969 which allowed many separated individuals to divorce and remarry.

In the past marriage rates have been higher in the USA and much lower in Sweden and Denmark. In recent years there have been falls in marriage rates in the USA, France, Belgium and West Germany comparable to those in Britain. In Sweden it has been estimated that among those aged 18 to 24 there are currently more cohabiting than married couples (Rimmer 1981).

Age at marriage

The so-called European marriage pattern, with a relatively late age of marriage and a relatively high proportion of unmarried women reaching the menopause, has been a characteristic of western Europe (i.e. west of an imaginary line drawn between Trieste and Leningrad). In eastern Europe and the United States age at marriage has tended to be younger and the proportion remaining unmarried to be lower (Glass 1974). However there was a universal decline in age at marriage in most countries after World War II. In 1931, 26% of women in the UK in the 20–24 year age group were married; in 1963 it was 60%. In 1931 the average age at marriage for women was 25.5; it declined to 22.6 years in 1971. Since then it has steadily risen to about 23 years for women (25.5 years for men; OPCS 1983). In the USA between the 1950s and late 1970s, the mean age of white women at first marriage rose from 21.4 to 23.0 years; for black women the increase was from 21.9 to 26.1 (Hofferth 1987) and according to Wyatt (1988), marriage is becoming less and less part of the plans of young black women in California.

In Britain since the early 1970s we have seen a marked decline in teenage marriages; by 30% during the 1970s and by at least 9% year since then (Griffin & Morris 1987). The rising age at marriage and falling marriage rate are in part attributable to increasing cohabitation. In 1979, in the 18–24-year age group 4.5% of women were cohabiting; in 1984 this had risen to 7.3%. As mentioned earlier, the proportion cohabiting prior to marriage has also risen substantially.

The earlier trend of younger marriage combined with a shorter birth interval and a modest increase in family size led to the general and substantial increase in birth rate which caused so much alarm. It bought to an end a trend which had halved the birth rate between 1870 and 1930. This remarkable earlier decline has been attributed to increased use of contraception, but this explanation is difficult to sustain in view of the more recent and more rapid increase in birth rate at a time when contraception was becoming much more effective and available. The birth rate increase reached its peak in 1964, however, and has been declining since. This is around the time that the main increase in premarital sexuality is thought to have got underway.

SEXUAL ACTIVITY DURING MARRIAGE

Much less attention has been paid by researchers to marital as compared to premarital sexuality, and we are largely dependent on the Kinsey data. The frequency of sexual intercourse in married couples, as found by Kinsey, is shown in Figure 4.10. It is seen to be highest in the younger age groups, as one might expect. There were only slight discrepancies between incidences reported by husbands and wives. The mean frequencies shown, however, conceal the very considerable variation which has been found in most studies. Gorer (1971) found less marked differences with age. Hunt (1974) concluded that there had been an increase in frequency of marital intercourse since Kinsey's study. But most of the other available evidence (e.g. Garde & Lunde 1980) does not suggest that there has been any major change in this area of human sexuality compared with that of the adolescent. Average frequencies of around twice a week are commonly found (Gorer 1971; Chester & Walker 1979). Frequency of love-making by men in different age groups was reported by Sanders (1987) from her Woman magazine survey (Fig. 4.11). As this is a self-selected sample, we must be cautious in extrapolating from the data. But the striking finding is that the frequency of two to three times per week was the most common for all age groups. Blumstein & Schwartz (1983) reported frequencies for

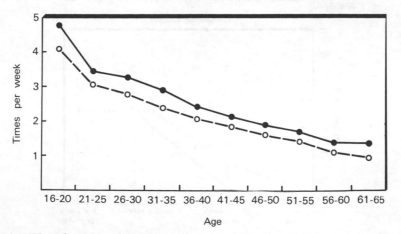

Fig. 4.10 Mean frequency of sexual intercourse per week, categorised by age, as reported by married men. (from the Kinsey data; Gebhard & Johnson 1979)
● = non-college males; ○ = college males.

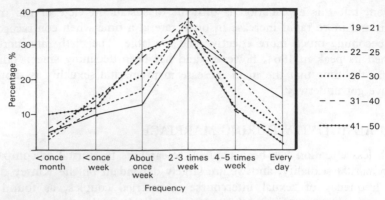

Fig. 4.11 Frequency of sexual intercourse by age group of men. (from Sanders 1987)

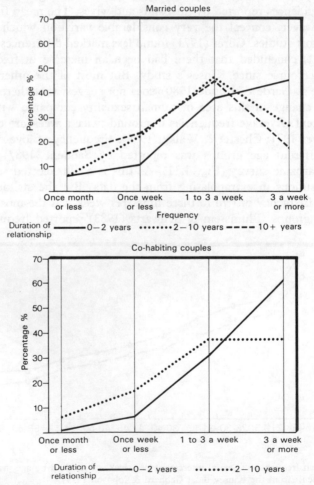

Fig. 4.12 Frequency of sexual intercourse in married and cohabitating couples by duration of relationship. (from Blumstein & Morris 1987)

married and cohabiting couples according to how long they had been living together (Fig. 4.12). This shows that frequency of sex declines markedly after the first 2 years. The cohabiting couples are more active sexually at all ages.

Comparable evidence from other cultures is hard to find. Ford & Beach (1952) in their survey of primitive societies concluded: 'In most of the societies on which information is available, every adult normally engages in heterosexual intercourse once daily or nightly during periods when coitus is permitted'. This would suggest that western societies are inactive by comparison, though there are far fewer cultural restrictions on intercourse in the modern world and it is difficult to judge the validity of such anthropological reports. Nag (1972), in an interesting paper comparing sexual activity in India and the USA, presents evidence from three groups of Indian women: two were Muslim and the third was Hindu. They all reported frequencies of intercourse well below the Kinsey figures for the USA for all age groups. The Hindus were somewhat lower than the Muslims and would have shown even lower frequency if the time for which coitus was forbidden had been taken into account. The extent of these restrictions varies from region to region but in some areas as many as 100 days per year may be excluded for religious reasons. Nag also stresses the Hindu, and to a lesser extent, Muslim belief that semen is a source of strength and should not be wasted. Carstairs (1967) gives us this description from a rural Hindu community:

> Every one knew that semen was not easily formed; it takes 40 days, and 40 drops of blood to make one drop of semen, but the process was variously described. Everyone was agreed on one point, that the semen is ultimately stored in a reservoir in the head, whose capacity is 20 'tolas' (6.8 ounces). Semen of good quality is rich and viscous, like the cream of unadulterated milk. A man who possesses a store of such good semen becomes a superman . . . celibacy was the first requirement of true fitness.

Carstairs reported that neurotic anxiety about semen loss or 'jirivan' was a common clinical problem. A more recent report from Sri Lanka shows that it has not lessened in importance (Kulanayagam 1979). Add to such beliefs the serious lack of privacy suffered by most married couples in India and the low rates of intercourse are not surprising.

Menstruation

One widespread restriction on sexual activity is that related to menstruation. In the majority of societies, the menstruating woman is considered unsuitable as a sexual partner, and in some cases there may be general rejection of the woman as 'unclean' during this phase of her cycle. Islamic religion regards the menstruating woman as impure, requiring ritual cleaning. Apart from not having intercourse, she is forbidden to touch the Koran, repeat a verse from it or enter a mosque (Bullough 1976). Hindu women are similarly ostracised when menstruating. Orthodox Jewish women still require a ritual bath after menstruation. In a WHO sponsored study of patterns of menstruation in 10 countries, Snowden & Christian (1983) found that almost all respondents believed that sexual intercourse should be avoided during menstruation. The UK, the only western country in the study, was an exception; just over half interviewed held that view, though the authors believed that in terms of actual practice the proportion would have been higher. In Whyte's (1980) cross-cultural study, only 10 of the 93 societies were free from menstrual taboos. Pietropinto & Simenaur (1977) asked their male subjects how they felt about sex during menstruation. About a third said they enjoyed it as usual; for the remainder it presented varying degrees of 'turn off' with 11% avoiding the partner completely at that time. It would be interesting to know if attitudes are changing in this respect and whether women feel differently to men about sex at this time. It is certainly not unusual for women to report feeling at their most sexy during their period (see Chapter 2).

Initiation of sex

Men have traditionally been the initiators in love-making (although according to Perper (1985) not in sociosexual interactions). Blumstein & Schwartz's (1983) study of American couples suggest that this is still predominantly the case. Only 12% of wives said they were more likely to initiate love-making and only 16% of the men said their wives were more likely to do so. In contrast, 51% of husbands usually initiated sex. This study found that many men often felt uncomfortable when their partner initiated, and by the same token men may feel guilty for failing in their *duty* to initiate sex. Not surprisingly, women found it more difficult than men to cope with refusal. This traditional pattern appears to be deeply rooted. Of interest was the finding that couples who were more equal in their initiation and refusal of sex were more likely to report a happy sex life (Blumstein & Schwartz 1983). The importance of the pattern of dominance in a marriage in determining sexual behaviour was postulated by Abernethy (1974) who suggested that female dominance inhibits heterosexual copula-tory behaviour, whereas male dominance facilitates it. This hypothesis has been challenged by Gray (1984) who, using the cross-cultural evidence from the HRAF, found that societies with high female power within marriage exhibited better, or certainly no worse, adjustment than societies with a low degree of female power. Societies with high female power tend to have open discussion of sexual matters, attach importance to foreplay, show less disapproval of female premarital sexual activity and allow women to initiate sex. They also tend to show less male fear of impotence and less evidence of male homosexual behaviour (though greater acceptance of it). It is an interesting idea that men would be sexually more functional if they were not expected to be sexually dominant.

Kissing

Kissing is seen by many couples as the height of intimacy, especially by women. Blumstein & Schwartz (1983) found that people kiss less during sex when they feel somewhat removed emotionally but still want physical release. It is remarkable how little attention has been paid to kissing in human sexual relationships. The Kinsey surveys assessed how often it occurred both premaritally and maritally (Gebhard & Johnson 1979) and reported it to be more frequent in higher educated groups. Ford & Beach (1952) described some primitive societies in which kissing was not a normal part of love-making, and others in which modified forms of kissing were used. Something akin to kissing has also been observed in primates. What is lacking is information on how people vary in their attitudes to and acceptance of kissing.

Coital positions

Coital positions predominantly used during intercourse vary across cultures but the commonest is the so-called 'missionary' position with the woman lying on her back and the man on top of her (Ford & Beach 1952). As previously mentioned, Kinsey found a social class difference in the variety of sexual activity. College-educated couples were more likely to use other positions, to make love in the nude and with the light on (Gebhard & Johnson 1979). There is reason to believe that these social class differences are lessening (Hunt 1974). Blumstein & Schwartz (1983) found that this balance of power in the relationship influenced the position adopted during intercourse. Couples with equitable relationships were more likely to use the female superior position; this was less likely in couples where the male was the dominant partner. Perhaps one of the most striking changes since the Kinsey survey is in the prevalence of oral sex. This now appears to be a more commonplace aspect of marital sexuality (Hunt 1974; Pietropinto & Simenaur 1977). Chester & Walker (1979) concluded from their survey that many women have a greater desire for cunnilingus than their partners are apt to satisfy. Blumstein & Schwartz (1983), however, found that oral sex was more important for sexual happiness for the male than for the female partner. Hunt (1974) has suggested that even more taboo types of sexual stimulation such as anal stimulation or intercourse have increased, particularly amongst the young.

Biting and scratching as a mutual form of stimulation are used quite frequently and a third to a half of Kinsey's subjects reported such experiences. The majority of these find the biting to be sexually arousing, presumably because it adds further intense stimulation when sexual arousal is already high.

In general the evidence indicates a weakening of taboos against unconventional types of sexual activity within marriage, a lessening of the working-class inhibitions and a generally greater tendency for couples to experiment and explore alternative methods of stimulation than was the case at the time of Kinsey's survey.

THE FATE OF MARRIAGE

The increase of marital breakdown and divorce is an international phenomenon, occurring in just about every country in which it has been studied. Most countries showed a rise after the Second World War, presumably reflecting the unstable nature of many wartime marriages; this was followed by a decline in the 1950s and a constant upward trend since 1960 (Dominion 1979a; Fig. 4.13). In England and Wales divorce became legally easier to obtain in 1971 with the divorce law reform. This was followed by

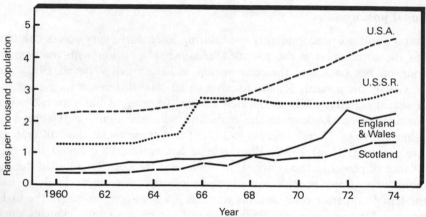

Fig. 4.13 Divorce rates: comparison of four countries 1960–1974.

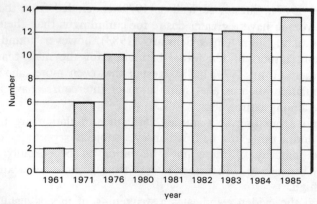

Fig. 4.14 Persons divorcing per 1000 married people in England and Wales. (from Griffin & Morris 1987)

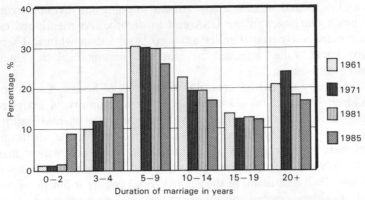

Fig. 4.15 Divorce rate by years of marriage, samples taken in 1961, 1971, 1981 and 1985.

a further rise in the divorce rate (Fig. 4.14). Further legislation in 1976 led to a similar increase in Scotland. If present trends continue, one in four of existing marriages are heading for divorce (Dominion 1979a). In the USA, the number of divorces has doubled since 1960 and nowadays one in three marriages end in divorce (Smith & Smith 1977). There has not been the same impact of legislation in the USA due to the variations in divorce laws from state to state.

Fifty per cent of divorces occur within the first nine years of marriage (Fig. 4.15). In the USA, the third year was found to be the peak year; in Sweden the maximum was reached after 4 years. In the USA, divorce has more than doubled since 1960 amongst couples married for 15 years or longer. In the UK, divorce rates peak between the age of 25 and 29 and there has been a continuing rise in the under-25 age group. Teenage marriages are particularly at risk for breakdown. Women married in their teens are four times as likely to divorce as those married when aged 25–29 (Rimmer 1981). The proportion of divorces involving children has also risen. In the USA, one child in seven is now being raised in a single-parent family (Smith & Smith 1977). In Britain the number of children involved in divorce rose from 82 000 in 1971 to 163 000 in 1978. However the current trend for divorce early in marriage and the trend to delay the first child may mean that in future a smaller proportion of divorces will involve children (Rimmer 1982).

The explanation for this universal trend is likely to be complex. Increasing divorce rates have been correlated with the falling age of marriage, rising life expectancy, decrease in the number of children and increased proportions of women in the labour market (Kunzel 1974; Murstein 1974). Changing expectations of 'individual growth' and the conflict between needs for closeness and for individual freedom have been implicated (Smith & Smith 1977).

In view of our earlier comparison of premarital sexuality and fertility of

American blacks and whites, it is pertinent to point out that approximately half of black marriages in the USA end in divorce. As mentioned earlier, there are more one-parent familes amongst blacks than whites. There is a generally lower value attached to marriage amongst black Americans particularly the males.

The social cost of marital breakdown in terms of health of both spouses and children is enormous (Dominion 1979b). Continuity of marriage, on the other hand, cannot be equated with happiness or mental health, and divorce is not the only criterion of marital failure. In the 1960s divorce statistics were registering only about half the total breakdowns of marriage (Dunnell 1979); this proportion will have risen following the changes in the divorce law. Full discussion of the related social factors is not possible here. We will consider some of the interpersonal processes involved in marital discord in Chapter 8 but at this point we will confine our attention to the possible role of sexual incompatibility and extramarital sex in marital breakdown.

Sexuality incompatibility

Gebhard (1978) summarised from the Kinsey data the types and frequencies of problems reported by their married respondents to be affecting their marriages. He confined his attention to white college-educated people reporting on their first marriage. This amounted to 1607 males and 1445 females. Only 8% reported trouble-free marriages. Those who married at a later age tended to have fewer problems than those who had married younger and for a longer period. Gebhard ranked the various types of problems according to their frequency of reporting. Sexual problems were the most common type for both sexes, and disagreement over coital frequency was at the top of both lists. More often it was the husband (20%) who wanted more sex rather than the wife (9%) but the wife's desire for more frequent intercourse was positively related to age, presumably reflecting the greater decline in sexual interest with age in the male than in the female. Problems with general sexual responsiveness were also common. Husbands were more likely to attribute this problem to their wives, while wives more likely to acknowledge this problem in themselves. The incidence of specific sexual dysfunction is discussed in Chapter 8. Sexual jealousy and extramarital activity were more likely to invoke the wife's concern about the husband's behaviour than the other way round.

From this evidence, it is apparent that sexual difficulties are an important source of marital stress. This may be class-related, however. Gebhard's sample is from the higher socioeconomic groups and a number of studies have found that concern with sexual incompatibility is more likely to be associated with divorce in middle-class than working-class couples (Smith & Smith 1977). As mentioned elsewhere, sexual dissatisfaction, particularly amongst women, is more prevalent in working-class marriages (Rainwater

1966) but may be regarded as less important than other factors. There is some evidence that a high sex drive in men has an adverse effect on marital adjustment, whereas in women it has a positive effect (Murstein 1974). Much of the evidence comes from relatively early studies and it is difficult to know to what extent this would apply nowadays.

Premarital sex and marital stability

In view of the major increase in premarital sexuality, discussed above, it is of some interest to consider the possible effects that such early experiences may have on later marital happiness. Several early studies (Davis 1929; Terman 1938; Locke 1951) found a weak but positive association between premarital chastity and later marital happiness. Various attempts have been made to account for these findings: that they are most noticeable in those societies which most condemn premarital sexuality; that those reluctant to permit premarital sex are also less likely to admit to marital unhappiness; that the important factor is the consistency between one's values and one's behaviour and those who are inconsistent premaritally are likely to have problems later, or simply that premarital permissiveness is related to other personality characteristics which are themselves more likely to lead to marital problems later. Nevertheless, Athanasiou & Sarkin (1974) making use of the questionnaire responses to the Psychology Today survey, attempted to control for some of these intervening variables and found that the weak but positive relationship between premarital chastity and marital adjustment persisted. The issue is complex but it seems that the statistical support for premarital virtue won't go away.

Extramarital sex

Clearly the relationship between sexual satisfaction and marital happiness is likely to be a two-way process (Clark & Wallin 1965; Gebhard 1966) and we will explore more closely the effects of marital discord on sexual function in Chapter 8. It is thus very difficult to establish to what extent marital breakdown actually results from sexual incompatibility. Similarly, it is not easy to decide to what extent extramarital sexuality is a result or a cause of marital disharmony. Extramarital sex may be tried by someone in an unhappy marriage to see if an alternative relationship is preferable (Walster et al 1978) and in this sense commonly occurs in the period preceding divorce. The available evidence certainly suggests that women are more likely to experience extramarital sex if they are unhappy in their marriage (Bell et al 1975) and this may be less obvious for men.

Social sanctions against extramarital sex are found in the majority of societies. In some, such as modern Islam, the punishment for offenders can be severe. In certain states of the USA adultery, to use the legal term, is still a criminal offence, though rarely prosecuted as such. It has certainly been used as grounds for divorce to the extent that in some areas couples will go to the trouble of having adultery witnessed to facilitate the divorce proceedings. Most primitive societies restrict extramarital sex and in the exceptions limits are usually set as to who can be involved (Ford & Beach 1952). In general the taboo against extramarital sex is greater than that against premarital sex. Another common if not universal characteristic is that extramarital activity by husbands is more accepted than that by wives. This is a part of the double standard considered earlier — an extension of the 'property value' of the wife. Broude & Greene (1980), in their analysis of 116 societies, found 43% in which extramarital sex was accepted for men but not for women, and only 11% where it was accepted for both men and women. The related aspect, which is probably important for the married man who is expected to take responsibility for the fathering and material welfare of his children, is the threat of cuckoldry, of being deceived by another man into rearing his child. This is an intriguing issue. There is an inescapable and fundamental sex difference in the reproductive consequences of extramarital sexuality. The male may see the surreptitious introduction of another man's child into his 'nest' as a serious attack on his honour or he may see it as a threat to the existence of his own offspring. How can he be sure that any of his children are his own? These two reactions may be different versions of the same thing, the first being a humanised version of a basic biological mechanism. It is of relevance that in animals where the male plays an active part in rearing or protecting the young, any threat to the fidelity of his mate, or any possibility that the offspring may be fathered by another male leads to strong action, such as rejection of the mate (Daly & Wilson 1978). We will return later to the possible biological implications or origins of male–female differences in sexual behaviour. But by the same token that threatens the cuckolded male, the offending male may gain in self-esteem or masculine status. Hence a man may engage in extramarital sexuality to bolster his self-esteem. Women may seek reassurance of their continuing attractiveness in the same way but the 'pay-off' is more complex for them and this may explain why for women extramarital sex is more likely to be used as a means of coping with an unsatisfactory marriage.

In the Kinsey data 34% of married men and 20% of married women had experienced extramarital sex (Gebhard & Johnson 1979). Kinsey considers it likely that these figures were an underestimate due to reluctance by some to admit to this behaviour. Hunt (1974) on the other hand has pointed out that Kinsey's figures are inflated by a disproportionate number of divorced people who for reasons already mentioned have a higher incidence of extramarital sex. What is interesting is that subsequent evidence does not show any appreciable change from these Kinsey figures. Hunt (1974) found very similar overall proportions. Garde & Lunde (1980) found that 13% of their 40 year-old Danish women had been unfaithful at some stage. In the Psychology Today survey (Athanasiou et al 1970) 40% of the males and 31%

of the females had had extramarital experience. This might indicate an increase, though this particular sample was likely to be more liberal in sexual behaviour than the Kinsey sample. Pietropinto & Simenaur (1977) found 43% of their married men had had extramarital experience. In Blumstein & Schwartz's (1983) study, 26% of husbands and 21% of wives admitted to extramarital sex. The percentages for the cohabiting couples were 33 and 30% respectively. The number of extramarital partners was higher for the men than for the women.

As far as the USA is concerned, there does not appear to be a major change in extramarital activity. However, there may be some change in relation to age and social class. Kinsey et al (1953) found that for men under 25 years, extramarital sex was more frequent amongst the less educated. For women the association was in reverse; for the over-25s the incidence was higher amongst the better educated. This pattern has not been noticeable in more recent studies (Hunt 1974; Pietropinto & Simenaur 1977), though Hunt did find an apparent increase amongst women under 25, bringing their level of extramarital experience more in line with the males. This is further suggestive evidence of a reduction in both social class and sex differences in sexual behaviour.

For the UK, less evidence is available. In Gorer's (1971) survey, only 8% of the married subjects admitted to extramarital sexual experience with twice as many men as women doing so. By comparison, this seems a very low figure. In a recent survey of men and women carried out for Woman magazine (Sanders 1985, 1987) 26% of men and 30% of woman admitted to extramarital experience. The number of extramarital partners was higher for the men similar to the finding of Blumstein & Schwartz (1983) in the USA. An Italian survey (Davis & Fabris 1980) reported 41% of men and 14% of women admitting to extramarital sex.

According to Kinsey, infidelity on the part of the wife was more likely to cause major marital problems than when the husband was involved. Obviously the effects of extramarital sexuality vary considerably with the circumstances. In the majority of cases the behaviour is unknown to the spouse. When discovered, reactions are likely to depend on the level and nature of the deceit involved, and whether the sexual activity was a casual 'one-off' encounter. A relatively long-standing extramarital relationship is obviously more traumatic to the marriage, not only because of the current threat to its emotional security, but also because the offended spouse has to reappraise a relatively long period of the past marriage as being quite different from what it was believed to be. An alternative to deceit is to be open about one's extramarital liaisons. The concept of the 'open marriage' has been popularised by the O'Neills (O'Neill & O'Neill 1972). They saw the possessiveness of the traditional 'closed' marriage as limiting personal growth and breeding insecurity through jealousy. They emphasised mutual caring through love rather than the reliance on institutional constraints. 'Freedom in open marriage does not mean freedom to "do your thing" without responsibility. It is the freedom to grow to the capacity of your individual potential through love — and one aspect of that love is caring for your partner's growth and welfare as much as your own'. They leave to the couple in the open marriage to choose whether to engage in extramarital sex or not. These are noble sentiments and in a way capture the essence of the problem of modern marriage. With the removal, or at least weakening, of the institutionalised supports for marriage, its success relies more and more on the special qualities of the individuals involved. Open marriage, particularly in its wider rather than specifically sexual sense, may well be an ideal to which we should aspire. But it does seem that for the majority of people it presents too many difficulties, at least if they aim to maintain a secure relationship on a life-long basis. The apparent need for the structural support of traditional marriage is suggested by the tendency for divorced people to remarry (unfortunately the divorce rate is even higher in these remarriages.) Most of us appear to need an external structure to our relationships to carry us through critical patches and to allow us to establish enough security to start behaving in a mutually constructive way. It is true that the powerfully destructive effect of sexual jealousy depends on the particular values attached to sexuality in the relationship. If we become comfortable with the idea of sex simply as a source of pleasure with people we like, then extramarital sex may become no more threatening than a game of squash with a neighbour's spouse. But in that case we will be losing the special intimacy that makes good sex a particularly binding force in the relationship (see Chapter 1). It is difficult to see how far our traditional need for sexual fidelity could be diminished without losing many of the advantages of sex in marriage.

Mate-swapping

An alternative to marital infidelity which has received much publicity in recent years is extramarital sexuality shared by both partners, usually known as 'mate-swapping' or 'swinging'. The common factor is that both partners participate, though this may mean swapping partners with another couple, participating in a foursome, or engaging in group sexual activity. It has been estimated that 1–2% of the American population has engaged in such activity at least once (Hunt 1974; Spanier & Cole 1975). There is a general tendency to maintain anonymity and secrecy which underlines the socially deviant nature of this behaviour. Evidence of the characteristics of 'swingers' is somewhat confusing and contradictory (Bartell 1970; Smith & Smith 1970). Wheeler & Kilman (1983), comparing 'swingers' with a group of 'non-swinging' married couples, found them to have more liberal attitudes to sex and greater sexual satisfaction than the controls. More surprisingly, the 'swingers' reported a greater need for social approval. Most people who have studied the phenomenon point out both advantages and disadvantages. Although it is assumed that participants are characteristically highly sexed, many find it difficult to perform predictably in group situations, particularly the men. Women involved commonly engage in homosexual activity with each other. Although it is said that it is usually the male partner who suggests the activity in the first place, it is apparently not unusual for the women to be more comfortable with the reality once it has occurred. Couples often report an improvement in their own sexual relationship as a result of 'swinging', and according to Bartell (1970), 'many swingers report an unsatisfactory sexual relationship prior to swinging'. The sharing of this dyadic form of deviance may provide a range of joint activities previously lacking to the couple. But Gagnon & Simon (1973) have well described the resulting radical alteration to the role of sex in the marriage: 'sex . . . binds the unit through its provision of sex to others, rather than in its provision to each other'. The authors go on to point out the advantage that swinging gives the male partner who 'now possesses an object which may be used in sexual trading' and the potential that the female has for 'going it alone' once started out on this course of action.

In one respect, this type of sexual freedom is reminiscent of earlier types of licentiousness such as the French love clubs and masques at the latter part of the 18th century (Murstein 1974) which were indulged in by the wealthy and otherwise bored. The main difference now is that married couples use this type of activity as a way of dealing with their marital boredom and although it is predominantly middle-class behaviour, it does not appear to be confined to the affluent. Nevertheless, it is a minority behaviour and there seems little prospect of it influencing the majority except perhaps in their fantasy lives.

SEXUAL FANTASY

The internal and private world of fantasy is an important part of an individual's sexual life, even if it only involves imaginary behaviour. Erotic imagery may have a sexually arousing effect and lead us to seek out real activity either in masturbation or with a partner. The relationship between sexual fantasy and sexual drive or appetite is complex (see p. 72) — to what extent should we see fantasy as a sexual stimulus or as a response to some internal state or external circumstance? Our fantasy lives provide us with an arena in which to rehearse our real activities. We discussed in Chapter 3 the possible importance of early sexual fantasies in determining our sexual preferences. Not infrequently the fantasies which were used early in an individual's sexual life retain some special erotic effect long after the content of the fantasy has any other current relevance. It is an intriguing but as yet unanswered question why in some individuals these specific fantasies retain their potency as conditioned erotic stimuli whilst in others the erotic fantasies change to reflect current sexual activities and interest. The scope that is possible in fantasy for an imaginative person may lead to imagery which is frightening in its effects or implications. The possibility that one may act out a fantasy can cause considerable anxiety. In some people, their early sexual fantasies developed at a time when their comprehension of sexuality was primitive and was influenced by immature anxieties or needs. These fantasies, retaining their erotic effect into adulthood, may later cause concern, suggesting to their user that he or she is seriously disturbed. Because fantasies can, and usually do, remain concealed, their frightening significance may continue unchallenged. Fantasies may be used to enhance or otherwise make more acceptable 'real' sexuality. As discussed in Chapter 10, identifying the discrepancies between an individual's real world and his or her fantasised, ideal world can be invaluable in helping people with sexual problems. Fantasies in their frequency, form or content may reveal interesting differences between males and females. There are therefore many reasons for taking sexual fantasies seriously. Unfortunately, because of the prejudice against introspection that has prevailed in experimental psychology for many years, it is only recently that attempts have been made to explore these phenomena and the available information is still sparse. (Wilson (1978) provides a useful review.)

THE INCIDENCE OF SEXUAL FANTASIES

An important distinction needs to be made between fantasies arising during the course of sexual activity, such as masturbation or intercourse, and those occurring at other times, such as daydreaming. Kinsey found that 84% of his male subjects were at least sometimes aroused by thinking of sexual activity — episodes they had already experienced or would like to experience. By contrast, 31% of the females insisted that they had never been aroused by such thoughts. Kinsey linked these findings to the belief that men are more likely to be sexually aroused at the beginning of a sexual encounter and before any physical contact with the female has occurred (Kinsey et al 1953). Hunt (1974) has attributed this sex difference to cultural factors as he found less difference between men and women in his study. However, he gave no figures and did not clearly distinguish between fantasies with and without sexual activity. Wilson (1980) did distinguish between daytime fantasies and fantasies during intercourse and masturbation. In both kinds, he found that men reported about twice as much erotic fantasy as women. Wagman (1967) found that men spent slightly more of their general daydreaming on sexual topics than did women. The content of this daydreaming, both sexual and otherwise, also fitted in with common stereotypes of male and female sexuality, with men using more aggressive, heroic and self-aggrandising and women more passive, narcissistic and affiliative themes. This general pattern has been found in a number of studies (Wilson 1980). Barclay (1973), in addition to finding such sex differences in content, also found that men described their fantasies with particular emphasis on visual aspects, whilst women emphasised accompanying emotions. Brown & Hart (1977) found that sexually experienced women reported twice as much fantasy as virgins, with the highest rates occurring in women between the ages of 21 and 35. There is some evidence that the better educated (or perhaps more intelligent) have richer fantasy lives (Crepault et al 1977; Pietropinto & Simenaur 1977). As most of the studies so far have used university students or middle-class subjects, there is a need for caution in extrapolating to the population in general.

Kinsey reported that 60% of his male subjects who masturbated always used fantasy during the act, and 10% never did so. For females, the percentages were 41% and 36% respectively. As stated earlier, the number of women who actively masturbated was also substantially lower than for men (40% and 93% respectively; Gebhard & Johnson 1979). Comparable findings were reported by Hesellund (1976) studying married couples and Garde & Lunde (1980) studying 40-year-old women.

In the Woman magazine survey of women (Sanders 1985) 50% of wives said they fantasised whilst making love; rather less than half of them did so regularly. Women who said they were completely satisfied with their relationship tended to use fantasies less often than those in unsatisfactory relationships. Sexual fantasies at other times or during masturbation were not reported. The commonest type of fantasy was of making love with a man known to the woman (40%). In 20% the favourite fantasy involved making love in a different or more exotic setting. Eight per cent described fantasies of rape or violence, though these were most likely to involve 'gentle' rape, the key element being the woman having no control over what was happening to her. In the male survey (Sanders 1987) most men said they used fantasies during masturbation and 37% during love-making. The favourite fantasy (18%) was making love with a different partner (not necessarily someone known to them), in a different situation (13%) and involving watching or being watched while making love (15%). Other favourites included being dominated or tied up (7%), other forms of masochism (5%) and raping a submissive woman (2%).

One of the more interesting studies is by Hariton & Singer (1974), though only married women were involved. These authors found that 65% of the women studied reported erotic fantasies at least some of the time during sexual intercourse with their husbands and in 37% such fantasies were common. Crepault et al (1977) in a group of 66 women found 14% who always, 39% who often and 47% who rarely or never used erotic fantasy during heterosexual activity. In neither study is there any clear indication how often the women fantasised when not involved in sexual activity. This distinction is relevant to the possible function or significance of erotic fantasies. Kinsey believed that fantasies led to the initiation of sexual activity, particularly in men. The fantasies can therefore be seen to reflect sexual drive. Giambra & Martin (1977) found that sexual fantasies were not only more frequent in men with high levels of coital activity, but declined with age so that in men after 65 they virtually disappear. Wilson (1980), on the other hand, found only a weak correlation between the use of fantasy and indicators of sexual drive in men. Crepault et al (1977) found that sexual fantasies in general were more common in women who masturbated and who started masturbating at an earlier age, suggesting that where sexual activity not dependent on a partner is concerned, fantasy and sexual drive may be related in women. In Wilson's study the women also showed significant correlations between the use of fantasy and self-reported sexual drive and orgasm frequency. Furthermore, their use of sexual fantasies was associated with general sexual satisfaction, whereas in the men it was not. Wilson therefore concluded that in men fantasies are manifestations of a sex drive that is not totally fulfilled whereas women seem to have more fantasies when their sex life is going well.

The role of sexual fantasy is not likely to be that simple, however. Hariton & Singer (1974), using factor analysis, identified four factors and associated types of women. Women scoring high on factor 1 tended to fantasise a great deal in general, using many sexual fantasies as well as other types of fantasy. These women showed personality features of aggression, exhibition, impulsivity, autonomy and dominance whilst scoring low on measures of nurturance and affiliation, two traditionally feminine traits. Their exploratory approach to sex was reflected in high frequencies of premarital and extramarital affairs, with the latter being apparently motivated more by curiosity than marital unhappiness. One is tempted to see these women as showing masculine rather than feminine characteristics, at least as far as our sex role stereotypes would indicate. The second group of women experienced sexual dissatisfaction or guilt and tended not to use enjoyable sexual fantasies. The third group were somewhat older, and reared in a more traditional background of sexual repression. They were generally satisfied with their sexual relations in marriage but used fantasies of sexual submission to enhance their enjoyment. Several studies have stressed the importance of forced compliance in women's fantasies and have sometimes used this evidence to suggest that masochism is a basic feminine trait. In this study, the evidence suggests that forced compliance may be used as a means of avoiding sexual guilt. In a sexually repressive environment, females may feel less guilty about responding sexually to a situation, albeit imaginary, for which they cannot be held responsible. (A similar theme is sometimes apparent in the histories of men who use masochistic fantasies.) The fourth group were unhappy with their marriages and used erotic fantasies, usually involving men other than their husbands, as if to compensate for their lack of sexual response to their partner.

It thus appears that the use of sexual fantasy by women can on the one hand reflect a general cognitive style, in which case the content of the fantasy is less important than the general tendency to fantasise. On the other hand, they may serve some specific sexual purpose, in which case the content of the fantasies is of particular relevance. It has been suggested that the huge market in 'soft porn' or erotic romances which are read (and written) predominantly by women portray the types of situation common in women's fantasies (Coles & Shamp 1984).

Comparable evidence for men is not yet available. Although many of the apparent differences between men and women may be culturally determined, there may be some of more basic psychobiological significance which would deserve further study.

RESPONSE TO EROTICA

Somewhere between overt sexual activity and sexual fantasy come the various forms of visual or literary erotica as sources of erotic stimulation. Their very tangible existence and considerable commercial exploitation in recent years has caused much concern about possible harmful effects and the need for control or censorship. In the USA this led to the Commission on Obscenity and Pornography which started in 1968 to direct and fund a series of research studies (Technical Reports of the Commission on Obscenity and Pornography 1970). This exercise was an interesting example of the misuse of science. The real issues of public concern were not, and probably could not be resolved by the types of research commissioned, though the general findings were reassuring as far as they went. In this respect the investigators could be criticised for drawing conclusions that went beyond the scope of the evidence. Even more striking, however, was the outright rejection of the commission's findings by the US government, presumably because the results were not in the desired direction. On emotive issues such as these, one cannot replace value judgements with scientific evidence, though hopefully our values will be at least influenced by such evidence. In the UK, Lord Longford, on his own initiative, set up a private enquiry into pornography in 1971 which, it could be said, was predestined to reach opposing conclusions to the US commission (Longford 1972). Later, a government-sponsored committee delivered its report, perhaps less biased than either of the previous two, but none the less controversial in its conclusions (Williams 1979).

The main concern of such inquiries is the possibility that pornography may have an undesirable effect on morals, or to put it more practically, on the behaviour of members of society, particularly the young. We must leave this question unanswered and possibly unanswerable. The possible relationship between pornography and sexual crime will be considered further in chapter 13.

But we can make use of the research to answer less emotive questions. For those people studied, mainly university students, what are the short-term effects of exposure to erotica? How do males and females compare in their responses? How do different types of erotica compare in their effects?

The short-term effects are much as one might expect. Erotica tends to induce a degree of sexual arousal which is often followed by a temporary increase in sexual activity, either masturbation or sex with the usual partner, and the effect is noticeable for no more than 1 or 2 days. There has been little evidence that new types of sexual activity, as depicted in erotica, have resulted, though they may have done so in fantasy (Yaffe 1972; Schmidt 1975; Bancroft 1978). It nevertheless seems inherently likely that exposure to a novel kind of sexual stimulation, if it is found to hold appeal for the observer and does not generate anxiety or guilt, may result in it being tried out eventually when the circumstances are right.

Of more interest is the comparison of male and female responses. Kinsey and his colleagues (1953) found a greater proportion of males than females reporting erotic responses to a variety of types of stimuli, though the differences were most marked for pornographic pictures. Little difference between the sexes was reported for responses to literature or films which were not explicitly erotic. As with other sex differences reported by Kinsey, they are much less noticeable in later studies; this is part of the general convergence of male and female sexuality that has already been mentioned. Gebhard (1973) has also suggested that the method of interviewing in the Kinsey study exaggerated the sex differences, especially for the less well educated women who were asked 'Does it get you hot and bothered?' when giving information about erotic responses.

Schmidt (1975) has summarised the results from a series of studies he and his colleagues carried out in West Germany. Females described them-selves as less sexually aroused than the males after pictorial and narrative stimulation but the differences were slight. The large majority of both men and women were aware of some physiological–sexual reaction during such stimulation. Emotional agitation or tension commonly followed in both women and men. There was no support for the widely held belief that women require evidence of affection in order to respond sexually. With erotic stories which excluded any expression of tenderness or affection, sexual responses were as great amongst women as men. Responses to films of rape did show some interesting sex differences, however. Both males and females reported a mixture of sexual arousal and strong aversion, but the women showed stronger emotional avoidance reactions. There was also evidence of a different type of emotional conflict: 'In women the rape film produced sexual arousal and by identification with the female victim, fears of being helplessly overpowered. In men, the conflict is more characterised by guilt feelings and dismay that they are stimulated by aggressive sexual activities, incompatible with their conscious ideals of sexuality'. The relationship between sexuality and aggression appears to be complex. But it is important and needs further understanding (see Chapters 2 and 13).

Schmidt went on to see if other sex differences in his results supported the 'projection-versus-objectification' theory of Money & Ehrhardt (1972). This proposes that a woman's sexual response to an erotic stimulus is dependent on her projecting herself into the picture, i.e. identifying with the woman in the scene, whereas men objectify the content, taking it out of the picture in order to have a relationship with it. Judging by the reactions of men and women to pictures of male and female masturbation, there was limited evidence in support of this interesting hypothesis. But the best test would require a situation in which the female subject could identify with a female relating to or being attractive to a sexual partner; solitary masturbation does not allow that. This potential sex difference is worthy of further study.

Kelley & Musialowski (1986) reported an interesting sex difference when studying the effects of habituation. Men were less likely to become habituated to erotic films if the participants in the films changed with repeated showing, whereas for women habituation was lessened by a change of sexual activity by the *same* participants.

In general, most other studies are in agreement with Schmidt's conclusions — that there are sex differences but they are much less than was suggested by the Kinsey findings. A limitation has been the reliance in most studies on self-report of sexual arousal. Those few studies which have measured genital response to erotic stimuli have produced further interesting sex differences. In general, men show higher correlations between self-report of sexual arousal and measures of genital response than do women (Heiman & Hatch 1981). Wincze et al (1976) found that normal and sexually dysfunctional women differed more in their subjective ratings of arousal than in their vaginal blood volume responses to erotic stimuli. This reminds us of the potentially greater feedback effect of genital responses in the male than in the female, discussed in Chapter 2. Because men are more confronted by their penile responses, they are less able to deny that they have responded sexually and hence may be less susceptible to social conditioning of sexual attitudes.

Another intriguing sex difference emerged in a study by Levi (1969). He showed erotic films to a group of 50 males and 50 females, together in a cinema. In addition, he collected urine from each of them before and after the film and measured the urinary catecholamine excretion as well as obtaining self-ratings of sexual arousal. Both male and female groups reported significant increases in sexual arousal, though the increase for the males was significantly greater than that for the females. Both groups showed increases in urinary adrenaline and noradrenaline excretion, but whereas for noradrenaline this was similar for the two groups, for adrenaline it was substantially higher in the men. The possibility that the autonomic nervous system and adrenal medullary responses to sexual stimuli are fundamentally different in the two sexes is of considerable interest and this finding deserves replication in a further study. Also of interest is the fact that whereas self-ratings of sexual arousal correlated with catecholamine excretion in the females, they did not do so for the males. One possible explanation is that the self-ratings of the males were more influenced by their degree of erection, whereas for the females they were influenced by their state of general arousal which was more likely to be determined by adrenal medullary activity.

Reactions to different types of erotic stimuli also show little evidence of sex differences, particularly when genital responses are measured. In most such studies films have been found to be more effective than slides or fantasies. But in the author's experience it is not unusual for a subject, either male or female, to feel more comfortable with and to give a higher subjective rating for a fantasy response than for a response to a film if the content of the film provokes any conflict.

PERSONALITY AND SEXUAL BEHAVIOUR

Considering the extensive work that has been carried out in the field of personality measurement, surprisingly little attention has been paid to the influence of personality variables on sexual behaviour. The main exception has been Eysenck (1976), who devised a questionnaire covering various aspects of sexual attitudes and behaviours (Eysenck 1971) and related the answers to his usual personality measures of extroversion–introversion (E), neuroticism (N) and toughmindedness (P). Extroverts are more sociable, impulsive, physically active, talkative, carefree, hopeful and hotheaded; introverts are more thoughtful, serious, unsociable, high-principled, controlled in their behaviour and less outgoing. Neuroticism is a tendency to show strong and easily elicited emotional reactions which tend to persist over a long period. The P factor measures male as opposed to female characteristics, which in extreme cases are manifested in psychopathic, hostile or sadistic behaviour.

Factor analysis of the sexual questionnaire responses produced 11 groups of questions labelled permissiveness, satisfaction, neurotic sex, impersonal sex, pornography, shyness, prudishness, sexual disgust, sexual excitement, physical sex and aggressive sex. These factors were not independent of one another and hence they were regrouped to produce two major independent factors which Eysenck called 'libido' (or sexual desire) and 'satisfaction'. He then found that extroverts were high on libido and tended to the positive end of the satisfaction factor. Introverts were at the low end of the libido factor, although they showed greater satisfaction at older age levels. 'Extroversion is more appropriate to youth'.

High neuroticism scorers complained more of sexual dysfunction of various kinds and reported high anxiety about sex (i.e. low satisfaction) whilst being high on the libido dimension. According to Eysenck, high N scorers show a conflict between their strong desires and equally strong inhibitions. High P scorers emerged as advocates of impersonal permissive sexual practices — the 'all's fair in love and war' attitude. They were high on libido, but rather low on satisfaction. Eysenck (1976) stressed the importance of genetic and biological factors in accounting for these contrasting types of personality and sexuality.

Other writers have criticised the strength of Eysenck's claims. Farley et al (1977), using different but comparable measures of personality and sexuality, concluded that there was a 'general lack of contribution of personality variables . . . to sexuality, as measured.' Schenk et al (1981), using Eysenck's measures of E and N, found no support for his conclusions in a study of married couples, concluding that the quality of the marriage was more important than personality variables in determining the sexual relationship. In a later study of *single* men (Schenk & Pfrang 1986) they found some support for the link between sexuality and extroversion but not neuroticism.

Frenken (1976), in developing his sexual experience scales which measure aspects of sexual attitudes as well as behaviour, drew comparisons with various measures of personality and found the predictive power of personality characteristics to be weak. Gender, age and frequency of church attendance were the best predictors of sexual behaviour.

Fisher & Byrne (1987) have developed a questionnaire about sexuality that measures what they call erotophilia–erotophobia. Authoritarian individuals tend to be erotophobic. Androgynous men and women (using Bem's (1974) measure of androgyny) tend to be more erotophilic than traditional sex role men and women. Erotophobic men generally tend to adhere more to the work ethic. In women erotophilia was negatively associated with achievement aspiration but positively with understanding.

More research is needed in this area, but thus far it would appear that established measures of personality only allow us to account for a small proportion of the variance in human sexuality.

COMPARISON OF MEN AND WOMEN

It is widely believed that men are fundamentally different to women in most aspects of their sex lives. They are assumed to have a higher sexual drive, to be more easily aroused sexually, to tolerate sexual abstinence less well, to see sex as a more important part of their lives, and to be polygamous by nature whereas women are monogamous. We have considered the evidence for these and other assumptions at various points in the book. Let us now draw the evidence together and summarise.

There is convincing evidence that over the past 25 years there has been a convergence between male and female sexuality, as shown in the onset and frequency of premarital sexuality and masturbation, patterns of marital sex and interest in and response to erotica. In most respects, this has meant that women have become more like men, but in some respects it may be the other way round, or there may be a convergence by both towards some middle ground. The shift away from the adolescent double standard towards sex as a manifestation of a loving relationship comes into this category. The speed and extent of this convergence can only be understood as a change in social influences, not as a change in the biological nature of women. But it does not follow from this that all behavioural differences between the sexes are culturally determined or that as far as their biological capacities are concerned, men and women, apart from the inescapable reproductive differences, are basically the same. We have already suggested various ways in which biological factors may enhance the differentiating effects of social factors. For example, the fact that young females are much less aware of their genital responses to sexual stimuli than are young males may make them more susceptible to social influences that aim to suppress their sexuality. For the male, his erect penis stands as a kind of monument to his biological sexuality. There are other ways in which biological differences facilitate cultural discrimination so that basic but modest sex differences become amplified and accentuated into sex role stereotypes. In any rational attempt to counter the undesirable consequences of such stereotyping, it is necessary to understand as well as we can the biological starting point. We are still a long way from doing this adequately; there remain many uncertainties, but let us consider some possibilities.

Do men have a higher sexual drive than women? The deficiencies of the concept of 'sexual drive' were discussed in Chapter 2. We need to distinguish between the capacity to respond to a sexual stimulus with sexual arousal and pleasure, and the tendency to seek out such a stimulus in the first place. This latter aspect is experienced as an appetite for sex. In the first respect, there seems little difference between men and women in their capacity to respond to sexual stimulation and arousal, and from the physiological point of view, in the speed of those responses. Women in fact appear to have a greater capacity for repeated orgasms than men. In terms of sexual appetite the question is more difficult to answer. If one determines the degree of sexual appetite by its manifestations in overt behaviour, then the association is confounded by whether men are more likely to or more able to initiate sexual activity than women. Part of the female's apparent reluctance to initiate has cultural origins; women once in an established sexual relationship find it easier to initiate love-making than those who are seeking a mate. At the courtship stage, the prevailing view of what is proper female behaviour is all-important. Even after marriage, however, there are still many women who continue to feel uncomfortable with the initiator role, or who are only able to deliver subtle cues to encourage their partners. Garde & Lunde (1980) asked their 40-year-old Danish women whether they experienced spontaneous libido and 32% said they did not. In all, 24% experienced it at least once a week, 41% once or twice monthly and 23% more rarely. There are no comparable data for men, but one might expect rather more spontaneous interest than these women appear to have. Is there a basic male–female difference in this respect? Is it biologically less important for women to experience spontaneous desire? Is it possible that the basic paradigm of female sexuality is to be submissive, and of the male, to be dominant, at least in a physical sense? Does the pattern that the majority fall into most easily and most comfortably have a biological basis?

The tendency for female fantasies to contain more submissive behaviour and the male more dominance is relevant here. The interesting theory that men objectify sexual stimuli, relating them to themselves as the sexual subject, whereas women identify with the object, is also relevant. The fact that men may quite frequently condition sexual responses to stimuli which are depersonalised (as in fetishism) whereas for women sexual stimuli are nearly always personalised (i.e. at least potentially part of an interpersonal relationship) may reflect the same pattern. For the young male, sexually relevant experiences are more likely to occur in the course of male type behaviour — the physical contact that accompanies rough and tumble play. The possibility that for many males sexual arousal occurs more easily when they are being physically dominant with their partner reminds us of the complex relationship between aggression and sexuality, and the homosocial rewards derived from heterosexual interaction by many adolescent males (see Chapter 13). Of course, much or even all of these differences could be accounted for by social learning, and the suggestion from the cross-cultural data that men are less anxious about sex in societies where the women typically are more dominant within marriage raises the possibility that social expectations which do not require the male to be sexually dominant may be best for the expression of male sexuality. But the striking similarity between many of these themes and the sexual behaviour patterns of our primate relatives should convince us that male/female stereotypes are not solely the product of human social structure.

Women do appear to tolerate, or at least experience, longer periods of sexual inactivity than men. This is noticeable from childhood onwards. Some of these interruptions in their sexual careers are linked to reproduction, as with pregnancy and lactation. But if women have in general less of a tendency to initiate sexual activity, whilst retaining the capacity to respond to the initiation of others, then this apparent sex difference would not be surprising. But earlier we considered Perper's (1985) view that it is women who control albeit subtly the sociosexual interaction. Perper believes that women are not only more in control, they are also more aware of what is going on. He goes further and suggests that women are much more open about their sexuality. The public expression of female sexuality, in our society at least, is legitimate. Men, he suggests, are much less open about their sexuality; they use allusive, indirect language to describe it; they are less comfortable revealing that they are sexual beings. This idea has many potential ramifications in our thinking about male–female differences and deserves further consideration.

Some of the more specific physiological differences could also have considerable repercussions on general male–female differences. Of particular interest is the difference in the relationship between orgasm and anxiety (see Chapter 8). Most women find orgasm more difficult to attain when they are tense or anxious. Men, by contrast, often find that their ejaculation (and hence orgasm) is accelerated by such psychological factors (though there are some important exceptions). It is interesting to speculate how much this particular difference accounts for the very differing patterns of sexual responsiveness through the lifespan. Males reach their maximum capacity for orgasm and ejaculation very soon after puberty. Females are much more variable and many do not realise their full potential until well into their 20s. There is some evidence of convergence here, perhaps because young girls now are able to feel more positive and less inhibited about their sexuality. But the important point is that guilt and anxiety do not have the same effects on the pattern of male adolescent sexuality.

There are further age-related changes, probably of a basically physiological kind, such as the increasingly long post-orgasm refractory period of the male and his reduced efficiency of erectile response which may interact with other aspects of masculinity in complex ways. The fact that males have this built-in spacing mechanism after ejaculation may have an important function in optimising fertility; the male needs a period of time to replenish his sperm count. The lack of any comparable spacing device in the female may simply reflect the lack of reproductive benefit of such a mechanism but the implications for male–female relationships, once females are able to realise their full orgasmic potential, could be considerable. This has led Sherfey (1966), for example, to suggest that men have found it necessary to control female sexuality for fear of being overwhelmed by it.

The idea that men are polygamous and women monogamous is perhaps the most intriguing and in social terms the most important of these issues. It is easy to see that the reproductive role of the female puts her into a special position. If she is going to find herself with the task of rearing children, she will have a powerful need to ensure that the father of her children will share some of the consequences, both in terms of child-rearing and controlling family size. In other words, she would prefer a situation in which the reproductive consequences of sexual behaviour were as important, or nearly so, for the man as for the woman. The polygamous male, sowing his seed freely, can only do so by dissociating himself from the reproductive consequences. Comparative studies have suggested that the polygynous pattern of the human male may have biological roots. Sexual dimorphism of size (i.e. the tendency for the male of a species to be larger than the female) is believed to be a consequence of sexual selection in which male competes with male for access to the female — the larger, hence stronger, male wins and reproduces himself. In primates those species which are sexually dimorphic show polygynous mating patterns; the gorilla is perhaps the most striking example. Monogamous primates such as the marmoset or gibbon are not sexually dimorphic. The human primate *is* sexually dimorphic, leading Short (1981) to postulate that as far as our biological heritage is concerned, man is polygynous, or at least serially monogamous by nature. Comparative studies of testis size to body weight ratio in primates have also led to some interesting conclusions. A high testis:body weight ratio indicates the capacity for high sperm production, which is necessary for a promiscuous male if he is to remain fertile after frequent ejaculations. Amongst the great apes, for example, the gorilla, which copulates infrequently, has a very low testis:body weight ratio; the chimpanzee, which copulates promiscuously whenever a female is in oestrus, has a very high ratio. Thus the testis:body weight ratio has been proposed as a biological indicator of the pattern of mating, i.e. single male versus multi-male (promiscuous). Harcourt et al (1981) presented data for 33 primate species supporting this hypothesis. On this basis the human primate is in the single male (i.e. non-promiscuous) part of the distribution — just!

There is a widespread tendency to reject evidence of this kind as being of no relevance to the human condition — a kind of modern day anti-Darwinism, fuelled by the women's movement. It is important that such cross-species evidence should be kept in perspective when interpreting human behaviour. Much of so-called sociobiology has been rightly criticised for its simplistic overdetermination. Clearly biological determinants can be readily obscured by social factors. But at the same time, it would seem imprudent to ignore or reject such evidence. There may be much we can learn from cross-species comparative studies, just as we must make as much use as we can of cross-cultural studies. Academic insularity is not a recipe for progress in understanding the complexities of human behaviour.

What will happen to female sexuality when the woman has complete control of her fertility? To what extent will the tables be turned, and a woman will feel able to delay conception until the circumstances are right for her, whilst men become threatened by the possibility that they may never be able to ensure their own offspring? Perhaps males will become the monogamous ones. Many of the changes in female sexuality documented here are related to the change in women's control over their fertility. But we are too much in the midst of this change to see clearly where it will lead. Is there a trend towards voluntary childlessness, one which would have very positive biological consequences? What effect would this have on the monogamous aspirations of the traditional woman? It would be interesting if at the end of it all we still found women were more prone to monogamy than men — but who knows?

Kinsey pointed out that in many respects women were much more variable in their sexuality than men, showing greater extremes of interest and activity. To some extent this could be accounted for by the greater need for men to fall within the norm to maintain their self-esteem. It may be easier for women to admit to having no interest in sex at all than it is for a man. But there are alternative explanations which are considered in Chapter 2 in an attempt to explain the more variable and less consistent evidence of hormone–behaviour relationships in women compared to men. Women may present a much more varied picture than men in both their actual and their potential sexuality.

REFERENCES

Abernethy V 1974 Dominance and sexual behavior: a hypothesis. American Journal of Psychiatry 131: 813–817

Armstrong E G 1978 Massage parlors and their customers. Archives of Sexual Behavior 7: 117–126

Asayama S 1976 Sexual behaviour in Japanese students: comparisons for 1974, 1960 and 1952. Archives of Sexual Behavior 5: 371–390

Athanasiou R, Sarkin R 1974 Premarital sexual behavior and postmarital adjustment. Archives of Sexual Behavior 3: 207–226

Athanasiou R, Shaver P, Tavris C 1970 Sex. Psychology Today 4 July: 39–52

Bancroft J 1978 Psychological and physiological responses to sexual stimuli in men and women. In: Levi L (ed) Society, stress and disease, vol 3. The productive and reproductive age. Oxford University Press, Oxford

Barclay A M 1973 Sexual fantasies in men and women. Medical Aspects of Sexuality 7: 205–216

Barry H III, Schlegel A 1980 (eds) Cross-cultural samples and codes. University Pittsburgh Press, Pittsburgh

Bartell G D 1970 Group sex among the mid-Americans. Journal of Sex Research 6 (2): 113–130

Beck S B 1978 Women's somatic preferences. In: Cook M, Wilson G D (eds) Love and attraction: an international conference. Pergamon, Oxford

Bell R R 1966 Premarital sex in a changing society. Prentice-Hall, Englewood Cliffs, New Jersey

Bell R R, Chaskes J B 1970 Premarital sexual experience among coeds, 1958 and 1968. Journal of Marriage and the Family 32: 81–84

Bell R R, Turner S, Rosen L 1975 A multivariate analysis of female extramarital coitus. Journal of Marriage and the Family 37: 375–384

Bem S L 1974 The measurement of psychological androgyny. Journal of Consulting and Clinical Psychology 42: 155–162

Blumstein P, Schwartz P 1983 American couples. Morrow, New York

Bone M 1986 Trends in single women's sexual behaviour in Scotland. Population Trends 43: 7–14

Boswell J 1980 Christianity, social tolerance and homosexuality. University Chicago Press, Chicago.

Brecher E M 1984 Love, sex and aging. A Consumer Union report. Little, Brown, Boston

Broude G J, Greene S J 1980 Cross-cultural codes on 20 sexual attitudes and practices. In: Barry H III, Schlegel A (eds) Cross-cultural samples and codes. University of Pittsburgh Press, Pittsburgh, pp 313–333

Brown J J, Hart D H 1977 Correlates of female's sexual fantasies. Perceptual and Motor Skills 45: 819–825

Bullough V L 1976 Sexual variance in society and history. Wiley, New York

Bury J 1983 Teenage pregnancies in Britain. Birth Control Trust, London

Cartwright A 1970 Parents and family planning services. Routledge & Kegan Paul, London

Chesser E 1956 The sexual, marital and family relationships of the English woman. Rox Publisher, New York

Chester R, Walker C 1979 Sexual experience and attitudes of British women. In: Chester R, Peel J (eds) Changing patterns of sexual behaviour. Academic Press, London

Christensen H R, Gregg C F 1970 Changing sex norms in America and Scandinavia. Journal of Marriage and the Family 32: 616–627

Clark A L, Wallin P 1965 Women's sexual responsiveness and the duration and quality of their marriages. American Journal of Sociology Sept: 187–196

Clement U, Schmidt G, Kruse M 1984 Changes in sex differences in sexual behavior: a replication of a study of West German students (1966–1981). Archives of Sexual Behavior 13: 99–120

Cochran W G, Mosteller F, Turkey J W 1953 Statistical problems of the Kinsey report. Journal of the American Statistical Association 48: 673–716

Coles C D, Shamp M J 1984 Some sexual, personality and demographic characteristics of women readers of erotic romances. Archives of Sexual Behavior 13: 187–210

Crepault C, Abraham C, Porto R, Couture M 1977 Erotic imagery in women. In: Gemme

R, Wheeler C C (eds) Progress in sexology. Plenum, New York

Daly M, Wilson M 1978 Sex, evolution and behaviour. Wadsworth, Belmont, California

Davis K B 1929 Factors in the sex life of 2200 women. Harper, New York

Davis R, Fabris G 1980 The sexual life cycle in a male-supremacist Catholic society: the case of Italy. In: Forleo R, Pasini W (eds) Medical sexology. Elsevier/North Holland, Amsterdam

Dion K 1981 Physical attractiveness, sex roles and heterosexual attraction. In: Cook M (ed) The bases of human sexual attraction. Academic, London, pp 3–22

Dominian J 1979a Definition and extent of marital pathology. British Medical Journal 2: 478–479

Dominian J 1979b Health and marital breakdown. British Medical Journal 2: 424–425

Dryfoos J G 1978 The incidence and outcome of adolescent pregnancy in the United States. In: Parkes A S, Short R V, Potts M, Herbertson M A (eds) Fertility in adolescence. Journal of Biosocial Science (suppl 5): 85–100

Dunnell K 1979 Family formation 1976. HMSO, London

Elwin 1968 The kingdom of the young. Oxford University Press, Oxford

Eysenck H J 1971 Personality and sexual adjustment. British Journal of Psychiatry 118: 593–608

Eysenck H J 1976 Sex and personality. Open Books, London

Eysenck H J, Wilson G 1979 The psychology of sex. Dent, London

Farley F, Nelson J G, Knight W C, Garcia-Colberg E 1977 Sex, politics and personality: a multidimensional study of college students. Archives of Sexual Behavior 6: 105–120

Farman-Farmaian S 1978 Socio-cultural aspects of age at marriage in the middle-east. Journal Biosocial Science (suppl) 5: 215–226

Farrell C 1978 My mother said . . . the way young people learn about sex and birth control. Routledge & Kegan Paul, London

Fisher W, Byrne D 1981 Social background, attitudes and sexual attraction. In: Cook M (ed) The bases of human sexual attraction. Academic, London pp 23–64

Fisher W, Byrne D 1988 Erotophobia–erotophilia as a dimension of personality. Journal of Sex Research (in press)

Ford C S, Beach F A 1952 Patterns of sexual behaviour. Eyre & Spottiswoode, London

Fox G L 1981 The family role in adolescent sexual behavior. In: Ooms T (ed) Teenage pregnancy in a family context. Temple University Press, Philadelphia

Fox G L, Inazu J K 1980 Patterns and outcomes of mother–daughter communication about sexuality. Journal of Social Issues 36: 7–29

Frenken J 1976 Afkeer van seksualiteit. English summary: pp 219–225. Van Loghum Staterus, Deventer

Gagnon J, Simon W 1973 Sexual conduct: the social sources of human sexuality. Aldine, Chicago

Gagnon J, Simon W 1987 The sexual scripting of oral genital contacts. Archives of Sexual Behavior 16: 1–26

Galton F 1883 Inquiries into human faculty and its development. Macmillan, London

Garde K, Lunde I 1980 Female sexual behaviour. A study in a random sample of 40 year old women. Maturitas 2: 225–240

Gebhard P H 1966 Factors in marital orgasm. Journal of Social Issues 22(2): 88–95

Gebhard P H 1973 Sex differences in sexual response. Archives of Sexual Behavior 2: 201–204

Gebhard P H 1978 Marital stress. In: Levi L (ed) Society, stress and disease, vol 3. The productive and reproductive age. Oxford University Press, Oxford

Gebhard P H, Johnson A B 1979 The Kinsey data. Saunders, Philadelphia

Giambra L M, Martin C E 1977 Sexual daydreams and quantitative aspects of sexual activity: some relation for males across adulthood. Archives of Sexual Behaviour 6: 497–505

Gillis J R 1985 For better, for worse. British marriages, 1600 to the present. Oxford University Press, Oxford

Glass D V 1974 Population growth in developed countries. In: Parry H B (ed) Population and its problems: a plain man's guide. Clarendon Press, Oxford

Gorer G 1971 Sex and marriage in England today. Nelson, London

Gray J P 1984 The influence of female power in marriage on sexual behavior and attitudes: a holocultural study. Archives of Sexual Behavior 13: 223–232

Griffin T, Morris J 1987 Social trends no 17. HMSO, London
Hagstad A, Janson A 1984 Sexuality among Swedish women around 40 — an epidemiological survey. Journal of Psychosomatic Obstetrics and Gynaecology 3: 191–204
Harcourt A H, Harvey P H, Larson S G, Short R V 1981 Testis weight, body weight and breeding system in primates. Nature 293: 55–57
Hariton E B, Singer J L 1974 Women's fantasies during sexual intercourse: normative and theoretical implications. Journal of Consulting and Clinical Psychology 42: 313–322
Haskey J 1983 Social class patterns of marriage. Population Trends 34: 12–25
Haskey J, Coleman D 1986 Cohabitation before marriage: a comparison of information from marriage registration and the general household survey. Population Trends 43: 15–17
Hatfield E, Walster G W 1981 A new look at love. University Press of America, Lanshaw, Maryland
Heiman J R, Hatch J P 1981 Conceptual and therapeutic contribution of psychophysiology to sexual dysfunction. In: Hayner S, Gannon L (eds) Psychosomatic disorders: a psychophysiological approach to etiology and treatment. Gardner, New York
Herdt G H 1981 Guardians of the flutes. McGraw-Hill, New York
Hertoft P 1977 Nordic traditions of marriage: the betrothal system. In: Money J, Musaph H (eds) Handbook of sexology . Excerpta Medica, Amsterdam
Hess E H 1965 Attitudes and pupil size. Scientific American 212: 46–54
Hessellund H 1976 Masturbation and sexual fantasies in married couples. Archives of Sexual Behavior 5: 133–147
Hite S 1976 The Hite report. Talmy Franklin, London
Hobbs A H, Lambert R D 1948 An evaluation of sexual behaviour in the human male. American Journal of Psychiatry 104: 758–764
Hofferth S L 1988 Trends in adolescent sexual activity, contraception and pregnancy in the United States. In: Bancroft J, Reinisch J (eds) Adolescence and puberty. Third Kinsey symposium. Oxford University Press, New York
Hotvedt M E 1988 Emerging and submerging adolescent sexuality: culture and sexual orientation. In: Bancroft J, Reinisch J (eds) Adolescence and puberty. Third Kinsey symposium. Oxford Univeristy Press, New York
Hunt M 1974 Sexual behavior in the 1970s. Playboy Press, Chicago
Hyman H, Barmack J E 1954 Special review: sexual behavior in the human female. Psychological Bulletin 51 (4): 418–427
Ineichen B 1979 The social geography of marriage. In: Cook M, Wilson G (eds) Love and attraction. Pergamon, Oxford
Jones E F, Forrest J D, Goldman N et al 1985 Teenage pregnancies in developed countries: determinants and policy implications. Family Planning Perspectives 17: 53–63
Kantner J F, Zelnick M 1972 Sexual experience of young unmarried women in the United States. Family Planning Perspectives 4: 9–18
Katchadourian H A 1985 Fundamentals of human sexuality, 4th edn. Holt, Rinehart & Winston, New York
Kelley K, Musialowski D 1986 Repeated exposure to sexually explicit stimuli: novelty, sex and sexual attitudes. Archives of Sexual Behavior 15: 487–498
Kinsey A C, Pomeroy W B, Martin C F 1948 Sexual behavior in the human male. Saunders, Philadelphia
Kinsey A C, Pomeroy W B, Martin C F, Gebhard P H 1953 Sexual behavior in the human female. Saunders,.Philadelphia
Klausner S Z 1964 Inferential visibility and sex norms in the middle East. Journal of Social Psychology 63: 1–29
Kolata G B 1974 !Kung hunter- gatherers: feminism, diet and birth control. New York Science 185: 932
Kulanayagam R 1979 Semen-losing syndrome. Journal of the Psychiatric Association of Thailand 24: 152–158
Kunzel R 1974 The connection between the family cycle and divorce rates: an analysis based on European data. Journal of Marriage and the Family: 379–388
Landis C et al 1940 Sex in development. Hoeber, New York
Lee J A 1976 Lovestyles. Dent, New York
Levi L 1969 Sympatho-adreno-medullary activity, diuresis and emotional reactions during

visual sexual stimulation in human females and males. Psychosomatic Medicine 31: 251–268

Levi-Strauss C 1969 The elementary structures of kinship. Beacon, Boston

Linner B 1967 Sex and society in Sweden. Pantheon, New York

Littlewood B 1978 South Italian couples. In: Corbin M (ed) The couple. Penguin, London

Locke H J 1951 Predicting adjustment in marriage. A comparison of a divorced and a happily married group. Holt, New York

Longford 1972 Pornography: the Longford report. Coronet, London

McCabe M P, Collins J K 1983 The sexual and affectional attitudes and experiences of Australian adolescents during dating: the effects of age, church attendance, type of school and socio-economic class. Archives of Sexual Behavior 12: 525–540

McCance C, Hall D J 1972 Sexual behaviour and contraceptive practices of unmarried female undergraduates at Aberdeen University. British Medical Journal ii: 694–700

Malinowski B 1929 The sexual life of savages. Routledge, London

Marshall D S, Suggs R C 1971 (eds) Human sexual behavior. Prentice-Hall, Englewood Cliffs, New Jersey

Masters W H, Johnson V E 1966 Human sexual response. Churchill, London

Mathews A M, Bancroft J H J, Slater P 1972 The principal components of sexual preference. British Journal of Social and Clinical Psychology 11: 35–43

Mead M 1929 Coming of age in Samoa. Jonathan Cape, London

Mcad M 1931 Growing up in New Guinea. Routledge, London

Mead M 1950 Male and female. Pelican, London

Money J 1977 Peking: the sexual revolution. In: Money J, Musaph H (eds) Handbook of sexology. Excerpta Medica, Amsterdam

Money J, Ehrhardt A A 1972 Man and woman, boy and girl. Differentiation and dimorphism of gender identity from conception to maturity. Johns Hopkins University Press, Baltimore

Mullan B 1984 The mating trade. Routledge & Kegan Paul, London

Murdock G P 1967 Ethnographic atlas. University Pittsburgh Press, Pittsburgh

Murstein B I 1974 Love, sex and marriage through the ages. Springer, New York

Murstein B I 1981 Process, filter and stage theories of attraction. In: Cook M (ed) The bases of human sexual attraction. Academic, London. pp 179–211

Nag M 1972 Sex, culture and human fertility: India and the United States. Current Anthropology 13: 231–238

Newcomer S F, Udry J R 1985 Oral sex in an adolescent population. Archives of Sexual Behavior 14: 41–46

O'Neill N, O'Neill G 1972 Open marriage. Owen, London

Perper T 1985 Sex signals: the biology of love. ISI Press, New York

Pietropinto A, Simenauer J 1977 Beyond the male myth. A nationwide survey. Times Books, New York

Rainwater L 1966 Some aspects of lower class sexual behavior. Journal of Social Issues 22: 96–108

Reiss I L 1964 Premarital sexual permissiveness amongst Negroes and whites. American Sociological Review 29: 688–698

Reiss I L 1969 Premarital sexual standards. In: Broderick C B, Bernard J (eds) The individual, sex and society: a siecus handbook for teachers and counselors. Johns Hopkins Press, Baltimore

Rimmer L 1981 Families in focus. Marriage, divorce and family patterns. Occasional paper 6. Study Commission on the Family, London

Robinson P 1976 The modernization of sex. Harper & Row, New York

Rosenblatt P, Anderson R 1981 Human sexuality in cross-cultural perspective. In Cook M (ed) The bases of human sexual attraction. Academic, London, pp 215–250

Rothman D, Capell P 1978 Teenage pregnancy in England and Wales: some demographic and medicosocial aspects. Journal of Biosocial Science (suppl) 5: 65–83

Rubin Z 1970 Measurement of romantic love. Journal of Personality and Social Psychology 16: 265–273

Russell D E H 1983 The incidence and prevalence of intrafamilial and extrafamilial sexual abuse of female children. Child Abuse and Neglect 7: 133–146

Sai F A 1978 Social and psychosexual problems of African adolescents. Journal of Biosocial Science (suppl) 5: 235–247

Sanders D 1985 The Woman book of love and sex. Sphere, London

Sanders D 1987 The Woman report on men. Sphere, London

Schenk J, Pfrang H 1986 Extraversion, neuroticism and sexual behavior: interrelationships in a sample of young men. Archives of Sexual Behavior 12: 31–42

Schenk J, Pfrang H, Rausche A 1981 Personality traits versus the quality of the marital relationship as the determinants of marital sexuality. Archives of Sexual Behavior 15: 449–456

Schlegel A, Barry H III 1980 Adolescent initiation ceremonies. A cross-cultural code. In: Barry H III, Schlegel A 1980 (eds) Cross-cultural samples and codes. University of Pittsburgh Press, Pittsburgh, pp 227–288

Schmidt G 1975 Male–female differences in sexual arousal and behavior during and after exposure to sexually explicit stimuli. Archives of Sexual Behavior 4: 353–366

Schmidt G 1977 Introduction, sociohistorical perspectives. In: Money J, Musaph H (eds) Handbook of sexology. Excerpta Medica, Amsterdam

Schmidt G, Sigusch V 1971 Patterns of sexual behavior in West German workers and students. Journal of Sex Research 7: 89–106

Schmidt G, Sigusch V 1972 Changes in sexual behavior among young males and females between 1960 and 1970. Archives of Sexual Behavior 2: 27–45

Schofield M 1965 The sexual behaviour of young people. Longman, London

Shepher J 1971 Mate selection among second generation kibbutz adolescents and adults: incest avoidance and negative imprinting. Archives of Sexual Behavior 1: 293–308

Sherfey M J 1966 The evolution and nature of female sexuality in relation to psychoanalytic theory. Journal of the American Psychoanalytic Association 14: 28–128

Short R V 1976 The evolution of human reproduction. In: Short R V, Baird D T (eds) Contraceptives of the future. Royal Society, London

Short R V 1981 Sexual selection in man and the great apes. In: Graham C E (ed) Reproductive biology of the great apes. Academic, London, pp 319–341

Shorter E 1973 Female emancipation, birth control and fertility in European history. American Historical Review 78: 605–40

Shorter E 1975 The making of the modern family. Basic Books, New York

Smith L G, Smith J R 1977 Divorce and remarriage: trends and patterns in contemporary society. In: Money J, Musaph H (eds) Handbook of sexology. Excerpta Medica, Amsterdam

Smith J R, Smith L G 1970 Comarital sex and the sexual freedom movement. Journal of Sex Research 6 (2): 131–142

Snowden R, Christian B 1983 Patterns and perceptions of menstruation. A WHO international study. Croom Helm, London

Sorensen R C 1973 Adolescent sexuality in contemporary America. World Publishing, New York

Spanier G B, Cole C L 1975 Mate swapping: perceptions, value orientations and participation in a mid-Western community. Archives of Sexual Behaviour 4: 143–160

Starr B D, Weiner M B 1981 The Starr–Weiner report on sex and sexuality in the mature years. McGraw-Hill, New York

Stone L 1979 The family, sex and marriage in England 1500–1800. Pelican, London

Tannahill R 1980 Sex in history. Hamish Hamilton, London

Tanner J M 1962 Growth at adolescence, 2nd edn. Blackwell, Oxford

Technical Reports of the Commission on Obscenity and Pornography, vol I–VII. 1970 US Government Printing Office, Washington

Tennov D 1979 Love and limerence: the experience of being in love. Stein & Day, New York

Tennov D 1980 The clarification of proximate mechanisms. Comment on D Symon's The evolution of human sexuality. Behavioral and Brain Science 3: 200

Terman L M 1938 Psychological factors in marital happiness. McGraw-Hill, New York

Terman L M 1948 Kinsey's sexual behavior in the human male. Some comments and criticisms. Psychological Bulletin 45: 443–459

Thompson E J (ed) 1977 Social trends no 8. HMSO, London

Trost J 1978 Married and unmarried cohabitation in Sweden. In: Corbin M (ed) The couple. Penguin, London

Udry J R 1974 The social context of marriage 3rd edn. Lippincott, Philadelphia

Udry J R, Talbert L M, Morris N M 1986 Biosocial foundations for adolescent female
    sexuality. Demography 23: 217–227
Vener A M, Stewart C S 1974 Adolescent sexual behavior in middle America revisited:
    1970–1973. Journal of Marriage and the Family 36: 728–735
Visotsky H M 1969 A community project for unwed pregnant adolescents. In: Pollak O,
    Friedman A S (eds) Family dynamics and female sexual delinquency. Science and
    Behavior Books, Palo Alto
Wagman M 1967 Sex differences in types of daydreams. Journal of Personality and Social
    Psychology 7: 329–332
Wallin P 1949 An appraisal of some methodological aspects of the Kinsey report. American
    Sociological Review 14: 197–210
Walster E, Traupmann J, Walster G W 1978 Equity and extramarital sexuality. Archives of
    Sexual Behavior 7: 127–142
Wheeler J, Kilman P R 1983 Co-marital sexual behavior: individual and relationship
    variables. Archives of Sexual Behavior 12: 295–306
Whyte W F 1943 A slum sex code. American Journal of Sociology 49: 24–31
Whyte M K 1980 Cross-cultural codes dealing with the relative status of women. In: Barry
    H III, Schlegel A 1980 (eds) Cross-cultural samples and codes. University of Pittsburgh
    Press, Pittsburgh, pp 335–361
Wiggins J J, Wiggins N, Conger J C 1968 Correlates of heterosexual somatic preference.
    Journal of Personality and Social Psychology 10: 82–90
Williams B 1979 Report of the committee on obscenity and film censorship. HMSO,
    London
Wilson G D 1978 The secrets of sexual fantasy. Dent, London
Wilson G D 1980 Sex differences in sexual fantasy patterns. In: Forleo R, Pasini W (eds)
    Medical sexology. Elsevier/North Holland, Amsterdam
Wilson G D, Nias D K B 1976 Love's mysteries. Open Books, London
Winch R F 1958 Mate-selection: a study of complementary needs. Harper, New York
Wincze J P, Hoon P W, Hoon E F 1976 Physiological responsivity of normal and sexually
    dysfunctional women during erotic stimulus exposure. Journal of Psychosomatic Research
    20: 445–451
Wolf A P 1970 Childhood association and sexual attraction: a further test of the
    Westermarck hypothesis. American Anthropologist 72: 503–515
Wyatt G E 1988 Factors affecting adolescent sexuality. Have they changed in 40 years? In:
    Bancroft, J, Reinisch J (eds) Adolescence and puberty. Third Kinsey symposium. Oxford
    University Press, New York
Yaffe M 1972 Research survey. Appendix V. In: Longford (ed) Pornography: the Longford
    report. Coronet, London
Zelnick M, Kantner J F 1977 Sexual and contraceptive experience of young unmarried
    women in the United States, 1976 and 1971. Family Planning Perspectives 9: 55–71
Zelnick M, Kantner J F 1980 Sexual activity, contraceptive use and pregnancy among
    metropolitan area teenagers 1971–79. Family Planning Perspectives 12: 230–237
Zelnick M, Shah F K 1983 First intercourse among young Americans. Family Planning
    Perspectives 15: 64–70

5

Sexuality and ageing

Human beings are living longer and longer as education, the quality of life and medical science reduce the impact of illness. Two consequences of this trend are that we have more elderly people who are healthy and more who are in need of care. The part these healthy old people will play in our society and the increasing needs of the very old and senile pose some of the most crucial issues facing western societies. The life expectancy for women averages 6 years longer than for men, at least in developed countries, so we find an increasing difference in the number of men and women in the older age groups (Fig. 5.1).

The role of sexuality in old age is thus becoming more relevant. There has been a widespread tendency to assume that old people are too old for sex. As we shall see, there is an undoubted decline in the sexuality of both men and women with advancing years. But this decline varies considerably in extent from person to person, and with the changes in the health and social characteristics of this age group, sexuality could well play a crucial part in the maintenance of their relationships and their quality of life. It thus becomes important to establish the relative contributions of physical illness, social attitudes and normal ageing to the declining trend.

CHANGES IN SEXUAL BEHAVIOUR WITH AGE

Kinsey et al (1948) in their volume on the male, concluded that 'from the early and middle years the decline in sexual activity is remarkably steady and there is no point at which old age suddenly enters the picture' (p. 227). For the female the authors painted a somewhat different picture. 'There is little evidence of any ageing in the sexual capacities of the female until late in life' (Kinsey et al 1953, p. 353). The number of really elderly people in their otherwise large samples was relatively small and the conclusions about the effects of late old age were drawn rather tentatively. However, this trend, at least as far as the male is concerned, has been shown consistently in a number of later studies. Most of these studies have involved unrepresentative samples; the most representative are the Baltimore Aging Project (Martin 1977) for men, and Hallstrom's (1973) epidemiological

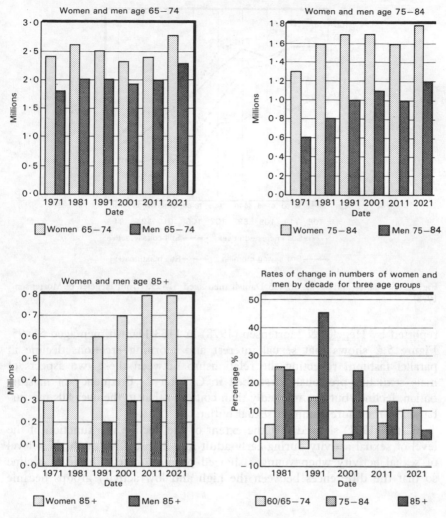

Fig. 5.1 Projected sex ratios of population in three age groups up to the year 2021, and rates of change for each sex by decade. (from Griffin & Morris 1987)

study of women before and after the menopause. Brecher's (1984) study is an example of an unrepresentative sample gleaned from the readers of a magazine, the Consumer's Union monthly Consumer's Report. This questionnaire study did, however, produce the largest amount of data for the older age groups and deserves consideration.

MALE SEXUALITY AND AGEING

A steady decline in the frequency of sexual activity was reported by Martin (1977) from the Baltimore Longitudinal Aging Study. Similar trends were

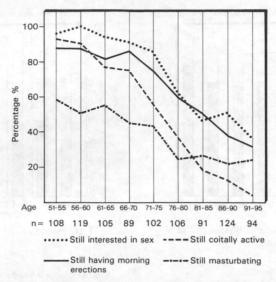

Age   51-55 56-60 61-65 66-70 71-75 76-80 81-85 86-90 91-95

n =   108   119   105   89   102   106   91   124   94

•••••• Still interested in sex   – – – Still coitally active

———— Still having morning   —•—•— Still masturbating
          erections

Fig. 5.2 Sexuality and ageing in 936 Danish men aged 51–95. (from Hegeler & Mortensen 1978)

reported by Hegeler & Mortensen (1978) in 1163 Danish men aged 51–95. Figure 5.2 shows that sexual interest and morning erections decline in parallel fashion, reflecting the relationship between these two aspects of male sexuality previously described in Chapter 2. Frequency of masturbation declines but less markedly than coitus so that in the over 80s masturbation is the more common sexual outlet.

Martin (1981) showed that the extent of the decline is a function of the level of sexual activity during early adult life. Those with the highest level of sexual activity when younger showed proportionately the least decline so that the differences between the high and low activity groups became

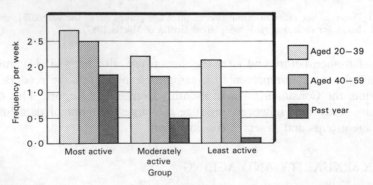

Fig. 5.3 Frequency of sexual activity at two different ages in three groups of older men categorised, according to their sexual activity in the past year, into most active, moderately active and least active. (from Martin 1981)

Table 5.1 Sexual changes decade by decade (from Brecher 1984)

	Percentage sexually active in age group		
	50s	60s	70s
All women (n = 1844)	93	81	65
All men (n = 2402)	98	91	79
Married women (n = 1245)	95	89	81
Unmarried women (n = 512)	88	63	50
Married men (n = 1895)	98	93	81
Unmarried men (n = 414)	95	85	75
	High enjoyment of sex (amongst sexually active; %)		
Women	71	65	61
Men	90	86	75

much more marked in the later years. This is shown graphically in Figure 5.3.

Brecher (1984) found similar changes (Table 5.1; Fig. 5.4) and also showed that the married and unmarried were very similar, with the latter showing only slightly greater decline. However in the over-70 age group, whereas 81% of the married were still sexually active, only 59% were having sex with their spouse. Presumably masturbation was being used as a substitute in a fair proportion. But although in some men, erectile problems may have led to cessation of joint sexual activity, these figures cast some doubt on the assumption of Kinsey et al (1953) and Martin (1981) that the decline in female sexuality is primarily a consequence of the decline in interest of the male partner.

Martin (1981) commented on the association between the duration of a sexual relationship and level of sexual interest. Several writers have

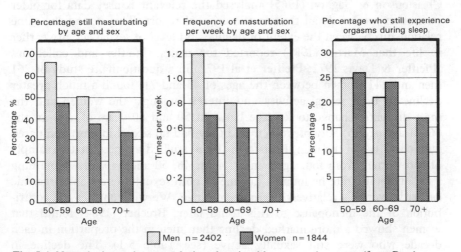

Men n = 2402   Women n = 1844

Fig. 5.4 Masturbation and orgasm during sleep in older men and women. (from Brecher 1984)

suggested that lack of novelty and boredom are important factors contributing to the age-related decline, as evidenced by the commonplace increase in sexual interest and activity with a new partner. However, as Martin points out, it is those men who are most active when younger who show the least decline, making a simple boredom explanation inadequate. The relationship between the time comfortable without sex and frequency of sexual activity is of particular interest. As we discussed in Chapter 2, when considering the determinants of sexual desire, the relationship between sexual abstinence and level of desire is much more complex than the relationship between the length of food deprivation and hunger. A large number of men interviewed in the Kinsey study were or had been inside a penal institution or stationed in remote outposts away from women. Many of these men, who had previously been sexually active, found their sexual desire diminishing in these sexually deprived environments, and sometimes it would disappear completely for months at a time. Martin concluded that the absence of appropriate erotic stimuli in the environment was a key factor — though this raises the interesting question why some men react to such deprivation in this way, whilst others do not; perhaps they are able to generate their own internal stimuli. Martin's argument breaks down when he uses these observations to account for the changes seen in the elderly. In fact this lack of erotic stimulation could result from the withdrawal of the spouse from active sexual participation or interest; thus, the male decline in interest depends at least in part on the decline of the women's sexuality, an interpretation that Martin, and Kinsey before him, rejected.

FEMALE SEXUALITY AND AGEING

Christenson & Gagnon (1965) analysed the relevant Kinsey data for older women in greater detail than in the original report. They found the same relationship between the extent of decline and level of sexual activity earlier in life that Martin (1981) reported for males. Pfeiffer and colleagues (Pfeiffer & Davis 1972; Pfeiffer et al 1972) in a questionnaire study of 261 men and 241 women between the ages of 45 and 71, found a much greater decline in both sexual activity and interest amongst the women and the most dramatic change took place between 50 and 60 years of age. In the 66–71 age group, 50% of women said they had no sexual interest compared with only 10% of the men. Hallstrom (1973) studied a representative sample of 956 women from four age bands — 38, 46, 50 and 54 years. Obtaining a 89% response rate he found a decline in both sexual interest and orgasmic capacity over this relatively narrow age range. We will consider the contribution of the menopause to this trend later. Brecher (1984) found that women showed a more marked decline than men in the proportion in each decade who were still sexually active (see Table 5.1). The decline in frequency of orgasm during sleep was similar for the two sexes, whereas amongst those who masturbated the frequency of masturbation remained stable in women, in contrast to the men who gradually declined to the same frequency as the women by the time they were over 70 (Fig. 5.4).

Christensen & Johnson (1973) looked closely at 71 women aged over 50 from the Kinsey sample who had never married. A third of them had been devoid of any erotic interest or activity throughout their lives. The remainder showed a decline in their sexuality similar to that observed in married and previously married women. The availability of sexual partners differs substantially for the two sexes in later life; it is more difficult for an older woman to obtain a new partner than for a man of similar age. Nevertheless the weight of evidence does suggest that ageing has a direct effect on the sexuality of women which is comparable if not as marked as that in men.

THE EFFECTS OF AGEING ON SEXUAL RESPONSE

In both sexes, as one gets older, there is a tendency for the speed and intensity of the various vasocongestive responses to sexual stimulation to be reduced (Masters & Johnson 1966).

In women, the vaginal lubrication response is slower and less marked. As we shall see, much of this change can be attributed to the decline in oestrogen following the menopause, but the reduction in lubrication continues well beyond the menopause. Brecher (1984) asked his respondents: 'How adequate is the vaginal lubrication you produce during sexual arousal?' The percentages reporting an adequate response for the three decades (i.e. 50s, 60s and over-70) were 48%, 35% and 23% respectively. There is a reduction in the tissue elasticity of the vaginal wall, leading to some shrinkage of the vaginal barrel. The effects of disuse are particularly marked in the vaginae of older women; shrinkage is accelerated by lack of vaginal intercourse. Non-genital changes such as breast enlargement and 'sex flush' become much less noticeable. The frequency of orgasm does not decline much in the older woman (Brecher 1984) but is associated with fewer contractions; in the over 60s the contractions may occasionally be painful (Masters & Johnson 1966). In general, and presumably because of a modified degree of pelvic congestion, the resolution phase following orgasm is much more rapid in the older woman.

In older men, erections not only take longer to develop, but may require more direct tactile stimulation; psychic stimulation becomes less and less sufficient. Tactile sensitivity, however, also declines. The period during which an erection can be sustained gets shorter and may only be a few minutes in those aged over 70. A man in this age group may have some difficulty regaining an erection if he loses it after a period of sexual arousal, even if he has not yet ejaculated. Erections on waking (and those occurring during sleep) and nocturnal emissions become less frequent (see p. 434). Scrotal and testicular changes become less marked. Pre-ejaculatory mucus

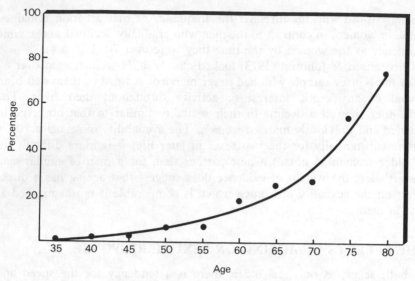

Fig. 5.5 Accumulative incidence of erectile dysfunction (more or less permanent). (Kinsey et al 1948)

secretion diminishes. Ejaculation becomes less powerful with fewer contractions and seminal fluid volume is reduced. The point of ejaculatory inevitability becomes more difficult to recognise since ejaculation becomes more of a one-phase than a two-phase process. The refractory period following ejaculation is at its briefest during adolescence and thereafter steadily declines, so that the older man may remain unresponsive for 24 hours or more. As with women, the resolution process becomes more rapid after orgasm (Kinsey et al 1948; Masters & Johnson 1966). In Brecher's (1984) sample of 2402 older men, 65% reported that their refractory period was longer; 50% took longer to get an erection; 44% said their erection was less rigid when fully erect and 32% were more likely to lose their erection during sexual activity.

Whilst this catalogue of decline may seem gloomy, it is important to realise that for most this process is extremely gradual, allowing a couple to adjust to a less intense, less frantic but not necessarily less enjoyable form of sexual activity. Nevertheless, the decline in erectile efficiency in men is reflected in an increasing incidence of erectile dysfunction with advancing age (Fig. 5.5) The relationship between the levels of sexual activity in early adulthood and old age, described by Martin (1981), also applies to erectile dysfunction. Martin found that of his least active group (i.e. those with the lowest level of sexual activity in early life) 75% had erectile problems in later life; of his moderately active group the figure was 46% and of his most active it was 19%. He also found that 21% of his least active group had long-term problems with premature ejaculation, as compared with only 8% of his most active group.

SEXUALITY AND HEALTH

As we shall see in Chapter 11, ill health of many kinds is associated with impaired sexuality and the elderly will be more susceptible to such effects than younger age groups. However, it is also clear that the decline in sexuality in older age is not dependent on poor health. Martin's (1981) study is of apparently healthy older men. Brecher (1984) concluded from his study that whilst respondents, both male and female, who were in poor health did show less sexual activity and enjoyment of sex, the effect of age was substantially greater than that of poor health. Further support for this conclusion is provided by Pfeiffer et al (1972) and Davidson et al (1982). It is also clear from this evidence that good health does not depend on sexual activity, as has sometimes been supposed (Martin 1981); many healthy old people are sexually inactive.

REPRODUCTIVE AND HORMONAL FACTORS

THE FEMALE MENOPAUSE

The reproductive span of women is quite different to that of men. Whereas both sexes attain fertility at roughly similar ages, men continue to be fertile into late life. Women, by comparison, have a relatively abrupt cessation of fertility around the menopause. The life cycle of reproductive hormones also differs in the two sexes. In men the gamete-producing and hormonal functions of the testis are relatively independent. A man can lose the capacity to produce sperm and continue with normal testosterone production from the Leydig cells. In women the ovarian hormone production is intimately associated with the growth of the follicle and maturation of the ovum at each menstrual cycle, as described in Chapter 2. Furthermore the ovary has a limited number of primitive ova present at birth, and these undergo some form of ageing so that follicles become increasingly resistant to gonadotrophic stimulation, to the point when ovarian activity and menstruation cease. This change is associated with a dramatic change in the ovarian output of steroids.

This is, however, a gradual process. The most discrete marker is the last menstrual bleed (literally the 'menopause') — an event which can only be identified in retrospect (by convention, a woman should have ceased to menstruate for at least a year before being considered post-menopausal; the average age for this event is 50 in the western world). This last menstruation is preceded by a gradual slowing down of ovarian responsiveness over a variable number of years, a process which continues for a time *after* the last menses, before the woman reaches a stable post-menopausal state. This transitional phase both preceding and following the last menses is often called the perimenopause. (For a review of the endocrine changes see WHO 1981.) The length of the follicular phase of the cycle gradually declines over two decades prior to the menopause with anovular cycles becoming more

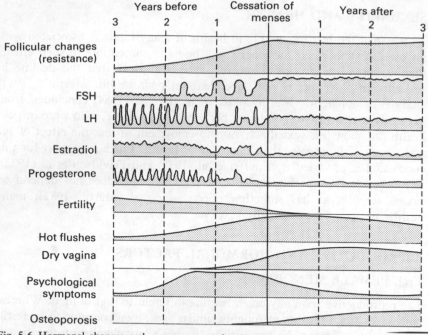

Fig. 5.6 Hormonal changes and symptoms associated with the menopause.

prevalent (3–7% of cycles between the age of 26–40; 12–15% between 41–50; Doring 1969). Metcalf & MacKenzie (1980) found that if cycles become irregular in the over-45 age group, approximately 50% will be anovular.

The overall cycle length tends to shorten, oestradiol levels decline and follicle-stimulating hormone (FSH) rises. By 1 year after cessation of menses, the level of FSH is 10–15 times higher than early follicular levels in younger women, and luteinising hormone (LH) is about three times higher.

The post-menopausal ovary virtually ceases to secrete oestradiol, although appreciable quantities of androstenedione and testosterone are produced by the ovarian stroma, and together with adrenal androgens provide an important source of oestrogen by peripheral aromatisation.

The symptoms most characteristic of the perimenopausal transitional phase are the vasomotor phenomena of hot flushes and night sweats. Their endocrine basis is not understood, and although typically the vasomotor symptoms will be suppressed by exogenous oestrogen administration, their severity is not correlated with circulating oestrogen levels. Other psychosomatic and relatively minor emotional problems are also prevalent during this phase (Jaszmann et al 1969; Hallstrom 1973; Ballinger 1975; Bungay et al 1980). Whether these have a hormonal basis is not known.

In contrast to these transitional phenomena, which are time-limited and presumably reflect some adaptation process in the brain, there are other symptoms which result if oestrogen levels fall too low after the menopause. The most convincing of these is vaginal dryness (Chakravarti et al 1979) which is an important cause of dyspareunia in this age group, though it only troubles a small minority of women (less than 10%). Presumably the majority produce sufficient oestrogen to maintain normal vaginal function. Insomnia, apart from the disturbance of sleep that results from night sweats, is a common post-menopausal problem that may respond to oestrogen replacement (Thomson & Oswald 1977). Urinary tract symptoms may be related to oestrogen deficiency. The most convincing long-term consequence of oestrogen lack is osteoporosis. The temporal relationships of these various hormonal changes and symptoms are shown graphically in Figure 5.6.

To what extent do these menopausal endocrine changes influence women's sexuality? As already mentioned, oestrogen lack is associated with vaginal dryness and atrophic vaginitis in about 8–10% of post-menopausal women (Hallstrom 1977). This causes discomfort or pain during intercourse and hence loss of interest and sometimes also of desire. Leiblum et al (1983) investigated the degree of vaginal atrophy and its relationship to sexual activity in post-menopausal women. They found that more sexually active women had less vaginal atrophy, raising the possibility that sexual activity protects the vagina, not simply by stretching it (masturbation also contributed to this apparent protective effect) but also by stimulating hormone production in some way; this is an interesting possibility which awaits evidence.

The most convincing evidence that the menopause per se contributes to the sexual decline in women comes from Halstrom's (1973) epidemiological study. He was able to demonstrate, by holding age constant in his analysis, that sexual decline was more marked in post-menopausal than premenopausal women. Further evidence of this kind comes from Pfeiffer et al (1972) and Bottiglioni & De Aloysio (1982), although Greene (1984), in reviewing this literature, concluded that the effect of the menopause is small when compared to the general effects of ageing.

The effect of the menopause may depend in part on the effect on vaginal function already discussed. But do hormonal changes lead more directly to a reduction in sexual desire, orgasmic capacity or enjoyment? Given the complexity of the role of hormones in female sexuality, described in Chapter 2, we should not expect any simple clearcut answer. As yet no study of the natural menopause and hormone replacement allows us to draw any firm conclusions, though McCoy & Davidson (1985) in a longitudinal study of post-menopausal women found no correlation between declining sexuality and declining oestrogen levels. Rather more substantial evidence comes from controlled studies of hormone replacement following hysterectomy and bilateral oophorectomy. This surgical menopause, as already described, produces more dramatic hormonal changes than the natural menopause, particularly in relation to androgens. Hence we may expect more clearcut evidence. As we shall see, the findings are of interest, but not straightforward.

The effects of oophorectomy and hormone replacement on female sexuality

Bilateral oophorectomy is sometimes carried out because of ovarian disease or in the management of hormone-dependent malignancies. Most commonly it is done as a preventive measure in women close to menopausal age who are undergoing hysterectomy, to ensure that they do not subsequently develop ovarian cancer, a particularly unpleasant form of malignancy. The justification for such an approach is that the post-menopausal ovary is of no real value and loss of the brief period of ovarian activity that would have preceded natural menopause can be counteracted with hormone replacement. This view is not shared by all gynaecologists and this approach remains controversial. Nevertheless in 1975 471 000 oophorectomies were performed in the USA, more than half of them in women under 45 years of age (Zussman et al 1981). The number may have declined somewhat since then.

A small number of controlled studies of hormone replacement therapy (HRT) following oophorectomy have been reported. Utian (1975), in a partially controlled study, found that oestrogen replacement benefited the dry vagina but not loss of libido. Dennerstein et al (1980) in a placebo-controlled study found that not only vaginal dryness but also sexual interest, enjoyment and orgasmic capacity were improved by oestrogen replacement, an effect which was reduced by the addition of a progestagen to the regime. Dow et al (1983) compared oestrogen implant with an oestrogen–testosterone combination in women who complained of loss of sexual interest following oophorectomy. They found that both regimes produced benefits indistinguishable in degree. In what is probably the best controlled prospective study so far, Sherwin et al (1985) compared androgen and oestrogen replacement following oophorectomy. They had four treatment groups — oestrogen–androgen combination, oestrogen alone, androgen alone and placebo. All women were assessed preoperatively and started on placebo, single-blind, following surgery. After 3 months they crossed over, double-blind, into one of the treatment groups. The results showed a beneficial effect of androgen, whether given alone or with oestrogen. The effects observed were on sexual motivation, i.e. sexual desire, arousal and number of sexual fantasies, and not on coital or orgasmic frequency. The authors were able to show that these behavioural variables covaried with plasma testosterone levels but not with oestradiol during the treatment period. Sherwin & Gelfand (1987) went on to study women on long-term hormone replacement following oophorectomy at least 2 years previously. One group was receiving a testosterone–oestradiol combination, a second oestradiol alone and a third no hormone replacement. The group receiving the androgen–oestrogen combination reported higher levels of sexual desire, sexual arousal and number of fantasies than the other two groups. Once again changes in these variables covaried with plasma testosterone levels but not with oestradiol. However, in contrast to the first study, an effect on coital frequency was also found. It is possible that these groups of women were different before starting on hormone replacement, and selected themselves because of their favourable response to the particular regime. This would be consistent with the hypothesis put forward in Chapter 2 that women vary in their patterns of hormone–behaviour relationships.

We can nevertheless conclude that hormonal changes following the natural menopause, and certainly following surgical menopause, may contribute to the sexual decline in a proportion of women. Both androgens and oestrogens may be involved, though not necessarily in the same women, and oestrogens may be relevant to sexual interest as well as vaginal response. As yet we have no idea of the proportions of women that come into these categories.

As with younger women, there are some apparent inconsistencies in the evidence reviewed here. One factor of possible importance, already discussed in Chapter 2, is the difference between studying women who present with established sexual problems, and those who are investigated before any such problems have developed. The studies of Dow et al (1983) and Sherwin et al (1985) differ in this way. It may be that the effects of hormones (or at least androgens) on sexuality are best demonstrated in women without existing sexual problems. This is relevant to the clinical role of hormone replacement in the sexual difficulties of women in this age group. Until we have further evidence we are obliged to use a trial-and-error approach in the hope of finding some women who benefit, but with the expectation that the majority will not, either with androgens or oestrogens. The risks associated with hormone replacement are still controversial and highly complex and are beyond the scope of this book. The possible effects on blood lipids are considered by Sherwin & Gelfand (1987).

THE MALE

Although ageing in the male reproductive system does occur, it is not comparable to the menopause in women. Decline in fertility, in so far as it occurs, is gradual. Hormonal changes are also gradual and very variable in degree. In male rodents the principal effects of ageing on reproduction are mediated via the hypothalamo-pituitary axis; in primates the principal changes may be in androgen receptors at the target organ, whereas in men, as we shall see, the testes show the most obvious decline (Davidson et al 1983).

A decline in the level of circulating testosterone in men as they get older has been reported in many studies. Harman (1983) in his review cites 16 such studies (e.g. Vermeulen et al 1972; Stearns et al 1976). Typically the decline is noticed from the age of 50 onwards. More recently the role that ageing per se plays in this decline has been questioned. Harman & Tsitouras (1980), in the Baltimore Longitudinal Ageing Project, found no significant decline in plasma testosterone in a group of essentially healthy old men. Comparable negative findings in healthy men were reported by Sparrow et al (1980). This led Harman & Tsitouras to conclude that this often reported decline is a function of ill health and not ageing. Since then Davidson et al (1982), Deslypere & Vermeulen (1984a) and Tsitouras & Hagen (1984); studying a group of healthy men with a different social background to the Baltimore subjects), have found further evidence of testicular decline which cannot be attributed to ill health.

There is comparable variability in the evidence of an increase in sex hormone-binding globulin (SHBG), reduction in free testosterone and increased oestradiol in the plasma (Harman 1983). A gradual increase in LH and FSH is a fairly consistent finding, but set against this is more recent evidence of changes at the hypothalamo-pituitary level, with increased sensitivity to negative feedback and the pituitary response to luteinising hormone-releasing hormone (LHRH) somewhat blunted (Myers & Bremner 1987). Also Deslypere & Vermeulen (1984b) have reported an age-related decline in androgens in the skin of the pubic and scrotal areas (and other tissues).

With the available evidence we can conclude that a decline in testicular function commonly occurs in men with advancing age, but is variable in degree. It is probably mainly a result of testicular ageing, although a rise in SHBG and testosterone-binding and a relative failure of the hypothalamo-pituitary axis to drive the testis also contribute.

What is the relevance, if any, of these changes to the decline in sexuality in older men? As yet there is little evidence relating androgens to behaviour in the same individuals. Vermeulen (1979) found some indication that the two processes were correlated. Davidson et al (1982), whilst demonstrating a decline both in testosterone and sexuality in a group of healthy men, found that although both trends correlated with age they did not correlate with each other when age was controlled. Tsitouras et al (1982), having showed that their healthy old men did not have significantly lowered testosterone levels, divided them into three groups of high, moderate and low sexual activity. Of these three, the high activity group had significantly higher testosterone levels. In other words, relatively slight differences in testosterone within the normal range were associated with differing levels of sexual activity. The authors also found that when they divided their men into those with and without erectile problems, these groups did *not* differ in testosterone levels, reinforcing the general view propounded earlier that androgens are necessary for sexual interest and activity but not erectile function per se.

As discussed in Chapter 2, the threshold for maximum testosterone effect on behaviour not only may vary between individuals but also fall well within the laboratory normal range. Hence it is conceivable that some older men experience a decline in testosterone to levels which are within the normal range but below their individual optimum for activating sexual interest. Any reduction in target organ or receptor sensitivity would add to this picture. Clearly it will not be easy to resolve this issue with correlational studies of this kind. The most convincing evidence is likely to come from controlled evaluation of the administration of exogenous androgens as reported by O'Carroll & Bancroft (1984). The main concern in pursuing such studies is that such administration may have adverse effects on blood lipids (Baker 1986) and on prostatic hypertrophy (Geller 1984). Against this is the possibility that exogenous androgens may protect older men against osteoporosis. But until we have such evidence the role of testosterone in the sexual decline of ageing men and the therapeutic value of testosterone replacement in such cases must remain uncertain.

PSYCHOSOCIAL FACTORS

We live in a society in which it is widely assumed that the elderly are normally asexual. It is also widely believed by health professionals that such negative attitudes to sexuality in the aged have an inhibitory effect on sexual expression in this age group. How important are such attitudes in explaining the sexual decline of the elderly? To what extent do old people cease sexual activity because they have been taught to regard it as inappropriate at their age?

Attitudes to sexuality in the elderly vary across cultures. Winn & Newton (1982) searched the Human Relations Area Files for relevant evidence from primitive societies. As usual with this source of anthropological data (see p. 201), evidence of sexual behaviour is often very limited, superficial or anecdotal, reflecting as much the observer's prejudices and expectations as those of the observed. Nevertheless Winn & Newton looked at the files on 106 societies. In 20 they found evidence of continuing sexual activity amongst old men, together with the shared expectation that this should happen. Not infrequently, anecdotes of sexual interaction between old men and young girls would be cited. There was evidence relating to elderly women from 26 societies, of which 22 revealed continuing sexual activity. There was often evidence of lessening sexual inhibitions in older women, leading them to be more openly expressive of their sexual wishes. Sexual relations between old women and much younger men were not unusual.

In some societies there were clearly negative attitudes to sexuality of the elderly, who were generally regarded as undesirable as sexual partners. The assumption is that we live in such a society. But there may be important differences in attitudes between the elderly themselves and younger adults (their children). Certainly the organisation of institutions for the elderly rarely recognises the sexual needs of their clients (White 1982). But the evidence that such attitudes restrict the sexual behaviour of the elderly living in their own homes is not great. Martin (1981) commented that he could not recall any research subject who had ceased sexual activity because of impropriety. On the other hand, the elderly of today may be relatively lacking in sexual knowledge since they have grown up in more sexually restrictive times. This ignorance may restrict their sexual activity in late life (White 1982). We live in a society which glamorises youth and its sexuality. This may inhibit old people from expressing or even talking about their sexuality because of the belief that they are no longer sexually attractive.

The relevance of social factors is evident in the finding of Hallstrom (1973) that the decline in sexuality in post-menopausal women is greater in the lower socioeconomic groups. This may reflect social influences on the quality of marriage rather than direct effects on sexuality (e.g. Rainwater 1966).

CONCLUSIONS

Whilst there is conclusive evidence of a decline in sexuality in both men and women with advancing age, the situation is changing and several factors are probably involved. People are healthier for longer and ill health is only one factor contributing to the decline. Changes in reproductive hormones may play a part, at least in some cases. Normal ageing, by mechanisms which are not understood, appears to alter the physiology of sexual response to some extent. This is not necessarily a disadvantage; love-making can become less frantic and more given over to intimacy. But concern over declining performance can be considerable and in its turn do more damage to the sexual relationship than the ageing itself. Preparedness to seek help when problems do arise may be lessened by the assumption that they are too old for it anyway. But attitudes are changing and the publication of popular reports such as Brecher's (1984) Love, Sex and Aging, and the Starr–Weiner report (1981) have brought into the open the fact that many old people continue to enjoy sex.

Elderly couples with sexual problems often benefit from sexual counselling. Paradoxically they sometimes present easier problems than younger couples because although their problems are long-standing, ignorance and inhibited attitudes may be important factors which are often more responsive to good counselling than the more deep-rooted sexual anxieties of some younger couples. The principles of counselling are basically the same, whatever the age of the couple, and we will consider these in detail in Chapter 10.

REFERENCES

Baker H W G 1986 Hormone replacement therapy in men — endocrine aspects. In: Dennerstein L, Fraser I (eds) Hormones and behaviour. Elsevier, Amsterdam, pp 423–432
Ballinger C B 1975 Psychiatric morbidity and the menopause. Screening of a general population sample. British Medical Journal 3: 344–346

Bottiglioni F, De Aloysio D 1982 Female sexual activity as a function of climacteric conditions and age. Maturitas 4: 27–31

Brecher E M 1984 Love, sex and aging: a Consumer's Union report. Little, Brown, Boston

Bungay G, Vessey M, McPherson C 1980 Study of symptoms in middle life, with special reference to the menopause. British Medical Journal 281: 181–183

Chakravarti S, Collins W, Thom M, Studd J 1979 The relation between plasma hormone profiles, symptoms and response to oestrogen treatment of women approaching the menopause. British Medical Journal 1: 983–985

Christenson C V, Gagnon J H 1965 Sexual behavior in a group of older women. Journal of Gerontology 20: 351–356

Christenson C V, Johnson A B 1973 Sexual patterns in a group of older, never-married women. Journal of Geriatric Psychiatry 6: 80–98

Davidson J M, Kwan M, Greenleaf W J 1982 Hormonal replacement and sexuality in men. Clinics in Endocrinology and Metabolism 11(3): 599–623

Davidson J M, Gray G D, Smith E R 1983 The sexual psychoendocrinology of aging. In: Meites J (ed) Neuroendocrinology of aging. Plenum, New York, pp 221–258

Dennerstein L, Burrows G D, Wood C, Hyman G 1980 Hormones and sexuality: effect of estrogen and progestogen. Obstetrics and Gynecology 56: 316–322

Deslypere J P, Vermeulen A 1984a Leydig cell function in normal men: effect of age, life style, residence, diet and activity. Journal of Clinical Endocrinology and Metabolism 59: 955–962

Deslypere J P, Vermeulen A 1984b Influence of age and sex on steroid concentration in different tissues in humans. Abstracts of 7th international congress of endocrinology no 572. Excerpta Medica, Amsterdam

Doring G K 1969 The incidence of anovular cycles in women. Journal of Reproduction and Fertility (suppl) 6: 77–81

Dow M G T, Hart D M, Forrest C A 1983 Hormonal treatment of sexual unresponsiveness in post-menopausal women; a comparative study. British Journal of Obstetrics and Gynaecology 90: 361–366

Geller J 1984 Benign prostatic hypertrophy — current understanding of its pathogenesis. In: Labrie F, Proulx L (eds) Endocrinology. Excerpta Medica, Amsterdam, pp 909–912

Greene J G 1984 The social and psychological origins of the climacteric syndrome. Gower, Aldershot

Griffin T, Morris J 1987 Social trends no. 17. HMSO, London

Hallstrom T 1973 Mental disorders and sexuality in the climacteric. Scandinavian University Books, Goteborg

Hallstrom T 1977 Sexuality in the climacteric. Clinics in Obstetrics and Gynaecology 4: 227–239

Harman S M 1983 Relation of the neuroendocrine system to reproductive decline in men. In: Meites J (ed) Neuroendocrinology of aging. Plenum, New York, pp 203–219

Harman S M, Tsitouras P D 1980 Reproductive hormones in ageing men. 1. Measurement of sex steroids, basal luteinizing hormone and Leydig cell response to human chorionic gonadotrophin. Journal of Clinical Endocrinology and Metabolism 51: 35–40

Hegeler S, Mortensen M 1978 Sexuality and ageing. British Journal of Sexual Medicine 5(32): 16–19

Jaszmann L J B, Van Lith N, Zaat J 1969 The perimenopausal symptoms: the statistical analysis of a survey. Medical Gynaecology and Sociology 4: 268–277

Kinsey A C, Pomeroy W B, Martin C E 1948 Sexual behavior in the human male. Saunders, Philadelphia

Kinsey A C, Pomeroy W B, Martin C E, Gebhard P H 1953 Sexual behavior in the human female. Saunders, Philadelphia

Leiblum S, Bachman G, Kemmann E, Colburn D, Swatzman L 1983 Vaginal atrophy in the post-menopausal woman The importance of sexual activity and hormones. Journal of the American Medical Association 249: 2195–2198

McCoy N, Davidson J M 1985 A longitudinal study of the effects of menopause on sexuality. Maturitas 7: 203–210

Martin C E 1977 Sexual activity in the ageing male. In: Money J, Musaph H (eds) Handbook of sexology. Elsevier/North Holland, Amsterdam, pp 813–824

Martin C E 1981 Factors affecting sexual functioning in 60–79 year old married males. Archives of Sexual Behavior 10: 399–420

Masters W H, Johnson V E 1966 Human sexual response. Churchill Livingstone, London
Metcalf M G, MacKenzie J A 1980 Incidence of ovulation in young women. Journal of Biosocial Science 12: 345–352
Myers J S, Bremner W J 1986 Endocrine aspects of reproductive and sexual function in aging men. In: Dennerstein L, Fraser I (eds) Hormones and behaviour. Elsevier, Amsterdam, pp 389–395
O'Carroll R, Bancroft J 1984 Testosterone therapy for low sexual interest and erectile dysfunction in men: a controlled study. British Journal of Psychiatry 145: 146–151
Pfeiffer E, Davis G C 1972 Determinants of sexual behavior in middle and old age. Journal of the American Geriatric Society 20: 151–158
Pfeiffer E, Verwoerdt A, Davis G C 1972 Sexual behavior in middle life. American Journal of Psychiatry 128: 1262–1267
Rainwater L 1966 Some aspects of lower class sexual behavior. Journal of Social Issues 22: 96–108
Sherwin B B, Gelfand M M 1987 The role of androgen in the maintenance of sexual functioning in oophorectomised women. Psychosomatic Medicine 49: 397–409
Sherwin B B, Gelfand M M, Brender W 1985 Androgen enhances sexual motivation in females: a prospective cross-over study of sex steroid administration in the surgical menopause. Psychosomatic Medicine 47: 339–351
Sparrow D, Bosse R, Rowe J W 1980 The influence of age, alcohol consumption and body build on gonadal function in men. Journal of Clinical Endocrinology and Metabolism 51: 508–511
Starr B D, Weiner M B 1981 The Starr–Weiner report on sex and sexuality in the later years. Stein & Day, New York
Stearns E L, MacDonnel J A, Kaaufman B J, Lucman T S, Winter J S, Faiman C 1976 Declining testicular function with age. American Journal of Medicine 57: 761–766
Thomson J, Oswald I 1977 Effect of oestrogen on the sleep, mood and anxiety of menopausal women. British Medical Journal 2: 1317–1319
Tsitouras P D, Hagen T C 1984 Testosterone, LH, FSHG, prolactin and sperm in aging healthy men. Abstracts of 7th international congress of endocrinology, no 1951. Excerpta Medica. International Congress Series 652, Amsterdam
Tsitouras P D, Martin C E, Harman S M 1982 Relationship of serum testosterone to sexual activity in healthy elderly men. Journal of Gerontology 37: 288–293
Utian W H 1975 Effect of hysterectomy, oophorectomy and estrogen therapy on libido. International Journal of Obstetrics and Gynaecology 13: 97–100
Vermeulen A 1979 Decline in sexual activity in aging men: correlation with sex hormone levels and testicular change. Journal of Biosocial Science (suppl). 6: 5–18
Vermeulen A, Rubens R, Verdonck L 1972 Testosterone secretion and metabolism in male senescence. Journal of Clinical Endocrinology 34: 730–735
White C B 1982 Sexual interest, attitudes, knowledge and sexual history in relation to sexual behavior in the institutionalised aged. Archives of Sexual Behavior 11: 11–22
WHO 1981 Research on the menopause. Report of a WHO scientific group. Technical report series 670. WHO, Geneva
Winn R L, Newton N 1982 Sexuality in aging: a study of 106 cultures. Archives of Sexual Behavior 11: 283–298
Zussman L, Zussman S, Sunley R, Bjornson E 1981 Sexual response after hysterectomy–oophorectomy: recent studies and reconsideration of psychogenesis. American Journal of Obstetrics and Gynecology 140: 725–729

6

Homosexuality

A minority of individuals are sexually attracted to members of their own sex. The homosexual relationships that may result differ from heterosexual relationships in two obvious ways. First, they will not bear children and secondly, at least in our society, the individuals concerned will be subjected to social stigma. There may be other differences, some of which will be discussed later in this chapter.

As explained in Chapter 3, we do not understand why people develop either homosexual or heterosexual preferences though each is probably the consequence of a complex and variable set of influences in which biological factors interact with social learning, and in which cognitive learning, the uniquely human phenomenon, plays a particularly important role in the establishment of our sexual identities.

Our understanding has not been helped by the more or less universal emotional reaction to homosexuality. Whether an individual rejects homosexuals or regards them as victims of unjust repression, that individual's appraisal of evidence is likely to be biased. The person who is truly dispassionate and impartial on the subject is hard to find. Many aetiological theories of homosexuality have apparently been motivated by a need to absolve the homosexual of responsibility for his disposition, hence early ideas that homosexuality was a congenital anomaly (e.g. put forward in the 19th century by men such as Westphal and Lombroso) and therefore not a sin. (For a fuller discussion of this issue, see Bancroft 1974. A more recent example is to be found in Bell et al 1981. After an interesting study of possible childhood factors contributing to sexual preferences they conclude, on no real scientific grounds whatsoever, that sexual preferences are biologically determined.)

In Chapter 3 it was pointed out that exclusive homosexuality appears to be a uniquely human phenomenon and it was suggested that this stems from our tendency to categorise people as *either* homosexual *or* heterosexual. It is also clear that this form of social labelling varies considerably across cultures, and in some cultures the exclusive homosexual does not seem to exist or is at least rare. In many societies the label for such an individual does not occur in the language, i.e. it is not an emic concept. In this chapter

I will consider in more detail the cross-cultural evidence. By avoiding the tendency to view homosexuality only in terms of our own society's reactions, it soon becomes apparent that many of our widely held assumptions about the origins of homosexuality are a product of our social values rather than of objective appraisal of the evidence. However, some understanding of western society's reaction to homosexuality is necessary before we can begin to understand homosexuals as people in our society. The importance of this subject goes beyond the needs and rights of the millions of individuals who come into this category and affects us all, whatever our orientation. Homosexuality in particular provides us with a model of a sexual relationship which, although externally repressed, is in many ways relatively free from the constraints of conventional sexual morality. Society's attitudes to homosexuality, therefore, reflect the conflict that rages between the reactionary and the radical in sexual politics. Since the first edition of this book was published the picture has been dramatically and tragically changed by the AIDS epidemic, which is bringing about not only powerful reactions in the heterosexual community against homosexuals but also radical reorganisation by many gay men of their own lifestyles. Even before AIDS started to have its effects there were important changes in the attitudes and behaviour of gay people. We will consider some of these later in this chapter.

CROSS-CULTURAL ASPECTS

In Ford & Beach's (1952) classic text, Patterns of Sexual Behaviour, they reported that homosexuality was approved or tolerated in some form in 49 of the 78 relatively primitive societies studied. Female homosexuality was evident in 17. Blackwood (1985) has reported on 95 cultures in which female homosexuality or female-to-male transsexualism occurred. Broude & Green (1980) reported that of 70 societies for which there was sufficient data, homosexuality was present or common in 41%. The proportion of societies accepting homosexuality was about the same as that disapproving of or rejecting it. When accepted, it almost always coexists with heterosexuality in the same individual. In other words, in such a society, the person who is exclusively homosexual throughout his life is unusual. This evidence has been mainly gleaned from the Human Relations Area File, a collection of reports from anthropologists, travellers, writers, missionaries etc. The extent to which these files deal with homosexuality and the validity of any such information appearing in them varies considerably and will often reflect the prejudices or personal values of the individual making the report. Many of the societies described no longer exist in the same form (Hotvedt 1983). The number of detailed anthropological studies of homosexual behaviour is relatively small.

Carrier (1980), in his useful review, emphasised that the main sociocultural factors influencing attitudes to homosexuality were the attitudes to cross-gender behaviour and the availability of sexual partners. On the first issue, he divided societies into those that accommodated cross-gender behaviour and those that actively disapproved of it. In the accommodating societies, there is usually an expectation that a few individuals will be 'born that way', i.e. show cross-gender behaviour, and would be expected to interact sexually with someone of the appropriate gender. Thus a male showing feminine behaviour would be expected to relate sexually to a man and neither the behaviour nor the participants would be labelled as homosexual.

In disapproving societies, the negative reaction mainly comes from men towards other males showing cross-gender behaviour. In such societies gender roles are sharply dichotomised, there are often laws against cross-dressing and cross-gender behaviour is equated with homosexuality. Carrier (1980) cites Mexico as an example of such a machismo culture. In such societies it is relatively acceptable for a man to act as the 'insertor' in sexual contact with a cross-gender male, providing that is not the exclusive pattern of his sexual behaviour. Such behaviour can still be seen as an expression of male dominance. It is the 'insertee' who is stigmatised, who is seen to be anomalous in terms of gender, and who is 'letting the side down' for the male gender.

Availability of sexual partners becomes relevant when there are strong expectations of virginity at marriage, usually associated with complete segregation of the sexes prior to marriage. Homosexual behaviour is then more likely amongst the unmarried. Polygamy may result in lesbian relationships between the wives, as in the Azanda of Africa (Blackwood 1985).

In general, the prevailing patterns of sexual interaction in a society will reflect both the degree of sexual segregation (in some societies males and females lead separate existencies for most of their lives) and the degree of sexual stratification (i.e. the extent to which men hold superior power). Hotvedt (1983) discusses some of the factors influencing the organisation of such sexually dimorphic characteristics in early human societies. She notes that both sexual segregation and stratification are less evident in hunter–gatherer societies (of which the !Kung of the Kalahari desert remain one of the few existing examples), becoming more in evidence as societies become more horticultural (i.e. agriculture without the plough or irrigation) or pastoral (i.e. the herding of domesticated animals). Sexual stratification increases the likelihood of a link between masculinity and heterosexuality in the machismo culture. Segregation of the sexes increases the likelihood of homosexual behaviour which may be ritualised or institutionalised in some way. When segregation is coupled with sexual antagonism (i.e. hostility and mistrust expressed by each gender group towards the other) ritual intensification of masculinity and same-sex bonding is likely, as described by Herdt (1981) in a New Guinea Highland society. In that culture, the ingestion of semen is seen as a vital part of the process of developing masculinity. Boys and girls are segregated from late childhood. The boys spend most of their time thereafter in the men's houses where they are expected to enter into sexual relationships with the men and older boys whom they fellate and whose semen they ingest. At a later stage they may marry and initially sexual activity with the wife involves fellatio. They eventually move on to coitus, though typically it is a somewhat perfunctory act with little concern for the female's pleasure.

There are many variations on these themes of premarital and extramarital homosexuality, with varying degrees of ritual and masculinisation involved. Money & Ehrhardt (1972) give several examples, including the Marind Anim of New Guinea, where adolescents leave the parental home to be adopted by another married couple; the husband acts as mentor to the boy, the wife to the girl. Homosexual relations typically develop between the male mentor and the boy, though not apparently between the woman and the girl.

Herdt (1988) has proposed that the cross-cultural patterns of homosexuality can be categorised into three broad sociocultural types. In addition to the *gender-reversed* pattern, which we have already considered, he describes *role-specific* homosexuality (i.e. certain individuals in a society, such as the shaman or temple priest, who are expected to behave homosexually), and *age-asymmetric* homosexuality, when there is substantial age difference between sexual partners. It is this age-structured homosexuality which is the most common form across cultures and which was very much in evidence in Ancient Greece and the Ancient Far East. It provides the greatest fluidity of sexual orientation and the clearest example of how bisexual behaviour can persist into adulthood alongside normal marriage. It is also relevant that in many societies, and in Europe in the past, age-asymmetry also prevails or prevailed in heterosexual relationships. It is not clear how modern western homosexuality evolved from these more basic patterns, though there is evidence of all three types. The characteristics of the modern gay movement and its associated homosexual lifestyles are not readily seen in primitive societies, though there may have been comparable forms earlier in European history.

HISTORICAL ASPECTS

Any attempt to summarise, let alone evaluate the historical evidence is beyond the scope of this book. If anthropological data are subject to bias, historical accounts are probably more so.*

It is difficult, however, to refrain from commenting on Boswell's (1980) book, Christianity, Social Tolerance and Homosexuality. As a classical scholar with the ability to use the original sources he sets a standard of

---

* Bullough (1976) provides the most substantial source. Rattray Taylor (1954) and Tannahill (1980) provide popular and readable texts.

scholarship which will be hard to sustain. He is also extremely readable. But scholarship does not render him immune to bias in his interpretations. He is identified with the gay movement so at least his bias is likely to differ from those of many earlier historians.

In Boswell's view, gay people were not particularly distinguished from others in Roman society, and homosexual interest was regarded as an ordinary part of the range of human eroticism. The early Christian Church had little to say on the subject. Hostility to gay people became noticeable during the third to sixth centuries, for reasons which are not clear. During the early Middle Ages, therefore, gay people were rarely visible; there is no evidence of a homosexual subculture. The revival of city life in the 11th century was accompanied by the reappearance of gay literature and evidence of a substantial gay minority. 'Gay people were prominent, influential and respected at many levels of society in most of Europe and left a permanent mark on the cultural movement of the age, both religious and secular'. It was in the latter half of the 12th century that hostility to homosexuals appeared, first in popular literature and later in theological and legal writings. Boswell sees this as part of an increase in general intolerance of minority groups, e.g. non-Christians, heretics, Jews, leading to the rise of the Inquisition and the anti-witchcraft movement. This intolerance eventually became incorporated into religious teaching. He makes the point that religious belief is not the *cause* of intolerance of homosexuality but rather reflects the intolerance of its time.

NEGATIVE SOCIAL ATTITUDES IN WESTERN SOCIETY

In Western 'civilised' societies, homosexuality is more or less universally rejected. Both laws and attitudes vary but always on the negative side of neutral. In Scandinavia, Holland, Belgium and France, homosexual behaviour between consenting adults has not been illegal for a long time. Illinois was the first state in the USA to legalise such behaviour in 1962 and several other states followed suit. The law was changed in England in 1967. In Scotland, all types of male homosexuality remain illegal, though rarely prosecuted if taking place in private and not involving individuals below the age of consent. In the majority of cases, the law does not concern itself with female homosexuality, though there have been specific statutes against such behaviour in Austria, Greece, Finland and Switzerland, and in several states of the USA statutes are phrased in such a way as to make them applicable to both female and male homosexual contacts (Kinsey et al 1953).

But even in those countries with relatively liberal laws in relation to homosexuality, legal discrimination persists in various ways. In England and many of the US states, the age of consent for homosexuals is 21 compared with 16 for heterosexual acts. Although men may solicit women they may not solicit other men. Women may in fact solicit men providing it is not for the purposes of prostitution. 'Privacy' is defined in a much more restrictive sense for homosexual than for heterosexual acts. Homosexuality of any kind is still illegal for members of the armed forces and merchant navy. Penalties are more severe than for equivalent heterosexual offences (Freeman 1979).

When changes in the law have occurred, they have usually been associated with some recorded change in public opinion. The Wolfenden committee (1957) recommended a change in the English law in 1957. Shortly after this, a Gallup poll showed nearly 25% in favour of such reform. Eight years later, after a period of public debate, a national opinion poll showed 63% in favour of reform. However, 93% still saw homosexuality as a form of medical illness requiring medical treatment (Bancroft 1974).

Weinberg & Williams (1974) compared three different societies: the USA (represented by New York City and San Francisco), Denmark and Holland. They found that attitudes to homosexuality were more negative amongst the general population in the USA than in the other two countries. There was other evidence of greater tolerance of, and less discrimination against, homosexuals in the two European countries, the most favourable circumstances being in Holland, where government-backed agencies support the needs of the homosexual community.

However, it is important to note that homosexuality in Holland is still tolerated rather than accepted. Particularly amongst the working class, acknowledging one's homosexuality may still prejudice the chance of a job (Ramsay et al 1974). The Dutch use words which mean 'normal' or 'homo' when distinguishing between hetero- and homosexuality. Dutch homosexuals still tend to conceal their sexual preferences from their parents and consequently from many others. A question of crucial social significance is whether attitudes to homosexuality will ever be more positive than those found in countries such as Holland at present. Before attempting an answer, let us consider why negative attitudes exist in the first place. Many writers have been puzzled by the strength of this hostility. Several have commented on the similarities between anti-homosexual feelings and anti-Semitism. Certainly in Nazi Germany, many homosexuals went side by side with Jews into the gas chambers. Men have been executed for homosexuality in Iran in the last decade. A variety of explanations have been offered, some of which we will discuss briefly.

Hostility to alien minority groups

Homosexuality is a form of minority behaviour which, like many others, may be stigmatised by the majority and blamed for a variety of social problems. This is an example of scapegoating and reflects either fear or suspicion of the unknown and alien, or alternatively, allows members of the majority who are unsure of themselves to bolster their self-esteem by emphasising the shortcomings of such minorities. Heterosexuals who are unsure of their sexual competence or identity may bolster their self-confidence by attacking homosexuals. In a similar way, the poor whites may persecute black people to enhance their own self-esteem.

Distrust of homosexuals was shown in an American survey (Levitt & Klassen 1974). Nearly 60% of the respondents believed that the majority of homosexuals would be security risks in government jobs. About 40% believed that the majority of homosexuals tend to corrupt their co-workers. Three-quarters would deny a homosexual the right to be a clergyman, a school teacher or a judge and two-thirds would debar him from medical practice or government service. Nearly a half agreed that homosexuality, by corruption, could cause a civilisation's downfall, a view that has been expressed by historians in relation to ancient Greece and other social declines (Bullough 1976). Now we have a new threat to civilisation that is being attributed to homosexuals — the AIDS epidemic. This is of such importance that it will be considered more fully later in the chapter.

Defence against one's own homosexual potential

Hostility to homosexuality in others may be a form of defence against awareness or at least fear of homosexual tendencies in oneself. This is an example of the mechanism of defence known as 'reaction formation'. Homosexuals themselves commonly assume this to be the main cause of anti-homosexual feelings; this is an understandable riposte on their part. It is difficult to say how important or how common it is but a number of factors are relevant. According to the findings of Kinsey and his colleagues (1948), which will be discussed further below, more than a third of adult men have experienced orgasm during a homosexual encounter at least once. If so, there will be many who may fear a homosexual component in themselves. Also striking is the extent to which homosexual behaviour may occur in situations where the sexes are segregated. Thus in prisons, otherwise heterosexual men, deprived of their normal heterosexual outlets, may exploit homosexual contact, though they often sustain their heterosexual identity by adopting a humiliating or hostile attitude to their homosexual partners. We have already seen how common this is amongst primitive societies where sexual segregation is the norm. In such societies which are more accepting of homosexual behaviour than ours, this is regarded as part of normal sexual experience. Bullough (1976) has documented many examples through the ages where concern has been expressed about homosexuality occurring amongst both men and women in monastic and ostensibly chaste religious orders. The increased likelihood of homosexual relationships occurring in single-sex schools, particularly boarding schools, is widely believed. The potential for this so-called 'facultative' homosexuality does appear to be widespread. Recognition of this could well lead to an intense reaction formation in some individuals.

Opposition to 'unnatural' behaviour

Our sexual appetites do present us with important problems of self-control. With the exception of those of us who are endowed with little or no interest in sex, we all need some self-imposed constraints if only to avoid hurting or humiliating ourselves or others. The need for control has exercised the minds of theologians and the dictators of our morals for a long time.

Of particular relevance are the views of St Thomas Aquinas (1225–1274) who is widely regarded as a major influence on sexual morality in the western world. Aquinas considered lust in general to be a vice because it was in conflict with reason. But he also made the crucial distinction between sins against one's neighbour and other people, such as adultery, seduction or rape, and sins against nature. The latter were regarded as more serious because they were against God. Included in this category, and in order of grievousness, were bestiality, homosexuality, intercourse in unnatural position (only the missionary position was considered natural) and masturbation (Bullough 1976). Boswell (1980) who discussed the concept of 'naturalness' extensively in his book pointed out the difficulties Aquinas found in striving to maintain a logical coherence in his case.

This concept of the 'unnaturalness' of homosexuality crops up frequently even today. Many who are opposed to homosexuality justify their opposition in precisely these terms — it is 'unnatural', 'our bodies were not designed (by God) to be used in that way'. Hoffman (1968) argued persuasively that this recourse to nature, which in the past has been used to explain much of our environment, became redundant as scientific knowledge provided a preferable and more effective model to explain the phenomena around us. The abandonment of nature and the adoption of scientific explanation has often been a stormy process, as with the reaction to Darwin's ideas. But nowadays, nature as an explanatory model is only used when we are bereft of a scientific explanation or when, reacting to an emotive issue, we retreat from a rational point of view. Thus however intellectually appropriate the concept of sin against nature may have been at the time of Aquinas, it should now be regarded as at best a rationalisation of an emotional reaction.

Opposition to non-procreative sex

More rationally coherent is the opposition to sexual behaviour that is not procreative. In part, this reflects the reluctant acknowledgement by ascetics such as Aquinas that some sexual activity is essential for reproduction, though preferably devoid of any associated pleasure. Aquinas got into logical difficulties here also in regarding voluntary virginity as the 'crowning Christian virtue' (Boswell 1980). It has been suggested that opposition to any form of non-procreative sex may have stemmed from fears of population decline, but it is not clear to what extent such a fear would be articulated as such. There is more to say about non-procreative sex when discussing the particular role of the medical profession in determining social attitudes.

In recent years, the school of sociobiology has attempted to account for much of human social behaviour as a consequence of the evolutionary process. The disposition to certain types of social behaviour, it supposes, becomes established genetically when it proves to have survival or adaptive value. It is therefore of interest how sociobiologists have attempted to account for the continuation of homosexuality. According to their basic thesis, unless it has some biological function, it would have evolved out some time ago. Wilson (1978) in a well intentioned but misguided attempt to establish the 'naturalness' of homosexuality proposed the 'kin-selection' hypothesis. According to this, the existence of homosexual members of a family would contribute to the survival of that family by providing members unburdened with the responsibilities of parenthood. A hetero-sexual member, supported thus, would more effectively reproduce and at the same time transmit some of the genetic predisposition to homosexuality. Such an explanation must sound ironic to modern-day homosexuals who are so often alienated from their families. A variety of sociobiological theories of this kind have been proposed and are reviewed by Kirsch & Rodman (1977).

Threat to established social norms and sex role stereotypes

Social groups do need clear guidelines for what is acceptable behaviour. If these are lacking, social chaos is likely. Prescribed boundaries of acceptable sexual behaviour have usually been at the forefront of such institutionalised constraints. Once a form of behaviour, such as homosexuality, becomes regarded as outside these boundaries, there will be opposition to it.

An important example of this is when sexual behaviour threatens the norms of masculinity and femininity. We have already considered how important this relationship is in many societies. In western societies we see varying degrees of this machismo attitude which Carrier (1980) described for Mexico. For the male, homosexuality is seen as unmasculine and to a lesser extent female homosexuality is seen as unfeminine. Quite apart from the more genital aspects of homosexuality, physical expression of affection between males may be seen as unmasculine. Its occurrence in certain circumstances, such as the football field or under the influence of alcohol, perhaps suggests that the need for such expression exists amongst men but is normally inhibited. There is no doubt that much of the hostility towards homosexuality centres around the stereotype of the effeminate 'queen' or the 'butch' lesbian, even though, as we shall discuss below, such individuals are very much in the minority. Evidence from surveys shows that such attitudes are widespread. Negative attitudes towards homosexuality are often seen to stem from a need to maintain clear distinctions between male and female roles. Those who favour greater sexual equality are more likely to hold positive attitudes towards homosexuality (MacDonald & Games 1974). Although the stereotype of the male homosexual as effeminate prevails at the present time, historical evidence suggests that at other times homosexuality was seen not only as compatible with manliness but also with great courage. Plato suggested that the most formidable army in the world would be composed of lovers inspiring one another to deeds of heroism and sacrifice. The military effectiveness of the Dorian Greeks in Sparta and Crete is often attributed to such a factor, and the elite fighting corps at Thebes was traditionally grouped as pairs of lovers (Bullough 1976). Whether homosexuality bolsters the effectiveness of modern armies is not known, though clearly the official attitude of the military establishment towards homosexuality indicates that no such benefit is acknowledged (Williams & Weinberg 1971).

Association between 'abnormal' sexuality and other antisocial behaviour

Bullough (1976) pointed out the continuing tendency to attribute 'perverse' sexual practices to those who are non-conformist in other ways. Apart from the specific link between witchcraft and sodomy with the devil, a link with heresy was commonly made. One of the most intriguing examples was that of albigensianism, a heretical religious doctrine present in western Europe in the 13th and 14th centuries. This disapproved of procreation because it 'entrapped souls in evil matter'. Homosexual relationships were therefore not only sinless but a desirable way to avoid this entrapment (Boswell 1980). The Albigensians, believed to come from Bulgaria, were called Bulgars. The term 'Buggery' is a corruption of Bulgar and, according to Bullough, was originally used to describe heresy. The confusion of heresy with sexual deviance led to the current use of the term. Bullough goes on to suggest that perhaps sexual deviance was evident amongst some heretical groups, partly because it was a way of rejecting conventional social standards. These observations of the Middle Ages bring to mind the central role sexual morality plays in much radical political thought today, best exemplified in the writings of Marcuse. Sexual politics are fundamental to much of contemporary radical politics, as was hinted at earlier.

The position of women in society

The association between attitudes to homosexuality and the position of women in society has been commented on by various writers (e.g. Bullough 1976). Rattray Taylor (1954) proposed a relationship between the incidence of homosexuality and the degree of matriarchy or patriarchy prevailing at the time. In matriarchal societies, he suggests, there is a permissive attitude to sex and women are accorded a higher status. Incest is then the sexual behaviour most feared and condemned; homosexuality is tolerated and considered unimportant. In patriarchal societies, there is a more restrictive attitude to sex in general and women are considered inferior. Homosexuality (particularly of the male variety) is then much feared and condemned. This is a rather simplistic but attractive idea. Rattray Taylor went on to suggest that it is in the transitional periods between matriarchy and patriarchy that homosexuality will become most prominent and he implied that Ancient Greece represented such a transitional phase.

Ancient Greece does require special consideration. Bullough (1976) suggests that the Greeks tolerated or even encouraged homosexuality as long as it did not threaten the family. Women, whilst having low status in most respects, were regarded as having the supreme purpose of bearing children, especially sons. Alongside this reproductive family unit, the Greek men seemed to indulge in their love affairs with young boys as though it were a separate and perhaps even narcissistic exercise. From the many descriptions of this boy love, one is struck by the erotic identification the older man makes with a beautiful youth, as though he were trying to perpetuate or idealise his own youth. The comparison of this type of love with that between a father and his son is worthy of consideration. According to Boswell (1980), however, many Greeks viewed homosexual love as the only form of eroticism which could be 'lasting, pure and truly spiritual'. Plato believed that only love between people of the same gender could transcend sex. In fact throughout the period of history covered by Boswell's book the picture is presented of men valuing their love for each other more highly than any love between men and women. This must be set against the fact that romantic love was not regarded as a suitable basis for heterosexual marriage until well into the 18th century (Stone 1977). For further discussion of this issue see p. 246.

It is easy to see that in such a situation as existed in Ancient Greece, being exclusively homosexual would be regarded very differently and in fact it seemed to be relatively unusual and was probably considered pathological.

The reader may have noticed that more has been said about male than female homosexuality so far. This is because little has been written about the female in the past; in itself this emphasises the lowly position of women in society. It is also no doubt relevant that female homosexuality, or at least bisexuality, is finding much more expression in recent years as a result of the women's movement, as we will discuss below. Having been repressed by men for so long, it is not surprising that women will assert themselves by denying the sexual importance of men. Being a romantic in such matters, I hope that such a view does not take hold too strongly and that a better balance between men and women will prevail and allow heterosexuality to flourish.

SICKNESS OR SIN?

The role of the Church and the medical profession

So far we have discussed a number of factors which may underlie or serve to perpetuate anti-homosexual feelings. Before leaving the topic, let us consider two institutions in the western world which have played a particular part in fostering these negative attitudes: the Church and the medical profession.

The Church, acting as custodian of our morals, has often taken the lead in establishing explicit norms of sexual behaviour. Aquinas, and Augustine before him, must have had considerable and lasting influence. The Church's role has been complicated not only by the already mentioned association of heresy and sexual deviance, but also because of the difficulties the Church imposes upon its own members when chastity is required and sexual segregation follows. Religious values have gone through periods both of stagnation and of change and reform. As Boswell (1980) points out, the Church has by no means always been opposed to homosexuality, and when intolerance has arisen popular attitudes may have changed before those of the clergy. Nevertheless, sooner or later the Church has become a powerful instrument for imposing such attitudes, backed by the authority of religious doctrine.

At the present time, it is fair to say that the Christian Church is beginning actively to reappraise its attitudes to homosexuality. A more scholarly and less emotive reinterpretation of the Bible is contributing to this. Boyd (1974) has discussed some of these changes, particularly a reappraisal of the story of Sodom which has played such a central part in religious attitudes to homosexuality. The more recent interpretation sees the fate of Sodom as a punishment not for homosexuality but for meanness, arrogance and general wickedness. The homosexual interpretation was perhaps the product of Palestinian Jews in the second century BC, reflecting their contempt for the Greek culture which they associated with homosexual practices. However such reinterpretations must be seen as minority views held by a few churchmen. The majority view is persistently traditional. In 1974, the Board for Social Responsibility of the Church of England set up a working party to study the problem of homosexuality. It is noteworthy that the working party, after making a sincere attempt to reappraise the situation, came up with a report which, by traditional standards, was enlightened. And yet the Board found it necessary to dissociate itself from most of the conclusions of the working party, objecting in particular to any reinterpretation of the Scriptures (CIO 1979). However, we should not expect rapid change in such circumstances.

In 1987, as moral reaction to the AIDS epidemic gathered pace, the General Synod of the Church of England debated the issue of homosexuality amongst the clergy. Whilst some in the debate strived to maintain an attitude of tolerance, the conclusion reached was that overt homosexuality was unacceptable behaviour for a clergyman. The sinfulness of homosexuality, however committed or loving the relationship involved, was left in no doubt. If there had been signs of progress in the Church's adoption of more enlightened attitudes to homosexuality, this was certainly a set back.

The reaction of the medical profession to homosexuality was most prominent during the 19th century, though some crucial beliefs had already been clearly expressed in the 18th century, in particular, the medical rationale for the undesirability of non-procreative sex, namely that seminal discharge was dangerously wasteful of vital energy and should be restricted to necessary procreation (Bullough 1974). In 1838, Morrison, a psychiatrist at the Bethnal Hospital, described homosexuality as 'monomania with unnatural propensity' and concluded that 'being of so detestable a character it is a consolation to know that it is sometimes a consequence of insanity' (Hunter & MacAlpine 1963). This was an early example of 'sinful' behaviour becoming tolerated by labelling it as 'sickness'. By the mid-19th century this conflict between sin and sickness was in full swing, showing that the medical profession, as a cross-section of humanity, contained both the tough- and the tender-minded. The former saw mental disorders as a consequence of sin which should be treated as such; the latter, showing compassion for the underprivileged and deprived, aimed to avoid moral judgement of abnormal behaviour. The resulting medical compromise usually looked for organic pathology which would permit both the moral taint of familiar degeneration and acceptance that the tainted individual was not fully responsible for his own state. Homosexuality was treated in the same way, and came to seem less a consequence of insanity and more a congenital anomaly.

The extent to which supposedly scientific reasoning and moral values can become confounded is strikingly illustrated in the comments expressed at various times on the treatability of homosexuality. As effective treatment might imply that the condition is not innate but rather is acquired, this would reinforce the view that homosexuality is a sin. Hence any attempt to treat homosexuality has been vigorously opposed by those who are aiming to protect the homosexual from social stigma. This issue still prevails today (Bancroft 1974, 1975) and will be considered further in Chapter 10.

During the 20th century the attitudes of the medical profession have become less negative, reflecting a change of attitude in the general population. But in no way has the profession pioneered or even encouraged such a change. In the 1920s and 30s the mental hygiene movement succeeded in confusing mental health with morality, the 20th century equivalent of the moral strictures of the mid 19th century physicians. In 1955, the British Medical Association presented its evidence to the Wolfenden committee on homosexuality and prostitution. The following short extract will convey the prevailing views of the medical establishment at that time:

The attempts to suppress homosexual activity by law can only be one factor in diminishing this problem. The public opinion against homosexual practice is a greater safeguard and this can be achieved by promoting in the minds, motives and wills of the people the desire for clean and unselfish living . . . People who are mainly concerned with themselves and their sensations associate together and obtain from each other the physical and emotional experiences they desire. Personal discipline and unselfishness have little place in their thoughts. If this behaviour is multiplied on a national scale, the problem to society is apparent for widespread irresponsibility and selfishness can only demoralise and weaken the nature. What is needed is responsible citizenship where concern for the nation's welfare and the needs of others takes priority over selfish interest and self-indulgence.

In 1974, the American Psychiatric Association removed homosexuality from its list of pathological diagnoses (Bayer 1981) and this probably represents a majority view amongst the medical profession today — which must be regarded as progress, though in no way does it signify a generally accepting attitude to homosexuality. Many psychoanalysts persevere in their view of homosexuality as a sickness or a perversion.

With the prevailing attitudes towards homosexuality it would indeed be surprising if our scientific knowledge of homosexuality or homosexuals was not obscured or distorted or in many aspects deficient. But let us judge the evidence as best we can.

WHO IS GAY OR LESBIAN?

For reasons that should now be obvious, we may never know the true incidence of homosexuality in our society. It is worth asking whether that matters. Gagnon & Simon (1973) point out that numbers *are* relevant in influencing both public policy and the self-concepts of homosexuals themselves. It is more difficult to enforce laws against behaviour which is seen to be commonplace; it is easier to avoid labelling yourself as pathological if you know that you are in large company. Some major reappraisal of homosexuality undoubtedly followed Kinsey's findings, which we will discuss shortly. It became no longer possible to regard this behaviour in general as bizarre. But establishing whether the incidence is 4% or 10% is probably of much less importance than the realisation that vast numbers of people are involved.

As soon as you grapple with the question of incidence, you meet a conceptual problem — the incidence of what? Kinsey and his colleagues (1948) and other writers (e.g. Churchill 1967) have preferred to comment on the homosexuality of acts rather than people, and Kinsey proposed the Kinsey scale (Table 6.1) to stress that individuals range from those whose sexual acts are exclusively heterosexual to those who are exclusively homosexual, with all gradations in between. Recently a multi-disciplinary symposium was organised at the Kinsey Institute to reappraise the Kinsey

Table 6.1 The Kinsey scale (from Kinsey et al 1948)

Based on both psychological reaction and overt experience, individuals are rated for each specific age period as follows:
0. Exclusively heterosexual with no homosexual
1. Predominantly heterosexual, only incidental homosexual
2. Predominantly heterosexual, but more than incidentally homosexual
3. Equally heterosexual and homosexual
4. Predominantly homosexual, but more than incidentally heterosexual
5. Predominantly homosexual, but incidentally heterosexual
6. Exclusively homosexual

Scale (McWhirter & Reinisch 1988). One general conclusion was that Kinsey's motives for presenting this scale had been more political than scientific. He was clearly trying to counter the prevailing tendency to see people as *either* heterosexual *or* homosexual (the polarising influence discussed in Chapter 3). Robinson (1976) has already delivered a telling critique of Kinsey's logic in this respect, and there is no doubt that Kinsey and the Kinsey scale have seriously underestimated the importance of the individual's sexual identity.

Regardless of the proportion or extent of an individual's homosexual activity, whether he considers himself a homosexual or whether others do so will have an enormous influence on his life. Much distress and anxiety stems from uncertainty about one's identity and in a society which very much divides people into heterosexual and homosexual, regarding oneself as Kinsey 3 is not too relevant! We will therefore need to consider the deciding factors for how we label ourselves, whether it be as heterosexual or homosexual or bisexual. But first let us look at such evidence as we have about the incidence of homosexual behaviour.

Our information is largely confined to the Kinsey studies. The Kinsey ratings are briefly defined in Table 6.1. In their study of white males, Kinsey et al found that 37% had had some homosexual experience to the point of orgasm between adolescence and old age and 4% had been exclusively homosexual since adolescence.

Gagnon & Simon (1973) have suggested that these figures overestimate the incidence of homosexual behaviour because the total Kinsey sample included a disproportionate number of criminal and delinquent males whose homosexual activity may have been enhanced by time spent in penal institutions (in addition to other possible factors). They therefore reanalysed the original Kinsey data, concentrating on a group of 2900 young men who were in college between the years 1938 and 1950, the majority being under 30 at the time of the interview. They regarded this as a more representative sample, at least of that population.

They found that 30% had undergone at least one homosexual experience in which *either* the subject *or* his male partner attained orgasm but slightly more than half of these (i.e. 16% of the total) had shared no such experiences since the age of 15 and an additional third (9% of the total) had experienced all their homosexual acts during adolescence or only incidentally in their late teens. This left about 3% with extensive homosexual as well as heterosexual histories and 3% with exclusive homosexual histories.

These figures, though confined to college males aged 18–25, suggest a much lower incidence of homosexual behaviour than did the original Kinsey report. Gagnon & Simon (1973) do not believe that these figures would differ much in other educational or occupational groups except those with a high proportion of criminal careers.

A further reanalysis of the Kinsey data was presented by Van Wyk & Geist (1984). They summed up all the heterosexual and homosexual behaviour for each individual between the ages of 18 and 40, or the age at interview, whichever was earlier. They then computed a Kinsey rating from the ratio. This showed that 4.7% of men were in the range 4–6, and only 1.2% in the range 2–4. There was therefore a bimodal distribution.

Hunt's 1974 survey found that 1% of males were exclusively homosexual and 1% bisexual. Pietropinto & Simenauer (1977) in a large scale questionnaire survey of men found 1.3% to be homosexual and 3.1% bisexual. In a study of people aged over 50, 2.3% of an unrepresentative sample of 2402 men considered themselves to be homosexual, whilst 13% had had one or more homosexual experiences (Brecher 1984). Such figures, whilst apparently modest, indicate that large numbers of people are involved, running into millions when countries like the USA or the UK are considered.

In their study of women, Kinsey and his colleagues (1953) found a much lower incidence of homosexual activity than in men. Homosexual responses (with or without orgasm) had occurred in about half as many women as men, and contacts leading to orgasm in about a third as many. Moreover, there were only about half to a third as many of the females who in any age group were primarily or exclusively homosexual. In general, women who were single when interviewed showed a higher incidence of past homosexual activity than married women. Gagnon & Simon carried out a re-analysis of the female college students comparable to that of males mentioned above. Here the sex difference was even more striking. Only 6% had undergone at least one homosexual experience compared with 30% of the men; only 2% had had any significant amount of homosexual experience and less than 1% were exclusively homosexual. In Brecher's (1984) study of the over 50, 8% of 1844 women had had one or more homosexual experience. Interestingly the women (11%) were more likely than the men (8%) to say they had felt sexual attraction to someone of the same sex. According to this evidence, women appear to be less likely than men to act on recognised homosexual attraction.

There is no evidence available to suggest that the incidence of homosexual behaviour has increased in recent times. In fact, the Kinsey data suggest that it has remained relatively constant.

HOMOSEXUAL IDENTITY

Our sexual identity is an important part of our general identity and self-image, and needs to be stable for our well-being. Uncertainty about sexual identity often causes distress. In Chapter 3 I described three stages in the development of sexual identity: firstly, the pre-labelling stage, when early sexual experience occurs before we need to categorise ourselves in sexual terms. Then comes a stage of self-labelling, when we begin to ask the question 'What sort of sexual person am I?' Then there is the social labelling stage when the individual's social world reinforces one label or another. The labels we use, as discussed earlier in this chapter, are products of our particular social system. In western society the labels are *either* heterosexual *or* homosexual. Bisexual has not been a given label, though as we shall see that may be changing. Not surprisingly, the homosexual community prefers to have its own labels rather than use those imposed upon it by the heterosexual establishment. Thus the term 'gay' is now the favoured label — 'I am gay'. Heterosexuals are often reluctant to use this term and sometimes resentment is expressed that a general term from the English language has been purloined by the homosexual world and now cannot be used with its original meaning. Boswell (1980) has pointed out that the term 'homosexual' was coined in the late 19th century, whereas 'gay', or words close to it, have been used in this way for several centuries. He states: 'Most speakers use "gay" to describe persons who are conscious of erotic preference for their own gender'. In other words it is a self-assigned label and captures the essence of homosexual identity. Homosexual women, perhaps because they would rather be regarded separately, prefer to use the term 'lesbian'; 'gay' is predominantly used by men.

Whatever the precise label we use, the implications of assigning ourselves to a particular category of sexual orientation are substantial and go far beyond simple sexual partner choice. Apart from the negative consequences of being stigmatised, membership of such a 'club' can organise many aspects of your life — where you live and socialise, who you meet, and perhaps even what job you get (Hoffman 1968). Being heterosexual has no such consequences. But as Hooker (1967) pointed out, there is a range of homosexual 'clubs' that one can join. The gay bar is in many ways the most open and the most all-embracing. Those who frequent it have to a large extent publicly declared their homosexuality. Some bars specialise in certain types of identity, the effeminate 'queen' or the ultramasculine or 'S–M leather' set. But beyond these bars there is a range of social groups which permit varying degrees of concealment of one's homosexuality, or the maintenance of normal, straight public personas. Clearly the social setting will be chosen to meet the emerging identity of the individual and will in turn shape that identity. In particular, membership of such subcultures limits participation in other groups, especially re-entry into the heterosexual world.

One feature typifies the modern gay world. Presumably because it is outside the constraints of social convention it is in a state of more or less constant flux.

In fact the 1970s were a time of particularly rapid changes (Altman 1985). During that decade gay men became far more visible. The new style of gay man is 'masculine, non-apologetic about his sexuality, self-assertive, highly consumerist and not at all revolutionary, though prepared to demonstrate for gay rights'. Altman stresses the importance in the gay community of the emergence of a gay economy, so that advertisers talk of the gay market (and politicians of the gay vote). This public visibility and economic viability leads to the concept of the 'ethnic homosexual' — a minority which requires and deserves the same rights as other ethnic minorities. Altman cautions that as economic conditions decline homosexuals may once again become scape-goats for society's ills. He clearly had not foreseen the AIDS epidemic, of which more later.

Lesbians have gone through their own changes in a rather different way. There is much less of a lesbian economy, but whereas gay men have become relatively apolitical, similar to other relatively affluent consumer groups, lesbians have retained much more of a revolutionary fervour and have been closely linked with the women's movement. Nicholls (1986) described some of the contrasting developments amongst lesbians, with some imitating gay (or straight) men in their preoccupation with sexual pleasure, whilst others have somewhat retreated from the sexual aspect, seeing it as too much a reflection of the man's world. It is too early to see where these intriguing changes and experiments will lead.

The lesbian movement, particularly through its links with the women's movement, has presented us with evidence of the bisexual potential of women. The concept of bisexuality has for many years been somewhat threatening, particularly to gay men. There may be a tendency to regard the bisexual as in no man's land and hence more likely to have psychological problems. This seems a paradox as, given a liberal view of homosexuality, the ability to relate to people of either sex would seem to be an ideal, and one which is commonly realised in many other societies. Weinberg & Williams (1974) found no evidence that those who regarded themselves as bisexual suffered from any more psychological disturbances than others. But given the battle that has been waged against social stigma, there is an entirely understandable need by the gay community to defend their status as gay, and to see it as both natural and immutable. Hence they have reinforced the idea of 'once a homosexual, always a homosexual' or 'you are either straight or gay'.

The Kinsey data have given us an idea of how many people engage in homosexual acts at some stage and yet, as already mentioned, the pro-portion of their sample who can be regarded as bisexual is small. Humphreys (1970) studied males who sought sexual contact in public toilets and found that 54% of them were married and living with their families. Presumably they presented a heterosexual front to the world, but whether they regarded themselves as bisexual is not clear. Weinberg & Williams (1974) asked the respondents in their study to place themselves on the Kinsey scale. Only 4.4% of the American respondents and even less of the Dutch and Danish men rated themselves as Kinsey 3. Such individuals often describe a different quality to their hetero- and homosexual relationships. One patient of mine said: 'They are like red and white wine, I enjoy both but they taste different'. Such a pattern of bisexuality may be very different from that in which similar romantic sexual attachments are experienced with both male and female.

Blumstein & Schwartz (1976) have described that for many, sexual identity is an evolving and sometimes fluctuating issue. Certainly this has been increasingly evident amongst women (Bell & Weinberg 1978). Blumstein & Schwartz (1976) suggest that one of the factors contributing to bisexuality in women is identification with the women's movement. Not only does this foster close same-sex relationships, often with women who are already lesbian, but the sexuality of such relationships for otherwise heterosexual women allows them to dissociate themselves from men on ideological grounds. But in the last few years there has been evidence of an increasing tendency for men to experience bisexuality (Klein 1988). Is the traditional dichotomy of straight and gay beginning to fade, and if so what will be the social consequences?

WHAT ARE THEY LIKE AS PEOPLE?

As with most minority groups, homosexuals tend to be seen by the majority in terms of stereotypes. Much of the misunderstanding about homosexuality stems from these stereotypes and the failure to recognise that homosexuals are no less heterogeneous than heterosexuals. Male homosexuals are often seen as effeminate, working in jobs which are more suitable for women, or which at least require no 'masculine' attributes. Lesbians on the other hand tend to be classed as either 'butch' (masculine), or 'femme' (feminine). The view of female homosexuality in particular tends to be based on the heterosexual model. Homosexuals of both sexes are considered to be neurotic, with abnormal personalities and usually unhappy. To what extent do these stereotypes bear any resemblance to reality?

THE GENDER IDENTITY AND ROLE OF HOMOSEXUALS

Several studies have reported on the proportion of male homosexuals who show effeminacy. They range from 14–27% (Bancroft 1972), and the effeminacy is usually based on rather unsystematic observation. Satisfactory psychometric methods for assessing feminine or masculine attributes have been lacking (Bancroft 1974; Freund et al 1974) but studies by Siegelman (1972), Freund et al (1974) and Schatzberg et al (1975) have demonstrated significant differences between homosexual and heterosexual males in psychological measures of femininity or effeminacy. It is important to emphasise that such differences relate to a subgroup of homosexuals and that the majority are indistinguishable from the heterosexual population in this respect. There is even less evidence about the degree of psychological masculinity or femininity in lesbians (Kenyon 1974). Neither male homosexuals nor lesbians have been shown to have distinguishing characteristics in terms of body shape.

The possible importance of 'feminine' gender identity and role causing psychological problems will be considered below, but what is its relationship to the homosexual orientation per se? In Chapter 3 we suggested that uncertainty about gender identity during childhood and adolescence may be one factor contributing to homosexual development. Zuger (1978) and Green (1979) who followed effeminate boys into adolescence and adulthood found that a majority of them developed homosexual preferences. In retrospective studies of adult homosexual men and women there has been a consistent finding of reported gender non-conformity in the childhood of many of them (Saghir & Robins 1973; Siegelman 1974, 1978, 1979; Bell et al 1981; Grellert et al 1982). The importance of cross-gender behaviour in the homosexuality of many other cultures has already been emphasised. Harry (1983) presents evidence that this gender non-conformity of childhood largely disappears during the adulthood of gay men — what he calls 'defeminisation'. This childhood pattern is undoubtedly the most robust finding in the developmental histories of homosexuals and there has perhaps been a tendency to over emphasise its importance. Carrier (1986) has warned against this, pointing out that it is in a minority albeit a large one that this history is evident. Nevertheless, this association is striking and does require careful consideration.

Bieber et al (1982) suggested that a homosexual identity allows an escape from the demands of masculinity that many heterosexual males experience. Gagnon & Simon (1973) described how the young male homosexual, soon after acknowledging his homosexuality, often goes through a crisis of masculine identity during which he may adopt an effeminate identity or behaviour. They imply that in the majority, as this identity crisis is resolved the need to be effeminate recedes. It is as though the homosexuality conflicts with the prevailing criteria of masculinity until new criteria are adopted. Westfall et al (1975) described how effeminate behaviour is apparently exaggerated in social situations which provoke anxiety. Alternative ways of reacting to the 'demasculinising' effects of homosexuality are to emphasise other non-sexual forms of masculine behaviour or adopt patterns of sexual activity with an ultramasculine or aggressive quality.

Evelyn Hooker (1967) in her detailed study of male homosexuals suggested various ways by which this conflict between homosexual activity and masculine identity may be resolved. One way is to see a dichotomy between masculine and feminine and to place oneself in one category or the other; if in the masculine, this would require consistent sexual behaviour such as the exclusively 'insertor' role. A second solution is to see masculinity and femininity as a continuum, positioning oneself towards one end or the other. This, she suggested, was an unstable solution. The third was to regard homosexuality as a third gender identity, incorporating some masculine and feminine characteristics as well as having qualities of its own.

The heterosexual, whilst vulnerable to crises in gender identity, does have some advantages in this regard over the homosexual, mainly stemming from the relative stability fostered by long-term relationships such as marriage. Nevertheless there are many ways in which the heterosexual man or woman's sexual activity, like the homosexual's, may strengthen or weaken his or her gender identity.

The tendency for homosexual males, especially early in their homosexual development, to feel particular attraction to heterosexual males and the importance that many of them attach to the penis of their partner suggest that masculinity may be for them a basic ingredient in sexual attractiveness. This can be compared with much of early heterosexual attraction and experience, when reinforcement of gender identity and self-esteem is no less important, than sexual or interpersonal rewards per se (see Chapter 3).

In general, therefore, we should assume that sexual activity and gender identity are related in a complex and dynamic way. Although effeminate traits are evident in some male homosexuals, the stereotype of the effeminate homosexual is about as useful as the stereotype of the aggressive macho heterosexual male.

PERSONALITY

In 1974, the American Psychiatric Association removed homosexuality from its list of diagnoses, putting in its place 'sexual orientation disturbance' (Bayer 1981). 'This category is for individuals whose sexual interests are directed primarily towards people of the same sex and who are either disturbed by, in conflict with, or wish to change their sexual orientation. The diagnostic category is distinguished from homosexuality which by itself does not necessarily constitute a psychiatric disorder'.

How disturbed or unhappy are homosexuals? The mainstream of psychoanalysis continues to see homosexuality as a pathological state or perversion (see Rosen (1978) for psychoanalytic opinions). The point has been made frequently that most psychiatric opinion about homosexuality has been based on psychiatric patients with homosexual orientation rather than on a repesentative section of the homosexual community. Comments on their psychopathology should not therefore be seen as relevant to homosexuals in general. This is undoubtedly a valid and important point. Schofield (1965) in his study of homosexuals in different settings found that homosexuals who were undergoing psychiatric treatment had more in common with heterosexual psychiatric patients than they did with the other homosexual groups. Turner et al (1974) found that homosexuals seeking treatment to become heterosexual differed from homosexuals who had never sought such treatment on a number of measures of neuroticism.

Once again we have more evidence concerning male homosexuals than females. Siegelman (1972) found that although a group of non-patient homosexuals showed more neuroticism than their heterosexual controls, this difference disappeared when the homosexuals with evidence of feminine gender identity were excluded. He found this in both American and British subjects (Siegelman 1978). In other words, the neuroticism may be associated with effeminacy (or, as suggested earlier, the effeminacy may be part of a reaction of anxiety or insecurity).

Saghir & Robins (1973) found no difference between their homosexual and heterosexual male subjects in terms of depression and anxiety or psychosomatic symptoms. This study has been criticised on the grounds that they chose only single heterosexual subjects for their comparison group, who therefore were not typical of heterosexuals generally, whereas single homosexuals are the rule. Two other large scale studies did find some differences. Weinberg & Williams (1974) found their male homosexuals to be less happy than their heterosexual controls but to have no more psychosomatic symptoms. Bell & Weinberg (1978) found not only more psychosomatic symptoms, but also more loneliness, lower self-acceptance and more depression and suicidal ideas; 20% of their homosexual men had previously made a suicide attempt compared with 4% of their controls. They stressed that these differences were largely accounted for by certain subgroups of their homosexual population, but as they did not categorise their heterosexual subjects in a comparable fashion this point is of less importance.

The picture for lesbian women is similar although perhaps a little more cheerful. Saghir & Robins (1973) found their lesbian group to show more depression but to be relatively unaffected by it. Kenyon (1974) found lesbians to be more neurotic than their heterosexual counterparts. Two studies (reviewed by Riess et al 1974) suggested that lesbians may have stronger or more adaptive personalities than heterosexual women, at least in terms of independence. In Bell & Weinberg's (1978) study, the lesbian women reported less current happiness, lower self-esteem and more suicidal ideas. For questions such as these, the problem of appropriate and satisfactory comparison groups are formidable and we should bear this in mind when interpreting such studies. But it certainly seems likely that, whereas homosexuality is quite compatible with mental and physical health and happiness, it does increase the likelihood of problems. An important finding in Bell & Weinberg's study was that both their male and female homosexuals reported a higher incidence of seeking professional help in the past. Remembering Gagnon & Simon's (1973) observation of the temporary phase of effeminacy in young male homosexuals and the reported association between effeminacy and neuroticism, we should perhaps expect that transient periods of disturbance and unhappiness are more likely at some stage in the homosexual's life. To what extent that vulnerability is dependent on the prevailing negative social reaction to homosexuality is difficult to say but it probably accounts for a large part. Having said that, it is still probably unrealistic to anticipate the disappearance of such negative social influences. Consequently, it seems necessary to conclude that being a homosexual does have its problems, though for the more fortunate these problems can be satisfactorily overcome. The AIDS epidemic has added a whole new dimension to both the social stigma and personal problems of gay men. There is a sad irony about the use of the word 'gay' by the homosexual community. It is curiously effective in making 'straight' people feel uncomfortable, which may be part of its appeal, but it does not seem to be an accurate description of the homosexual's lot.

WHAT DO HOMOSEXUALS DO?

Whilst heterosexual couples can employ any of the sexual techniques available to homosexuals, they have in addition the essential heterosexual opportunity for vaginal intercourse. In fact, for many heterosexuals, this is both the biological and the social norm, other types of activity being consequently less acceptable. In the absence of any equivalent norm for homosexual interaction, the heterosexual model is commonly imposed as a further stereotype. Thus it is widely assumed that homosexual couples have one person taking the active or masculine role, the other the passive or feminine. Homosexuals, especially males, are also widely believed to be not only highly sexed, but promiscuous, seldom maintaining stable sexual relationships. Let us now examine these stereotypes more closely.

PATTERNS OF SEXUAL ACTIVITY

Masters & Johnson (1979) extended their laboratory observations of heterosexual activity to homosexual pairs and concluded that the physiological changes accompanying sexual arousal and orgasm were the same whether heterosexual or homosexual activity was involved. This comes as no surprise. Of more interest were some of the differences they reported. Established homosexual couples took their time during sexual activity, with considerable emphasis on the exchange of pleasure. Established heterosexual couples, on the other hand, were more goal-oriented and keen to 'get the job done'. Homosexuals not only communicated more openly with their partners, but they appeared to be more sensitive and responsive to their partners' needs, presumably reflecting the empathy that comes from being of the same gender. Whilst one should be cautious in generalising from this special laboratory setting to more normal sexual encounters, these observations suggest that in terms of sexual pleasure, homosexuals may have some advantages over heterosexuals.

This emphasis on mutual pleasure underlines the point that for most established homosexual couples the choice of sexual techniques is determined by this need for mutual pleasure, rather than conforming to predetermined active or passive roles. Hence there is usually a reciprocation or exchange of roles in the use of a variety of techniques.

Bell & Weinberg (1978) asked their male subjects about mutual masturbation, fellatio, rubbing bodies together and anal intercourse. Almost all of their subjects had engaged in most of these during the preceding 12 months. Fellatio in both the insertor and receptive role was the most frequent, followed by being masturbated, masturbating one's partner, the insertor role in anal intercourse, the receptive role and body contact in that order of frequency. Nearly all the men expressed a definite preference for one type of sexual activity. Being fellated was the most popular, and taking the active role in anal intercourse a close second (this order was reversed for the black male subjects). Only about 6% preferred the passive or insertee role in anal intercourse. In recent years there has been evidence of increasing experimentation with anal eroticism, involving for example 'rimming' (oral–anal contact), insertion of foreign bodies, 'water sports' (erotic enemas) and 'fisting' (inserting of the whole hand into the rectum). These practices, some of which carry a substantial risk of rectal trauma (Agnew 1986) have also become relevant to the risks of transmitting the AIDS virus (see below and Chapter 11).

For lesbian subjects (Bell & Weinberg 1978) the order of frequency of different types of sexual activity was as follows: mutual masturbation, cunnilingus (oral sex) and body rubbing (which was more common amongst the black women). Cunnilingus was the technique most favoured. Dildos (or artificial penises) for intravaginal stimulation do not appear to be widely used by lesbians.

The stereotype of the typically active or passive homosexual is once again relevant to only a small minority. The avoidance of certain roles or techniques may be a way of concealing sexual dysfunction (e.g. confining oneself to the receptive role in either fellatio or anal intercourse) and, as Masters & Johnson (1979) have pointed out, it is easier for the homosexual male to conceal erectile or ejaculatory dysfunction than it is for the heterosexual male. The avoidance of or the preference for specific techniques may also reflect the psychological or gender significance of the behaviour rather than simply its sensual quality. Hence the recipient role in intercourse may be avoided by those who are threatened by its 'feminine' implications.

Hoffman (1968) describes the compulsive 'fellator' who is driven to find a masculine, virile male to fellate, often involving himself in considerable risk in the process. This activity, Hoffman suggests, is a method, albeit unconsciously motivated, of incorporating the masculinity of the man being fellated — in the manner of a sacramental feast (reminiscent of the ritualised fellatio described earlier in this Chapter). Such activity, he says, often occurs at times when the individual's self-esteem has been lowered. In general, this reflects the importance that male homosexuals attach to their partner's penis, and possibly to their semen, as mentioned earlier. There are of course equivalent, if qualitatively different, forms of heterosexual activity. The heterosexual male may assert his masculinity in a variety of sexual ways, usually at the expense of his female partner. Of particular interest is the humiliation of the woman through anal intercourse (see the critique of Norman Mailer by Kate Millet (1969)).

PATTERNS OF SEXUAL RELATIONSHIPS

It is unfortunately inevitable that, because homosexuals are designated according to their sexual preferences, they will be seen very much in sexual terms. One consequence of this is that they are often assumed to be highly sexed and preoccupied with sexual matters. Whilst there is no direct comparison of the levels of sexual interest of hetero- and homosexuals, the findings of Bell & Weinberg (1978) suggest that homosexuals show a range of sexual interest similar to heterosexuals, with males more likely to express high interest than females. The average heterosexual will nevertheless be struck by the extent to which sex in the homosexual world precedes relationships, often being quite detached from any interpersonal relationship of even the most transient kind. Perhaps the extreme example of depersonalised sex is the hole in the wall between public lavatory cubicles, allowing the penis of a man on one side of the wall to be fellated by a man on the other side, all entirely anonymously. The gay steam baths where men pass from one sexual encounter to another is unlike any form of heterosexual experience available to the vast majority of 'straight' individuals. Several studies have shown that many homosexual men have had large numbers of sexual partners during their sexual careers, much more so than would be expected in the heterosexual population. Such studies have also consistently found that lesbian women have had far fewer partners than their male counterparts and are more likely to be at any time in a loving relationship. The evidence does therefore suggest that, by heterosexual criteria, homosexual men tend to be promiscuous and lesbians much less so. This raises the interesting possibility that this promiscuity is more to do with maleness than with homosexuality. If men, as is often assumed to be the case, tend to be more promiscuous than women then the heterosexual version of the male has to contend with the restraining influence of his female partner. The homosexual male has no such constraint. On top of that is the fact that for the homosexual there is no social encouragement of stable sexual relationships — if anything, the reverse (see Chapter 5 for a discussion of polygamy).

In Chapter 3 we considered sexual development and the incorporation of our sexuality into loving dyadic relationships. In the homosexual's world, sex outside such relationships is more or less institutionalised, at least for the males. But homosexual men and women are not, as we have already stressed, preoccupied with sex and they have the same needs for loving relationships and companionship as anyone else. How difficult is it for them to achieve such relationships without the social reinforcement of marriage encountered by heterosexuals? Probably the best evidence on this point comes from two studies. Bell & Weinberg (1978), using factor analysis of many of the variables from their interview study, produced a typology of homosexuality; the same types emerged for their male and female subjects.

1. *Close-coupled.* These seem to be comparable to the happily married faithful heterosexuals, living contentedly in a stable relationship with little sexual activity outside the relationship. They presented themselves as a particularly happy and well-adjusted group by any standards.
2. *Open-coupled.* Here the stable relationship was associated with a fair amount of 'extramarital' sexuality. Though not as well adjusted as the close-coupled, the males of this category seemed better able to cope with this lifestyle than the lesbians — perhaps further evidence of the woman's needs for a monogamous relationship.
3. *Functionals.* These individuals were not in stable relationships and enjoyed a wide variety of sexual partners. They tended to be the most highly sexed group and were also somewhat younger. Presumably a proportion of them move into other categories as they get older. Once again, the male in this category seems to have less problems than the female.
4. *Dysfunctionals.* Individuals in this category conformed very much to the stereotype of the unhappy homosexual. They tended to have recurring problems in their sexual relationships, often with sexual dysfunction and frequently feeling unhappy with their homosexual identities.
5. *Asexuals.* Comparable to the dysfunctionals, these individuals are characterised by a low level of sexual interest and hence are more inclined to live solitary existences.

The proportions of males and females found in these categories are shown in Table 6.2. It will be seen that more than a quarter of each sex were unclassifiable by this method. In addition, the lesbians included a much higher proportion of the close-coupled, underlining once again that they are less promiscuous than the males. Although this study was published in 1978 the data were collected prior to 1970. As already mentioned, the 1970s were a time of major change in the gay world. We must therefore be cautious in extrapolating from this evidence to gay relationships in the late 1980s.

Table 6.2 Typology of homosexuality (from Bell & Weinberg 1978)

	Males (n = 686) (%)	Female (n = 293) (%)
Close-coupled	10	28
Open-coupled	18	17
Functional	15	10
Dysfunctional	12	5
Asexual	16	11
Unclassifiable	29	28
Total	100	100

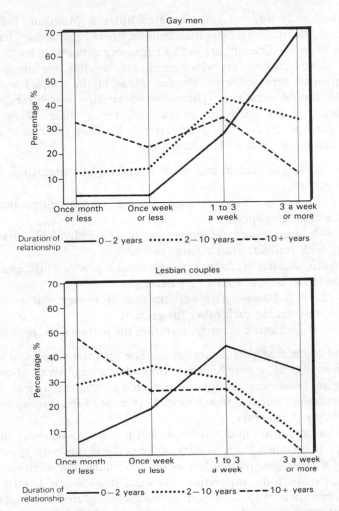

Fig. 6.1 Frequency of sexual activity in gay and lesbian couples by duration of relationship. (from Blumstein & Schwartz 1983)

In Blumstein & Schwartz's (1983) study of American couples, gay male and lesbian couples were included. The reported frequency of love-making in these couples according to the duration of the relationship is shown in Figure 6.1. The authors found that initiation of love-making can be a problem, particularly for lesbian couples. They suggested that the woman's tendency to feel uncomfortable with the sexual aggressor role contributes to the relatively low frequency of sex in lesbian relationships (see p. 254 for further discussion of initiation of love-making). They also found that lesbian couples were more likely to separate if one partner became sexually involved outside the relationship. The lesbians seemed less able than gay men to keep 'extramarital' sex on a casual basis.

A further study was published by McWhirter & Mattison (1984), who interviewed 156 established gay male couples whose relationships had lasted from 1 to 37 years. The authors used a friendship network to locate couples and interviewed all contacts who agreed. Neither this nor the other two studies involved representative samples. Many of the couples were interviewed on several occasions. They showed various joint lifestyles: some lived together, some apart but in the same town, while others lived in different parts of the country. McWhirter & Mattison described six stages in the evolution of these male relationships:

1. year 1, *blending* (merging, limerence, equalising of partnership, frequent sexual activity);
2. year 2–3, *nesting* (home-making, finding compatibility, decline of limerence, ambivalence);
3. years 4–5, *maintaining* (reappearance of the individual, risk-taking, dealing with conflict, establishing tradition);
4. years 6–10, *building* (collaborating, increasing productivity, establishing independence, dependability of partner);
5. years 11–20, *releasing* (trusting, merging of money and possessions, constructing, taking each other for granted);
6. 20 years on, achieving security, restoring the partnership, remembering.

The end of the first year is a common time for male couples to split up. Expectations of fidelity were high but this was defined in terms of emotional commitment. Sexual exclusivity was expected by the majority at the start of the relationship but this soon changed. In most of the couples there was an assumption of equality.

This is an interesting in-depth study, but it is impressionistic; there was no attempt to establish the reliability of method and one must question the validity of their stages, particularly as regards timing and duration. Nevertheless this raises some interesting ideas and it would be fruitful to test them out in a more systematic and methodologically rigorous study of gay and heterosexual as well as lesbian stable couples. It is interesting to speculate how they might differ.

AIDS

When the first edition of this book was published AIDS was not an issue. Now it hangs over the gay world like a deadly cloud. AIDS is a fatal viral illness which in the western world until recently was mainly transmitted during male homosexual activity. For the first few years of the epidemic in the west it was seen as a gay disease. Soon it became apparent that other groups were being infected either by contaminated blood products (e.g. haemophiliacs) or, in the case of intravenous drug users, by sharing needles. Through these sources and through bisexual men the disease is now becoming established in the heterosexual community. The medical aspects of AIDS will be considered in more detail in Chapter 11. Here we will consider its impact on the gay world, an impact which is only beginning to gather momentum. It is difficult to see where it will end.

The impact on gay men is twofold. First it is killing them. In gay communities such as in New York and San Francisco there are few members who have not already suffered bereavement of a close friend or lover. Secondly, it is beginning to refuel anti-gay feeling in the heterosexual community. As the realisation grows that this major epidemic will increasingly involve heterosexual people, hostility to gay people is likely to escalate. Already there have been attempts to isolate AIDS victims in a manner reminiscent of the medieval leper colonies.

To a considerable extent the response of the gay community in the USA and Europe has been responsible and constructive. Gay people have taken the initiative in setting up education campaigns to promote safe sex as well as organising counselling services for AIDS victims. Unfortunately the group most likely to introduce the virus to heterosexual communities, the drug users, are by the nature of their habit much less likely to react in a constructive and responsible fashion. They have already embarked on a self-destructive pattern of behaviour.

There are three types of 'victims' needing counselling. First, the person with the active disease — a particularly unpleasant form of recurrent illness which is invariably fatal. The second category has an AIDS-related condition (ARC); here the prognosis is uncertain. Third is the person who is simply seropositive (i.e. has antibodies to the HIV virus in his blood indicating that he has been infected at some stage and may well still be carrying the active virus.) This last category poses counselling problems of a unique kind. (There are some similarities to when syphilis was rife.) The seropositive individual has an unknown likelihood of contracting the fatal disease after an uncertain time interval, which could be several years. Throughout that time he is assumed to have the capacity to infect other people. It is difficult to overestimate the continuing psychological trauma of such a state of affairs.

Research is in progress to investigate the relationship between type of sexual activity and risk of infection, and some preliminary results have been reported. Thus in a longitudinal Dutch study (Tielman & van Grieusven 1986) it has so far been shown that certain types of sexual activity (in particular passive anal intercourse) are associated with positive serology. (The reason why, together with other evidence, will be discussed in Chapter 11.) The number of sexual partners per se is not predictive of positive serology, except indirectly through its association with types of sexual practice. Cannabis use was found to be associated with infection. In a New York study (Martin 1986), 745 gay men were asked about their sexual activity before and since they learnt about AIDS. Substantial changes in the pattern of their sex lives were shown as a result of fear of contracting the disease. There was a reduction by 82% in the number of 'extradomestic' partners (i.e. outside the home); by 80% in oral–anal sex; 80% in episodes of ingesting the partner's semen, either orally or anally; 68% in anal–genital and 60% in oral–genital sex and 50% reduction in episodes of kissing. This study has also found that men who have experienced bereavement due to AIDS were significantly more fearful of contracting the disease themselves, producing a state of distress which may well contribute to their morbidity.

So far there have clearly been dramatic changes in the sexual activity of gay men as a result of this epidemic (see p. 596). The previous value attached to casual sex is bound to lessen, with greater emphasis on stable relationships. The impact on gay lifestyle is likely to be considerable and we are at an early stage of this radical process. The reaction of the non-gay community may well influence this process negatively if public hysteria gains a hold.

CONCLUSIONS

It should by now be clear that there are only two things that homosexuals have in common: their sexual preference for members of their own sex and their stigmatisation by the heterosexual majority. For a while it seemed that they had their own awful disease, but that was a temporary phase. The prevailing stereotypes of homosexuality are unhelpful and tell us more about heterosexual attitudes to homosexuality than the real homosexual world. Unfortunately we will see prejudice and bigotry being inflamed and hardened by the threat of AIDS.

People with homosexual preferences have always had more than their fair share of problems, and we will be discussing ways of helping them later in this book. But there are important lessons for heterosexuals to learn from the gay and lesbian communities, not only about sexuality but also the effects of social processes on human relationships. Ironically, at a time when the polarisation of homo- and heterosexuality is beginning to weaken, and when bisexuality is becoming more a part of human experience, the AIDS threat will tend to drive these two sections of society apart. It is to be hoped, nevertheless, that some good may come of this disease, both for gay men and for people in general. But the price for any long-term benefits is likely to be very high.

REFERENCES

Agnew J 1986 Hazards associated with anal erotic activity. Archives of Sexual Behaviour 15: 307–314
Altman D 1985 What changed in the 70s? In: Gay Left Collective (eds) Homosexuality: power and politics. Allison & Busby, London, pp 52–63
Bancroft J 1972 The relationship between gender identity and sexual behaviour: some clinical aspects. In: Ounsted C, Taylor D C (eds) Gender differences: their ontogeny and significance. Churchill Livingstone, Edinburgh
Bancroft J 1974 Deviant sexual behaviour: modification and assessment. Clarendon Press, Oxford

Bancroft J 1975 Homosexuality and the medical profession: a behaviourist's view. Journal of Medical Ethics 1: 176–180

Bayer R 1981 Homosexuality and American psychiatry: the politics of diagnosis. Basic Books, New York

Bell A P, Weinberg M S 1978 Homosexualities. A study of diversity among men and women. Mitchell Beazley, London

Bell A P, Weinberg M S, Hammersmith S K 1981 Sexual preference: its development in men and women. Indiana University Press, Bloomington

Bieber I, Dain H J, Dince P R et al 1962 Homosexuality: a psychoanalytic study. Basic Books, New York

Blackwood E 1985 Breaking the mirror: the construction of lesbianism and the anthropological discourse on homosexuality. Journal of Homosexuality 11: 1–18

Blumstein P W, Schwartz P 1976 Bisexuality in women. Archives of Sexual Behavior 5: 171–182

Blumstein P, Schwartz P 1983 American couples. Morrow, New York

Boswell J 1980 Christianity, social tolerance and homosexuality. University of Chicago Press, Chicago

Boyd K 1974 Homosexuality and the church. In: Loraine J A (ed) Understanding homosexuality — its biological and psychological bases. MTP, Lancaster

Brecher E M 1984 Love, sex and aging. A Consumer Union report. Little, Brown, Boston

British Medical Association 1955 Memorandum on homosexuality drawn up by a special committee of the British Medical Association BMA, London

Broude G J, Green S J 1980 Cross-cultural codes on 20 sexual attitudes and practices. In: Berry H III & Schlegel A (eds) Cross-cultural samples and codes. University of Pittsburg Press, Pittsburg, pp 313–334

Bullough V L 1974 Homosexuality and the medical model. Journal of Homosexuality 1: 99–110

Bullough V L 1976 Sexual variance in society and history. Wiley, New York

Carrier J M 1980 Homosexual behavior in cross-cultural perspective. In: Marmor J (ed) Homosexual behavior; a modern reappraisal. Basic Books, New York, pp 100–122

Carrier J M 1986 Childhood cross-gender behavior and adult homosexuality. Archives of Sexual Behavior 15: 89–93

Churchill W 1967 Homosexual behavior among males. Hawthorn, New York

CIO 1979 Homosexual relationships. A contribution to discussion. CIO Publishing

Ford C S, Beach F A 1952 Patterns of sexual behaviour. Eyre & Spottiswoode, London

Freeman M D A 1979 The law and sexual deviation. In: Rosen I (ed) Sexual deviation. Oxford University Press, Oxford

Freund K, Nagler E, Langevin R, Zajac A, Steiner B 1974 Measuring feminine gender identity in homosexual males. Archives of Sexual Behavior 3: 249–260

Gagnon J, Simon W 1973 Sexual conduct: the social sources of human sexuality. Aldine, Chicago

Green R 1979 Sex-dimorphic behaviour development in the human — pre-natal hormone administration and post-natal socialisation. In: Sex, hormones and behaviour. Ciba Foundation Symposium 62. Excerpta Medica, Amsterdam

Grellert E A, Newcomb M D, Bentler P M 1982 Childhood play activities of male and female homosexuals and heterosexuals. Archives of Sexual Behavior 11: 451–478

Harry J 1983 Defeminisation and adult psychological well-being among male homosexuals. Archives of Sexual Behavior 12: 1–20

Herdt G H 1981 Guardians of the flutes. McGraw-Hill, New York

Herdt G H 1988 Contemporary cross-cultural views on sexual orientation and homosexuality. In: McWhirter D, Reinisch J (eds) Homosexuality/heterosexuality; the Kinsey scale and current research. Second Kinsey symposium. Oxford University Press, New York (in press)

Hoffman M 1968 The gay world. Basic Books, Southport

Hooker E 1967 The homosexual community. In: Gagnon J H, Simon W (eds) Sexual deviance. Harper & Row, London

Hotvedt M 1983 Gender identity and sexual orientation: the anthropological perspective. In: Schwartz M F, Moraczewski A S, Monteleone J A (eds) Sex and Gender. A theological and scientific inquiry. Pope John Center, St Louis, Missouri, pp 144–176

Humphreys R A L 1970 Tearoom trade. Aldine, Chicago

Hunt M 1974 Sexual behavior in the 1970s. Playboy Press, Chicago
Hunter R, MacAlpine I 1963 Three hundred years of psychiatry. Oxford University Press, London
Kenyon F E 1974 Female homosexuality — a review. In: Loraine J A (ed) Understanding homosexuality. MTP, Lancaster
Kinsey A C, Pomeroy W B, Martin C E 1948 Sexual behavior in the human male. Saunders, Philadelphia
Kinsey A C, Pomeroy W B, Martin C E, Gebhard P H 1953 Sexual behavior in the human female. Saunders, Philadelphia
Kirsch J, Rodman J 1977 The natural history of homosexuality. Yale Scientific Magazine 51 (3): 7–13
Klein F 1988 The need to view sexual orientation as a multivariable, dynamic process. In: McWhirter D, Reinisch J (eds) Homosexuality/heterosexuality; the Kinsey scale and current research. Second Kinsey symposium. Oxford University Press, New York (in press)
Levitt E E, Klassen A D 1974 Public attitudes towards homosexuality. Journal of Homosexuality 1: 29–43
MacDonald A P, Games R C 1974 Some characteristics of those who hold positive and negative attitudes towards homosexuals. Journal of Homosexuality 1: 9–27
McWhirter D P, Mattison A M 1984 The male couple. How relationships develop. Prentice-Hall, New Jersey
McWhirter D P, Reinisch J (eds) 1988 Homosexuality/heterosexuality; the Kinsey scale and current research. Second Kinsey Symposium. Oxford University Press, New York (in press)
Martin J L 1986 Psychological, social and serological correlates of sexual behavior change among gay men: a life stress and illness perspective. Paper at 11th Annual Conference, International Academy of Sex Research. Amsterdam, Netherlands
Masters W H, Johnson V E 1979 Homosexuality in perspective. Little, Brown, Boston
Millet K 1968 Sexual politics. Sphere, London
Money J, Ehrhardt A A 1972 Man and woman, boy and girl. Johns Hopkins University Press, Baltimore, pp 125–145
Nicholls M 1986 Sexual behavior of lesbians and its implications for female sexuality. Paper presented at 11th Annual Meeting of the International Academy of Sex Research. Amsterdam, Netherlands.
Pietropinto A, Simenauer J 1977 Beyond the male myth. A nationwide survey. Time Books, New York
Ramsay R W, Heringa P M, Boorsma I 1974 A case study: homosexuality in the Netherlands. In: Loraine J A (ed) Understanding homosexuality: its biological and psychological base. MTP, Lancaster
Rattray Taylor G 1954 Sex in history. Ballantine, New York
Riess B F Safer J, Yotive W 1974 Psychological test data on female homosexuality: a review of the literature. Journal of Homosexuality 1: 71–85
Robinson P 1976 The modernisation of sex. Harper & Row, New York, pp 42–119
Rosen I 1978 Sexual deviation (2nd edn). Oxford University Press, Oxford
Saghir M T, Robins E 1973 Male and female homosexuality: a comprehensive investigation. Williams & Wilkins, Baltimore
Schatzberg A F, Westfall M P, Blumetti A B, Birk L C 1975 Effeminacy I. A quantitative rating scale. Archives of Sexual Behavior 4: 31–42
Schofield M 1965 Sociological aspects of homosexuality. A comparative study of three types of homosexuals. Longman, London
Siegelman M 1972 Adjustment of male homosexuals and heterosexuals. Archives of Sexual Behavior 2: 9–25
Siegelman M 1974 Parental background of male homosexuals and heterosexuals. Archives of Sexual Behavior 3: 3–18
Siegelman M 1978 Psychological adjustment of homosexual and heterosexual men: a cross national replication. Archives of Sexual Behavior 7: 1–12
Siegelman M 1979 Adjustment of homosexual and heterosexual women: a cross-national replication. Archives of Sexual Behavior 8: 121–126
Stone L 1977 The family, sex and marriage in England 1500–1800. Weidenfeld & Nicholas, London

Tannahill R 1980 Sex in history. Hamish Hamilton, London

Tielman R A P, van Grieusven G J P 1986 The impact of AIDS on homosexual lifestyle. Paper at 11th Annual Conference, International Academy of Sex Research. Amsterdam, Netherlands.

Turner R K, Pielmaier R, James S, Orwin A 1974 Personality characteristics of male homosexuals referred for aversion therapy: a comparative study. British Journal of Psychiatry 125: 447–49

Van Wyk P H, Geist C S 1984 Psychosocial development of heterosexual, bisexual and homosexual behavior. Archives of Sexual Behavior 13: 505–544

Weinberg M S, Williams C J 1974 Male homosexuals: their problems and adaptation. Oxford University Press, New York

Westfall M P, Schatzberg A F, Blumetti A B, Birk C L 1975 Effeminacy II. Variation with social context. Archives of Sexual Behavior 4: 43–52

Williams C J, Weinberg M S 1971 Homosexuals and the military: a study of less than honorable discharge. Harper & Row, New York

Wilson E O 1978 On human nature. Harvard University Press, Cambridge, Massachusetts

Wolfenden J 1957 Report of the committee on homosexual offences and prostitution. Cmnd 247. HMSO, London

Zuger B 1978 Effeminate behavior present in boys from childhood: 10 additional years to follow up. Comprehensive Psychiatry 19: 363–369

7

Other sexual minorities

A tendency in much medical writing on sex is to regard particular forms of sexual behaviour as either normal or pathological. We have already emphasised how misled medical opinion has been by generalising from homosexuals who seek medical help. There are other individuals whose sexual behaviour is not regarded as normal but who usually do not seek medical help to cure their condition. Attitudes to sexual behaviour are sufficiently emotive that any behaviour which is not regarded as normal will tend to be seen as abnormal in a derogatory way. All these types of behaviour therefore share in common social stigma; they are regarded as deviant. We have discussed at some length the implications of this stigma for the homosexual. Let us now consider the concept of deviance in a more general sense.

THE CONCEPT OF SEXUAL DEVIANCE

Deviance is behaviour that contravenes the norms of society. These norms combine the institutionalised norms or laws and the internalised and shared norms or mores. Deviance is sometimes defined in terms of statistical abnormality or of psychopathology. The statistical criteria tell us nothing of the value of or the problems associated with a particular form of behaviour. The criteria used to define psychopathology may be no more than medical rationalisation of the social criteria, as we have seen in relation to homosexuality. The first sociological definition is however valid and important as it confronts us with the social stigma which plays such an important negative part in the lives of deviant individuals. Unfortunately, the term 'deviant' has grown to have pejorative connotations, so that when using it one may be accused of expressing a negative value about the particular behaviour or individual. This is unfortunate as the concept of deviance is essential to our proper understanding of the plight of these individuals in society. Perhaps an alternative term without this tendency to misinterpretation can be found; sexual stigma is one possibility, sexual minority behaviour is another.

Gagnon & Simon (1967) drew an important distinction between three types of sexual deviance. The first they called *normal deviance*; this encompasses behaviour such as masturbation, premarital intercourse, oral sex, which whilst frowned upon and even in some parts of the world still legally proscribed, are nevertheless carried out by large numbers of people. Maybe such behaviours are becoming progressively destigmatised* and in the past would have been regarded as more deviant. The other two types distinguish between behaviours which are associated with particular subcultures (such as the homosexual subcultures) called *subcultural deviance* and those which are not (such as exhibitionism or incest), called *individual deviance*. The existence of a subculture with which the deviant individual can identify may be crucial to his well-being and adaptation. It makes the difference between having a social group within which one feels normal and feeling at all times abnormal and stigmatised. Such subcultures are far from static, however, and are constantly evolving and changing, reflecting the social attitudes of their time. In the mid 19th century, homosexuals had little opportunity for finding a homosexual subculture; now there is an international network of such organisations. Not all homosexuals are prepared to identify with these groups and they may remain isolated, but the option is there. Other types of deviant sexuality have generated their own organisations or subcultures and are continuing to do so. There are now well established organisations of transvestites and transsexuals, and to a lesser extent of fetishists and sadomasochists.

An interesting example is paedophilia or sexual attraction to children. In the late 1970s, a group called the Paedophilia Information Exchange (PIE) was formed. But the prevailing social antagonism to paedophilia was such that any public meeting of this group generated considerable public hostility. Plummer (1979) likened this to the public reaction to homosexuality in the past, and it is conceivable that attitudes to this form of behaviour will become more tolerant, or at least less extreme as time goes on. O'Carroll (1980), a member of PIE, has made a serious but in my view unsuccessful attempt to defend the paedophiliac's sexual preference.

Gagnon & Simon (1967) call the individual type of deviance 'pathological'. It is clear, however, that social rather than medical criteria determine membership of this category and that these criteria are changing.

In this chapter we will consider four forms of sexual behaviour which come into the subcultural category: fetishism, sadomasochism, transvestism and transsexuality. Whilst the incidence of these behaviours is difficult or impossible to establish, they are not rare and medical help is not requested by most people involved in them. (The transsexual, as we shall see, does typically seek medical help but this is in order to normalise deviance rather than cure it.) It is nevertheless slightly arbitrary which behaviours we include in this chapter and which we leave to the clinical part

---

* A statement by Mrs Alison Adcock to the General Synod of the Church of England, 1979: 'A masturbator is more harmlessly and less anti-socially occupied than a smoker, a toper, or a compulsive consumer of confectionery.' Observer, 11 November 1979.

of the book. Rape, incest, paedophilia, exhibitionism, voyeurism and related behaviours will be dealt with in the chapter on sexual offences because they most commonly come to the professional's attention through the legal system.

We have considered homosexuality separately, not only because it is numerically of much greater significance but also because, alone amongst the deviant forms of sexuality, it basically involves a sexual relationship. Theoretically, therefore, homosexuality should allow incorporation of sexual responsiveness into loving dyadic relationships, no less than heterosexuality, and hence be no less capable of the sexual maturity alluded to in Chapter 3. As far as the forms of sexual activity discussed in this chapter are concerned, mature sexual relationships, if they are to be attained, will be in spite of these preferences which in their various ways are opposed to the stability and security of the sexual dyad. Understanding of these forms of sexual behaviour, however, is likely to increase our understanding of human sexuality in general and they are therefore of some theoretical importance.

FETISHISM

As described in Chapter 3, the sexual response system becomes conditioned to respond to various kinds of stimuli. These sexual signals usually serve to attract us to a suitable partner as well as to initiate sexual interaction. If we are successful in our sexual development, we are eventually able to sustain a relationship with a suitable partner in spite of the distractions of other sexual signals all around us.

Usually these sexual signals involve physical characteristics of the potential partner. Visual signals of this kind may be more important to the male than to the female. Males often show preference for particular parts of the female (or male) body, e.g. for breasts, buttocks or legs (for a review of this evidence see Bancroft 1978). To some extent preferences for the parts of the body may be culturally determined. In the west, the large breast, sexually fashionable during the war years, seems to have given way to more modest breast size as a cultural sex symbol. In China, until recently, the 'lotus' or bound foot had a special sexual appeal (Money 1977). When are such specific attributes to be regarded as fetishes?

The word 'fetish', which from its Portuguese origins implies an artistically created artefact, also conveys a special symbolism or magical meaning — the love token or erotic icon. But we should consider such detachable tokens of the loved one alongside the physical attributes or body parts already mentioned. The fetishistic quality is a graduated one. The concept becomes more relevant as the subject becomes more preoccupied with the signal itself and less concerned with the associated partner. The fetish becomes more problematic as it serves to weaken rather than strengthen the sexual bond with the sexual partner and, in its most extreme form, makes the sexual partner, as a person, completely redundant.

There are three principal categories of sexual signal or stimulus to consider:

1. a part of the body;
2. an inanimate extension of the body, e.g. article of clothing;
3. a source of specific tactile stimulation (e.g. the texture of a particular form of material).

Parts of the body or partialism

This category overlaps most obviously with the normal, but interest in specific body parts may override any interest in the rest of the person or the body as a whole. Von Kraft-Ebbing (1965) gives a rich account of fetishes in the 19th century and there are some interesting differences with modern fetishism which presumably stem from changing attitudes to sexuality. He described hand fetishes as common at that time. He relates this to a preoccupation with masturbation and a transfer from one's own masturbating hand to that of a girl. The infrequency of hand fetishism nowadays (this author has never seen a case) and possibly the greater frequency of predilection for more intimate parts of body, e.g. top of a woman's thigh or buttocks, may reflect a very different degree of public body exposure in recent times compared with the late 19th century. Some fetishes have a bizarre quality. Sexual attraction to lame women or female amputees featured in Von Kraft-Ebbing's account and is still seen nowadays (Marks et al 1970).

Inanimate extensions of the body

Articles of clothing, boots and shoes are perhaps the commonest type of fetish. The use of women's clothes as fetishes overlaps with transvestism and will be considered further below.

Specific textures

One of the most common fetishes at the present time is rubber, particularly clothing made out of rubber. Other materials are leather and shiny black plastic. In Von Kraft-Ebbing's time, furs, velvets and silks were the popular textures.

Chalkley & Powell (1983) found 48 cases of fetishism referred to the Maudsley Hospital over a 20-year period (0.8% of all referrals). Only one was female (a lesbian with a fetish for breasts). Of the men, 15% showed partialism (mainly for legs). The remainder involved articles of clothing: 15% footwear, 23% rubber items. Seventeen men had one fetish, nine had two and the remaining 22 had three or more (to a maximum of nine different fetishes). In all, 25% of this group stole their fetish articles.

Gosselin & Wilson (1980) reported on 87 members of the Mackintosh Society for rubber fetishists and 38 members of the Atomage correspondence club for leatherites. They also contacted 133 members of a sadomasochistic club and 285 members of the Beaumont society for transvestites and transsexuals. Using the Eysenck personality questionnaire they found all four groups tended towards introversion and neuroticism, though none of the four had mean scores within the clinical range. Their social backgrounds were fairly unremarkable and they came from a normal socioeconomic cross-section.

There is general agreement that fetishism is rare in women (Kinsey et al 1953). Apart from the case cited above, Stoller (1982) describes three cases of fetishistic transvestism in women.

THE DETERMINANTS OF FETISHISM

It is widely believed that fetishism results from the specific conditioning of sexual response to particular stimuli. In the male, the capacity for classical conditioning of erections to unusual stimuli has been demonstrated experimentally (Rachman & Hodgson 1968; Bancroft 1974) and it may be that erection is a peculiarly conditionable response. This may depend in part on the obviousness of penile erection so that cognitive processes may mediate in linking a sexual response to specific stimuli (e.g. 'that object produced an erection, it must have sexual significance'). The absence of any equivalent obvious genital response in the female may account for the lack of such fetishistic learning. A simple conditioning model is not sufficient, however. Other factors must operate to maintain the response. It has been suggested that, as with other sexual preferences, masturbation and orgasm in response to the fetish object will serve to reinforce and maintain the association (McGuire et al 1965). But it remains a puzzle to the learning theorist why some stimuli become discriminately reinforced, whilst in other cases there is a generalisation of learning which allows sexual preferences to evolve and to mature with experience. This is a question of fundamental importance. Is it reflecting some peculiarity of learning or does it indicate problems when trying to incorporate sexual responses into dyadic relationships, resulting in greater isolation of the individual's sexuality? It is also far from clear why certain stimuli are more likely to be conditioned than others. It may be that learning at an early age, before any mature concept of sexuality has developed, permits more bizarre associations to develop, but it is nevertheless tempting to assume that the fetish object has some significance beyond that of a randomly conditioned stimulus.

The psychoanalytic theorists have no doubt on that matter. The fetish object represents to them a penis, a protection against castration or a denial of the penisless state of the woman (Freud 1927). Greenacre (1979), a current psychoanalytic authority, considers that fetishism is invariably associated with a very severe castration complex.

The majority of fetishes can be understood as an extension of the loved one which perhaps acquires special importance if there are other factors or causes of anxiety blocking the development of a more appropriate sexual relationship. In some instances, fetishes are exceedingly bizarre and cannot be understood as extensions of the body and are more likely to be associated with some neurological abnormality such as temporal lobe epilepsy. In such cases, the stimulus can be seen as more random, the abnormality being in the disturbance of learning.

Gosselin & Wilson (1980) in their study of 'rubberites' found that the interest in rubber originated between the ages of 4 and 10. From the ages of their subjects they concluded that many of them would have developed this interest around the early stages of the Second World War. They therefore speculated that such anxiety-provoking circumstances, combined with an often absent father and overprotective mother plus a lot of rubber articles in use at that time, provided the ingredients for this particular fetish to flourish.

Further consideration will be given to the origins of fetish objects in the section on transvestism. Whilst we must remain uncertain of their origins, the various factors influencing the development of sexual preferences discussed in Chapter 3 are likely to be relevant in these cases also.

SADOMASOCHISM

The sexual response to the infliction of pain, psychological humiliation or ritualised dominance or submission is the basis of sadomasochism. The sadist plays the active (i.e. inflictor) role in order to be sexually stimulated; the masochist, the passive role (i.e. the inflicted). The submission is commonly manifested through various forms of bondage, which involves being tied up or constrained so that you are at the mercy of your assailant, and unable to protect yourself. The terms 'sadism' and 'masochism' tend to be used very loosely to cover any situation where an individual seems to gain some reward from hurting or dominating another person or being hurt or dominated. We are concerned here with such behaviour in which the rewards are clearly sexual and for which the terms 'sadism' and 'masochism' were originally coined by Von Kraft-Ebbing.

Whereas fetishism is a more or less exclusively male concern, the sex difference with sadomasochism is not so clearcut. Fantasies of being raped or being forced into sexual activity are used by many women during masturbation or intercourse (Wilson 1978). The use of mild bondage or flagellation as a form of sexual game may not be uncommon in either sex (Comfort 1972). But the more serious use of sadomasochistic sexual activity appears to be less common amongst women (Spengler 1977). This perhaps reflects the difference between fantasy and reality. Whereas rape may have an exciting quality in fantasy, it is not likely to be enjoyed in reality; similarly with the infliction of pain. The reality of such an experience may be unacceptable, not just because of the pain, but because of the negative effects such interaction has on the sexual relationship.

Moderate pain inflicted as an expression of high arousal is perhaps more acceptable. The commonest form of this is the love bite. This phenomenon is widespread amongst mammals. Kinsey et al (1953) found that 55% of women and 50% of men interviewed had responded erotically to such bites during love-making. By contrast, only 12% of women and 22% of men had responded erotically to sadomasochistic stories. Sexual assaults, in which the infliction of pain or suffering is carried out for sexual purposes, seem to be rare although sadomasochistic fantasies are not uncommon amongst rapists or those convicted of sexual assault (Gebhard et al 1965) and in some cases the sadistic fantasies become acted out to the point where a sadistic assault or murder occurs. (MacCulloch et al 1983). We will consider this aspect further in the chapter on sexual offences.

Once again, we have very little evidence of the extent of more ritualised sadomasochistic practices. One study has been reported by Spengler (1977). He sent questionnaires in response to contact advertisements used by sadomasochists seeking partners and also distributed them to members of sadomasochistic clubs. He stressed the difficulty in making such contacts and the apparent high need to maintain secrecy. His response rate was low — 28%. He expressed the view that, apart from the prostitutes who provided a special service for sadomasochists, women were more or less absent from this sadomasochistic world. As we shall see below, Breslow et al (1985) reached a different conclusion.

The relative paucity of women creates an obvious difference between the sadomasochistic worlds of homosexuals and heterosexuals. Homosexual sadomasochists have each other as partners and are much more likely to be associated with other sadomasochists in clubs or to attend sadomasochistic parties. The heterosexual sadomasochist relies to a greater extent on prostitutes. He may still associate with other sadomasochists, however. Contact by correspondence or reading sadomasochistic magazines is common and a number of Spengler's heterosexual respondents had male friends who shared their sadomasochistic interest. The heterosexual sadomasochistic subculture is therefore a mutual support group; for the homosexual, on the other hand, it is also a source of sadomasochistic partners.

The respondents to Spengler's questionnaire were relatively affluent, and all over 20 years of age; 30% were exclusively heterosexual, 38% exclusively homosexual. They showed a high divorce rate and those who were married indicated the unacceptibility of their sadomasochistic practices to their wives.

The frequency of sadomasochistic activity was relatively low (median five occasions per year), with the homosexuals having more opportunities. The majority were prepared to take either the active or passive role, enabling them to adapt to various partners (this tendency is also shown in sado-masochistic fantasies; Wilson 1978). The majority were not exclusively sadomasochistic and only 15% required sadomasochistic stimulation before they could experience orgasm. Exclusive sadomasochistic interest was more likely in those with masochistic preferences. The commonest practices were flagellation, with whip or cane, and bondage. The additional use of fetish objects (leather clothes and boots) was also common.

The reported age at which sadomasochistic interest was acknowledged varied considerably; in 17% it was 13 years or younger but in 43% it was after the age of 20. A total of 90% of this group had never sought medical help and the large majority were quite happy with their sadomasochistic tendencies, particularly if they had established contact with a sadomasochistic subculture.

Breslow et al (1985) persuaded two sadomasochistic magazines to include a questionnaire for their readers. They received 182 replies, of which 72% were male and 28% female. Of the women, 12 of the 52 were prostitutes. This implies a larger population of female non-prostitute sadomasochistics than has previously been acknowledged. A comparison of the two sexes revealed that men recognised their interest at an earlier age than women, who tended to be introduced to sadomasochism by a sexual partner. This sample reported a greater frequency of sadomasochistic activity than was reported by Spengler's group, and the women had been about twice as active as the men with more partners in the preceding year, perhaps reflecting the greater demand for female partners. The two sexes did not differ in their preferences for dominance or submission, and showed equal interest in rubber and leather regalia (a possible challenge to the assumption of the absence of female fetishism). The women did show a greater preference for bondage.

THE DETERMINANTS OF SADOMASOCHISM

The relationship between aggression and sexual behaviour is complex but in general they interfere with one another. Most animals need to curb their aggression to allow sexual behaviour to occur satisfactorily (Hinde 1974). The destructive effect that anger and resentment have on human sexual relationships will be discussed in Chapter 8. The role of aggression in sexual assaults is discussed in Chapter 3. Sexually receptive and submissive responses are often used by primates to appease aggression from another animal (although the animal seeking to appease can be either male or female, sexual submission is only likely to succeed when the aggressor is male). A psychoanalytic view which is reminiscent of this biological tendency has been put forward by Glasser (1979). He sees aggression as basically destructive; by sexualising the aggression and turning it into sadism, destruction is avoided — the object of the aggression is maintained as a source of pleasure rather than destroyed. This is an intriguing if not entirely convincing idea. Whilst the masochist on this basis may feel relief at finding an escape from destruction, it is not clear why for him the experience should be sexually exciting.

Closely related to aggression is dominance and this has more direct relevance to sadomasochism. A fundamental and intriguing question is whether male dominance is biologically necessary or even desirable for satisfactory sexual interaction other than in the form of the posture adopted during coitus. What is beyond dispute is that in most cultures sexual dominance is seen to be one hallmark of masculinity, part of the sex role stereotype; similarly, female submission or at least passivity is seen as a feminine characteristic. Not only does sexual dominance carry weight as a gender characteristic, it also provides one of a variety of ways for one human being to dominate another. When women are seen as the 'property' of men, then sexual domination by the man is one way of asserting dominance over his female partner. An extension of this process is political rape, e.g. of white women by militant and angry black men in a white-dominated racist society. The rape that follows conquest during war time suggests that the sense of power and dominance that victory brings enhances or triggers the male's sexual response, so that rape becomes another expression of the dominance with its own physiological rewards (Brownmiller 1975; see Chapter 12 for fuller discussion).

The role of dominance in sadomasochism, however, is complicated by the ease with which it can be replaced by submission. The sadist who is unable to dominate may be quite prepared to submit as a masochist. This is more difficult to understand unless we see that the sexualisation has divorced the behaviour from dominance in its more general sense. In other words, dominance and submission in highly ritualised forms become types of sexual stimuli. If that is so, then it is perhaps a further example of the peculiar conditionability of sexual responses which allows them to develop, over a time, an existence of their own. The search for dominance may nevertheless have involved the individual in a specific learning process in the first place.

But what of the initial search for submission? For the female, this would again conform to the sex role stereotype; but why submission for the male? Of potential importance is the abrogation of responsibility. The passive participant, particularly if coerced into participation by physical force or authority, cannot be held responsible for that participation. If sex is associated with guilt, this may be a powerful method of permitting sexual response. This could well account for the sexually arousing effects of fantasies of sexual dominance in the adolescent girl. It may account for some such responses in males also. A corollary of this is that punishment given at the time of the crime in some way condones the crime, hence the reinforcement of a sexual response during the receipt of corporal punishment.

But there is still need for a further ingredient; the sexual effects of painful stimuli. The very common occurrence of painful stimuli in the form of love bites reminds us that they are at least compatible with sexual response. The effect of sexual arousal is to increase the threshold for painful stimuli. That being so, the non-specifically arousing effect of the injury may contribute to the state of sexual arousal.

These attempts at explaining the origins of sadomasochism have been highly speculative. Nevertheless, the need for dominance, the psychological significance of passivity, the sexualisation of anger and the arousing effects of pain in certain situations may interact and through the peculiarly conditionable nature of our sexual responses provide the ingredients for that ritualised form of sexual stimulation we call sadomasochism.

THE POLYMORPHOUS PERVERSE

Although the various kinds of sexual preference discussed in this chapter are scattered fairly widely through the population, they have a striking tendency to occur together. The existence of one of these minority preferences (with the exception of homosexuality) greatly increases the likelihood of one or more of the others. Gosselin & Wilson (1980) in their survey of fetishists, sadomasochists and transvestites, found it was common for fetishism to coexist with either of the other two patterns. Interest in bondage is apparently common amongst transvestites (Buhrich & Beaumont 1981), though Croughan et al (1981) found that sadomasochistic tendencies were unusual in their group of transvestites. Occasionally there is a startling variety of unusual sexual preferences affecting the same individual — who is sometimes known as 'polymorphous perverse'.

The frequency of these associations is of theoretical importance. It suggests that the conditions necessary for the development of one type of preference may facilitate the development of others. This potential may stem from some characteristic of the individual's nervous system, which underlies sexual learning, e.g. the capacity for conditioning sexual responses to a variety of stimuli. Alternatively, it may reflect difficulties in the interpersonal domain, which make it difficult for the individual to incorporate his sexuality into a dyadic relationship. Lacking the framework for sexual expression that such a relationship normally provides, other varieties of sexual expression are given free rein.

We should keep an open mind on this issue, but careful study of these associations may prove to be an important source of understanding of these otherwise curious forms of human sexual expression.

TRANSVESTISM AND TRANSSEXUALISM

Dressing up in clothes of the opposite sex or 'cross-dressing' has a fascination for most of us. It occurs in most societies and throughout history. It has been institutionalised in various ways, but especially as a form of entertainment. Although in recent times cross-dressing in the theatre has been mainly used for comic effect, burlesque and pantomime, it has had more serious use in the past, and like the mask, can create intriguing illusion. Cross-dressing is widespread outside the theatre and is the common theme in various aspects of sexual behaviour which we need to consider. The sexual significance of cross-dressing is complex, as we shall see, but it is appropriately regarded as a sexual minority behaviour and organisations of cross-dressers are now to be found in many countries. In the UK, the Beaumont Society is such a group, providing opportunities for its members to cross-dress in company as well as providing support and counsel.

We have very little understanding of the origins or determinants of this behaviour. As with homosexuality and some other aspects of human sexuality, our confusion has been increased by the need of most workers to find a common cause or to evolve a simple diagnostic typology in the medical manner. Throughout this book we return to this problem and the need to understand human sexual behaviour as a consequence of dynamic processes in our individual developments.

To introduce some attempt at order, four typical but contrasting examples of cross-dressing individuals will be described. Each example emphasises a particular aspect of the phenomenon.

1. *The fetishistic transvestite*. This is a man (probably never a woman) who wears female clothes as fetish objects. The clothes are sexually arousing and usually wearing them leads to masturbation. Cross-dressing in this case is a sexual act.
2. *The transsexual*. This is a man (or woman) who believes himself (or herself) to be a woman (or man), or has a strong desire to be accepted as such in spite of his or her anatomy. In this case, cross-dressing is part of the process of expressing one's preferred gender. There is no more sexual significance to the cross-dressing in this case than there is when a woman wears normal women's clothes. Both the male and the female transsexual are likely to seek medical help to alter their bodies to be consistent with their psychological gender.
3. *The double-role transvestite*. This is usually a man who spends part of his life as a normal heterosexual male and part dressing and passing as a woman. Cross-dressing is usually similar to that of the transsexual but there is no desire to change sex permanently. This person wants to maintain both options.
4. *The homosexual transvestite*. This is a man or woman who is sexually attracted to members of the same sex and who cross-dresses but with less intention of being considered of the opposite sex. This cross-dressing is not necessarily fetishistic and is often in the form of caricature rather than serious impersonation.

These four examples demonstrate the three principal dimensions of the cross-dressing experience: the fetish component; the cross-gender identity and role and sexual orientation or preference. Most of the variety of cross-dressing behaviour can be accounted for by interaction of these three dimensions. We will consider them more closely as we discuss the various aetiological or developmental theories.

INCIDENCE

It is impossible to assess the incidence of cross-dressing behaviour. There is good reason to believe that it is far from rare. The Beaumont Society in the UK has approximately 500 members and advises about as many transvestite enquirers each year (Brierley 1979). In the USA, Prince & Bentler (1972) sent postal questionnaires to the 1300 subscribers of a magazine called Transvestia. They were presumed to be transvestites. Some 540 (approximately 40%) returned the questionnaires. There are probably a much larger number of individuals who cross-dress secretly.

The person who is most likely to contact the medical profession is the transsexual who seeks anatomical change in the form of hormone effects or surgery. After the case of Christine Jorgensen was publicised in the early 1950s, revealing that as far as outward appearances are concerned surgical re-assignment can be surprisingly effective, Hamburger (1953) received more than 400 letters from individuals in various parts of the world wanting a sex change. In Baltimore during the first 3 years of the gender identity clinic, more than 1000 letters were received and many more telephone enquiries (Meyer et al 1971).

Estimates of the incidence of people seeking sex re-assignment have ranged from 1 in 100 000 (for males) to 1 in 400 000 (for females; Pauly 1974). Hoenig & Kenna (1974) estimated a prevalence in the UK of male-to-female transsexuals as 1 in 33 000, and female-to-males as 1 in 108 000. More recently, Ross et al (1981) estimated a prevalence of 1 in 37 000 in Sweden and 1 in 24 000 in Australia for biological males, and 1 in 103 000 and 1 in 150 000 for these two countries for biological females. By contrast, Bullough (1975) found that in the popular literature over the past 200 years reports of women passing as men are much more common than the other way round. He attributes this to the assumed inferiority of women and hence the greater significance of successful male impersonation. The greater scope for surgical re-assignment for the male-to-female (see Chapter 10) and the greater stability of female-to-male transsexuals (see below) may also contribute to the discrepancy in those seeking surgery. We should keep an open mind about the sex ratio; there may be important differences in the determinants of male and female transsexualism.

Attempts to assess the personality of cross-dressers demonstrate the same problems found in the studies of homosexuality. Those contacted through clinics showed more personality disturbance than those contacted through transvestite organisations (see Brierley (1979) for a review). Members of these organisations show a median age in the 30s (32% of the Beaumont Society membership is over 40).

Several writers have commented on the difficulty in assessing retrospective histories of transvestites, particularly those with transsexual tendencies who may have an understandable need to distort their past life to make it more consistent with their present gender identity. An example of an account of early childhood changing as the individual becomes more transsexual has been given elsewhere (Bancroft 1972). Findings from questionnaire studies should therefore be interpreted with caution.

Prince & Bentler (1972) found that 14% of their Transvestia readers started cross-dressing before the age of 5, 40% between the ages of 5 and 10, 37% between 10 and 18, and 8% after 18 years (similar findings were reported by Buhrich & McConaghy 1977). What we do not know is the incidence of cross-dressing in children who do not become established cross-dressers later in life. Half of these questionnaire respondents had always kept their cross-dressing a secret, whereas about one-third had cross-dressed in public. Three-quarters of this group described feeling a different person when cross-dressed; 14% were considering sex re-assignment surgery and 5% were taking hormones. Buhrich & McConaghy (1977) studied members of an Australian transvestite club and compared them with patients attending their transsexual clinic. Although, as one would expect, the clinical population showed more features of transsexualism, there was a considerable overlap, with approximately one-fifth of the club members wanting sex re-assignment surgery and a similar proportion of the clinic attenders experiencing fetishistic arousal to cross-dressing. Although these workers used these findings to claim that transvestism and transsexualism were distinct clinical entities, their results and those of other workers indicate that cross-dressing behaviour occurs on a continuum, with at one end the clearly defined fetishistic transvestite, on the other the committed full-time transsexual. Factors which may influence an individual's position on this continuum will become clearer when we consider the possible determinants of these behaviours.

THE PERSONALITIES OF CROSS-DRESSERS

Brierley (1979) has reviewed various studies of personality in transvestites. The usual conclusion is that in general they do not differ in any characteristic way from 'normals'. There was some evidence of rigidity. Randell (1959) regards transvestism as a form of obsessional compulsion. There are crucial differences between this form of behaviour and compulsive behaviour in its usual psychiatric sense, but it may be that there is an increased incidence of obsessional personality traits in these individuals.

In most of the studies reviewed by Brierley, the number of transvestites with transsexual tendencies is not stated but is probably low. In other studies of clinic populations of transsexuals (i.e. those seeking sex re-assignment), there is more evidence of personality disturbance (Hoenig et al 1970; Langevin et al 1977). Walinder (1967) found such disturbance to be more marked in male than in female transsexuals and other authorities have reached similar conclusions (Dixen et al 1984). According to Pauly (1974) the cross-gender role behaviour of male transsexuals is more exaggerated than it is with female transsexuals.

The impression from the available evidence is that transvestites without transsexual tendencies show a level of intelligence and career achievement which is often above average, whereas transsexuals, perhaps because of the many practical difficulties associated with their chosen role, are of lower socioeconomic status than average (Hoenig et al 1970).

THE SEXUAL RELATIONSHIPS OF CROSS-DRESSERS

In Prince & Bentler's (1972) series of transvestites, more than three-quarters had been married and about two-thirds were still married at the time of the study. Three-quarters were parents. A comparable proportion was reported from members of the Beaumont Society and Brierley (1979) has concluded that transvestites do not differ from the general population in these respects. A fair proportion have problems in their marriage, not infrequently as a consequence of their cross-dressing. What is perhaps more surprising is that a sizeable proportion maintain reasonably stable marriages in spite of this behaviour.

It may be that if the cross-dressing is limited, confined to private places and does not involve more obvious transsexual tendencies, a marriage might adapt to it. There seems little doubt, however, that once the transsexual urge takes over, the marriage is put under considerable strain. Those whose transsexual tendencies declare themselves at a relatively early stage are less likely to get married and in those who do marital breakdown is common, particularly with female transsexuals (Hoenig et al 1970).

It is the author's clinical impression that transvestite behaviour, having become established typically during adolescence, often largely disappears during the early stages of a heterosexual relationship. When problems arise in the relationship or marriage, particularly sexual difficulties, the urge to cross-dress returns and over a number of years may fluctuate as the success of the marital relationship varies. This would support the idea that the fetishistic type of cross-dressing in particular is an alternative form of heterosexual behaviour which becomes redundant if normal heterosexuality is working well. We should therefore be cautious in assuming that marital breakdown with transvestites is primarily a consequence of cross-dressing. It is interesting to speculate how many more men might indulge in cross-dressing if they failed in normal heterosexual relationships.

In the case of the transsexual we have two kinds of relationship to consider. First, as above, the relationships formed whilst living in their original gender role (these may be either hetero- or homosexual) and secondly those established in the transsexual role. This latter kind is of special interest as it confronts us with the particular needs of the partner.

Green (1974) provides vivid descriptions of some of these girl- and boyfriends. Once again, it seems as if the relationships of the female-to-male transsexuals are more stable, though their girlfriends have usually experienced some difficulty with normal heterosexual relationships and often are seen to be looking for a 'man without a penis'. Their sexual activity is usually characterised by the transsexual taking an active role and the girlfriend avoiding direct stimulation of the male's breasts or genitalia as if to avoid this incongruent anatomical evidence (Pauly 1974). In spite of such limitations, these relationships can be surprisingly satisfactory and stable (Fleming et al 1985).

The male-to-female transsexual is less likely to find a stable partner but it does happen and it can be surprisingly effective when relatively normal sexual intercourse is made possible by the surgical creation of a vagina. The male transsexual after penectomy can often continue to experience orgasm (Bentler 1976). We will consider below the role that these partners might play in influencing the transsexual to seek re-assignment.

POSSIBLE DETERMINANTS OF TRANSVESTISM AND TRANSSEXUALISM

A variety of theoretical explanations for this behaviour have been put forward and each will be considered in more detail. In the process, the very heterogeneous nature of this form of behaviour will become clear.

Biological factors

There is as yet no evidence of a genetic mechanism underlying transvestism or transsexualism. Although occasional transsexuals may be found to have abnormal sex chromosomes (e.g. XXY karyotype), this is the exception and simply reminds us that individuals with such sex chromosome anomalies are somewhat prone to abnormal sexual development of various kinds (see Chapter 3).

Claims were recently made that transsexualism is an abnormal Hy-antigen phenotype (Eicher et al 1979; see p. 153). This improbable suggestion has been laid to rest by Wachtel et al (1986) and probably resulted from faulty methodology.

In view of the importance of prenatal androgens to gender identity development, as shown in individuals with adrenogenital syndrome or androgen-insensitivity syndrome (see Chapter 3), there has been an understandable search for endocrine abnormalities in transvestites and transsexuals. So far, for male-to-female transsexuals, no such mechanisms have been clearly identified, though there have been some suggestive findings (e.g. Boyar & Aiman 1982). In Chapter 3 we considered Dorner's claims that male homosexuals have abnormal positive feedback responses of the hypothalamic pituitary system, which are more suggestive of the female brain. He has made similar claims for male-to-female transsexuals (Dorner 1979). However, his findings in transsexuals were not replicated by either Goodman et al (1985) or Gooren (1986).

With female transsexuals, the story is somewhat different. Although the majority show no evidence of physical or endocrine abnormalities, a number of studies have now reported raised testosterone levels (Sipova & Starka 1977), menstrual irregularities or evidence of polycystic ovarian disease (Futterweit et al 1986). Seyler et al (1978) reported some evidence of impaired positive feedback in female-to-male transsexuals, but this was not found by Gooren (1986). More research on the relevance of endocrine abnormalities in female-to-male transsexuals is needed, though it is clear that such abnormalities are not *necessary* for transsexual development. A particular caution is required in investigating such cases to ensure that any endocrine abnormalities are not due to the surreptitious use of exogenous hormones.

Several studies have reported a high incidence of epilepsy or abnormal electroencephalograms (EEGs) in transsexuals (Hoenig & Kenna 1979). The possible relevance of this remains obscure as the majority of transsexuals show no such abnormalities. It is possible, however, that some consti-tutional neurological abnormality may predispose the individual to abnormal sexual or gender learning. Hoenig & Kenna also question whether the link may be through hyposexuality (i.e. low sex drive). There is an increased incidence of hyposexuality in temporal lobe epileptics (see Chapter 11) and this could predispose to abnormal sexual learning. Many male-to-female transsexuals have a low sex drive though this is often a consequence of exogenous oestrogens. EEG abnormalities were more common in the female transsexuals, however (Hoenig & Kenna 1979), and they are not particularly prone to low sex drive.

At the present time, biological mechanisms sufficient to account for either transvestism or transsexualism are yet to be found, though there may be some instances, particularly of female transsexuals, where some predis-posing mechanism is involved.

Social and cultural factors

In Chapter 6 we considered the universal occurrence of cross-gender behav-iour in human societies and how cultures differed in the way they reacted to this behaviour (Carrier 1980). There is evidence that such cultural factors influence the prevalence of such behaviour. Goldman & Goldman (1982), in their cross-cultural study of the sexual thoughts of children, found that 5% of boys and 9.5% of girls expressed aversion to their biological sex. This reaction peaked in adolescence with 30% of 13-year-old boys in Australia and 20% in the USA expressing such feelings, which by contrast were virtually absent in Sweden. The implication is that the more rigid the sex role stereotypes in a society the greater the likelihood of this gender discomfort. Whilst at first sight this may seem paradoxical, it is not difficult to see how such rigid expectations could generate anxiety and insecurity about gender identity, for which transsexual ideas would offer one method of coping. Ross et al (1981) have suggested that this cultural factor leads to greater numbers of transsexuals seeking help in Australia than Sweden. And Ross (1983) reported that gay men in Australia identified themselves more strongly as feminine than their counterparts in Sweden.

Thus, though the universal occurrence of cross-gender behaviour across a wide variety of cultures points to some early or even biological influence, these apparent cultural contrasts in prevalence emphasise the role social factors may play in the later development and expression of such behaviour.

Early childhood influences

The importance of social learning in gender identity development was discussed in Chapter 3. In seeking an explanation for abnormal gender identity development amongst transvestites and transsexuals, we have two principal sources of evidence: the study of children with disturbed gender identities and the retrospective accounts of childhood from adult transvestites and transsexuals (or their parents). As yet these two sources of evidence must be regarded separately. But as time goes on, there will be an increasing number of children with disturbed gender identity who are followed through into adulthood and in whom the importance of these childhood experiences will become more obvious.

Feminine boys

Richard Green (1976) has made a special study of these children, comparing them with normal children. Typically they show a marked interest in cross-dressing (three-quarters of them starting before their fourth birthday, all by their sixth), choose female roles in make-believe games, prefer playing with girls' toys, especially dolls, avoid rough and tumble sports and tend to be loners, relating better to girls than to other boys. They are often particularly adept at play-acting. Green gives a list of factors which are sometimes found in the upbringing of these boys and which may have some aetiological significance. As yet, it is not possible to say whether any of these factors are necessary or sufficient or even causative and they occur with considerable variability. His list is as follows:

1. Parental indifference to feminine behaviour in a boy during his first year. In about 50% of Green's cases, help was sought by parents because of pressure from outside the family (e.g. school). Paradoxically when parents are concerned about the behaviour, the mother is likely to show more concern than the father.
2. Parental encouragement of feminine behaviour during the first years. In

about 10% of cases, the mother wanted a daughter so badly she tended to see her baby son as a girl.

3. Repeated cross-dressing of a young boy by a female. About 15% of these mothers cross-dressed their sons; less frequently sisters or grandmothers were responsible.

4. Maternal over-protection of a son and inhibition of boyish or rough and tumble play. Bieber et al (1962), in their psychoanalytic study of homosexuality, identified maternal over-protectiveness as a characteristic of their 'close binding–intimate' mothers (see p. 181). Presumably this parental attitude is likely to operate by undermining masculine identity.

5. Excessive maternal attention and physical contact, resulting in lack of separation and 'individuation' of boy from his mother. This is the mechanism regarded by Stoller (1979) as of fundamental importance in childhood transsexualism, though Green could only find evidence of it in about 20% of cases.

6. Absence of or rejection by father. A third of the feminine boys were separated from their father before the age of 4. In general when fathers were present, the boys were more likely to be closer to their mothers than were the control boys. Rekers et al (1983) studied 46 boys attending a child gender clinic and found that for 67% the biological father was absent, and when a father or father substitute was in the home 60% of these were 'psychologically absent'. These workers have laid much greater emphasis on the lack of father. As Green points out, it is difficult to interpret this relationship. A boy may feel rejected when his father finds it easier to relate to an older brother with more developed masculine aptitudes. Conversely the father may feel rejected by a son when he is disinterested in masculine things. Detachment of the father could be secondary to the gender identity problem. There is also some evidence from the retrospective accounts of adult transvestites that their fathers were more dependent, affiliative and less aggressive or dominant in relation to the mothers than in heterosexual control families (Newcomb 1985), whilst male transsexuals remember their fathers as 'deficient in caring and more over-protective, as though discouraging their sons' independence and autonomy' (Parker & Barr 1982).

7. Physical beauty of a boy, influencing adults to treat him in a feminine manner. About a third of the feminine boys were pretty children.

8. Lack of male playmates during early years of socialisation. About one-third of boys were deprived of the opportunity for contact with male peers. In other cases, avoidance of male peers reflected existing gender identity problems.

Green failed to find any difference in the pattern of parental role division (e.g. who was dominant, and in which sphere) between the families of his feminine and his normal boys. This is not surprising as in many cases the feminine boys have normally masculine brothers. The one factor which

Green regarded as close to a necessary variable the lack of discourage-ment of the feminine behaviour for an appreciable period of time and presumably during crucial periods of gender identity development. This has been true in nearly every family he has studied. Green is continuing to follow these boys into adulthood (Green 1979, 1985). The gender identity disturbance may persist and so far it appears that the most likely outcome is the development of homosexual preferences (about 40% at preliminary follow-up). Adult transsexualism has occurred infrequently in the studies of Zuger (1978) and Lebovitz (1972). As yet, most of the boys in Green's study are still relatively young and it may be that as they get older the trans-sexual role will become more likely if those who appear now as homosexual are unable to make a satisfactory homosexual adaptation (see below).

The retrospective accounts of adult males

In Prince & Bentler's (1972) group of Transvestia readers (an unknown proportion of whom had transsexual wishes) more than 80% reported being brought up normally as a boy. Benjamin (1966) stated that in 56% of his 122 cases of adult male transsexualism, there was no evidence of condi-tioning (i.e. parental encouragement of feminine behaviour) during child-hood. The majority of transsexuals (i.e. those seeking sex re-assignment) report preferences for female company and interests during childhood (Green 1974), though by no means all do. Nearly a half of Green's group of 30 adult male transsexuals reported a normal male self-concept during childhood.

Tomboy girls

Young girls with typically boyish interests are considerably more common than their male counterparts. Such behaviour is also regarded as more acceptable and hence parents seldom seek help for this problem. Paradox-ically we therefore have less systematic information about tomboys than we have about the much less common 'cissy'. Green has started a prospective study of tomboys and a comparison group of non-tomboys (Green et al 1982). So far, whilst the two groups of girls differed considerably in behav-iour such as sex-typed preferred toys, gender of peer group, participation in sports, roles taken in playing house and the stated wish to be a boy, there were few discernible differences in their families.

In contrast to the effeminate boy who usually carries into adulthood considerable problems relating to his gender identity, the tomboyish girl seldom has any difficulty in adapting to an adult female role. This also usually applies to those girls who are masculinised due to endocrine abnor-malities (see Chapter 3) although they may continue to show some typically male characteristics, putting careers before marriage or preferring male-type clothes.

A substantial majority of adult female transsexuals report a marked degree of tomboyism during childhood (Green 1974; Pauly 1974). A disturbed parental relationship is also commonly reported, the majority with a weak or depressive mother or an aggressive, excessively masculine and often alcoholic father. Encouragement by both parents of masculinity in the daughter appears to be common (Pauly 1974). It may be that the family constellations typically found in these cases serve to reinforce masculine traits which are in any case common amongst girls, but in these particular cases this may lead to more marked gender identity disturbance. Such family influences are not always found however and should not be considered necessary for transsexual development.

Sexual learning

The role of learning and conditioning in the development of fetishes has already been discussed. The fetish component of male cross-dressing is common, particularly during adolescence when the pattern of erotic responsiveness is being established. Typically the pubertal boy discovers that women's clothes have an erotic effect. They are an obvious extension of a woman's body and in the case of underclothes have been in contact with her genitalia. Frequently the clothes used belong to the boy's mother or sister and may reflect guilt-ridden, incestuous feelings. The fetish effect of the clothing may be enhanced by the texture of the material, particularly when worn next to the boy's own body. Starting off as an erotic aid to masturbation, the simple fetish object, by being worn, initiates the process of female role identification. Though this is difficult to understand, it may be that given certain types of imagination, one's own body can be used to create 'another person' with more effect than by using fantasy alone. Certainly the descriptions of fetishistic cross-dressers suggest the 'creation of a woman' and it is unusual for them to imagine involvement of that woman with another man. This emphasises the heterosexual orientation of the majority of fetishistic cross-dressers, but also increases the likelihood that the sexually arousing effect is dependent on producing this doppelgänger sexual partner (Bancroft 1972).

It may also be that such a boy is already sensitised to female identification. The fetish object is chosen not only because of its sexual significance but also because it appeals to an already established cross-gender tendency. Thus Buhrich & Beaumont (1981) and Buhrich & McConaghy (1985) found that 50% of fetishistic transvestites had been cross-dressing before the behaviour had obvious sexual connotations. They divided their fetishistic transvestites into two groups according to whether they reported early transsexual ideas. Interestingly, these two groups did not differ in the frequency of early pre-fetishistic cross-dressing.

A third mechanism has been suggested by psychoanalytic theorists. The cross-dressing is seen as a defence against the threat to the boy's masculinity and in particular the threat of castration. The act of cross-dressing in the presence of an erect penis is thought to serve that purpose (Stoller 1979). This explanation is difficult to accept. The cross-dressing itself must pose a threat to the boy's masculinity, as we will discuss below. In addition, the majority of fetishistic cross-dressers imagine themselves during cross-dressing as women with a vagina and breasts. Whatever they may be doing with their penis, they usually do not want to emphasise it or look at it (Bancroft 1972).

Whatever the factors that initiate this behaviour, the sexually arousing effect of cross-dressing serves to perpetuate the pattern. Typically it leads to masturbation and orgasm following which the spell is broken and the clothes removed immediately, often with a degree of disgust or other negative feelings.

The male fetishistic cross-dresser may continue to show a very simple fetish pattern just using or wearing one article of female clothing (usually underwear) or he may use more and more as time goes on until he becomes intent on creating as convincing an illusion of a woman as possible. With time, he may even move out of the fetish pattern and become primarily concerned with cross-gender identification. Such a shift will be discussed further.

The importance of sexual orientation

One of the most confusing issues in the literature on transsexualism is the sexual orientation of the transsexual or transvestite. If a male transsexual has sex with another male, is that a homosexual act or is it revealing the transsexual's heterosexual orientation? This confusion, much of it semantic, amongst professionals working in the field gives us a clue to the potential confusion that often exists in the transsexuals themselves. How an individual reacts to the possibility of being homosexual or heterosexual may play an important part in determining the transsexual experience.

In Chapter 3 we considered the ways in which gender identity may influence sexual preference; how for example lack of confidence in his masculinity may make it more difficult for a male to develop rewarding heterosexual relationships and thereby increase the likelihood of developing homosexual interest; how concern about masculinity may be reduced by adopting a homosexual role for which the criteria of masculinity are different. Now we should consider how sexual preferences may affect our gender identity.

A large majority of fetishistic transvestites regard themselves as heterosexual; they *may* enjoy fantasies in which they relate sexually to men but only if they are seeing themselves as women at the time. Usually they are sexually attracted to women and, as already indicated, many of them have enjoyed heterosexual relationships. By contrast, a fair proportion of those who seek re-assignment, in whom fetishistic arousal is not the principal motive for cross-dressing, may regard themselves as homosexual. Bentler (1976) studied a group of 42 male-to-female transsexuals following sex reassignment surgery. Approximately a third considered themselves homosexual before the operation, a third heterosexual and a third were categorised as asexual (they had not experienced enjoyable sex with a woman but were not homosexual, though half of them regarded themselves as heterosexual in spite of lack of experience). Almost all of these individuals considered themselves heterosexual following sex re-assignment.

A number of writers have suggested that avoidance of homosexuality is an important determinant of transsexualism. Let us consider the ways in which that might operate. In its most striking form, there may be a need to avoid a homosexual identity from the start. This is most often observed in the female transsexual who typically is aware of a normal or strong sexual attraction to females from late childhood or early adolescence (Pauly 1974). Commonly there is a rejection of these homosexual feelings and a flight into heterosexuality. Sexual relationships with boys are tried out but invariably found unsatisfactory. The resistance to accepting a homosexual identity continues however and they are likely to choose as sexual partners girls who have had no previous homosexual experience. By regarding themselves as boys they can then maintain a heterosexual identity, the previous existence of masculine interest and mannerisms making this a more feasible solution. The transsexual role is thus serving the primary purpose of permitting the desired sexual relationship. During love-making, direct stimulation of the transsexual's breasts or genitalia by the partner is usually avoided, to minimise this tangible evidence of anatomic femaleness (Pauly 1974).

This sequence of events, whilst apparently common amongst female transsexuals, is much less so amongst males. If the men have passed through a fetishistic cross-dressing phase, they are likely to have developed clear heterosexual attraction to women and often rewarding heterosexual relationships. In these men, the primary need underlying the transsexual wish is for a female identity. Following from that is the natural heterosexual desire to have a sexual relationship with a man, the final and possibly the most crucial proof of their femininity if it can be done with a new vagina. Such male-to-female transsexuals will usually prefer to delay any sexual activity until they have acquired a vagina.

Part of the puzzling difference in the importance of sexual orientation between male and female transsexuals may stem from the stereotypes of male and female sexuality. The stereotyped female is likely to regard herself as a sexual object; being sexually attractive to her partner is more important than her own sexual feelings. Conversely for the stereotyped male, being sexually attracted to women is a more fundamental component of maleness. Transsexuals have an understandable tendency to conform to stereotypes. Of relevance to this point is Bentler's (1976) observation that the previously heterosexual transsexuals he studied are more likely to see sex primarily as a means of pleasing the partner.

Problems of gender identity

Apart from the primary disturbance of gender identity which may be the basis for cross-dressing or transsexualism (e.g. as with the child transsexual), difficulties with the assigned gender role may eventually encourage the adoption of an alternative gender. Thus the individual who has struggled to maintain a successful masculine identity may feel that adoption of female identity would be a release from these pressures. In the traditional world, where men are expected to be in a position of superiority over women, less is expected of women and it may be assumed that change from male to female will 'reduce the disparity between expectation and performance' (Prince 1978).

Meyer (1974) described the 'ageing transvestite', a male who is depressed following long-standing internal struggles between his male and female identities. Such men may have exhibited the dual role, but with chronic difficulty. Giving up the male identity, often at a time of waning masculine powers, may be a desperate form of coping.

Fleming et al (1985) found evidence that the rejection of the assigned sex role is more marked in male-to-female than in female-to-male transexuals; this is further evidence of different mechanisms operating in these two forms of transsexualism.

The transvestite–transsexual shift

Although some authorities have regarded fetishistic transvestism and transsexualism as distinct entities, there is increasing recognition not only of their co-existence but also of the tendency for the fetishistic transvestite to become more transsexual as time goes on (Benjamin 1966; Bancroft 1974). This may be, as Benjamin suggests, a reflection of the latent transsexualism in that individual. An alternative explanation is worth considering. Whatever its origins, repeated cross-dressing with more and more effective impersonation of the female is likely to undermine the masculine gender identity of these men. It is not unusual for the individual, prior to the transsexual stage, to go through phases of excessively masculine activity (Jan Morris is an example), as if to compensate for the demasculinising effects of cross-dressing. In some cases it would seem the battle is lost, the female role becomes not only a desirable state in its own right, but a refuge from the struggle with maleness. The ageing transvestite described above perhaps shows a late variety of this process.

Often accompanying this shift is a change in the sexual component of the cross-dressing. The initial post-orgasmic state, sometimes characterised by disgust but usually with a strong wish to remove the clothes as quickly as possible, gives way to a period of peace and calm, in which wearing the clothes is enjoyed for non-sexual reasons. The cross-dresser 'just feels right'. The next stage is for the sexual component more or less to disappear and the non-sexual cross-dressing to take over. In some cases, this desexualisation could be a result of exogenous oestrogens but this is unlikely to account for all. Whatever its origins, such desexualisation can serve to reduce some of the tension the transvestite experiences in his marital or sexual relationships. The often increasing wish to incorporate the cross-dressing into the marital sexual relationship can pose considerable strains on the wife. Unfortunately the desexualisation may lead to withdrawal from the sexual relationship altogether in preference for the female role and this brings its own strains on the marriage.

There would seem to be two end-points to this shift. The first is the dual role transvestite for whom the fetish component has largely receded and who is able to maintain a reasonable balance between male and female existence. For some this remains a stable state for a considerable time, perhaps indefinitely. To the second end-point, the progression is inexorable, the transsexual urge taking over the individual's life more and more completely, usually resulting in a break-up of the family, loss of job and other major upheavals. I have likened this previously to a psychological malignancy because of its unstoppable destructive effect, often in a person with a remarkably normal previous adaptation (Bancroft 1974). Whether this shift is a psychological consequence of the repeated fetishistic cross-dressing or whether it reflects some other obscure process is not understood. Buhrich & Beaumont (1981), in making their distinction between 'nuclear' and 'marginal' fetishistic transvestites, see the latter group as having tendencies to transexualism preceding the fetish component. Whilst this might be the case, it is also important to remember the doubts about the retrospective accounts of adult transsexuals who have an understandable need to describe their childhood in ways which make sense and justify their current status.

Transsexualism as a psychotic illness

The conviction often held by transsexuals that they really are members of the opposite sex in spite of their anatomy has been likened to a delusional belief and transsexualism itself seen as a form of psychosis. Transsexuals, particularly male transsexuals, often have disturbed personalities. This is only to be expected when one considers the identity confusion they have endured, often during crucial stages of their personality development. Occasionally an obviously psychotic illness develops of either schizophrenic or affective type. Sometimes transsexual manifestations may show themselves for the first time during a florid psychotic illness or simply be symptoms of that illness. But the incidence of such associations is no more than you would expect in any other psychologically vulnerable group. Occasionally a depressed state may aggravate the wish for sex re-assignment as part of a nihilistic rejection of the individual's previous identity (Meyer 1974). In the large majority of transvestites and transsexuals, therefore, no support for a psychotic basis for the condition can be found (Hoenig & Kenna 1979).

The iatrogenic effect of surgery

Much of the conceptual confusion in this field stems from the fact that surgical sex re-assignment has become in some sense a reality. Prior to this being so, the person with gender identity confusion would have been less likely to see change of sex as a real alternative. With the possibility of surgery, however remote, not only is this a potential solution to a chronic problem but one which is seen to require only passive co-operation on the individual's part. An unrealistic expectation of the help to be derived from the surgical procedures is an important factor in the failures following sex re-assignment. But it is nevertheless understandable that such a tangible and dramatic process as sex re-assignment surgery should be seen as an escape route from a chronically disturbed or unrewarding existence. As a result, people who seek sex re-assignment are a very heterogeneous group. A tendency to call them transsexuals because of their wish for surgery has created a spurious homogeneity. Sex re-assignment with or without surgery is an end-point or at least a choice for people with very different developmental histories. They simply have in common the belief that escaping from one sex into the other will improve their lot.

CONCLUSIONS

We have recognised the very heterogeneous nature of cross-dressing behaviour and the variable developmental histories that precede it. We have also considered a range of possible determinants, some or all of which may be involved. A variable combination of these factors presumably creates the heterogeneity. Let us therefore try to summarise. One point which has emerged repeatedly from the evidence is an important difference between males and females. For the male, the two most important factors appear to be firstly, the search for a female identity and secondly, a fetishistic response to women's clothes. If the latter predominates, we have the typical fetishistic transvestite; if the former, the transsexual. An interaction between the two may however lead to a gradual change over time. The fetish pattern may remain throughout the individual's sexual life, or the cross-gender role may assume greater and greater importance, leading either to the relatively stable dual role position, or to the full transsexual position, with its unremitting desire for sex change. The third mechanism which may be involved is the need to maintain a heterosexual and avoid a homosexual identity. This may give further impetus to the search for sex change so that the desired sexual relationship with a man can be achieved whilst maintaining heterosexuality.

In the female transsexual there is no fetishistic component. The other two components predominate. Typically, the development of a relatively masculine identity in childhood is associated with sexual attraction to women. Whereas in the majority of such women this progresses to an adult homosexual role (with or without cross-dressing), in some, the homosexual identity is unacceptable either to the woman herself or to her partner. The transsexual position then provides a solution, albeit an extremely difficult one. In both the male and female, biological factors may facilitate such development, either affecting gender identity development or sexual learning. At the moment such factors seem to be more relevant to the female than to the male. There is much still to learn about this puzzling behaviour. In the meantime, we should keep an open mind about its causation.

REFERENCES

Bancroft J 1972 The relationship between gender identity and sexual behaviour: some clinical aspects. In: Ounsted C, Taylor D C (eds) Gender differences: their ontogeny and significance. Churchill Livingstone, Edinburgh

Bancroft J 1974 Deviant sexual behaviour: modification and assessment. Clarendon Press, Oxford

Bancroft J 1978 Psychological and physiological responses to sexual stimuli in men and women. In: Levi L (ed) Society, stress and disease, vol 3. The productive and reproductive age. Oxford University Press, Oxford

Benjamin H 1966 The transsexual phenomenon. Julian Press, New York

Bentler P M 1976 A typology of transsexualism: gender identity, theory and data. Archives of Sexual Behavior 5: 567–584

Bieber I, Dain H J, Dince P R et al 1962 Homosexuality: a psychoanalytic study. Basic Books, New York

Boyar R, Aiman J 1982 The 24 hour secretory pattern of LH and the response to LHRH in transsexual men. Archives of Sexual Behavior 11: 157–170

Breslow N, Evans L, Lamgley J 1985 On the prevalence and roles of females in the sado-masochistic subculture: report of an empirical study. Archives of Sexual Behavior 14: 303–318

Brierley H 1979 Transvestism. A handbook with case studies for psychologists, psychiatrists and counsellors. Pergamon Press, Oxford

Brownmiller S 1975 Against our will. Men, women and rape. Simon Schuster, New York

Buhrich N, Beaumont T 1981 Comparison of transvestism in Australia and America. Archives of Sexual Behavior 10: 269–282

Buhrich N, McConaghy N 1977 The discrete syndromes of transvestism and transexualism. Archives of Sexual Behavior 6: 483–496

Buhrich N, McConaghy N 1985 Preadult feminine behavior of male transvestites. Archives of Sexual Behavior 14: 413–420

Bullough V L 1975 Transsexualism in history. Archives of Sexual Behavior 4: 561–572

Carrier J M 1980 Homosexual behavior in cross-cultural perspective. In Marmor J (ed) Homosexual behavior: a modern reappraisal. Basic Books, New York, pp 100–122

Chalkley A J, Powell G E 1983 The clinical description of 48 cases of sexual fetishism. British Journal of Psychiatry 142: 292–295

Comfort A 1972 The joy of sex. Quartet, London

Croughan J L, Saghir M, Cohen R, Robins E 1981 A comparison of treated and untreated male cross-dressers. Archives of Sexual Behavior 10: 515–528

Dixen J M, Madderer H, Maasdam J V, Edwards P N 1984 Psychosocial characteristics of applicants for evaluation for surgical gender reassignment. Archives of Sexual Behavior 13: 269–276

Dorner G 1979 Hormones and sexual differentiation of the brain. In: Sex, hormones and behaviour. Ciba Foundation Symposium 62. Excerpta Medica, Amsterdam, pp 81–101

Eicher W, Spoljar M, Cleve H, Murken J D, Richter K, Stengel-Rutkowski S 1979 HY antigen in transexuality. Lancet ii: 1137–1138

Fleming M, MacGowan B, Costos D 1985 The dyadic adjustment of female to male transsexuals. Archives of Sexual Behavior 14: 47–56

Freud S 1927 Fetishism. Complete works. Standard edition 21: 175 Hogarth Press, London

Futterweit W, Weiss R A, Fagerstrom R M 1986 Endocrine evaluation of 40 female to male transsexuals: increased frequency of polycystic ovarian disease in female transsexualism. Archives of Sexual Behavior 15: 69 — 78

Gagnon J H, Simon W 1967 Sexual deviance. Harper & Row, New York

Gebhard P, Gagnon J, Pomeroy N, Christenson C 1965 Sex offenders. Harper & Row, New York

Glasser M 1979 Some aspects of the role of aggression in the perversions. In: Rosen I (ed) Sexual deviation, 2nd edn. Oxford University Press, Oxford

Goldman R, Goldman J 1982 Children's sexual thinking. Routledge & Kegan Paul, London

Goodman R E, Anderson D C, Bu'lock D E, Sheffield B, Lynch S S, Butt W R 1985 Study of the effect of estradiol on gonadotrophin levels in untreated male to female transsexuals. Archives of Sexual Behavior 14: 141–146

Gooren L 1986 The neuroendocrine response of luteinising hormone to estrogen administration in the human is not sex specific but dependent on the hormonal environment. Journal of Clinical Endocrinology and Metabolism 63: 589–593

Gosselin C, Wilson G 1980 Sexual variations: fetishism, transvestism and sado-masochism. Faber & Faber, London

Green R 1974 Sexual identity conflict in children and adults. Duckworth, London

Green R 1976 One hundred and ten feminine and masculine boys: behavioural contrasts and demographic similarities. Archives of Sexual Behavior 5: 425–446

Green R 1979 Childhood cross-gender behavior and subsequent sexual preference. American Journal of Psychiatry 136: 106–108

Green R 1985 Gender identity in childhood and later sexual orientation: follow up of 78 males. American Journal of Psychiatry 142: 339–341

Green R, Williams K, Goodman M 1982 Ninety-nine 'tomboys' and 'non-tomboys': behavioural contrasts and demographic similarities. Archives of Sexual Behavior 11: 247–266

Greenacre P 1979 Fetishism. In: Rosen I (ed) Sexual deviation. Oxford University Press, Oxford

Hamburger C 1953 The desire for change of sex as shown by personal letters from 465 men and women. Acta Endocrinologica 14: 361–375

Hinde R A 1974 Biological bases of human social behaviour. McGraw Hill, New York

Hoenig J, Kenna J C 1974 The prevalence of transsexualism in England and Wales. British Journal of Psychiatry 124: 181–190

Hoenig J, Kenna J C 1979 EEG abnormalities and transsexualism. British Journal of Psychiatry 134: 293–300

Hoenig J, Kenna J, Youd A 1970 Social and economic aspects of transsexualism. British Journal of Psychiatry 117: 163–172

Kinsey A C, Pomeroy W B, Martin C F, Gebhard P H 1953 Sexual behavior in the human female. Saunders, Philadelphia

Langevin R, Paitich D, Steiner B 1977 The clinical profile of male transexuals living as females vs. those living as males. Archives of Sexual Behavior 6: 143–154

Lebovitz 1972 Feminine behavior in boys. Aspects of its outcome. American Journal of Psychiatry 128: 1283–1289

MacCulloch M J, Snowden P R, Wood P J W, Mills H E 1983 Sadistic fantasy, sadistic behaviour and offending. British Journal of Psychiatry 143: 20–29

McGuire R J, Carlisle J M, Young B G 1965 Sexual deviations and conditioned behaviour: a simple technique. Behaviour Research and Therapy 3: 185–190

Marks I, Gelder M, Bancroft J 1970 Sexual deviants 2 years after electric aversion. British Journal of Psychiatry 117: 173–186

Meyer J 1974 Clinical variants among applicants for sex reassignment. Archives of Sexual Behavior 3: 527–558

Meyer J K, Knorr N J, Blumer D 1971 Characterization of a self-designated transexual population. Archives of Sexual Behavior 1: 219–230

Money J 1977 Peking: the sexual revolution. In: Money J, Musaph H (eds) Handbook of sexology. Excerpta Medica, Amsterdam

Newcomb M D 1985 The role of perceived relative parent personality in the development of homosexuality, heterosexuality and transvestism. Archives of Sexual Behavior 14: 147–164

O'Carroll T 1980 Paedophilia: the radical case. Peter Owen, London

Parker G, Barr R 1982 Parental representation of transsexuals. Archives of Sexual Behavior 11: 221–230

Pauly I B 1974 Female transsexualism. Archives of Sexual Behavior 3: 487–526

Plummer K 1979 Images of pedophilia. In: Cook M, Wilson G (eds) Love and attraction. Pergamon Press, Oxford

Prince V 1978 Transsexuals and pseudo transsexuals. Archives of Sexual Behavior 7: 263–272

Prince C V, Bentler P M 1972 Survey of 504 cases of transvestism. Psychological Report 31: 903–917

Rachman S, Hodgson R 1968 Experimentally induced 'sexual fetishism': replication and development. Psychological Record 18: 25–7

Randell J 1959 Transvestism and transsexualism. British Medical Journal 2: 1448–1452

Rekers G A, Mead S L, Rosen A C, Brigham S L 1983 Family correlates of male childhood gender disturbance. Journal of Genetic Psychology 142: 31–42

Ross M W 1983 Societal relationships and gender roles in homosexuals. Journal of Sex Research 19: 273–288

Ross M W, Walinder J, Lundstrom B, Thuwe I 1981 Cross-cultural approaches to transsexualism: a comparison between Sweden and Australia. Acta Psychiatrica Scandinavica 63: 75–82

Seyler L E, Canalis E, Spare S, Reichlin S 1978 Abnormal gonadotrophin secretory responses to L RH in transsexual women after diethystilbestrol priming. Journal of Clinical Endocrinology and Metabolism 47: 176–183

Sipova I, Starka L 1977 Plasma testosterone values in transexual women. Archives of Sexual Behavior 6: 477–481

Spengler A 1977 Manifest sadomasochism of males: results of an empirical study. Archives of Sexual Behavior 6: 441–456

Stoller R 1979 Gender disorders. In: Rosen I (ed) Sexual deviation. Oxford University Press, Oxford

Stoller R 1982 Transvestism in women. Archives of Sexual Behavior 11: 99–116

Von Kraft-Ebbing R 1965 Psychopathia sexualis. Translation by Klaf F S. Stern & Day, New York

Wachtel S, Green R, Simon N G et al 1986 On the expression of HY antigen in transexuals. Archives of Sexual Behavior 15: 51–68

Walinder J 1967 Transsexualism: a study of 43 cases. Scandinavian University Books, Goteborg

Wilson G D 1978 The secrets of sexual fantasy. Dent, London

Zuger B 1978 Effeminate behavior present in boys from childhood: 10 additional years of follow up. Comprehensive Psychiatry 19: 363–369

8

Sexual problems

Previously in this book when considering homosexual behaviour, transsexualism and other varieties of sexual preference, we have emphasised the need to distinguish between those who attend clinics, seeking help for a sexual problem, and those who do not. We must do the same when considering the ordinary range of heterosexual difficulties. Why do some people seek professional help, whilst others do not? A satisfactory sex life is not an 'all or nothing' phenomenon — there are varying degrees of satisfaction as well as varying types of problem. The more severe the problem, the more likely that help will be sought. But other factors also play a part. How much stigma is attached to exposing your sexual inadequacy? Does it mean you are psychiatrically disturbed if the clinic you attend is in a psychiatric hospital? You may have been led to believe that sexual problems are the result of serious personality difficulties and will only be helped by lengthy psychotherapy. You may be frightened of having to perform sexually in front of a therapist. You may feel more comfortable discussing this aspect of your life if you are from the same social class or background as the professional involved. The decision to seek professional advice for a sexual problem is a difficult one for the majority of people. The attitude of the professional to whom they first speak is probably crucial. In medical clinics and general practice, if the clinician asks questions about sex routinely rather than waiting for the patient to raise the subject, twice as many sexual problems are reported (Burnap & Golden 1967).

On the other hand, for some couples the sexual problem with its physical connotations may be less threatening than a marital or interpersonal problem; the sexual relationship may become the scapegoat for other difficulties in the relationship and physical methods of treatment may be requested and preferred.

THE INCIDENCE OF SEXUAL PROBLEMS

IN THE GENERAL POPULATION

To what extent do people experience difficulties in their sexual relationships? Sexual problems are not restricted to modern societies. Broude &

Greene (1980), in their analysis of 50 pre-industrial societies, found that fear and concern about impotence and reliance on magical cures were evident in 80% of the societies.

The impossibility of establishing the true incidence of any aspect of sexual behaviour in the general population, even in modern society, was stressed in Chapter 4. Kinsey's two major surveys (Kinsey et al 1948, 1953) come closest to succeeding. Of their male sample, 1.6% had 'reached more or less permanent erectile impotence', with the incidence rising with increasing age so that by the age of 70, 27% came into this category (see Fig. 5.5). Some 35% of men reported 'incidental impotence' (i.e. infrequent or justifiable) and 7.1%, 'more than incidental' (Gebhard & Johnson 1979). In Gebhard's (1978) analysis of marital problems from the Kinsey interviews, only 1.7% of the husbands reported erectile impotence as a problem, though 3.9% of the wives did so. Nearly 6% of the men regarded premature ejaculation to be a problem. Kinsey and his colleagues emphasised the rarity of ejaculatory failure (0.15%) but this has been disputed by other workers (e.g. Hunt 1974).

The decline in male sexual responsiveness with age is apparently accompanied by a decline in sexual interest. In general, therefore, the ageing process does not necessarily lead to sexual dissatisfaction, though for some couples the man's response may decline at a time when the woman's responsiveness and interest are still increasing, leading to sexual tensions. Further discussion of sexual problems of the elderly is found in Chapter 5.

The female dysfunction that has received most attention is inability to achieve orgasm. Kinsey et al (1953) reported that a woman's ability to experience orgasm increased gradually from puberty. In the later teens, nearly a half of their subjects had not yet experienced orgasm and by the mid-30s there were about 10% who remained incapable of this experience. Gebhard (1978) found that 16% of wives considered themselves to have a problem achieving orgasm. Hunt (1974) reported 15% were 'never or almost never' orgasmic whereas Fisher (1973), Terman (1951), Garde & Lunde (1980a) and Hagstad & Janson 1984 gave figures of 5, 8, and 4% respectively. Fisher has emphasised that for those women who are orgasmic, the majority are not invariably so during love-making and the consistency of their orgasmic attainment does not seem to determine their satisfaction with the sexual relationship (a similar conclusion was reached earlier by Chesser (1956). Dyspareunia (i.e. painful intercourse) was reported by 2.6% of Gebhard's (1978) wives whereas insufficient vaginal lubrication was mentioned by less than 1%. Hagstad & Janson (1984) in their survey of 444 Swedish women aged 37–46 years found that 6% experienced deep and 7% superficial dyspareunia.

The uncertain relationship between sexual dissatisfaction and sexual dysfunction has been highlighted in a study by Frank et al (1978). In a questionnaire given to 100 married couples, covering most aspects of marriage, they looked at three separate aspects of the sexual relationship:

1. *Sexual dysfunction*, which for the men included erectile and ejaculatory difficulties and for the women meant difficulty getting or staying excited, reaching orgasm too quickly and difficulty or inability to reach orgasm.
2. *Sexual difficulties*, a heterogeneous collection including inability to relax, lack of interest in sex, distaste or revulsion, too little foreplay, too little tenderness after intercourse, factors which were not dependent on efficiency of sexual performance but rather reflected subjective feelings during love-making or the nature of the sexual interaction.
3. *Dissatisfaction with the sexual relationship* — a global self-assessment.

A number of interesting findings emerged. A fifth of the women and a third of the men were sexually dissatisfied. Some degree of sexual dysfunction was reported by nearly two-thirds of the women (mainly difficulty in getting excited) and 40% of the men (mainly premature ejaculation). Similarly, a higher proportion of women than men reported sexual difficulties (mainly difficulties in relaxing and a lack of interest). Sexual dissatisfaction was more highly correlated with the presence of sexual difficulties than with sexual dysfunction, particularly in the men.

These results raise two important issues. First, they indicate that sexual dysfunction to some degree is common, and secondly that other aspects of the sexual relationship may be more important in causing dissatisfaction and hence lead to requests for professional help. We must be cautious, however, in generalising from this interesting study. The sample of marriages is not representative of any particular population; it was obtained by asking for volunteers from various social groups (e.g. rotary clubs, night school classes) and agreement to participate varied from 5% in some groups to 50% in others. The subjects were predominantly middle class and ostensibly happy (volunteers whose marriages were working were asked for), though it became apparent that in some cases the person volunteering was not aware of the dissatisfaction of his or her partner. But it is noteworthy that Nettelbladt & Uddenberg (1979), in a study of 58 married Swedish men, found a very similar pattern.

One of the better attempts at achieving a representative population sample in recent years has been that of Frenken (1976) in developing the sexual experience scales (SES) in Holland (see Chapter 5). The SES include four scales — sexual morality, psychosexual stimulation, sexual motivation and attraction to marriage. The sexual motivation scale is most relevant here, reflecting the individual's engagement in or avoidance of sexual behaviour. A total of 12% of the men and 9% of the women clearly avoided sexual activity but a further 14% of men and 33% of women showed weak avoidance. The factor analysis of the individual items revealed two factors comprising the sexual motivation scale: firstly, the ability to enjoy sexual interaction and to become sexually aroused and secondly, the ability to experience and to be satisfied with orgasm. It is of some interest that these two factors were found to be relatively independent of each other. In all,

26% of men and 43% of women indicated problems with enjoyment and arousal and a further 9% of women expressed actual aversion; 12% of men and 33% of women indicated difficulty or dissatisfaction with orgasm with a further 5% of women being anorgasmic.

Another study with a good representative sample is reported by Garde & Lunde (1980a), who interviewed 40-year-old Danish women and found that 35% reported having sexual problems. The nature of the problems were not clearly defined, but 15% 'had too little motivation', 7% 'derived nothing from intercourse' whilst 6% 'felt it to be an "obligation"'; 11% wished to obtain advice whilst 5% wanted 'sexological treatment'.

Two studies of marriage, one American (Levin & Levin 1975), the other British (Thorns & Collard 1979), have found that between 12 and 20% of young wives were dissatisfied with their sexual relationship. A number of other studies, usually involving highly unrepresentative samples, often respondents to questionnaires included in magazines, have been published (e.g. Hite 1976; Tavris & Sadd 1977). The short-comings of such data have been discussed in Chapter 4. A summary of some relevant findings from some of these studies is given in Table 8.1.

Table 8.1 Incidence of sexual problems reported in magazine surveys

	Dissatisfaction			Sexual dysfunction
Athanasiou et al (1970)				
Psychology Today (USA)				
Questionnaire n = 20 000		M	F	*Female*
M 47%: F 53%	Unsatisfactory	23%	18%	20% 'never or almost
Mainly young, well educated	Very unsatisfactory	8%	9%	never' orgasmic
Politically liberal				
Chester & Walker (1979)				
Woman's Own (UK)				
Questionnaire n = 10 000	*Female*			*Female*
(2289 analysed)	Bit dissatisfied	20%		Orgasm during
All female, ⅔ under 30	Very dissatisfied	12%		intercourse
Not biased to higher social				Rarely 17%
classes but ⅔ employed				Never 19%
Woman (3 November 1979) (UK)				
Questionnaire + interview	*Male*			*Male*
33% of 750	Disappointed	5%		Never have trouble
All males				making
				love 75%

Two reports by Sanders (1985, 1987) based on questionnaires in Woman magazine are noteworthy. The first report is of surveys directed at women, the second at men. About 15000 women and 5000 men returned the questionnaires; from this response they selected samples which were representative of age and regional distribution through the UK. In both cases respondents were asked about sexual problems in themselves or their part-

Table 8.2 Incidence of sexual problems in married couples as reported by female and male respondents to Woman questionnaires (Sanders 1985, 1987)

	Female respondents (%)	Male respondents (%)
Problems for women		
Low sexual interest	22	21
Difficulty with orgasm	11	7
Problems for men		
Low sexual interest	11	15
Difficulty with orgasm	1	1
Premature ejaculation	8	9
Erectile problems	8	7

ners. A total of 59% of the women had experienced sexual difficulties in their relationships at some stage while 23% were currently doing so; the percentages for male respondents were 49% and 19% respectively. The percentages of married respondents who had experienced specific sexual problems at some stage in their marriage are given in Table 8.2

These various studies do show some consistency where male problems are concerned. The greater variability in percentages for women may reflect differences in definition.

INCIDENCE IN CLINIC POPULATIONS

In a study of first attenders at a psychiatric clinic (i.e. people with no previous psychiatric treatment), 25% reported sexual/marital difficulties; 12% wanted and were considered suitable for sexual/marital therapy, while the remainder had psychiatric problems of greater importance or other reasons for not wanting this type of help (Swan & Wilson 1979). Unfortunately, no attempt was made to distinguish between sexual and non-sexual marital problems.

Levine & Yost (1976) sampled the women attending a gynaecological clinic in the USA. They approached 75 women and interviewed 59 (21% refused). This population was exclusively black and working-class. In all, 17% reported some sexual dysfunction and 28% had sexual problems. Once again, there was a variable relationship between sexual dysfunction and sexual dissatisfaction. Indifference to sex was the most frequent problem in those without specific dysfunctions.

Frenken & Van Tol (1987) interviewed a sample of Dutch gynaecologists about their practice during the preceding week: 7.2% of cases had presented with a sexual problem. The most common problems were dyspareunia and loss of sexual desire. Slag et al (1983) surveyed 1180 men attending a medical outpatient clinic and found 34% to have erectile problems. The association between sexual dysfunction and different medical conditions will be considered in more detail in Chapter 11.

An Edinburgh family planning clinic population was surveyed by questionnaire (Dickerson et al, unpublished data). One thousand consecutive women attenders were given an anonymous questionnaire and 750 completed it (25% refusal). In all, 12% said they had a sexual problem and 8% were uncertain. (An identical percentage was found in a smaller pilot survey 2 years earlier; Begg et al 1976.) Once again the existence of sexual dysfunction was a poor predictor of the acknowledgement of a problem (e.g. only a third of the anorgasmic women considered they had a problem). The best predictor was a lack of interest in sexual activity. Questions about communication or other non-physiological aspects of the sexual relationship were not asked. This population was by definition sexually active, but not representative of sexually active women. Their mean age was 26.5 years; 63% were unmarried, 68% had no children and we know from other studies that this type of family planning clinic population is skewed towards the middle class.

Golombok et al (1984) interviewed a random selection of 30 men and 30 woman attending their general practitioner for non-sexual problems. They were aged 18–50 years. A total of 20% of the women and 10% of the men had difficulty becoming sexually aroused; 7% of the women were anorgasmic, 17% with their partner. Some 20% of the men had premature ejaculation and 7% had erectile problems on most occasions (none had complete erectile failure). In spite of those various difficulties 97% of the men and 77% of the women said they were satisfied with their sexual relationship.

THE RELEVANCE OF SOCIAL CLASS

There are several reasons to pay attention to the relationship between social class and sexual problems. As we shall see in Chapter 10 our current approach to counselling such problems derives from a middle-class model. The interaction between sexuality and marital satisfaction may vary with social and economic factors. Cultural factors of this kind may determine not only the extent to which the woman sees sex as something with which she has to barter but also the extent to which the male uses his sexual relationship to bolster his masculinity (see Chapters 3 and 4).

Kinsey et al (1953) and Chesser (1956) found that women's orgasmic capacity was positively associated with both educational attainment and social class. Terman (1951) had not found these associations. Kinsey also noted briefly: 'At lower educational levels, it is usual for the male to try to achieve an orgasm as soon as possible after effecting genital union. Upper levels more often attempt to delay orgasm'. This tendency could well contribute to the aforementioned social class differences in females. Slater & Woodside (1951) still found in British working-class marriages the Victorian idea that sexual responsiveness in the wife was hardly expected and, if particularly marked, it should be disapproved of.

The most important study in this respect is that of Rainwater (1966). He found a much lower proportion of working-class women had a positive attitude to their sexual relationship than middle-class women (20% of the lower-lower class women rejected sex; only 3% of the middle-class women did so). Rainwater went on to relate these factors to the nature or quality of the marriage. He found that a key factor was the degree of segregation in the marriage; those marriages where husband and wife had very little non-sexual interest or activities in common were much more likely to have a sexually dissatisfied wife. Such segregated marriages were much more frequent in the working class. Schmidt (1977), in comparing his data from West Germany with that of Rainwater, has emphasised that the most striking differences are between the unstable and stable working classes; the differences between the stable working classes and the middle classes are relatively minor. The unstable working classes are characterised by lack of regular or secure employment, no vocational training and residence in slum areas.

Garde & Lunde (1980b) contrasted the highest and lowest status in their Danish women and found a marked difference in the incidence of sexual problems and orgasmic capacity; the lowest status women were at a disadvantage in several respects.

We will need to return to this issue when considering more closely the causes of sexual problems. The relationship between sexual dissatisfaction and marital dissatisfaction, though complex, is of crucial importance (Clark & Wallin 1965).

CLINICAL PRESENTATION OF SEXUAL PROBLEMS

It should now be obvious that sexual dissatisfaction and sexual dysfunctions occur with a frequency that would overwhelm the health services if they all presented for help. Many are presumably not sufficiently important to the individuals concerned to justify taking such a difficult step. But there will be others who are denied such help because it is unavailable or inaccessible.

Because of the psychosomatic nature of sexual problems, they may be presented in a wide variety of clinical settings. The discomfort of the clinician in talking about sexual problems and the lack of training in dealing with them is therefore a major factor in determining how these problems present or whether they are presented at all (Burnap & Golden 1967). One can only speculate on the number of patients who set out to seek advice for their sexual difficulty but fail because of the discouraging response from the clinician involved. The family planning clinic, because of its obvious sexual connotations, is an important setting. Hospital specialities that are obviously likely to encounter sexual problems are gynaecology, urology, infertility services and psychiatry, but as we shall see in Chapter 11, sexual problems are commonly associated with a number of medical and surgical problems (e.g. diabetes, multiple sclerosis). The majority of patients with sexual problems, however, approach their GP in the first instance and he is the commonest referral source for most sexual problem clinics (Bancroft & Coles 1976). The ability for patients to refer themselves to specialist clinics varies from one centre to another. For those who find their GP unsympathetic or difficult to approach or who wish to retain confidentiality, self-referral is important.

PEOPLE WHO ATTEND SEXUAL PROBLEM CLINICS AND THEIR PROBLEMS

In spite of the uncertain and variable association between dysfunction and dissatisfaction discussed above, the clinical literature on sexual problems has been predominantly oriented to the dysfunctions. Problems have been categorised in terms of genital and orgasmic responses. In recent years, the most influential study has been that of Masters & Johnson (1970). They classified their female cases as orgasmic dysfunction (primary or situational) and vaginismus and their male cases as primary and secondary impotence, premature ejaculation and ejaculatory incompetence. Although their categories have been widely adopted, there has been an increasing awareness amongst sex therapists that they are unsatisfactory. Kaplan (1974), emphasising the need to distinguish between arousal and orgasmic phases, suggested the term 'general sexual dysfunction' to cover inhibition or difficulty with the arousal phase, preferring it to the earlier pejorative term 'frigidity'. Sharpe et al (1976) took this re-classification a stage further and suggested a distinction between disturbances of arousal, orgasm and the resolution phase, disturbances of the perceptual component (anaesthesia), impaired satisfaction, problems stemming from ignorance and false beliefs, and sociosexual distress. Whilst this was an admirable scheme in theory, the authors did not go on to demonstrate its practical usefulness by applying it to a series of actual cases. If they had, they would have had problems in allocating the majority of individuals to any one category.

In spite of a substantial and growing clinical literature in this area, there have been very few descriptions of clinic populations. What are the problems which present at sexual problem clinics and with what frequency? Masters & Johnson's series is of treated cases, and we do not know the number or nature of those cases which are initially referred but not accepted. The powerful selection criteria make their population, as they acknowledge, a highly selective one.

In Edinburgh there is a clinical service for sexual problems, co-ordinated by the Edinburgh Human Sexuality Group and staffed by trained sexual counsellors from a variety of disciplines. Clinics are situated in:

1. gynaecology outpatient clinic;
2. psychiatric hospital annex;
3. health centre and family planning clinic;
4. small district general hospital;
5. local marriage guidance centre.

The referrals to this co-ordinated service have been analysed for a 3-year period, 1981–1983 (Warner et al 1987). There were 1194 referrals during that

Table 8.3 Principal problems of men and women presenting at a sexual problem service in Edinburgh. (Problems of those presenting as couples, both with problems of equal importance, are not included)

Male problems	%	Female problems	%
Low sexual interest	7	Low sexual interest	35
Lack of enjoyment	1	Lack of enjoyment	12
Other orgasmic problems	5	Orgasmic dysfunction	7
Dyspareunia	1	Dyspareunia	11
Erectile failure	50	Vaginismus	13
Premature ejaculation	13	Sexual aversion	3
Problems relating to			
homosexuality	3	Problems relating	
Transsexualism	4	to homosexuality	0.2
Sexual deviance	2	Transsexualism	2
Sexual offences	3		
Miscellaneous	12	Miscellaneous	15
Total	100		100
	(n = 533)		(n = 577)

time. The percentage of males presenting was 45% and of females 48%. In 7% both partners had problems and presented as a couple. In all, 56% of cases were referred by GPs, 10% were self-referred, while the remainder came from a variety of agencies, including hospital consultants. The types of problems presented are shown in Table 8.3.

For men, erectile dysfunction is clearly the most commonly presented problem, whilst low sexual desire is relatively infrequent, and it is rare for men to complain principally of lack of sexual enjoyment. In women low sexual interest is the most common. Together with lack of enjoyment this is comparable to the general sexual dysfunction category used by Kaplan (1974).

Table 8.4 lists the problems regarded as most important in each case; however, more than one problem can coexist in the same individual. In this table we see how these various common types of problem relate to one another. In the Edinburgh survey it was possible to specify up to five problems, ranked in order of importance, for each individual. The first ranked problem is shown as the main complaint. The second column in Table 8.4 shows the percentage of presenters for whom the complaint was indicated amongst the five choices, and second and third rank problems are also shown. In men we see that premature ejaculation is an additional problem in 15% of men with erectile failure, whereas erectile problems were present in 18% of men with premature ejaculation as their main problem. A third of men with low sexual interest also had erectile failure. Amongst the women we see a strong association between low interest and low enjoyment, though in part this reflects a common difficulty in women in making a clear distinction between the two. We see that more women have orgasmic dysfunction as a secondary problem than as the main complaint, so that in all, 20% of women have this difficulty to some extent. This nevertheless

Table 8.4 The commonest types of sexual problems in men and women attending a sexual problem clinic, showing the main problem, associated problems (ranked second or third), and the percentage for whom a problem was listed amongst the first five. (from Warner et al 1987)

Male presenters

Problem	Main complaint (n = 535) % of total	Problem listed (max. 5) (n = 615*) % of total	Associated problem ranked second or third (% of row)				
			Low interest	Low enjoyment	Erectile failure	Premature ejaculation	Other orgasmic problem
Low interest	6	16		13	32	12	
Erectile failure	50	54	11			15	
Premature ejaculation	13	24			18		

Female presenters

Problem	Main complaint (n = 577) % of total	Problem listed (max. 5) (n = 657*) % ot total	Associated problem ranked second or third (% of row)				
			Low interest	Low enjoyment	Orgasmic dysfunction	Dyspareunia	Vaginismus
Low interest	36	49		50	16	13	
Low enjoyment	12	38	46		24	18	
Orgasmic dysfunction	7	20	20	24			
Dyspareunia	11	20	20	27			
Vaginismus	14	15		10		17	

*In this column, men and women presenting as couples are also included, producing a larger n.

seems a low proportion when we recall Kaplan's (1974) statement: 'By far the most common sexual complaints of women involve the specific inhibition of the orgastic reflex'. Either there are differences in the presentation of these problems between the USA and the UK, or Kaplan has used this definition in a very broad way.

The most striking impression from these tables is the extent to which men complain principally of problems with their genital responses (i.e. erection or ejaculation) whereas women predominantly complain of lack of interest or enjoyment, i.e. the subjective quality of the sexual experience. To some extent this is inevitable as the fulfilment of coitus depends more on the genital response of the male than of the female. But it is also likely that other factors, such as differing expectation and the different significance of sexual performance on the self-esteem of men and women, contribute to this major sex difference of self-presentation (Bancroft 1984).

There are important relationships between sexual problems and age. In general male presenters are older than female (Fig. 8.1); of the men, those presenting with premature ejaculation are younger than those with erectile dysfunction (Fig. 8.2) In a study of normal married couples, erectile failure was the only sexual dysfunction to be correlated with age, an association that has been reported in other clinic studies (e.g. Bancroft & Coles 1976; Milne 1976). We will return to that issue later. The age distributions for the main types of female problem are shown in Figure 8.3. The bimodal distribution for orgasmic dysfunction may reflect the different age of presentation of primary and secondary problems; unfortunately this survey did not make that distinction. The bimodal distribution for dyspareunia, with a second peak in the older age group, reflects the post-menopausal causes of this problem (see p. 291).

An earlier study of 200 referrals to a sexual problem clinic in Oxford, based in a psychiatric hospital, reported comparable findings (Bancroft & Coles 1976). The most noticeable differences were the higher percentage

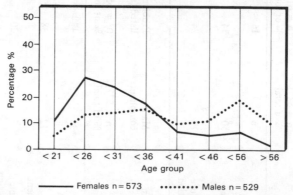

Fig. 8.1 Age distribution of men and women presenting at sexual problem clinics in Edinburgh. The two distributions differ; $p<0.001$. (from Warner et al 1987)

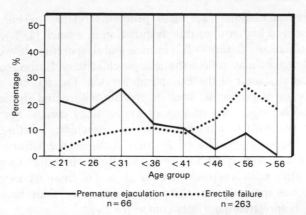

Fig. 8.2 Age distribution of men presenting with erectile failure and premature ejaculation. The two distributions differ; $p<0.001$. (from Warner et al 1987)

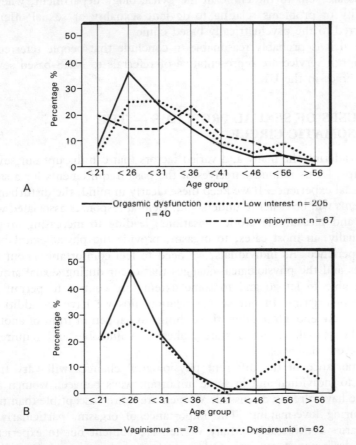

Fig. 8.3A & B Age distribution of women presenting with five different complaints at sexual dysfunction clinics. (from Warner et al 1987)

of premature ejaculation (23%) and problems related to homosexuality (12%) in men, and higher orgasmic dysfunction in women (18%), and lower percentages of erectile failure (42%) in men and dyspareunia in women. The last two differences may reflect the less psychiatric and more surgical and gynaecological character of the Edinburgh service. There is still a tendency for certain types of problems, such as erectile failure and dyspareunia, to be referred to non-specialist urology or gynaecology clinics. Some patients are certainly reluctant to attend a clinic in a psychiatric setting. Segraves et al (1982) followed the fate of 76 men with erectile failure who were referred from a urology clinic to a sexual dysfunction clinic in a psychiatric department. Only 62% accepted the referral, and of those who were advised to have sex therapy only one-third accepted, more than half of whom dropped out before treatment was completed.

In Edinburgh there are differences in the pattern of referrals to the differently situated clinics. Thus 70% of cases of dyspareunia and 44% of vaginismus are sent to the clinic in the gynaecology department, whereas the majority of problems relating to deviant sexuality or sexual offences were referred to the psychiatrically based clinic.

In general it is probably reasonable to conclude that people referred to the Edinburgh service are representative of referrals to NHS-based sexual problem clinics in the UK.

THE CAUSES OF SEXUAL PROBLEMS — THE PSYCHOSOMATIC CIRCLE

Before considering the many and varied factors that can disrupt our sexual relationships, let us remind ourselves of the basic requirements for a satisfactory sexual experience. If we keep these clearly in mind, the disturbances and problems will be easier to understand. Genital responses associated with enhanced and pleasurable erotic sensations, leading to increasing arousal and eventually, in most cases, to orgasm, provide the physiological basis for the experience. As individuals, we need to feel comfortable about our own bodies and the physiological changes that occur during sexual arousal and to be able to let go and to some extent lose control to permit the experience of orgasm. In our sexual relationships we have an additional need to feel safe enough to allow these things to happen in front of another person. The sexually aroused state makes us vulnerable and requires a lowering of our defences.

The importance of the different physiological changes will vary from individual to individual and in some important ways between women and men, as we have already discussed. Women are more susceptible than men to pain during love-making. The importance of orgasm, particularly in women, varies considerably. Many women are content not to experience orgasm, at least not every time. Others are put under pressure from their partners to 'come' as if it were a test of the male's potency. As mentioned earlier, women's expectations of orgasm (and men's expectations of their partner's orgasm) have probably increased over the past two or three decades as a result of the media and changing attitudes to female sexuality. The man tends to assume that he will ejaculate during love-making and often regards this as the end of active proceedings. The women is less likely to assume that her orgasm brings love-making to a halt; this in part reflects the differences in the post-orgasmic refractory period in the two sexes (see p. 77) but is not simply a physiological difference. For the woman, orgasm is a challenge to let go and lose control; for the man, the challenge is to keep control to some extent to avoid ejaculating too quickly. The implications of this particular and seemingly physiological contrast between the sexes have not been fully recognised.

Sexual function is a prime example of a psychosomatic process, and it is essential to keep this in mind when striving to understand the problems. In Chapter 2 we considered the psychosomatic circle of sex (see Fig. 8.4) and the ways in which physiological and psychological processes interact.

When we speak of causes of sexual dysfunction, we are usually referring to negative factors operating at some specific point in this circle. The consequences of such factors can only be understood by considering their effects in the whole circle, not just at the point of action. Furthermore, such factors may lead to continuing effects in the system after they themselves

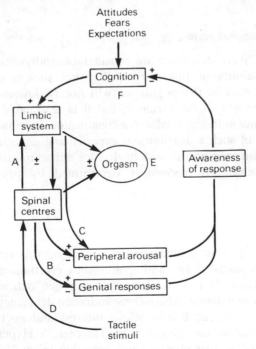

Fig. 8.4 The Psychosomatic Circle of sex, showing the six points at which aetiological factors will be considered.

have ceased to operate. Thus the effect of a drug or too much alcohol or a local cause of pain on either the vagina or the penis may initiate a reverberating process of anxiety and failure which continues long after the initial precipitant has ended. This is the essence of the psychosomatic approach as well as the system theory approach to any complex interacting system.

Let us therefore break into the psychosomatic circle at various points and consider the negative factors operating those points. Some of the disease processes involved are of sufficient importance that they will receive special attention later, but at this stage it is desirable to develop some overall perspective. In Figure 8.2 we have indicated six such points (A–F) in arbitrary order and we will consider each one in turn.

A. THE LIMBIC SYSTEM — SPINAL CENTRES COMPLEX

This is the 'black box' of our sexuality. We know very little of its workings and yet it provides the substrate for our sexual behaviour. But, as discussed in Chapter 2, the arousability of this system determines to a large extent whether we respond to sexual stimuli with purposeful sexual behaviour; it probably provides a basis of what we experience as sexual appetite or call sexual drive. The following are factors that may influence this system adversely, though our lack of knowledge permits only vague or hypothetical causal relationships.

Innate or constitutional factors

It is inherently likely that there are considerable individual differences in the basic arousability of this system. Whether such a characteristic is normally distributed in the population will not be known until we have some satisfactory way of measuring it, but it is reasonable to assume that there will be some individuals who, for constitutional or innate reasons, are at the extremes of such a distribution, experiencing either abnormally low or high arousability within this system. It does not seem justified to assume that these extremes are necessarily determined by psychopathological factors.

Hormones

In Chapter 2 we presented evidence that in the male central arousability, as manifested in sexual desire and spontaneous erections during sleep, is androgen-dependent. It is thus clear that androgen deficiency will cause impairment of sexual desire. Also *relative* androgen deficiency in ageing men may contribute to the decline in sexual interest and nocturnal erections commonly reported in that age group (see Chapter 5). Hyperprolactinaemia in men produces a similar effect to androgen deficiency.

From women presenting with sexual dysfunction there is a remarkable lack of endocrine data. But, as discussed in Chapter 2, the evidence we do have of the role of hormones in female sexuality is remarkably inconsistent and often contradictory. There is some evidence that once sexual problems become established in women, the psychological ramifications may obscure any hormone–behaviour relationship that does exist (see p. 120). At the moment we can do little more than suggest that in some women androgens and/or oestrogens influence sexual interest and arousability and that in such women hormonal deficiency may contribute to sexual problems.

Drugs

The effects of drugs on sexual response are often considered to be peripherally mediated, but central effects may be important, particularly with those drugs altering cerebral amine metabolism (see Chapter 2 for evidence of central pharmacological effects on sexual behaviour and Chapter 11 for details of different drugs in clinical use which may be responsible). Drugs which block the effects of androgens (i.e. anti-androgens) or lower the level of free testosterone in the blood (e.g. anti-convulsants) may be expected to produce effects similar to androgen deficiency.

Alcohol

Whereas raised blood alcohol levels are associated with impaired sexual responses, probably through central inhibitory effects, the effects of alcohol abuse are complex because of the interpersonal and social consequences. These will be discussed more fully in Chapter 11.

Generalised metabolic disturbance

It is well known that sexual appetite and arousability are frequently impaired during disease states that produce generalised metabolic disturbance (e.g. after severe trauma, or during toxic or infective states). In some instances (e.g. renal dialysis; see p. 567) more specific metabolic disturbances may be implicated, although in general we have little understanding of the mechanisms involved. It is possible that these effects may be mediated in the limbic system.

Mood disturbance

Although mood will influence sexuality through cognitive processes, it is becoming increasingly clear that there is a more basic, possibly biological link between depressive illness and loss of sexual desire. The fact that in men sleep erections, a measure of central arousability, are impaired in states of low sexual desire, depression and androgen deficiency, raises the possibility that there may be some biochemical mechanism common to all three phenomena (see p. 76).

Neurological abnormalities

Any functional disturbance of the limbic system or spinal cord may affect sexual function. It is difficult to predict what sexual effects will be produced by any particular lesion or abnormality (see p. 575). There is a common association between temporal lobe epilepsy and hyposexuality (i.e. low arousability and appetite) and this will be considered in more detail in Chapter 11.

B. GENITAL RESPONSES

Genital responses in both the male and the female rely predominantly on vasocongestion (See Chapter 2). The function of the pelvic muscles, particularly in women, is also relevant. Let us consider possible pathological processes in the male and female separately.

Erectile failure in men

In Chapter 2 it was noted that erection is a consequence of a sequence of responses involving the brain, spinal cord, peripheral nerves and local vasculature. In addition awareness of a lack of erectile response can adversely affect this system by means of psychological mechanisms (see p. 128). Thus it is obvious that a variety of factors can intervene at different points in this complex system, all producing failure of erection. Often more than one mechanism is involved. Disease or damage to the peripheral nerves controlling the penile vasculature or damage to the vascular mechanisms themselves are the most common and probably the best understood aetiological factors. But, as we shall see in Chapter 11, injury or disease of spinal cord can result in erectile failure. Also it is becoming clear that central mechanisms, as described above, may contribute, at least as far as spontaneous erections are concerned. The case study reported on p. 99 illustrates how loss of sexual appetite and spontaneous arousal may lead to erectile failure as a result of psychological mechanisms, in particular from fear of failure.

Ageing is associated with a decreased efficiency of the erectile response; speed of erection and in particular responsiveness to psychic stimuli decline (Solnick & Birren 1977). The older male usually requires more tactile stimulation of the penis. The mechanisms underlying this change are not understood, but presumably a more extreme form of this normal ageing process could lead to erectile failure.

We have already seen the strong association between age and erectile dysfunction in clinical populations. To some extent this must reflect the greater likelihood of pathological factors, such as arterial disease, in older men.

Vascular disease

Disease causing narrowing or obstruction of the arteries of the pelvis and penis is becoming increasingly recognised as a cause of erectile failure. The evidence for this is discussed in more detail in Chapter 9 and 11.

The existence of arteriovenous 'leaks' causing erectile failure has been reported by Ebbehøj & Wagner (1979). As the establishment of a full erection (and the associated high pressures within the corpora cavernosa) depends on effective shutting down of venous drainage, any leak in the system will impair the response. The cause of such leaks is not clear — they could result from vascular anomalies or possibly following penile trauma. Surgical occlusion of the leaks is apparently an effective treatment. It is not known how common such a condition is, as it can only be diagnosed with appropriate angiography. As it is treatable, it deserves wider attention. It has been reported as a cause of importance in bulls (Ashdown & Gilanpour 1974).

Neurological deficits

Any condition which interferes with the nerve supply to the erectile tissues, whether a pathological process, trauma or the consequences of surgery, may result in erectile problems. It is important to emphasise that our knowledge of the neural control of erection is incomplete and it is therefore difficult to be certain which nerves may be involved and precisely what effects their damage would produce. The possible role of autonomic neuropathy in causing erectile problems in diabetes and the sexual effects of multiple sclerosis and spinal injuries will be considered in greater detail in Chapter 11. The extremely variable anatomical distribution of the pelvic nerves makes it very difficult for the surgeon operating in the pelvis to be certain of avoiding damage to the erectile supply.

Priapism

Though a rare cause of erectile failure, this is a condition of theoretical relevance to the pathophysiology of erection as well as constituting a surgical emergency. Priapism is a persistent and often painful erection. It is of theoretical interest because only the corpora cavernosa and not the corpus spongiosum or glands are involved. This indicates that the erectile mechanisms affected are found in the cavernosa but not in the other erectile tissues. The clinical importance of priapism is that unless it is relieved within 24 hours or so, there is a considerable likelihood of permanent erectile failure resulting. This is thought to result from the fibrin deposition and eventual fibrosis that follows a prolonged period of anoxic venous stasis (Hinman 1960). Many causes for priapism have been suggested and most articles on the subject provide a long list of associated conditions (Shackman

1974). Considering the rarity of priapism, it would seem appropriate to regard its cause as unknown, though its association with various blood dyscrasias may prove to be important. The corpora cavernosa develop much higher pressures during erection than do the spongiosum and glans and are mainly responsible for the stiffness of a full erection. The specialised vascular structures (described on p. 56) are more abundant in the cavernosa and it is possible that some interference with their normal functioning underlies the condition. Simple aspiration of the cavernosal blood is not effective in relieving the priapism, which suggests that a simple pressure effect on the venous return is not responsible. Only when normal circulation through the cavernosa has been established for 3–4 days does the problem resolve; some biochemical or relatively long-term vasomotor effect may therefore be involved. Successful surgical treatment depends on anasto-mosing the cavernosa to the spongiosum or glans. If the anastomosis spon-taneously closes too early, the priapism returns (Wellwood et al 1972). If, on the other hand, it remains open indefinitely, then normal erection will not occur as the anastomosis will constitute a form of arteriovenous leak, as we described above. In some cases the anastomosis has to be closed surgically to prevent this happening (Ebbehøj & Wagner 1979).

The recent use of intracavernosal injections of smooth muscle relaxants in the diagnosis and treatment of erectile failure has resulted in prolonged erection, in some cases similar to priapism. This has been effectively reversed pharmacologically (with adrenergic drugs such as metaraminol) and pharmacological treatment is now probably the first line of attack in the treatment of spontaneous priapism (Brindley 1984).

Peyronie's disease

This condition interferes with normal erection causing a deformity of the erect penis, which can be embarrassing or painful, and sometimes inter-fering with ejaculation. The condition is thought to start as a vasculitis in the connective tissue between the tunica albuginea and the corpus caver-nosum. This leads to a progressive fibrosis of surrounding tissues producing, typically, a palpable plaque in the dorsum of the penis (Smith 1966). The penis bends towards the side of the lesion during erection, presumably because of unequal filling pressures in the two corpora caver-nosa. Although penile trauma and non-specific urethritis have been impli-cated, the cause is unknown. It has been suggested that it is increasing in incidence and the subclinical forms of the condition may be quite common (Smith 1969). A wide variety of treatments have been tried, vitamin E and potassium p-amino benzoate (Potaba) being the most widely used (Rhind 1987). However, no rational therapy is likely to become available until a better understanding of the aetiology is obtained. In cases where there is a simple bend of the erect penis in one direction, the deformity can often be corrected by a simple surgical procedure called Nesbit's operation (Bailey et al 1985).

Hormonal deficiencies

As mentioned earlier, erectile failure developing in the presence of androgen deficiency or hyperprolactinaemia is most likely to result from a psychological reaction to the hormonally induced loss of sexual interest.

Varicocele

The veins of the testes and epididymis form an anastomosing plexus, the pampiniform plexus, as they lie within the spermatic cord. Varicosity of this plexus is called varicocele and is relatively common (occurring usually on the left side). This condition is usually symptom-free, though it is well recognised as a cause of infertility in men, possibly due to the consequent rise of local temperature or to its effects on testosterone production. Raboch & Starka (1973) found in a study of infertile men that those with varicocele had lower plasma testosterone levels than those who were otherwise normal. They did not differ in terms of sexual activity, however and varicoceles are not usually regarded as relevant to sexual function.

There is no evidence that other scrotal swellings, such as hydrocele or spermatocele, are associated with impaired sexual function, though hydrocele, which can grow to a considerable size, could cause embarrassment or even interfere mechanically with normal coitus.

Drugs

As yet there is no unequivocal evidence of specific pharmacological interference with the peripheral erectile mechanisms except in the case of ganglion blockers. We will discuss this point further when we deal with the sexual side-effects of drugs.

Local causes of painful intercourse in the male

Although pain is a much more common problem for the female, it can arise in the male and affect sexual functioning in a similar way. Painful retraction of a foreskin which is too tight may be experienced during the first attempt at intercourse or may become a problem with tightening or scarring following inflammation or local infection. Small tears in the frenum of the foreskin may occur during vigorous intercourse or masturbation and become exquisitely painful. Any painful lesion or inflammation of the penis may be relevant, herpetic infections being one of the more common causes. Pain may be experienced during intercourse with deformities of the penis that cause bending or bowing during erection. Such deformity is commonly associated with hypospadias (a congenital anomaly in which there is incomplete development of the penis and the urethra opens at some point along the underside of the penis). This bending is sometimes called 'chordee'. It may arise with Peyronie's disease or following penile trauma when damage to part of the erectile tissue and scarring result in asymmetrical erection (Masters & Johnson 1970).

Hypersensitivity of the glans penis following orgasm and ejaculation is common. This may be so extreme that the man fears ejaculation occurring. This obviously can have a powerful inhibitory effect on his sexual performance and enjoyment.

The young male quite commonly experiences an aching sensation, usually in the testicular or inguinal region, following prolonged periods of sexual arousal not resolved by ejaculation. The discomfort presumably results from vasocongestion and is fairly quickly relieved following ejaculation.

Genital responses in the female and the causes of painful intercourse

The failure of genital response in the female and pain during intercourse are so intimately related that we must consider them together.

Failure of vaginal lubrication may cause soreness and irritation during intercourse or afterwards. Inadequate vasocongestion of the labia and vaginal opening makes vaginal entry not only more difficult but often painful. Failure of the uterine elevation and vaginal ballooning that normally accompanies intense sexual arousal may lead to deep discomfort or pain as the cervix is buffeted by the thrusting penis. The experience of pain, or its anticipation, will in turn inhibit, through the psychosomatic circle, these normal responses so that a negative sequence reverberates.

Oestrogen deficiency, whether following menopause or oophorectomy or during lactation, is associated with a vaginal wall that is thinner, relatively atrophic and lubricates poorly. The association of these factors commonly causes vaginal soreness. Whether oral contraceptives sometimes interfere with normal vaginal lubrication directly is not clearly established (see Chapter 12). Radiotherapy for pelvic malignancy is likely to render the vaginal wall severely atrophic and more susceptible to trauma.

Vasocongestion of the female genitalia is functionally and physiologically similar to erection in the male. In spite of this, we have no evidence of the effects of peripheral vascular disease or of peripheral nerve lesions on these responses in women (see Chapter 11).

Vaginal inflammation and infection

Acute infection of the vagina, whether due to bacteria, *Trichomonas*, *Monilia* or genital herpes, is painful. It is more important to realise that following acute infection the normal lubrication response may continue to be impaired. Subclinical or low grade infection is also common (see Chapter 11).

Other sources of vaginal irritation are sensitivity reactions to contraceptive creams, rubber, deodorants or underclothes made from man-made fibres. A tendency to douche the vagina excessively, by lowering the normal acidity may paradoxically render the vagina more susceptible to bacterial infection. Women with diabetes are prone to get vulval irritation and soreness, usually associated with monilial infection.

Deep pelvic responses

Little is known about local causes of failure of the ballooning of the vaginal vault and uterine elevation, partly because the normal physiology of these changes is not understood. It was suggested on p. 62 that smooth muscle fibres in the paravaginal and uterine supportive tissues may be responsible. Interference with the function of these fibres, as with adhesions or fibrosis, may be relevant. A retroverted uterus may be associated with painful intercourse, perhaps because of the resulting inadequacy of uterine elevation and greater susceptibility to coital buffeting.

Drugs

The possibility that certain drugs interfere with the vasocongestive or smooth muscle responses during sexual arousal in women has to be considered, although as yet no evidence is available.

Perivaginal and pelvic musculature

The muscles of the pelvic floor that surround the vagina as it leaves the pelvis (the levator ani and in particular the pubococcygeus) may cause problems in two ways. Some degree of tone in these muscles is probably desirable and if they are too lax intercourse may be less satisfactory for both partners. If the muscles are too tense, they make vaginal entry difficult, painful or impossible — a condition known as vaginismus (see Fig. 2.13).

It has been suggested that deficient tone in these muscles is associated with problems of arousal and orgasm in women (Kline-Graber & Graber 1978). Hartman & Fithian (1972) have advocated Kegel's exercises for improving the tone. As yet, there is no convincing evidence either that deficient tone impairs sexual enjoyment or that these exercises improve it. Levitt et al (1979) have presented some normal data on intravaginal pressures as measured by the Kegel perineometer and have shown that the muscle tone is reduced, as one would expect, by vaginal childbirth.

The opposite condition, spasm of the vaginal muscles (including the superficial perineal strap muscles as well as the levator ani) or vaginismus, presents a psychosomatic paradox. In one sense, the psychosomatic circle is clearly relevant; the experience or even the anticipation of pain on vaginal entry may cause these muscles to contract, occluding the vaginal opening and causing further pain when penetration is attempted.

In some cases of vaginismus, the onset can be clearly related to a painful episode such as rape or a traumatic gynaecological examination. But the substantial majority of cases of vaginismus are primary in nature, i.e. the problem was evident at the first attempt at intercourse (late-onset cases, particularly after childbirth, are unusual but do occasionally occur) and usually the woman concerned has had previous difficulty inserting or has been reluctant to insert anything, such as her own finger or a tampon, into her vagina.

The paradox is that there are many women who experience pain on vaginal entry for one reason or another, or have experienced vaginal trauma and yet do not develop vaginismus. Similarly, although there are some well described psychological factors associated with vaginismus which may well serve to aggravate or perpetuate the problem (and these will be considered later), they are not exclusive to vaginismus. It is therefore necessary to conclude that these women have a particular tendency to react to vaginal entry with muscle spasm. What underlies this predisposition is not known. It may indicate a pattern of responding that was learnt and established relatively early in life.

A corollary of this is the fact that the majority of women would welcome the ability to contract these muscles in a controlled way to enhance their grip on the penis during intercourse, yet for most this voluntary contraction is far from easy. When we consider the tightness and more or less total occlusion of the vaginal canal that results from vaginismus, it is also surprising that such spasm does not occur after the penis is inserted. 'Locking' during intercourse, which is a characteristic of canine coitus, appears to be exceedingly rare amongst humans (Kräupl-Taylor 1979), though occasionally a case is reported, usually termed 'penis captivus' (e.g. Melody 1977).

In its simplest form, the muscle spasm is limited to the vaginal muscles. In other cases, fear of vaginal penetration, such as during an attempt at vaginal examination, may lead to a more extensive muscle spasm, in particular of the thigh adductors, making even external contact with the genitalia impossible. In extreme cases, this leads to arching of the back as if the woman were trying to flee from the couch. Women with vaginismus also present a very broad range of difficulty from the therapeutic point of view. Many cases are easy to help with minimal reassurance, education and simple techniques of vaginal dilatation (see p. 486). These are perhaps examples of a relatively simple conditioned response. Other cases show associated psychopathology which may present some of the most formidable tasks for the sex therapist. In such cases, the vaginal spasm appears to be serving a much more general cause (see p. 394).

Other causes of pain in the vulval region

Difficulty and pain with vaginal entry may occasionally be due to a genuinely small and non-distensible vaginal opening, particularly in women who first attempt intercourse late in life. A rigid hymen may cause problems and hymeneal bands may remain concealed but are a cause of sharp pain on vaginal entry (see p. 42).

Retention cysts of Bartholin's glands may cause pain, particularly later during sexual arousal, when they would normally secrete and when pressure inside the cyst increases. A cyst may also be tender, particularly if it becomes infected (i.e. Bartholin's abscess).

An important and often over-looked cause of pain is tender scarring following either episiotomy or vaginal repair operations (see Chapter 11). The fourchette, the fold of skin at the posterior end of the vestibule, may, as a result of surgical repair, be unduly prominent and liable to be caught by the penis during vaginal entry. Sometimes, careful examination will reveal a localised tender or inflamed area (see p. 418).

Other causes of deep pain during intercourse

A variety of pelvic pathology may cause pain during intercourse, particularly during deep thrusting. Pelvic inflammatory disease, prolapsed ovaries and endometriosis are amongst the more common (see p. 420 and gynaecological text for a full description of these conditions).

C. NON-GENITAL PERIPHERAL AROUSAL

The various bodily and cardiovascular changes accompanying the genital responses were described in Chapter 2. Little attention has been paid to the problems associated with these in either men or women. The cardiovascular demands during arousal are of clinical importance in both men and women with cardiovascular disease, particularly ischaemic heart disease, and we will consider this more fully in Chapter 11. The increased motor tone and generalised body movement, as well as the adoption of various positions during coitus, may present problems for people with painful skeletal or arthritic conditions which, as with genital pain, may result in general inhibition of response.

The importance of these non-genital responses for sexual satisfaction is difficult to judge. There is some evidence that the rise in blood pressure can be blocked by drugs without impairing enjoyment of the act (Fox 1970).

D. TACTILE STIMULATION

The perception of touch, like other perceptual processes, is highly complex, relying not merely on sensory input, but also on central regulation of that input. Interference with afferent sensory nerve supply, as in peripheral nerve or spinal lesions, interferes with this important source of sexual excitation. More puzzling are cases of apparent genital or erotic anaesthesia, where erotic stimulation is hardly perceived, though pain sensitivity is not impaired. The most likely but unproven cause of such a condition is some psychologically determined central suppression of sensory input. In its simplest form, the anticipation of pain may result in such suppression. Fear of sexual arousal or its consequences may also be responsible.

Also puzzling is the hyperaesthesia which sometimes occurs; tactile stimulation leads to an intense sensation which is unpleasant rather than pleasurable, though the difference may be subtle. This is most commonly experienced with the clitoris or glans penis after orgasm (as mentioned above) but may occur elsewhere, especially in the anterior abdominal wall, leading to unpleasant spasm of the abdominal wall muscles. Although there are some neurological causes of hyperaesthesia, it is probable that most examples result from psychological interference with the perceptual process. This assumption is strengthened by the relatively common observation of a reduction in the hyperaesthesia during psychological treatment when the patient becomes more relaxed and less apprehensive during lovemaking.

In Chapter 2 we discussed the role that androgens play in penile sensitivity in many animals, due to their effect on penile spines. Human males do not have such spines, but the possibility that androgens affect tactile sensitivity of both the penis and the clitoris must be considered. Enhanced clitoral sensitivity following administration of androgens has been reported, but usually with large (i.e. pharmacological) doses and it is not clear whether this is a central affect dependent on greater arousability and erectability of the clitoris. As yet, there is no satisfactory evidence on this point, either in the male or the female.

Decrease in tactile sensitivity of the penis with age has been reported (Edwards & Husted 1976) and may contribute to the general decline of sexual response and behaviour with advancing years.

E. ORGASM AND EJACULATION

In the male

We concluded earlier that whilst orgasm and emission are normally linked, they are potentially separable. A combination of orgasmic muscle contraction and emission is responsible for ejaculation.

Delayed or absent ejaculation

Unfortunately, there has been a tendency to ignore the orgasm component when studying disturbances of ejaculation. Thus Whitelaw & Smithwick (1951), reporting on the sexual effects of sympathectomy, found permanent loss of ejaculation in roughly half of men when the first three lumbar roots were removed. However, they did not say whether the capacity for orgasm remained. Higgins (1979) in his review of the literature on the sexual effects of spinal cord injuries, found similar confusion, though it would appear that both ejaculation and orgasm are rare after such injuries. Brindley & Gillan (1982) found the bulbocavernosus or (as they prefer to call it) the glandi-pudendal reflex to be absent in two out of nine men with complete primary ejaculatory failure. A high incidence of ejaculatory failure is reported as a side-effect of anti-adrenergic hypotensive drugs, such as guanethidine and bethanidine. But usually no comments are made about orgasm (see Chapter 11). Money & Yankowitz (1967), by contrast, described drug-induced 'dry run orgasms' (i.e. orgasms without emission and no apparent evidence of retrograde ejaculation into the bladder). Thus it seems possible that emission and orgasm can be differentially affected by drugs and neurological lesions and more attention needs to be given to this possibility.

Retrograde ejaculation and other disturbances in the timing and co-ordination of the ejaculatory process can occur, and are sometimes reported as early sexual symptoms of diabetes. Such disturbance is often linked with other evidence of bladder dysfunction, which reminds us of the complex interaction of sexual and bladder mechanisms during ejaculation.

It is also likely that drugs may affect the orgasm component more directly, though presumably by a central mechanism. Chlormipramine and monoamine oxidase inhibitors sometimes produce failure of orgasm and ejaculation as a side-effect and have been used as a method of treating premature ejaculation (see Chapter 10).

Androgens undoubtedly have an important role in permitting normal ejaculation in males. Inability to ejaculate (and usually to experience orgasm) is one of the first sexual consequences of androgen withdrawal and is rapidly restored with androgen replacement (Skakkebaek et al 1981).

Premature ejaculation

Although it is often stated that premature ejaculation can be caused by local pathological states, such as prostatitis or urethritis (Kaplan 1974) no evidence of such causation is available. Nor do we know of any evidence of drugs causing premature ejaculation. But whilst it is difficult to identify local physical causes, we should be cautious in attributing the problem solely to psychological factors.

There is a natural tendency for most young males to ejaculate quickly and the longer the period since last ejaculating, the quicker it is likely to be. On p. 365 we considered the sociological factors influencing whether a male seeks to delay his ejaculation.

With increasing sexual experience greater control over ejaculation usually develops. This is partly because of the dampening effects of the ageing process and also because of the lessening of novelty that comes particularly with a stable sexual relationship. But some process of learnt control is probably necessary. It is in this aspect that males differ from one another, with some failing to learn. At the present time, the best theoretical explanation for this acquired control is that the man learns to recognise when he is getting close to the point of ejaculatory inevitability so that he can temporarily reduce the level of stimulation and allow his arousal to subside a little. It may be that for some men this aspect of autonomic function is peculiarly difficult to control — they have over-excitable and too easily triggered 'ejaculation centres'. There are a variety of psychological factors that might interfere with the learning process, perhaps by impairing the man's ability to discriminate and identify this crucial point of impending physiological response. Anxiety, whether specifically related to sex or not, is especially prone to aggravate the problem. We shall return to this later when discussing the sexual effects of various emotional states, but it is relevant at this point to ponder on the rather contrasting effects that anxiety has on emission and orgasm.

The impulsive, inexperienced young man may ejaculate rapidly and enjoy the experience. As soon as he starts to worry about this rapid response, i.e. to anticipate premature ejaculation, two consequences follow. He will tend to ejaculate even more quickly and his associated orgasm will become less and less intense and pleasurable. It is as though anxiety excites emission and inhibits orgasm. Eventually premature ejaculation gives way to premature emission with minimal orgasm. In extreme cases, the orgasmless emission can occur while the penis is still flaccid.

As shown on p. 369, there is a strong association between premature ejaculation and erectile failure. Typically, a man with lifelong problems of ejaculatory control develops erectile problems in middle age. The nature of this association is not understood. A persisting inability to relax during love-making because of the need to delay ejaculation may render the individual more vulnerable to the effects of performance anxiety. But there may be other explanations and we should keep an open mind on this point.

It is also necessary to distinguish between genuine and apparent premature ejaculation. In men with physical impairment of erectile response, the time required for stimulation to produce an adequate erection may be prolonged whilst the amount of stimulation required to produce ejaculation remains the same. Hence the interval between achieving an erection and ejaculating shortens, suggesting premature ejaculation when in fact the problem is delayed erection (Michal 1982).

Painful ejaculation

The unpleasant hyperaesthesia of the glans that may follow ejaculation has already been mentioned. Pain during ejaculation can be due to strictures of the urethra and if there is infection in the bladder, seminal vesicles, prostate or urethra, intense burning immediately following ejaculation may occur. With gonococcal infection this pain can be severe. Such symptoms call for bacteriological investigation and appropriate therapy. Other types of prostatic disease may cause ejaculatory pain (Masters & Johnson 1970).

Orgasm in the female

Considering our lack of knowledge of the neurophysiological basis of orgasm in either male or female, it is not surprising that there is very little to say about local or physical causes of orgasmic failure in women. Raboch & Bartak (1981) found that late menarche was associated with less frequent or absent orgasm in adult life. These authors (1983) also found a similar negative association between orgasmic capacity and age at first sexual intercourse. Brindley & Gillan (1982) found that anorgasmic women who had absent or impaired bulbocavernosus (glandi-pudendal) reflexes were unlikely to respond to psychological treatment, suggesting that a neurological deficit underlay their problem. The effect of anxiety is to inhibit or delay orgasm, hence the self-perpetuating effect of performance anxiety which perversely delays the woman's orgasm whilst aggravating her partner's premature emission.

The effect of spinal cord injury on female orgasm is even less clear than in the male. Evidence of possible effects of drugs on female orgasm is lacking though, as in the male, the opiates may have a direct inhibitory effect on orgasm, and there, have been a number of case reports of other drug effects (Segraves 1985). Similarly the role of hormones in female orgasm is not known. Apart from the possible role of steroids such as testosterone and oestradiol, peptides such as oxytocin may play a part in causing the uterine contractions that accompany orgasm. There is as yet no evidence of specific orgasmic difficulty as a result of hormone deficiencies.

Pain associated with orgasm does occur in some women and can be sufficiently severe to make them fearful of orgasm. Usually the pain is experienced in the pelvis or lower abdomen and is probably related to muscle spasm. Some descriptions suggest a uterine location, others rectal or colonic. Local causes of such pain have not been identified and further work is need on this relatively common and troublesome complaint.

Headaches associated with orgasm

Three types of headache have been described in association with sexual activity, all more common in men (Rose & Petty 1982). The first type, sometimes called 'coital cephalgia', develops before orgasm and is a dull aching bilateral pain, associated with contraction of neck and facial muscles, comparable to the pain of tension headache. The second type, benign orgasmic cephalgia, typically occurs in the minutes before or after orgasm, and is a sharp, explosive, usually unilateral headache. It may be delayed for 1–2 hours after orgasm. It is often associated with a history of migraine, and, like migraine, is unpredictable in its occurrence. The third type has been called 'malignant orgasmic cephalgia' and is caused by a subarachnoid haemorrhage occurring during sexual activity. Lundberg & Osterman (1974) found six cases of subarachnoid haemorrhage in a series of 50 patients with coital headache.

F. PSYCHOLOGICAL FACTORS AND ASSOCIATED EMOTIONAL STATES

It is widely believed that psychological factors are the commonest and most important factors disrupting normal sexual responses. Anxiety is given pride of place by both psychoanalysts and behaviourists and its possible effects have already been mentioned on a number of occasions. Anger, hostility and resentment are also regarded as crucial. The importance of mood to sexuality is becoming recognised. The consequences of becoming a spectator rather than a participant during love-making or of becoming unduly aware of how you or your partner are responding is also believed to have a negative effect. The relationships between these psychological processes and sexual response were examined in detail in Chapter 2 and found to be complex.

Anxiety

Few would disagree that anxiety is commonly present in those experiencing sexual failure. In one study the fear of failure and fear of being ridiculed were the most commonly reported types of anxiety (Cooper 1969a). But anxiety may not necessarily *cause* sexual failure; it may simply accompany it. Thus if a sexual encounter is perceived as threatening, the result may be a direct inhibition of sexual response together with the experience of subjective anxiety. The inhibition and the anxiety share a common cause, but one is not causing the other. This reintroduces the concept of *neurophysiological inhibition* first discussed on p. 68. The association of excitatory and inhibitory mechanisms is fundamental to much of central nervous system activity. The precise link between the psychological threat and the activation of such inhibitory mechanisms is not understood but it does not require the existence of manifest anxiety. This would explain why reducing anxiety pharmacologically does not necessarily solve the problem. In such cases, it is the underlying threat that needs to be reduced so that both anxiety and inhibition decline and sexual function returns. Obviously anxiety generated by the sexual failure can add to the picture and may interfere by means of the disruptive effects discussed earlier (see p. 128).

Once we acknowledge direct inhibition of sexual response as a basic mechanism, it follows that in certain circumstances sexual responses may be inhibited in order to *avoid* anxiety, when sexual activity or response itself is threatening. Thus if we call performance anxiety 'fear of failure', we can call this further type of anxiety 'fear of success' (Bancroft 1980).

The role of anxiety in sexual dysfunction may therefore be varied and complex. It may have direct disruptive effects on sexual response, it may act as a signal of an underlying sexual threat or it may motivate the avoidance of sexual activity.

Anger

The role of anger and resentment needs to be looked at in a similar way. Anger as an autonomic state may directly interfere with sexual response — for some it may be physiologically impossible to be angry and sexually aroused at the same time. Psychologically, it certainly makes some of the basic requirements for satisfactory sexual interaction difficult to attain, such as the preparedness to be open and vulnerable and the ability of both partners to feel safe. But there are some individuals (probably a minority) whose sexual responses may be facilitated by anger or at least unimpaired by it (see Chapter 2). Certainly sex may be used as a means of expressing anger and conversely avoidance of or inhibition of sexual responses may be motivated by a need to hurt the partner. Anger may be a reaction to sexual difficulties in either one's self or one's partner and, as with performance anxiety, serve to compound the problem. As yet, we have no reason for linking anger with any particular type of sexual dysfunction but, as with anxiety, it is commonly present in many cases of sexual failure.

Mood

The importance of mood as a determinant of sexuality has only recently been acknowledged. Schreiner-Engel & Schiavi (1986) have found an association between loss of sexual desire and a history of depressive illness in both men and women. This link may reflect common biochemical mechanisms (see p. 130). But obviously mood has important effects on how we think about ourselves — whether we feel attractive, desirable, worthy of love etc.

Awareness — the spectator role

The fourth mental state that we have mentioned is that of self-awareness or the spectator role. Awareness of sexual failure leads to what we have called performance anxiety and this has also been regarded as of causal significance in a simplistic way. It is perfectly possible that there are some individuals who are particularly susceptible to the negative effects of feedback or awareness of their own response. But once again it is necessary to consider the particular significance of the feedback to those individuals when understanding its effect. Certain types of 'spectatoring' may be sexually stimulating (see p. 131).

Simple assumptions about the effects of various mental states on sexual function are therefore unwarranted and have the disadvantage of leading us into simplistic or naive methods of treatment.

THE ORIGINS OF PSYCHOLOGICAL PROBLEMS

If simple assumptions about the direct effects of emotional states are to be avoided, we should also beware of making simple causal connections between identifiable psychological problems and sexual failures. In the course of therapy, as we shall see later, psychological problems or threats are often identified but we can seldom be certain of their relevance to the sexual dysfunction. We may discuss them, remove some of the guilt, tension or anxiety associated with them and subsequently see the sexual problem improve. We may therefore consider it likely that the problem was relevant but we can never be sure because so many other things are going on at the same time during treatment. Nevertheless we follow the common-sense principle that anything which interferes with comfort and security during a sexual encounter is likely to impair sexual responses. As yet there is very little good evidence of the associations between particular types of psychological problems and specific types of sexual dysfunction and we must rely largely on clinical experience. Kaplan (1974) provides a rich source of such experience and many case illustrations. We must be prepared to find subsequently that many of our more precious assumptions prove to be misleading. But with these limitations in mind let us look at some of the more common reasons for feeling anxious, guilty, tense, angry or depressed in our sexual relationships.

Throughout we will be dealing with the complex interaction between knowledge or information and personal values. In any emotive area, these two can never be completely separated. Also ever-present is an interaction between factors in the current situation and those from the past. This can also be seen as an interaction of intra- and interpersonal problems. Intrapersonal problems stem from the individual's earlier experience and affect not only attitudes and feelings about sex but also ability to communicate and to manage anger and intimacy. Interpersonal problems are the difficulties two people have in adjusting in their relationship — the interplay of their two sets of intrapersonal problems.

Misunderstandings and ignorance

Simple lack of knowledge about the elementary anatomy and physiology of sex can lead to problems. A couple may have interfemoral intercourse, thinking that vaginal entry is taking place. Attempts at vaginal intercourse may be abandoned because they have been directed at the rectum rather than the vagina. It is nevertheless important to be cautious about attributing too much to simple ignorance. Whereas learning of sexual technique is normally necessary, even amongst animals, failure to learn may stem from more than lack of appropriate education. Acknowledging ignorance may be easier for some people than acknowledging fear or guilt. Sometimes the change that follows a simple provision of information is as much a consequence of the 'permission' that implicitly accompanies that information.

A particularly important form of misinformation is the false or unhelpful assumption of what is 'normal' and hence desirable. Norms about frequency of sexual intercourse may impose pressures on a couple who lag behind the national average. It is commonly believed to be normal for both partners to reach orgasm at the same time; anything else is failure. The woman who requires clitoral stimulation for orgasm may believe herself to be abnormal or, if she has read the relevant psychoanalytic literature, immature. Certain positions during intercourse may be seen as normal, anything else as 'kinky' and hence unacceptable. A couple may not realise that their strong liking for oral sex is widely shared and fear that they are in some way peculiar for enjoying it.

As a couple gets older, they may misinterpret the male's normal decline in erectile responsiveness as evidence of loss of love or sexual failure, still regarding it as normal that a man should get a full erection without his partner touching his penis. The man may believe that each time he ejaculates he is losing some of his irreplaceable life-energy. Many more commonly held and damaging beliefs could be cited.

Unsuitable circumstances

The middle-class, reasonably affluent sex therapist usually has an image of good sex which, if it doesn't involve making love under a warm sun on a tropical beach, at least requires privacy and comfort. All too often, less affluent sexual partners have neither privacy nor comfort for their love-making. Living in over-crowded conditions, they often have children sleeping in the same room or able to hear much of what happens through the walls. What private space they can find is often cold and uncomfortable. It is important to recognise these situational factors which may be of primary importance.

The affluent also suffer from unsuitable circumstances. Pressure of work may seriously interfere with their sex life, which becomes squeezed into those few minutes remaining between a full and exhausting day and a fitful sleep. The rejuvenation of sexual feelings that so often happens on holiday is testimony to the negative effects of our day-to-day pressures. Our sexual relationships, if they are to flourish, have to be nourished with adequate time in the right circumstances.

Bad feelings about sex

When we consider the adult silence and implied taboo that surrounded the subject of sex during the childhood of so many of us, it is not surprising that children develop and harbour peculiar or primitive fears or beliefs about sex that remain in adult life because they are not challenged. Most commonly we learn to view sex as wrong, naughty, dirty or even evil. Such strong negative values may be incompletely resolved when we start our sexual relationships and serve to temper or even inhibit what should be spontaneous pleasures. We may feel that sexual pleasure is always wrong or we may feel sufficiently unsure about it that we must conceal its occurrence from everyone (except possibly our partner). We certainly must not be seen, or even heard, indulging in any form of sexually pleasurable activity. On no account must we give our children any reason for thinking that we enjoy sex and so on.

Identifying sex as bad may have other results. Some people learn to enjoy sex in spite of the 'bad' image by confining sexual pleasure to 'bad' or at least illicit relationships. Illicit sex is exciting; respectable sex, as part of a good, loving relationship is unacceptable. Sometimes in such cases part of the excitement stems from the risk involved of getting caught or being found out. We must not forget the variable ways in which human beings learn to associate emotional states with sexual response. Sexual pleasure may be unacceptable in a loving relationship which is too closely identified with the child–parent relationship, particularly when Oedipal anxieties have not been resolved. Although I do not accept the almost ubiquitous role Oedipal feelings are assigned by most psychoanalysts, they are probably important in some cases. It may be that when an especially close father–daughter or mother–son relationship leads to active denial of the sexuality involved, trouble is to be expected in the subsequent marriage.

In recent years there has been an increasing awareness of sexual abuse during the childhood of adults presenting with sexual problems. This will be dealt with more fully in Chapter 13. Such abuse can vary from incidents which are tantamount to violent rape by parents, siblings or others outside the family, to those in which the child participated with some pleasure or at least curiosity. There are various repercussions in adulthood. A sense of betrayal that one has been exploited or used by someone in a position of influence or trust results in anger and a need for retribution. Often the story was not told by the child for fear that this would lead to a break-up of the family, for which the child would feel responsible; this later leads to intensification of the anger. In some cases the child tried to tell someone what had happened and was not believed, a particularly damaging form of betrayal by other adults apart from the offender. Often there is guilt that as a child one must have encouraged or colluded with the behaviour in some way, particularly if at any stage the incidents had been enjoyed. It is particularly difficult to acknowledge the occurrence of any sexual feelings in such situations, however unimportant, in the face of the extreme public reaction to any form of child sexual abuse which denies that children are capable of sexual feelings or interest.

For these various reasons the adult who has suffered such experiences may have difficulty acknowledging his or her sexual feelings in adulthood or is unable to feel sufficiently secure in a sexual relationship to let down defences.

Sex may be seen as disgusting rather than bad. Disgust is a puzzling emotion. Lazarus (1966) has suggested that it is a combination of approach and avoidance. If we simply want to avoid something, we feel frightened of it, but if we have strong mixed feelings about it we may feel disgust. Although unproven, and possibly unprovable, this is an interesting idea. Not infrequently it is the disgusted patient who seems to show the most dramatic breakthrough of sexual pleasure, which would support Lazarus's idea. Disgust may be directed specifically at the penis or the vagina, the vaginal smell or the ejaculate or vaginal fluid. It may occur in those who learned to associate sex and excretion, particularly those who are generally fastidious about their body cleanliness. This type of disgust, reflecting a more general personality characteristic, may be rather different in its origins, as it is often more difficult to resolve.

It is important to remember that in a state of sexual arousal we may tolerate or even enjoy sensations or smells that in a non-aroused state we might find somewhat offensive. Sexual disgust may therefore arise or become established when there are other factors blocking normal sexual arousal. In those instances, it is obviously of secondary importance.

Sexual arousal may threaten our need for *self-control*. Some people who have not experienced orgasm may have an image of it which is threatening. Others have experienced orgasm during masturbation and feel unable to allow such abandonment to happen in front of another person. This may reflect a general need to 'keep control', particularly in the sort of person who never likes getting ruffled or showing too much emotion. In others the fear may stem from the intensity of sensation involved and the extent of loss of control experienced. They may dislike their physical appearance during orgasm; they may fear losing control of bowel or bladder function. They may be aware of becoming vulnerable, not only because momentarily they are unable to protect themselves, but also because they may lay themselves open to ridicule or rejection by their lover.

In Fisher's (1973) study of female orgasm, he found one particular feature which distinguished between women with high and low orgasmic attainment. 'The low orgasmic woman . . . feels that people she values and loves are not dependable, that they may unpredictably leave her. She seems to be chronically preoccupied with the possibility of being separated from those with whom she has intimate relationships'. These women tended to have detached or absent fathers during their childhood and adolescense. Fisher suggested that their difficulties in letting go for orgasm resulted from their fear of losing contact with the loved one. Certainly, for many people orgasm means 'taking off' for a few moments on a solitary 'trip'. Those who are only comfortable with sex as an expression of love may enjoy the shared experience of the earlier stages of love-making and feel uncomfortable when they find themselves moving into this solitary phase. Such a reaction may not completely prevent orgasm, but may temper its intensity.

Sexual pleasure may be feared as a road to promiscuity. This is particularly likely to be a problem for a woman who may feel that if she lets herself go and really enjoys sex, she will have difficulty in controlling herself and become promiscuous. In some cases, she may have passed through a relatively promiscuous phase earlier in her development. After a stage of sexual restraint she enters a reasonably stable and respectable marriage but at the expense of loss of sexual abandonment. Any attempt to recapture earlier sexual enjoyment may bring fears of returning promiscuity.

Sex may be feared as painful or dangerous. For women in particular, fear may become a self-fulfilling prophecy because of the resulting muscle spasm, as discussed above. Such fear may originate from an earlier traumatic sexual experience such as rape or a painful gynaecological examination. It may stem from irrational beliefs about the physical harm that will result from entry of the penis, because the vagina is thought to be too small or to open in a rather vague manner into the abdominal cavity.

Fear of pregnancy of an understandable and rational kind has probably succeeded in spoiling more sexual relationships than any other single factor. In the days before effective birth control was available, and when there was a comparatively high maternal and infant mortality, it was perhaps surprising that women were able to develop relaxed, enjoyable sexual relationships at all. Much of the emergence of female sexuality in the past few decades must be attributed to the liberating effect of modern contraception. There are nevertheless some women for whom sex cannot be comfortably separated from reproduction. Only when there is some risk of conception are they able to enjoy sex. If such a woman is also fearful of the practical consequences of having more children then she is certainly likely to have difficulty in her sexual relationship.

Fear of venereal disease may be adaptive during casual sexual encounters but sometimes, as a form of phobia, it may act as an obstacle to any sexual relationship. Unfortunately we must expect a new wave of phobic reactions in the wake of the AIDS epidemic (see p. 598).

Neurotic disposition and secondary gain: when dealing with sexual phobias, inappropriate beliefs and persistent misunderstandings, we have to ask why the problem often continues in spite of actual experiences or the availability of information which should counter it. Why, for example, does a woman persist in believing that some unspecified harm will result from vaginal intercourse when she is reassured to the contrary by authoritative medical opinion? As with most neurotic fears, we must consider two types of explanation. First, a neurotic disposition, difficult to explain or account for but which is associated with inappropriate learning of anxiety responses. Secondly, the use (presumably unwittingly) of the fear for other purposes — so-called 'secondary gain'. Thus the avoidance of intercourse because of irrational fears may serve the purpose of avoiding the mature adult sexual role that intercourse in some way symbolises. This has relevance to some cases of vaginismus, where sexual arousal from petting is enjoyed but intercourse resisted. One or both partners may be trying to maintain a more child-like role without the responsibilities of adulthood (and certainly parenthood). The sexual problem is then a manifestation of a much broader personality difficulty. Similarly, intercourse may be avoided because it represents the consummation of a marriage for a person who is very ambivalent about the relationship. Such instances provide the sex therapist with some of the most difficult therapeutic problems.

Bad feelings about oneself

Our vulnerability during sexual encounters and our need to feel safe and secure have already been emphasised. It thus follows that we are less likely to feel safe and comfortable when relating to a sexual partner if we are feeling bad about ourselves — if we have low self-esteem. This may be specifically related to body image; we may feel uncomfortable with our bodies, dislike their shape, thinking they are too fat or too thin or just not attractive. This is probably more often an issue for women, who rely so much more on their physical appearance for their self-esteem than men do. Self-esteem may be generally low, as when depressed. If a man is experiencing failure in his job, he feels less effective, less potent as a man and this can adversely affect his sexual relationship. Sometimes the problem is compounded by a need to reassert himself sexually when he is failing to do so in other ways — a return to the adolescent use of sex as a self-esteem booster. Sometimes low self-esteem is best understood as a symptom of a depressive illness.

Bad feelings about one's partner.

There are two emotions which cause havoc with sexual relationships: resentment and insecurity. Often the two are closely related, with insecurity resulting in behaviour which makes you or your partner feel resentful and vice versa.

Anger is a normal emotion which is bound to arise from time to time in any close relationship. We should expect anger to interfere with our sexual feelings — it would be surprising if we could feel angry with and make love to a person at the same time. Some couples may use sex as a way of making up after a row, which usually means that they have already started to resolve their angry feelings when their love-making starts. Others seem able to dissociate sex from other aspects of their relationship with surprising effect, though one wonders what sex means to them in interpersonal terms. For most people, anger and good sex are incompatible though there may be important exceptions, as discussed in relation to sexual assaults in Chapter 13. What is particularly important for sexual problems is the existence of chronic unresolved resentment. It is often striking how much couples fail to recognise the link between some long-standing feeling of hurt or resentment and a decline in their sexual relationship. This stems from one of the links between anger and insecurity. For many people, full acknowledgement of the extent of their resentment is too threatening as it may lead to the loss of their partner or rejection.

We thus have to look at this problem from two viewpoints — the factors in the 'here and now' which provoke or precipitate anger and insecurity and the characteristics of the individuals concerned which make it difficult for them to deal appropriately with these angry feelings when they arise. Let us consider some of these background personality factors first.

Relationships with parents

Most people would agree that the relationships we have with our parents influence to a large extent how we relate to other people and, not surprisingly, to our sexual partners. Our abilities to put trust in the relationship — to feel secure — reflect our childhood relationships with parents, though it is important not to jump to the conclusion that any failure in this respect is necessarily the fault of the parent. The loving parent–child relationship is a two-way process, and in some cases, the detached rejecting parent may be reacting to a lack of the emotional reward that most children give so spontaneously. Problems over control, such as when a mother dominates her son emotionally or is demanding of love from him, may result in a tendency to withdraw from loving relationships to avoid being swamped further. We have already considered the daughter who has felt let down or rejected by her father, and who has problems feeling safe in other relationships with men. Conversely, a continuation of a child-like emotionally dependent relationship between daughter and father and a failure of adequate separation and independence developing during late adolescence may make it more difficult to accept the responsibilities of an adult relationship during marriage. There are many other ways in which the parent–child relationship affects the marriage through what psychoanalysts call 'transference'.

Communication

The ability of a couple to cope with the inevitable vicissitudes of a long-term relationship depends to a great extent on their methods of communication. This involves the communication of both information and feelings which together allow us to assert ourselves and to protect ourselves as two individuals in a relationship. We shall consider such processes more closely when dealing with treatment as these principles provide much of the basis of effective counselling. Ineffective communication not only sustains but also often aggravates problems. How common it is to find couples conforming to a stereotype of the nagging wife who is only too ready to communicate (i.e. complain) and the silent husband who withdraws into his long-suffering shell. An imbalance of this kind has powerfully destructive effects — the husband feels increasingly resentful about being nagged while, the wife, in addition to her burning resentment, feels herself increasingly trapped in this unattractive role of the nagging woman, lowering her self-esteem even further. Dealing inappropriately with anger is often the crux of the problem. Some of us grow up learning to avoid outward expression of anger if at all possible — 'one shouldn't wear one's heart on one's sleeve'. Others fear that if they get angry they might lose control and some irreversible physical or psychological harm would result. Others are reluctant to acknowledge the intensity of their anger towards the person they believe they do or should love. Often, such individuals have seldom if ever experienced full-blown anger in a key relationship and so have not learnt that relationships can indeed survive such storms.

Misinterpretation of a response as motivated by anger when it in fact stems from fear often leads to an escalation of resentment between the couple. One of the fundamental reactions to being hurt is to be able to express that hurt *at the time*. The cause of the hurt is then clear. This is what we mean by self-protection. Both individuals in a pair need to do this, and to expect the other to do the same.

Such is the seedbed of marital discord. Let us look at some of the interpersonal problems that take root and then take their toll on the sexual relationship.

PATTERNS OF MARITAL DISCORD AND BREAKDOWN

There has been much attention paid to the various phases of the marriage cycle and the different types of problem associated with them. One of the clearest and clinically most useful accounts has been presented by Dominian (1985) and I will make use of his description in the following summary.

Marriage can be seen to have three phases: the first lasts approximately 5 years (typically from age 25 to 30); the second is the next 20 years or so, covering the growth of the family unit as well as personal growth of the individual spouses; the third phase, from age 50 onwards, is the postfamily, 'empty nest' phase, when ageing and sometimes physical disability require adjustment. At each phase the relationship functions in five dimensions: social, emotional, sexual, intellectual and spiritual. Each of these dimensions may lead to problems.

Phase 1 — the first 5 years

During this period there are important tasks of separation from both family and premarital friends, organisation of household arrangements, the management of money, commitment to work and to leisure. Any of these aspects may reveal that one or other of the partners is not ready or willing to make the commitment to the relationship that marriage, in its conventional form, demands. We are living in an age when many of the traditional views about marriage are being challenged, mainly by women because they have least to gain from the old view of marriage and most to gain from appropriate change. Nevertheless, expectations still abound and often those of husband and wife do not coincide.

The bartering approach to marriage is a common cause of problems. The assumption is made that in return for material security and companionship the wife will provide sex. If she feels she is missing out on her side of the bargain she will be less inclined to provide sex, or at least her enjoyment of it. Her sexual pleasure becomes a form of currency and both partners suffer the consequence of its withdrawal.

The traditional expectation of wife as home-keeper and child-rearer, often held firmly by both partners, may place the modern wife at a disadvantage compared with her husband. She becomes cut off from her peer group (in particular her previous work-mates); she may be relatively isolated in a semi-rural housing estate, reliant on inadequate public transport. More often than not she is separated from her own mother and extended family and if she has more than one child of pre-school age, there are demands on her patience and resources that are seriously underestimated in our society. This is a stressful time and yet both she and her husband are inclined to the view that she has everything she has always wanted — a home of her own, little children and a loving husband. Her reaction to this situation may make her feel a failure and hence even more depressed than the circumstances already warrant. She will certainly find herself unduly dependent on her husband, who will seem to be much more self-sufficient. Unless he is perceptive and responsive, he will not meet her needs and the seeds of resentment and low self-esteem are sown.

If both partners recognise the size of the wife's task during this early parenting phase of marriage, then mutual support may see them through and sex can continue to provide a powerful binding force in their relationship. Unfortunately, for many couples, there are also needs for basic adjustment in the sexual relationship in these first few years.

Whilst some people decry sex education on the grounds that sex is 'doing what comes naturally', most higher mammals require a fair amount of learning, usually by trial and error, before they are predictably competent in their sexual activity. Humans are no exception. The majority of young couples, particularly those with a minimum amount of previous sexual experience, have a lot of finding out to do, not just about each other but also about themselves, before their sexual relationship settles down to be comfortable and predictably enjoyable.

For some couples, this period of sexual adjustment goes badly, either because of other interpersonal problems, or because of specific difficulties in coping with their sexual responses. The commonest and probably most important example is when the man has a tendency to ejaculate too quickly, and the woman is a little slow to respond. Each may worry about this discrepancy, further aggravating the problem. Premature ejaculation becomes established and the woman gradually loses interest in sex as her way of coping with repeated frustration and disappointment. All too often the problem is tolerated for many years but eventually becomes inextricably tangled with other causes of resentment in the relationship. Once again, poor or inhibited communication (which may be specifically related to sexual matters) has served to turn what should be a normal developmental stage into a chronic difficulty. Sometimes the couple will seek help at an early stage and often benefit from simple counselling with surprising ease.

For those who have established a satisfactory sexual relationship prior to marriage, it is not unusual to experience a sexual decline in the first year or two of marriage. The traditionalist might say that they are paying the price for foregoing premarital chastity but their premarital experience has shown them how good sex can be; it provides a discomforting contrast. Usually in such cases, sex was better before marriage because it was not taken for granted, and for many women was a means of expressing their love. After marriage they are 'contracted to provide it'. In a comparable way the man may, after marriage, feel under pressure to perform sexually.

The first 5 years are the commonest time for marital breakdown to occur.

Phase 2 — the next 20 years

When two young people get married, they still have a great deal of development and growth as individuals ahead of them. After the first phase of adjusting to one another, they may have substantial social changes to cope with, either upwards with career improvement, or downwards with unemployment, problems with alcohol or even chronic illness. The parental role creates its own demands and can lead to tension in the marriage in a variety of ways. Parenting adolescent children, when anxieties about sexuality are often paramount, may have repercussions on the sexuality of the marital relationship.

We have already discussed the ways sex is used to bolster our self-esteem during adolescence — to feel sexually admired is to feel good. The need for this type of reassurance may not only continue into early marriage but will recur at times when, for other reasons, our self-esteem is low. The woman may feel that her physical attractiveness, previously so important to her, is now waning as she gets older. The man in a similar way may feel less virile or less attractive as he sees younger men moving into the ascendancy. Either may then look for reassurance either in overt extramarital affairs, or more commonly by flirtations which, whilst not involving overt sex, may nevertheless be threatening and hurtful to the partner.

Often crises, either for the individual or the relationship, are followed by important stages of personal growth and maturity. Sometimes progress for one partner can be threatening for the other, who may try to resist such change. Of particular importance is the move from traditional dependence of the wife to a state of independence as she establishes a role for herself in her own right which does not depend on being a mother or someone's wife. Increasing recognition of the importance of such changes in the lives of women, particularly in their 30s and 40s has led to popular accounts such as The Cinderella Complex (Dowling 1982), which describes how women have to overcome a basic fear of being on their own before they can risk developing a sense of independence — 'The fear . . that if we really stand on our own feet, we'll end up stranded — unwomanly, unlovely, unloved'.

Phase 3 — from 50 onwards

Most commonly this phase starts with the departure of children from the family home — the 'empty nest'. The presence of children may have provided a powerful reason for the marriage continuing and also served to obscure basic problems in the marriage. With the children gone, these problems become apparent.

Physical changes have to be dealt with. The woman has her menopause to cope with: not only the end of her fertility, which may have been important to her self-esteem, but also troublesome physical or emotional changes as she goes through the transition from pre- to post-menopause. Men are increasingly likely to encounter physical problems, which have their direct effects on sexual function and demand major adjustments to their self-image (see Chapter 5).

THE CLASSIFICATION OF SEXUAL DYSFUNCTION — THE PSYCHOSOMATIC CIRCLE REVISITED

Most texts on clinical sexology consider the aetiology of sexual dysfunction under the types of classification discussed on p. 368. In this chapter I have deliberately avoided this approach, concentrating instead on the psychosomatic circle and so emphasising the need to consider each aspect of the circle in any individual case. Thus whilst physical processes may be important, the psychological component should always be assessed.

These psychological factors also defy categorisation. Although the psychoanalytic literature abounds with descriptions of specific psychological factors leading to particular types of sexual dysfunction (e.g. Main 1976;

see also Kaplan 1974 for many examples), it is difficult to find satisfactory evidence supporting such specific causal links.

People with sexual dysfunction experience distress, though it is often difficult to know to what extent this is a cause or a result of the sexual dysfunction (Derogatis & Meyer 1979). Gender identity problems may be relatively common amongst men with sexual dysfunction (Bancroft 1978; Derogatis & Meyer 1979) but in an apparently non-specific way. Eysenck (1976) found high neuroticism in all types of male and female sexual dysfunction examined by him.

No convincing psychological profile has yet emerged of the man with erectile dysfunction. Munjack et al (1981) found that such men were more psychologically disturbed than sexually normal controls but were not different in this respect from other types of psychiatric patient. It is possible that high neuroticism in such cases is as much a consequence as a cause of the sexual difficulty.

Cooper (1968) found that, compared with other types of male sexual dysfunction, premature ejaculation was more likely to be associated with evidence of neuroticism. Retarded ejaculation has been linked with various kinds of psychological inhibition (Masters & Johnson 1970) but once again there have been no satisfactory studies to test this possibility (Munjack & Kanno 1979).

With female sexual dysfunction, Cooper (1969b) found high neuroticism in women with sexual aversion and vaginismus. A number of descriptions of women with vaginismus have been forthcoming but they lack consistency. Ellison (1972) stresses the importance of ignorance in such women. In contrast, Duddle (1977) found no difference in the level of sex education (or religious belief) between a group of women with vaginismus and a comparison group of family planning clinic attenders. Friedman (1962) gave colourful cameos of three types of women involved: the sleeping beauty who presents ignorance and naivety as a defence and has to be wakened into sexual activity; the Brunhilde who sees sex as a battle in which she has to protect her virtue or virginity and unfortunately wins; and the queen bee who is more interested in getting pregnant than having sex. Unfortunately Friedman does not tell us how common each type is and what proportion of women with vaginismus can be placed into any of these categories. The partners of women with vaginismus are often commented on as passive or lacking in assertiveness. But we cannot say that this is more likely than with other types of sexual dysfunction. It is possible that, as vaginismus is usually a primary problem leading to non-consummation of marriage, the more assertive partners are intolerant of the situation and leave the marriage before treatment is sought.

Fisher (1973) in his study of female orgasm failed to find differences between women with high and low orgasm potential on a large variety of variables, including such things as parental attitudes to sex, religious beliefs and impulsivity. The one difference of interest has already been discussed:

the tendency for the low orgasmic women to be insecure in their relationships and to have had a detached relationship with their father. These predominantly negative findings were supported by Munjack & Staples (1976).

There are two common types of sexual problem which impose particular demands on the sex therapist: erectile dysfunction and low sexual desire.

Erectile dysfunction poses a problem because of the increasing recognition that physical factors are commonly involved, probably more so than in any other type of sexual problem. The evaluation of possible physical disease becomes an important part of assessment and will be considered in more detail in the Chapter 9, when a comprehensive programme of investigation of erectile dysfunction will be considered.

LOW SEXUAL DESIRE

Low sexual desire is a widely used term which covers a very heterogeneous collection of problems and aetiologies requiring very varied treatment approaches, and hence more careful initial clinical analysis and investigation than is necessary for most other types of problem. The various aetiological factors relevant to loss of sexual desire have been considered at different stages of this chapter. Because of the importance of the subject I will briefly summarise them here. The concept of sexual desire or appetite was looked at closely in Chapter 2, when it was emphasised that this essentially experiential concept can be looked at through three 'windows': the cognitive; the affective and the neurophysiological.

Psychological causes

What are the mechanisms that allow psychological processes to interfere with sexual desire? Cognitive processes may interfere with normal sexual desire by relabelling stimuli as non-erotic which would normally be regarded as erotic, or focusing attention on non-erotic or anti-erotic aspects of the situation and hence impeding the normal escalation of the cognition–arousal interaction. Perhaps in some way psychological processes can directly inhibit our desire or appetite. The concept of inhibition is fundamental to neurophysiology. Much of the function of the central nervous system depends on a balance between excitatory and inhibitory signals; the sexual system is probably no exception. The post-ejaculatory refractory period in the male, when there is total unresponsiveness to sexual stimulation and absence of any sexual desire, probably results from active inhibition of the limbic system associated with post-orgasmic 'after-discharges'. It is feasible that some such neurophysiological mechanism mediates between cognitive processes and active inhibition of sexual arousability and its subjective correlate, sexual desire. But at present we can do no more than speculate on such matters. We can however consider the variety of psychological processes which may be involved.

Avoidance of anxiety

The prospect of sexual activity may threaten for a variety of reasons, e.g. failure of sexual response and resulting humiliation (fear of failure); fear of the consequences of sexual activity, such as retribution, guilt or shame (fear of success); fear of loss of control; fear of the consequences in terms of the relationship, e.g. rejection, intimacy or commitment to a relationship towards which there may be considerable ambivalence. Active inhibition of desire may serve to avoid the anxiety provoked by such threats.

Anger and other emotions

The inhibition of sexual desire is a powerful way of expressing anger or hostility to the partner. Probably more frequently, the existence of unresolved anger may simply be incompatible with sexual desire for that person. Other strong emotional states, such as anxiety, fear or disgust, may also serve to block sexual desire by being both incompatible and overwhelming. This is the basis of the 'reciprocal inhibition' approach to treatment when it is assumed that by actively reducing the competing emotion, such as anxiety, the overwhelmed sexual desire is allowed expression.

Non-acceptance of sexual identity

For some individuals the acknowledgement of their sexual desire and the fantasies that manifest it has disturbing implications for their sexual identity. They may be unable to accept that they are homosexual or their principal fantasy may suggest some violent side to their nature. The absence of sexual desire may allow such concerns to be put on one side.

Separation of love and sexuality

One of the most crucial aspects of sexual development is the integration of our sexuality into our loving dyadic relationships. Some individuals find this process difficult, perhaps because of unresolved Oedipal fears or from other sources of learning that one should not be sexual with someone worthy or love. This not infrequently shows itself as a loss of sexual desire when a sexual relationship becomes committed e.g. at engagement or marriage.

Scapegoating

This may occur when it is easier to attribute avoidance of sexual interaction to lack of desire, a state for which one cannot be held responsible, than to admit 'I don't want a sexual relationship with you' or 'I find your body offensive'.

Non-psychological causes

Constitutional

Obviously we have to assume that there will be normal variation and that some individuals, for constitutional reasons, fall at the extremes of the distribution. Some such constitutional factors may be genetically determined, e.g. target organ responsiveness to hormones.

Hormonal

Abnormal hormonal states are occasionally the cause of low sexual desire. Androgen deficiency has already been described, though in younger men this is an unusual cause. In older men relative androgen deficiency may be more common. There is a decline in both sexual desire and androgen levels with advancing age, and there is some evidence that these two phenomena may be causally related (see p. 293). The other principal hormone shown to have sexual effects in men is prolactin. Hyperprolactinaemic states in men are also rare but they are usually associated with loss of sexual interest and often with erectile dysfunction. It is probable that the effect of the high prolactin is similar to the effect of androgen deficiency; loss of desire is the primary effect and erectile problems are a psychogenic reaction to this change.

Metabolic

In any state of disturbed metabolism, as with illness or trauma, there is likely to be a loss of sexual desire. In most cases the specific reason for this is not understood, although in some circumstances, such as renal dialysis, specific biochemical mechanisms have been implicated (see p. 567).

Pharmacological

Drugs are also likely to have varied effects. There may be direct central inhibitory effects on sexual desire, or less specifically, sedation which interferes with normal sexual arousability. Alternatively direct pharmacological interference with sexual responses such as erection may result in psychological reactions leading to loss of desire.

Mood disturbance

The importance of mood has already been emphasised, and may influence how we view a sexual situation, or how we see ourselves as sexual beings.

In women we have found sexual feelings to be strongly related to general well-being, varying during the menstrual cycle (see p. 108) and there is no reason why men should not show a comparable relationship. Sexual desire is commonly though not invariably reduced during depressive and enhanced during hypomanic illnesses and persistent loss of sexual desire often starts at the time of a depressive illness, continuing after the mood has returned to normal (Schreiner-Engel & Schiavi 1986).

CONCLUSIONS

The message should now be proclaimed loud and clear that typologies of sexual dysfunction, at least with our present state of knowledge, simply serve to obscure the varied and often unique ways in which individuals and couples present with sexual problems. Only if we attempt to understand the interaction between the psychic and somatic processes in each individual do we begin to obtain a picture of therapeutic relevance. With few exceptions the precise type of dysfunction tells us relatively little about the approach to treatment we should use or the problems we are likely to encounter on the way.

PROBLEMS RELATED TO HOMOSEXUALITY

In the Edinburgh Survey for a 3-year period 1981–84 (Warner et al 1987), 18 men (out of 535) and one woman (out of 577) presented at clinics with problems relating to homosexuality. This contrasts with the 12% of males and 1–2% of females presented at the Oxford clinic 8–9 years earlier (Bancroft & Colen 1976) and reinforces my clinical impression that the number of people seeking help in relation to homosexuality has decreased over the past 20 years. Probably most of this reduction in attendance at heterosexually oriented sexual problem clinics is in those seeking treatment for their homosexuality. What is not clear is how many gay men or lesbian women would welcome help for sexual problems with their homosexual relationships.

Bell & Weinberg (1978) placed 12% of their male homosexuals and 5% of the lesbians into the dysfunctional category, with psychological problems related to their sexuality. They also found that their homosexual subjects sought professional help more often than heterosexuals (see p. 319) but the help homosexuals are likely to receive is strongly influenced by the attitudes of professionals to homosexuality. In one anonymous survey of American doctors, three-quarters of respondents admitted that their medical management of a patient would be adversely affected by knowledge of his or her homosexuality (Pauly & Goldstein 1970). Many homosexuals find that whatever their problems (medical or psychological) a heterosexual doctor is likely to attribute them in some way to their homosexual lifestyle. This must have a powerfully discouraging effect on their attempts to seek appropriate help. In Masters & Johnson's (1979) study of homosexuality, more than half of the couples or individuals who were treated by them had sought treatment for their sexual problem previously and of those, about three-quarters had been refused help, many more than once.

There are now an increasing number of professionals who are keen to offer help to homosexuals either as couples or as individuals. But we are left with a legacy of understandable suspicion in the homosexual community. There are various counselling organisations intended specifically for homosexuals or other sexual minorities which provide an important service in this respect, but it is difficult to know to what extent they meet the needs of this part of the population. The Albany Trust, a voluntary counselling organisation in London, had about 440 people contact them during 1978. Of these, about 35% were homosexual or bisexual (Albany Trust, personal communication).

The sexual problems related to homosexuality can be roughly divided into two types — sexual problems (e.g. dysfunction) affecting homosexual relationships, and dissatisfaction or concern with being homosexual or a desire to establish heterosexual relationships.

The first type of problem — the ordinary sexual difficulties of homosexuals — seldom presents at sexual problem clinics. Paff (1985) has reported on the types of sexual dysfunction in gay men seeking treatment from therapists identified with the gay movement. Broadly speaking, their problems are similar to those of heterosexual men, with some interesting differences. Aversion towards anal sex is one charactistically gay male problem, whereas premature ejaculation seems to be less common than amongst heterosexual men.

Masters and Johnson (1979), during a 10-year period, received requests for help from 54 male and 13 female homosexuals who were wanting conversion to heterosexuality. They were only accepted for treatment if they presented with an opposite-sex partner. More noteworthy is the fact that during the same 10 years they saw 81 homosexual couples (56 male and 25 female) seeking help for sexual dysfunction. In this group, there were only two cases of premature ejaculation and none of ejaculatory incompetence. The remainder all complained of erectile failure, though four were also sexually aversive. All the females were categorised as 'anorgasmic'. We have already commented on Masters and Johnson's use of this term (see p. 367). These authors made the interesting observations that whereas 'sexual fakery' is common amongst heterosexual women and rare amongst heterosexual men, homosexual men could conceal their sexual dysfunction (e.g. erectile failure) by restricting themselves to a servicing or passive role, and provided they were only involved in casual sexual relationships, could avoid confrontation with their sexual inadequacy. (Paff (1985) commented that erectile problems were less likely to occur during casual encounters.) Amongst the lesbians who were usually in committed relationships, sexual fakery was less common than amongst heterosexual women. Masters & Johnson attributed this in part to the lesbian's ability to admit orgasmic difficulty to her partner with less loss of face than her heterosexual counterpart.

Masters & Johnson approached the treatment of their dysfunctional homosexual couples in much the same way as with their heterosexual pairs. The implication is that the psychological problems are basically similar, or at least respond to the same style of approach. We will consider treatment methods both for the dysfunctional homosexual couples and the individual seeking conversion to heterosexuality more closely in Chapter 9.

Clearly, there are consequences of homosexual stigmatisation with which heterosexuals do not have to contend. But it remains an interesting question whether there are interpersonal problems that are specifically homosexual. Wilson (1977) offers a series of translations of 'what the individual's unconscious is most often pantomiming' in cases of homosexual impotence. Each one is strikingly reminiscent of many heterosexual relationships. Wilson then refers to a 'sameness problem', a tendency to over-emphasise shared traits whilst overlooking the differences between each other. Although this concept needs further clarification, it does raise a potentially important issue. The heterosexual couple, in working out and maintaining their individual identities within the relationship may rely a great deal on male–female differences to accommodate the differences between them. A homosexual pair cannot do that.

A common psychoanalytic idea is that homosexuals have problems in existing as separate individuals (Rosen 1978). Separation anxiety is thus seen as a causal factor in the development of homosexuality. Considering that such psychoanalytic explanatory theories are usually based on retrospective studies of adults, it is equally likely, if not more so, that separation anxiety may be a consequence of the homosexual role. We should not underestimate the power of the social institution of marriage in alleviating fears of isolation. The homosexual is not only lacking in that external support to his relationships, he also has to contend with a variety of factors that serve to undermine those relationships. The male tendency to polygamous relationships (see p. 274) when tempered by the more monogamous nature of women gives the serial monogamy of the heterosexual world a greater chance. For the male homosexual, there is no such constraint and the bilateral polygamous tendencies of male homosexual relationships may present particular problems.

PROBLEMS RELATING TO TRANSSEXUALISM AND OTHER TYPES OF SEXUAL DEVIANCE

TRANSSEXUALS

Almost invariably a transsexual seeking help from a sexual problem clinic is wanting medical assistance in the form of hormones and sex re-assignment surgery. In the USA, a numer of gender identity clinics have been established which provide a specialist service for transsexuals and combine the professional skills of psychologists, psychiatrists, endocrinologists and surgeons. They tend to attract patients from a wide area, making assessment of incidence difficult (see Chapter 7). In the UK, specialist clinics have not developed to the same extent. There are one or two in the London area and an occasional one outside London.

Some transsexuals seeking help have brief contacts with a series of clinics because, with often quite disturbed personalities, they seek unrealistic and immediate solutions and move from one clinician to another as soon as they fail to get what they demand. Others are prepared to stay with a particular clinic in a relatively long-term attempt to resolve their problems, provided that they feel confident that the clinician is intent on helping them achieve a satisfactory sexual role re-assignment and is not just playing for time. Such patients pose considerable demands on clinical resources and their management will be considered in Chapter 10.

OTHER FORMS OF DEVIANT SEXUALITY

During a 3-year period in the Edinburgh Sexual Problem Clinics only 12 men and 1 woman came into this category.

Occasionally a cross-dresser, a fetishist or a sadomasochist will present asking for help to modify or remove his particular sexual preference. More often he will present with his partner as a result of the marital tension their sexual activity has produced. The wife may be putting him under pressure to seek treatment or the man may be hoping that the therapist can persuade the wife to accept, or at least tolerate, the deviant pattern. Such cases can often be seen primarily as relationship problems and their management will be discussed in Chapter 10.

The sexual offender, who comes into contact with the helping professions as a consequence of criminal proceedings against him, presents a special case. He will be considered separately in Chapter 13.

REFERENCES

Ashdown R R, Gilanpour H 1974 Venous drainage of the corpus cavernosum in impotent and normal bulls. Journal of Anatomy 117: 159
Athanasiou R, Shaver P, Tavris C 1970 Sex. Psychology Today 4th July 39–52
Bailey M J, Yaude S, Walmsley B, Pryor J P 1985 Surgery for Peyronie's disease. British Journal of Urology 57: 746–749
Bancroft J 1978 Gender identity and sexual dysfunction in the male. In: Levi L (ed) Society, stress and disease, vol 3. The productive and reproductive age. Oxford University Press, Oxford
Bancroft J 1980 Psychophysiology of sexual dysfunction. In: van Praag H M, Lader M H, Rafaelson O J, Sachar E J (eds) Handbook of biological psychiatry. Dekker, New York, pp 359–392
Bancroft J 1984 Interaction of psychosocial and biological factors in marital sexuality — differences between men and women. British Journal of Guidance and Counselling 12: 62–71

Bancroft J, Coles L 1976 Three years experience in a sexual problems clinic. British
    Medical Journal 1: 1575–1577
Begg A, Dickerson M, Loudon N B 1976 Frequency of self-reported sexual problems in a
    family planning clinic. Journal of Family Planning Doctors 2: 41–48
Bell A P, Weinberg M S 1978 Homosexualities. A study of diversity among men and
    women. Mitchell Beazley, London
Brindley G S 1984 New treatment for priapism. Lancet July 28th 220
Brindley G S, Gillan P 1982 Men and women who do not have orgasms. British Journal of
    Psychiatry 140: 351–356
Broude G J, Greene S J 1980 Cross-cultural codes on 20 sexual attitudes and practices. In:
    Berry H, Schlegel A (eds) Cross-cultural samples and codes. University of Pittsburgh
    Press, Pittsburgh, pp 313–333
Burnap D W, Golden J S 1967 Sexual problems in medical practice. Journal of Medical
    Education 42: 673–680
Chesser E 1956 The sexual, marital and family relationships of the English woman. Rox
    Publisher, New York
Chester R, Walker C 1979 Sexual experience attitudes of British women. In: Chester R,
    Peel J (eds) Changing patterns of sexual behaviour. Academic Press, London
Clark A L, Wallin P 1965 Women's sexual responsiveness and the duration and quality of
    their marriages. American Journal of Sociology 71: 187–196
Cooper A J 1968 'Neurosis' and disorders of sexual potency in the male. Journal of
    Psychosomatic Research 12: 141–144
Cooper A J 1969a A clinical study of 'coital anxiety' in male potency disorders. Journal of
    Psychosomatic Research 13: 143–147
Cooper A J 1969b Some personality factors in frigidity. Journal of Psychosomatic Research
    13: 149–155
Derogatis L R, Meyer J K 1979 A psychological profile of the sexual dysfunctions.
    Archives of Sexual Behaviour 8: 201–224
Dominian J 1985 Patterns of marital breakdown. In: Dryden W (ed) Marital therapy in
    Britain, vol 1. Harper & Row, London
Dowling C 1982 The Cinderella complex: woman's hidden fear of independence. Fontana
Duddle M 1977 Aetiological factors in the unconsummated marriage. Journal of
    Psychosomatic Research 21: 157–60
Ebbehøj J, Wagner G 1979 Insufficient penile erection due to abnormal drainage of
    cavernous bodies. Urology 13: 507–510
Edwards A E, Husted J R 1976 Penile sensitivity, age and sexual behaviour. Journal of
    Clinical Psychology 32: 697–700
Ellison C 1972 Vaginismus. Medical Aspects of Human Sexuality 6(8): 34–54
Eysenck H J 1976 Sex and personality. Open Books, London
Fisher S 1973 The female orgasm. Basic Books, New York
Fox C A 1970 Reduction in the rise of systolic blood pressure during human coitus by the
    β-adrenergic blocking agent — propranolol. Journal of Reproduction and Fertility
    22: 587–590
Frank E, Anderson C, Rubinstein D 1978 Frequency of sexual dysfunction in 'normal'
    couples. New England Journal of Medicine 299: 111–115
Frenken J 1976 Afkeer van seksualiteit. English summary: Van Loghum Slaterus, Deventer
    pp 219–225.
Frenken J, Van Tol P 1987 Sexual problems in gynecological practice. Journal of
    Psychosomatic Obstetrics and Gynaecology 6: 143–155
Friedman L J 1962 Virgin wives. Tavistock Publications, London
Garde K, Lunde I 1980a Female sexual behavior. A study in a random sample of 40 year
    old women. Maturitas 2: 225–240
Garde K, Lunde I 1980b Social background and social status; influence on female sexual
    behaviour. A random sample study of 40-year-old Danish women. Maturitas 2: 241–246
Gebhard P H 1978 Marital stress. In: Levi L (ed) Society, stress and disease, vol 3. The
    productive and reproductive age. Oxford University Press, Oxford
Gebhard P H, Johnson A B 1979 The Kinsey data: marginal tabulations of the 1938–1963
    interviews conducted by the Institute for Sex Research. Saunders, Philadelphia
Golombok S, Rust J, Pickard C 1984 Sexual problems encountered in general practice.
    British Journal of Sexual Medicine 11: 210–212

Hagstad A, Janson P O 1984 Sexuality among Swedish women around 40 — an epidemiological survey. Journal of Psychosomatic Obstetrics and Gynaecology 3: 191–204

Hartman W E, Fithian M A 1972 Treatment of sexual dysfunction. Center for Marital and Sexual Studies, Long Beach

Higgins G E 1979 Sexual response in spinal cord injured adults: a review. Archives of Sexual Behavior 8: 173–196

Hinman F Jr 1960 Priapism; reason for failure of therapy. Journal of Urology 83: 420–428

Hite S 1976 The Hite report: a nationwide study of female sexuality. Dell, New York

Hunt M 1974 Sexual behavior in the 1970s. Playboy Press, Chicago

Kaplan H S 1974 The new sex therapy. Brunner/Mazel, New York

Kinsey A C, Pomeroy W B, Martin C E 1948 Sexual behavior in the human male. Saunders, Philadelphia

Kinsey A C, Pomeroy W B, Martin C E, Gebhard P H 1953 Sexual behavior in the human female. Saunders, Philadelphia

Kline-Graber B 1978 Diagnosis and treatment procedures of pubococcygeal deficiencies in women. In: Lo Piccolo J, Lo Piccolo L (eds) Handbook of sex therapy. Plenum, New York

Kräupl-Taylor F 1979 Penis captivus — did it occur? British Medical Journal ii: 977–78

Lazarus R S 1966 Psychological stress and the coping process. McGraw Hill, New York

Levin R J, Levin A 1975 Sexual pleasure. The surprising preference of 100 000 women. Redbook Magazine September: 51–58

Levine S B, Yost M A 1976 Frequency of sexual dysfunction in a general gynaecological clinic: an epidemiological approach. Archives of Sexual Behavior 5: 229–38

Levitt E E, Konovsky M, Freese M P, Thompson J P 1979 Intravaginal pressure assessed by the Kegel perineometer. Archives of Sexual Behavior 8: 425–430

Lundberg P O, Osterman P O 1974 The benign and malignant forms of orgasmic cephalgia. Headache 14: 164–165

Main T F 1976 Impotence. In: Milne H, Hardy S J (eds) Psychosexual problems. Crosby Lockwood Staples, London

Masters W H, Johnson V E 1970 Human sexual inadequacy. Churchill, London

Masters W H, Johnson V E 1979 Homosexuality in perspective. Little, Brown, Boston

Melody G F 1977 My most unusual sexual case. A case of penis captivus. Medical Aspects of Human Sexuality ii: 111

Michal V 1982 Arterial disease as a cause of impotence. Clinics in Endocrinology and Metabolism 11(3): 725–748

Milne H B 1976 The role of the psychiatrist. In: Milne H, Hardy S J (eds) Psychosexual problems. Crosby Lockwood Staples, London

Money J, Yankowitz R 1967 The sympathetic inhibiting effects of the drug Ismelin on human male eroticism, with a note on Melleril. Journal of Sexual Research 3: 69–00

Munjack D J, Kanno P H 1979 Retarded ejaculation: a review. Archives of Sexual Behavior 8: 139–150

Munjack D J, Staples F R 1976 Psychological characteristics of women with sexual inhibition (frigidity) in sex clinics. Journal of Nervous and Mental Diseases 163: 117–23

Munjack D J, Oziel L J, Kanno P H, Whipple K, Leonard M D 1981 Psychological characteristics of males with secondary erectile failure. Archives of Sexual Behavior 10: 123–132

Nettelbladt P, Uddenberg N 1979 Sexual dysfunction and sexual satisfaction in 58 married Swedish men. Journal of Psychosomatic Research 23: 141–147

Pauly I, Goldstein S 1970 Physician's attitudes in treating male homosexuals. Medical Aspects of Human Sexuality 4: 26–45

Paff B A 1985 Sexual dysfunction in gay men requesting treatment. Journal of Sexual Marital Therapy 11: 3–18

Raboch J, Bartak V 1981 Menarche and orgastic capacity. Archives of Sexual Behavior 10: 379–392

Raboch J, Bartak V 1983 Coitarche and orgastic capacity. Archives of Sexual Behavior 12: 409–414

Raboch J, Starka L 1973 Reported coital activity of men and levels of plasma testosterone. Archives of Sexual Behavior 2: 309–16

Rainwater L 1966 Some aspects of lower class sexual behavior. Journal of Social Issues 22: 96–108

Rhind J R 1987 Peyronie's disease. British Journal of Sexual Medicine 14: 16–19

Rose F C, Petty R G 1982 Sexual headache. British Journal of Sexual Medicine 9: 20–21

Rosen I 1978 Sexual deviation, 2nd edn. Oxford University Press, Oxford

Sanders D 1985 The Woman book on love and sex. Joseph, London

Sanders D 1987 The Woman report on men. Sphere, London

Schmidt G 1977 Working class and middle-class adolescents. In: Money J, Musaph H (eds) Handbook of sexology. Elsevier, North Holland

Schreiner-Engel P, Schiavi R 1986 Lifetime psychopathology in individuals with low sexual desire. Journal of Nervous and Mental Diseases 174: 646–651

Segraves R T, 1985 Psychiatric drugs and orgasm in the human female. Journal of Psychosomatic Obstetrics and Gynaecology 4: 125–128

Segraves R T, Schoenberg H W, Zarins C K, Knopf J, Camic P 1982 Referral of impotent patients to a sexual dysfunction clinic. Archives of Sexual Behavior 11: 521–528

Shackman R 1974 Priapism. British Journal of Sexual Medicine 1: 6–10

Sharpe L, Kuriansky J B, O'Connor J F 1976 A preliminary classification of human functional sexual disorder. Journal of Sex and Marital Therapy 2: 106–114

Skaakebaek N E, Bancroft J, Davidson D W, Warner P 1981 Androgen replacement with oral testosterone undecanoate in hypogonadal men: a double blind controlled study. Clinical Endocrinology 14: 49–61

Slag M F, Morley J E, Elson M K et al 1983 Impotence in medical clinic outpatients. Journal of the American Medical Association 249: 1736–1740

Slater E, Woodside M 1951 Patterns of marriage. A study of marriage relationships — the urban working classes. Cassell, London

Smith B H 1966 Peyronie's disease. American Journal of Clinical Pathology 45: 670–677

Smith B H 1969 Subclinical Peyronie's disease. American Journal of Clinical Pathology 52: 385

Solnick R L, Birren J 1977 Age and male erectile responsiveness. Archives of Sexual Behavior 6: 1–10

Swan M, Wilson L J 1979 Sexual and marital problems in a psychiatric outpatient population. British Journal of Psychiatry 135: 310–14

Tavris C, Sadd S 1977 The Redbook report of female sexuality. Delacorte, New York

Terman L M 1951 Correlates of orgasm adequacy in a group of 556 wives. Journal of Psychology 32: 115–172

Thorns B, Collard J 1979 Who divorces? Routledge & Kegan Paul, London

Warner P, Bancroft J and members of the Edinburgh Human Sexuality Group 1987 A regional service for sexual problems: a 3-year study. Sexual and Marital Therapy 2: 115–126

Wellwood J M, Bultitude M I, Rickford C, Lea Thomas M 1972 The role of corpus-saphenous by-pass in the treatment of priapism. British Journal of Urology 44: 607–611

Whitelaw G P, Smithwick R H 1951 Some secondary effects of sympathectomy: with particular reference to disturbance of sexual function. New England Journal of Medicine 245: 121–130

Wilson B 1977 Counselling the male homosexual. In: Money J, Musaph H (eds) Handbook of sexology. Excerpta Medica, Amsterdam

9

Assessing people with sexual problems

The clinician or sex therapist will be confronted with sexual problems in a variety of settings, as we shall see in Chapter 11. The approach taken will vary according to the setting and the expectations of the patient, though in *every* case it is important to facilitate comfortable unembarrased discussion of sexual topics with the patient.

In this chapter I will focus on one particular setting — the specialist clinic for sexual problems. This may be found in a variety of situations. The common feature is that the patient or couple will have been referred or have referred themselves for help with a sexual problem. In other words, the sexual nature of the problem has already been declared when the patient is first seen.

In Chapter 8 the increasing recognition of the role of physical factors in sexual dysfunction, especially in the male, was emphasised. It is now clear that in any sexual problem clinic there should be easy access to someone medically qualified who can carry out a physical examination and organise other types of physical investigation when indicated; preferably someone trained in sex therapy or at least who is comfortable talking about sex. As far as male sexual dysfunction is concerned there has been a growth of interest in a variety of investigative techniques, though as yet most of these tests are available only in a few centres. Only very recently have such procedures become available in National Health Service hospitals. Unfortunately there has been a notable shortage of rigorous research aimed at evaluating the cost-effectiveness and clinical usefulness of such techniques (LoPiccolo 1985). I will provide an overall framework of assessment in which such procedures are given a potential place. And in the latter part of the chapter I will consider each of the main procedures in closer detail. In chapter 8 the psychosomatic nature of sexuality was emphasised. My attention to physical methods of investigation in this chapter in no way detracts from the importance of psychosomatic interactions. Unfortunately much of the recent literature on the subject, especially concerning male dysfunction, is preoccupied with distinguishing between organic and psychogenic aetiology. It is important to assume that both types of factor

412

are likely to be involved in each case. It is a question of assessing the relative importance of each, how they interact and how this affects prognosis and the most suitable form of management.

THE OBJECTIVES OF THE INITIAL INTERVIEW

In most busy clinics time is limited. In our Edinburgh clinics we usually allow 1 hour for initial assessment. At the end of that time a number of practical decisions have to be made. The main purpose of the interview, therefore, is to obtain the information necessary for those decisions. Is couple therapy or another form of psychological treatment indicated? The therapist needs to consider whether focusing on the sexual relationship is appropriate (see Chapter 10) and whether both partners are sufficiently committed to improving the relationship to make counselling worthwhile. In order for the couple or individual patient to reach that decision they must have a reasonable idea of what treatment involves and what sort of commitment they would be making if they were to accept treatment. It may be appropriate for them to make their decision before leaving the clinic. If they have any uncertainties they should be encouraged to go away and discuss the matter together and then let the therapist know their decision. A fair proportion do not accept such offers of treatment, often for reasons which are not clear.

Is a physical examination required? Are physical methods of investigation needed? Many sex therapists take the view that a thorough physical examination is mandatory in every case (e.g. Kolodny et al 1979). I do not accept this view. The type of extensive examination advocated by Kolodny and his colleagues is time-consuming and expensive. There is as yet no evidence to indicate that the routine use of such examinations for every person presenting with a sexual problem would justify the cost and other practical disadvantages involved. There are many cases where counselling can proceed without such an examination, particularly when relationships appear to be of primary importance. But it is important for both medical and non-medical clinical staff to have guidelines as to when physical examination and investigations *are* indicated.

Genital examination has two purposes; diagnostic and educational or therapeutic. For the first, medical training is necessary and in many cases specialist skills such as those of gynaecologist or urologist are required. For educational or therapeutic purposes, on the other hand, such as explaining to a woman her genital anatomy, helping her to explore it and perhaps showing her how to insert dilators, a suitably trained non-medical therapist may be entirely suitable. It should always be made clear to the patient in those circumstances that the examination is not being used for medical diagnostic purposes.

414 HUMAN SEXUALITY AND ITS PROBLEMS

THE INITIAL ASSESSMENT INTERVIEW

Sex therapists vary in how they manage this first interview, particularly when seeing a couple. The couple may be interviewed together or separately. The method used in our clinic will be described here.

The first few minutes are intended primarily to establish rapport and to set the patient or couple at ease. At this stage both partners are seen together. The contents of the referral letter are discussed to check that it is correct and to give patients an idea of what the therapist already knows about them. Their feelings about coming to the clinic are then explored. This often gives an opportunity to express anxiety, embarrassment or ambivalence.

For couples the next stage of the interview is carried out on an individual basis. One of the partners, usually the one without the presenting problem, is asked to wait outside. After about 20 minutes they change round and the last 10 minutes or so of the interview are used to see the couple jointly again.

During the course of the individual interview the following points are covered:

1. The precise nature of the sexual problem. Often the problem presented by the patient or referring agency turns out to be misleading, e.g. 'erectile impotence' may, after careful enquiry, prove to be severe premature ejaculation, with erection being lost after ejaculation but before vaginal entry. The level of sexual desire or spontaneous interest should also be established.
2. The history of the sexual problem. The early stages in the development of a problem are often of crucial significance to treatment. It is common to find in the history of women presenting with loss of sexual interest or impaired sexual responses that they were responsive at an early stage of the relationship but were repeatedly frustrated by their partners' premature ejaculation. This not only indicates a need for help with the ejaculation problem but also serves to establish a less one-sided view of the couple's difficulty. Were there particular times of change in the sexual relationship and if so what was going on in their lives at those times?
3. The nature of the general relationship (if a stable sexual relationship exists) and other details of the immediate family and children. It is of particular importance to assess the extent of marital disharmony. Although it may be difficult at this stage to know whether marital tension is the cause or the result of the sexual problem, it will influence the couple's ability to work together in joint counselling.
4. Psychiatric history: the recognition of depression is important. Its relevance to sexual desire has already been emphasised (p. 375). If too severe, it may interfere with counselling and more specific treatment of depression may be indicated first. However, it is important to recognise

that depressed mood is commonly a reaction to marital or sexual difficulties, and by acknowledging the importance of those difficulties and tackling them directly, considerable improvement in mood may result. This can be a difficult judgement for the clinician, but there is a tendency, particularly for women, to collude with the partner in seeing themselves as suffering from a depressive illness rather than reacting to an unhappy marital situation. This can further lower the woman's self-esteem or intensify her depression. The therapist should be careful not to fall into this trap.

5. Medical history. Evidence of recent health (e.g. exercise) or illness is important. Particularly careful enquiry should be made of any drugs being used and for how long. Earlier medical history is also often important in understanding the early stages of a sexual problem, e.g. did if first become noticeable after a transient physical illness or accident?

6. Contraceptive history. Contraceptives may interfere with sexual enjoyment in a variety of ways (see Chapter 12) and may occasionally be the principal cause of the problem. A reappraisal of suitable contraception is therefore appropriate at this stage. Also, in many couples with severe sexual difficulties, contraception may have been abandoned as unnecessary. In such cases the couple should be advised to reorganise a suitable method before embarking upon sex therapy. Sometimes, when the couple is also keen to start a pregnancy, they may be reluctant to use any contraception for that reason. We encourage them to do so nevertheless, explaining that it is more sensible to concentrate on improving the sexual relationship first, without other possible complications of pregnancy or fear of pregnancy.

7. Attitudes to the sexual problem and possible treatment. By the end of the initial interview patients' attitudes and expectations about the nature of the problem and suitable treatment should be apparent. They may prefer to see their problem in physical terms and deny the importance of psychological factors. This will determine the acceptability of different treatment methods: counselling, particularly involving the partner, may be rejected on those grounds. The attitude of the partner is also crucial. Is he or she prepared to accept any responsibility for tackling the problem? Sometimes strong rejection by partners of any involvement in treatment may indicate some fear that they have problems they would rather not acknowledge. Special efforts by the therapist may then be required gradually to win the trust and confidence of the partner. In such cases, decisions about treatment may need to be delayed until further interviews have been completed.

The therapist should always be cautious in concluding that a patient is insufficiently motivated for psychological treatment. Often the only way such motivation can be properly determined is to make an offer of treatment and see if it is accepted. Sometimes what appears to be poor motivation is in reality ambivalence. Time may be needed to work through the ambivalence before a clear commitment to treatment emerges.

Let us now consider in more detail some of the more important points that need to be covered when assessing first women and then men. An exhaustive history is usually not required at the initial interview, particularly when it seems likely that sex therapy is to be involved. Often the best time to obtain more sensitive information is during the course of treatment when obstacles to behavioural change make such information more immediately relevant (see p. 470). It is also worth remembering that in the course of such an interview a great deal of highly confidential and sensitive information can be obtained which does not turn out to be of any relevance to the patient's management. It is therefore an ethical requirement that as far as possible we obtain no more information than seems to be appropriate and relevant at each stage of our intervention.

ASSESSING THE WOMAN

What attitude does the woman have to her body? Is she comfortable with nakedness? Does she have a particular concern about weight and is there evidence of abnormal eating patterns?

Does she feel spontaneous sexual desire? This usually requires more careful questioning of women than of men, as women are less likely to express their desire in explicit sexual approaches (though subtle proceptive cues may be evident). It is often necessary to make the clear distinction between spontaneous desire and desire which is part of a response to the partner's love-making. Does she feel attracted to others, apart from her regular partner? Does her sexual desire vary predictably with her menstrual cycle?

How does she experience menstruation? Does she have substantial perimenstrual mood change? If so, what effect does this have on her relationship? How does she cope with her periods? Are they heavy or painful? Does she use tampons? Such questions sometimes throw considerable light on a woman's attitudes to her genitalia. Has she been having other gynaecological problems, in particular vaginal infections, soreness or discharges?

A history of pain or soreness during sexual activity requires careful questioning. The history is often highly informative. Does her vagina lubricate during love-making? When is the pain experienced? Is it on initial entry of the penis, easing once the penis is inserted? Is it felt at the introitus or deeper in the vaginal barrel? Is it brought on by deep thrusting? Does the vagina feel sore after intercourse and for how long? Is the pain related to posture during love-making? Does she have a tendency to back pain and if so does she get backache after sexual intercourse?

Does she usually experience orgasm during love-making? If so, is this an enjoyable experience for her? Questions about orgasm often lead to hints that direct clitoral stimulation is required. This should be made explicit and appropriate reassurance given. Is there any indication of performance anxiety about orgasm? Does she masturbate on her own? (Attitudes to masturbation are often informative.) What sort of lover is her husband? Does he have problems with erection or does he ejaculate too soon? How sensitive is he to her needs? How does she feel about *his* body; does she mind touching or caressing his genitalia?

Were her early sexual experiences positive ones? This is an opportunity to invite information about sexual abuse during childhood or adolescence, though some women only feel safe enough to reveal such experiences once they have established a secure therapeutic relationship.

Indications for physical examination of the female

1. A complaint of pain or discomfort during sexual activity.
2. Recent history of ill health or physical symptoms apart from the sexual problem.
3. Recent onset of loss of sexual desire with no apparent cause.
4. Any woman in the peri- or post-menopausal age group with a sexual problem.
5. History of marked menstrual irregularities or infertility.
6. History of abnormal puberty or other endocrine disorder.
7. When the patient believes that a physical cause is most likely, or suspects there is something abnormal about her genitalia.

The timing of the physical examination is important. For women who are particularly apprehensive about being examined it may be appropriate to delay until a more secure therapeutic relationship has developed, though in such cases it should be made clear that an examination needs to be carried out at some stage.

Physical examination of the female

Whilst a general physical examination, including cardiovascular system, central nervous system, respiratory system etc. is often necessary, it is the genital examination which is of special relevance to the sexologist and which requires our particular consideration.

The psychological reaction of the patient to such an examination may give important information in addition to the direct results of the examination itself. As described in Chapter 11, such reactions provide the essence of the Balint approach to treatment. We do not see the examination as having such a crucial part to play as this, but there is no doubt that additional information of a psychological kind is often forthcoming. More important is the impact that the whole procedure has on the relationship between the examining doctor and the patient, particularly if the doctor is also the therapist.

If the examination is carried out in a sensitive manner it may have a constructive, positive effect on the therapeutic relationship. If carried out insensitively it may make treatment with that particular therapist difficult if not impossible.

How the examining doctor maintains his own comfort in this situation may be crucial. Some adopt an attitude of indifference to the patient's sexuality, deflect any reference to the topic with hearty jocularity, or deter it with an aloof aseptic clinical approach. Some tend to heavy-handedness during genital examination, to ensure that gentleness of touch is not mistaken for a caress. If the examination is to achieve its aims, however, it must be conducted in a gentle, relaxed, unhurried but thorough manner. Touching apart, an adequate sexological examination also calls for close and detailed visual inspection of the genitalia, in a manner which is not a customary part of clinical routine, when a cursory glance is usually regarded as more appropriate than a prolonged gaze. Opportunities should be taken to explain details of the patient's anatomy and physiology during the examination process. The use of a mirror can be valuable at this stage.

There is therefore a need to combine the sensitivity and perceptive awareness of the trained therapist with the physical expertise of gynaecologist or urologist.

Genital examination of the female

Many women have described vaginal examinations as distasteful, embarrassing and physically uncomfortable experiences, from which they have emerged feeling demeaned or sullied — an experience which detracts from their sense of sexual self-respect. In contrast, the aim during the examination of a patient with sexual dysfunction should not be merely to avoid inflicting discomfort and embarrassment but also to contribute to the therapeutic process, endorsing the patient's sexuality and enhancing her sense of sexual self-assurance.

In western cultures, the doctor should usually maintain eye contact and relevant conversation with the patient during the vaginal examination. But he should also be sensitive to the patient's cultural and personal background. For example, women from traditional Muslim or Hindu cultures may prefer to conceal their faces behind a sari or sheet during the examination, or if their face is exposed, may adopt an expression of exaggerated distaste, as if to demonstrate their respectability. The style of the examination therefore requires to be adapted to the individual patient.

Good lighting from an adjustable source is important. If during examination the patient's abdomen and thighs are kept covered by a draping sheet, she will be more ready to abduct her thighs widely, which is essential if the examination is to be comfortable and informative. When a self-lubricated disposable plastic glove is worn, it is rarely necessary to use more than a trace of lubricating jelly, providing that the labia minora are gently held apart by the fingers of the left hand, thus everting their moist medial surfaces while the examining finger or speculum is introduced.

In these circumstances, it is advisable to use a smaller than normal size of bivalve speculum such as a Brewer's or Cusco's. It should be near body temperature and the blades should be lubricated with a thin film of jelly. The handle of the speculum should be directed posteriorly to ensure minimal contact with the more sensitive areas of the clitoris and urethral meatus. Besides, only with the handle in this position is it possible to keep the instrument to its full depth within the vagina when opening the blades, minimising the stretching of the introital ring, which is especially sensitive in nulliparous women.

To inspect adequately the vaginal aspects of a perineal scar the speculum should be gently rotated through 90° before withdrawal so that the blades are spread laterally and the length of the vaginal wall is exposed to view posteriorly. In this way small tags of tender granulation or ridges of scar tissue are not overlooked.

When a patient has previously experienced pain during intercourse or attempted penetration, she will often show evidence of tension when examination is in prospect, i.e. she will be less willing to abduct her legs widely, or tend to draw away when the vulva is touched and may grimace when even gentle vaginal examination is attempted. The muscles surrounding the lower vagina will be found to be in spasm, and the medial margins of the levator ani muscle will be prominent. In these circumstances, successive steps of the examination should be conducted gradually, with continuing verbal encouragement and reassurance.

In women with vaginismus and marked spasm of the perivaginal muscles (see p. 381) entry of the examining finger may be impossible, and any attempts to insert it painful. In severe cases marked tensing of body musculature with arching of the back and firm adduction of the thighs gives an early indication of the diagnosis as well as preventing access to the vaginal area. Patience and sensitivity are then essential. Vaginismus can only be properly diagnosed by vaginal examination. It will not be apparent if examination is carried out under general anaesthesia, a procedure sometimes used in these circumstances. In cases when vaginismus seems likely from the history and considerable apprehension about an examination is expressed by the woman it may be advisable to delay examination until a more trusting relationship with the therapist has been established. Even so, it should be made clear at the start that an examination will eventually be necessary. In women with a marked aversive response to examination, it can be carried out in steps on a number of occasions. First, the patient is assured that only visual examination of the vulva will be involved, requiring abduction of her thighs. On the second occasion, the doctor's finger will simply be placed in the opening of the vagina but not inserted — and so on. This procedure, in addition to being gradual, demonstrates firmness combined with trustworthiness on the part of the doctor.

In women who complain of pain at the vaginal opening when insertion of the penis is attempted, the following local causes should be looked for at examination (see p. 383 and Chapter 11 for further details):

1. Hymeneal remnants. The hymen may have stretched but be intact or incompletely ruptured. A persistent arc or web of hymen may be present, particularly anteriorly below the urethral orifice. Even though the hymen has been completely disrupted, polypoidal tags of hymeneal skin may persist and become oedematous and tender, causing considerable discomfort if lubrication is inadequate or if vaginal infection (e.g. thrush) is present.
2. Post-partum scarring (see Chapter 12). Pain may result from extensive scarring due to a ragged tear; from introital narrowing due to the thin web-like fourchette (dashboard perineum); from retained suture material causing indolent infection; from granulation tissue or epithelial bridges on the vaginal aspect of the scar.
3. Inflammatory conditions (see Chapter 11). These include acute vulvo-vaginitis due to *Trichomonas* or *Monilia*. Itching of the vulva is usually a feature. With herpes genitalis, the vesicular lesions and shallow ulcers may be so small as to escape notice, but are disproportionately tender. Genital warts are common, usually multiple and often involve the cervix as well as the vulva. With Bartholin's cyst or abscess a diffuse swelling is usually unilateral and occupies the posterior third of the labium majus.
4. Atrophic change (see Chapter 5). This is encountered in post-menopausal, oestrogen-deficient women, especially when nulliparous. The introitus becomes narrowed, the epithelial surfaces are thin and tender and there is impaired lubrication.
5. Other causes in older women. A urethral caruncle, a small granulomatous excrescense at the urethral orifice, is usually exquisitely tender and is an occasional cause of dyspareunia in older women. Postoperative scarring or tender granulation tissue may result following pelvic floor repair (colporrhaphy).

When considering possible causes of pain on deep penetration or thrusting, it is important to remember the elongation of the vagina and elevation of the uterus which normally occur during sexual arousal. Deep discomfort may be due to an impairment of this normal functional response or to pelvic pathology or a combination of both.

1. Pelvic inflammatory disease. Infection may involve the adnexa (salpingitis) or the pelvic connective tissue (parametritis). There will be deep tenderness on palpation in the lateral fornices and on displacement of the cervix. It is worth noting here that cervical erosions, which are common, are *not* a manifestation of pelvic infection and are not a cause of dyspareunia.
2. Endometriosis. Even small deposits of endometriosis, if located (as they very often are) in or near the pouch of Douglas, will usually cause

intolerable pain during coitus. The tender nodules can often be felt on vaginal examination.

3. Uterine retroversion (see Chapter 2). The vast majority of patients with retroversion of the uterus do not experience pain during intercourse unless there is some additional complicating feature such as prolapsed ovary in the pouch of Douglas, retroversion fixed by adhesions or retroversion with impaired arousal and therefore no uterine elevation. Apart from the body of the retroverted uterus, other swellings in the pouch of Douglas, such as a low-lying fibroid or a fixed ovarian tumour, can similarly cause discomfort.

4. Vaginal vault scarring. The normal ability of the vaginal vault to dilate during sexual arousal may be impaired by scarring resulting from a deep cervical laceration at the time of delivery, or from hysterectomy. In the latter case, granulations may also be present at the site of the vault suture line.

In some women discomfort during coitus is not experienced at the introitus, nor on full penetration, but during coital movement, which causes pain in the vaginal walls at an intermediate depth.

1. Vaginal infection (thrush or *Trichomonas*) may be present in mild form without associated vulvitis. Frictional contact with the vaginal walls during thrusting elicits the discomfort and the woman is often left with the sensation of post-coital rawness for several hours. The diagnosis is based on microscopic examination of the vaginal fluid.

2. Oral contraceptives. It is possible that in some women oral contraceptives, particularly those with a relatively high progestagenic component, may cause vaginal dryness and consequent discomfort. Also women using steroidal contraceptives may be more vulnerable to active infection by *Monilia* present in the vaginal flora.

3. Vaginal obstetric scars. If an episiotomy has been sited too far laterally or a vaginal laceration has extended to the middle third of the lateral vaginal wall, the resulting scar will overlie the inner margin of the levator ani muscle. This area is particularly sensitive (and can also be an important source of erotic stimuli), so that severe dyspareunia is likely and will be localised to the affected side of the vagina.

Involvement of the partner during physical examination

Many sex therapists advocate the involvement of the partner during the educational part of the physical examination. Many couples find such an experience difficult to accept and it is questionable whether, as a routine part of assessment, the advantages outweigh the disadvantages. But with careful selection this procedure can be beneficial, with each partner undergoing examination in the presence of the other, and with open discussion of anatomy and function. The objectives are to educate and inform, to correct misinformation and to alleviate feelings of shame or aversion towards the genitalia. It is not desirable, however, to have only one partner examined in this way.

Laboratory investigations

The most important investigation in women is for evidence of vaginal infection and the most appropriate form of chemotherapy. The clinical value of hormonal measurement in the assessment of female sexual dysfunction remains very uncertain. It is possible to establish whether the woman is ovulating by the measurement of progesterone in the blood during the second half of the cycle, or more thoroughly by collecting early morning urine two or three times a week and measuring the oestrogen- and pregnanediol-to-creatinine ratios. Raised gonadotrophins at times other than mid-cycle may indicate a failing, perimenopausal ovary when menstruation is still occurring. A low level of testosterone may be found. But in none of these cases can we predict response to hormonal therapy which therefore has to be used on a trial-and-error basis. It may be sensible to establish a hormonal baseline *before* giving exogenous hormones. Hyperprolactinaemia may be associated with loss of sexual desire in women (see p. 116) and although non-sexual problems such as infertility or amenorrhoea are more likely to lead to clinical investigation in such cases, there are some hyperprolactinaemic women in whom the sexual problem is the only issue which concerns them.

The presence of deep dyspareunia warrants a full gynaecological assessment which may include laparoscopy or ultrasound.

Special investigations of sexual response in women

Very little attention has been paid to the diagnostic use of psychophysiological techniques in female sexual dysfunction, and these techniques rarely play a part in normal clinical management. This may change in the future. The measurement of episodic vaginal blood flow changes during sleep (discussed on p. 77) may prove to be of relevance in assessing the neurophysiological substrate of sexual desire in women, as the measurement of nocturnal penile tumescence (NPT) does in men; however, this awaits demonstration. The diagnostic significance of vaginal responses to erotic stimuli in the waking state is not yet clear. (Readers interested in the application of psychophysiological techniques to the assessment of sexually dysfunctional women should refer to Wincze et al 1976, 1978; Morokoff & Heiman 1980).

Sacral evoked responses have been shown to be impaired in women with orgasmic dysfunction, particularly those who are unresponsive to psychological treatment (Brindley & Gillan 1982). This procedure is described below.

ASSESSING THE MAN

There is a particular need to distinguish between problems of ejaculation, erection and sexual desire. Premature ejaculation is sometimes mistaken for an erectile problem because of the rapid loss of erection that follows it. Late-onset premature ejaculation may be secondary to erectile failure, perhaps as a result of the performance anxiety engendered by the erectile problem. Also, with erectile impairment, the time taken to elicit an erection may be prolonged, whereas that required to produce ejaculation is not. This can give the impression of premature ejaculation (Michal 1982). Careful questioning is necessary to distinguish between these various situations.

How soon after premature ejaculation can the man become aroused again? When ejaculation occurs quickly as a result of high arousal and with a long interval since his last ejaculation, it is usually possible for arousal to return in a relatively short time, at least during that same love-making session. When premature ejaculation is accompanied by performance anxiety, the post-ejaculatory refractory period tends to be complete and very prolonged.

Absent or delayed ejaculation also requires careful description. Does the problem occur only in the presence of the partner (e.g. is he able to ejaculate normally when masturbating on his own)? Or is it only a problem intravaginally (i.e. can he ejaculate outside the vagina during love play with his partner)? Does he get seminal emissions during sleep? Relatively frequent 'wet dreams' in a man who is unable to ejaculate when awake strongly suggest the action of psychological inhibition. Does orgasm occur without ejaculation (a 'dry run' orgasm may be drug-induced or due to a neurological deficit), or is there evidence of retrograde ejaculation (e.g. cloudiness of the first urine passed after orgasm)?

In assessing erectile problems, establish whether full erection can occur in any situation or at any stage during love-making. If so, at what stage does it start to fail? Loss of erection on attempting vaginal entry usually has a psychological explanation, although rarely it can result from a postural effect in someone with vascular disease and the 'pelvic steal' syndrome. Are erections painful or deformed in any way, suggesting Peyronie's disease?

Erections present on waking in the morning or during the night are evidence of normal sleep erections. The diagnostic significance of sleep erections will be discussed more fully later in this chapter, but the presence of full erections on waking is suggestive of a predominantly psychogenic causation. Segraves et al (1987) concluded that the differences which best distinguished between men with psychogenic and organic impotence were: the presence or absence of full waking erections, and the occurrence of full erections during masturbation and in non-coital situations (e.g. spontaneously or during foreplay). However it should be stressed that whereas the occurrence of full erections in these situations is of good diagnostic value, their absence is less helpful as it can be associated with both psychogenic and organic factors.

The assessment of sexual desire is somewhat easier in men than in women, as it is more readily manifested as a desire to initiate love-making. But the main difficulties are deciding whether a loss of sexual desire preceded or followed some other sexual dysfunction, such as erectile failure, and distinguishing between desire and concern about sexual performance, which can become a preoccupation. Loss of desire following erectile failure is of little help diagnostically; it is likely to be an understandable response to the genital failure. But loss of sexual desire which clearly preceded other dysfunctions may have important causes, such as hormonal deficiency, which need to be identified. In such cases the erectile failure can then be a psychological response to the loss of desire (see p. 99). As discussed in Chapter 8, the aetiology of loss of sexual desire is complex and heterogeneous and may require much more careful history-taking than is often necessary with other types of sexual problem.

The man's attitude to his general health may be important. Concern about sexual function is sometimes part of a general hypochondriacal pattern. Concerns about body image are sometimes important, but less often, it seems, than with women. The use of tobacco and excessive alcohol are potentially important factors (see p. 566).

The occurrence of pain during sexual activity needs careful enquiry. Where is the pain experienced? Is it in the glans, shaft of penis or elsewhere in the groin or scrotum? Is it a pain, a soreness to touch or an unpleasant hypersensitivity? At what point during the sexual response sequence does it occur? Is it associated with ejaculation, or does it occur with prolonged arousal and then is relieved by ejaculation? Is there ever blood in the ejaculation? Is it a skeletal pain associated with movement or posture during sexual intercourse?

Indications for physical examination of the male

Indications for physical examination in men include the following:

1. Recent history of ill health, or physical symptoms apart from the sexual problem.
2. Complaint of pain or discomfort associated with sexual activity.
3. Recent onset of loss of sexual desire with no apparent cause.
4. Any man aged over 50 with sexual problems.
5. Past history of abnormal puberty or other endocrine or genital problem (e.g. mumps orchitis, torsion of the testicle etc.).
6. When the patient believes a physical cause to be most likely, or is in some way concerned about his body or genitalia (e.g. penis too small, or bent, difficulty retracting the foreskin).

Genital examination of the male

In general, the comments about the need for sensitivity to the patient's feelings when examining women also apply to examination of men. In both cases this is particularly important when the examining doctor is of the opposite sex. Genital examination can be carried out with the man either lying or standing.

The size and consistency of the testes should be assessed. Normal adult size is 15–25 ml, approximately 4 cm in length. The presence of scrotal swellings, such as hydrocele or spermatocele, should be noted. Large swellings may be a cause of embarrassment or mechanical problems during sexual activity. They may also conceal testicular pathology. Varicoceles, nearly always on the left, are easy to identify and may be clinically relevant to sexual function (see p. 379).

The shaft of the penis should be examined by palpation. Penile arteries can often be palpated between thumb and index finger. Indurated plaques in one or other corpora cavernosa may be felt, probably indicating Peyronie's disease (see p. 378) or indurated scarring following penile trauma.

In uncircumcised men, the foreskin should be examined carefully. Can it be fully retracted? Are there any sites of tenderness, resulting from small tears? Torn or tight foreskin (phimosis) may cause pain during intercourse. Difficulty in replacing the retracted foreskin may indicate a tendency to paraphimosis when following coitus the tight collar of foreskin remains withdrawn, causing swelling and pain in the glans. Unfortunately it is not always possible to assess these problems with the penis not erect.

Pain during intercourse may also be caused by infection under the foreskin (balanitis) or genital thrush or herpes (see Chapter 11).

Pain accompanying ejaculation is sometimes a symptom of chronic prostatitis, vesiculitis or epididymitis. In such cases, a rectal examination is indicated, though often no such cause for the pain can be found. It is important to remember that rectal examination can be an unpleasant and demeaning experience for both men and women and should be carried out with sensitivity and care. The opportunity can be used however to assess anal tone and saddle innervation in response to light touch and pinpoint, as an assessment of sacral reflexes. Also the bulbocavernosus reflex is an indicator of intact pudendal nerve function (see p. 447). It is elicited by squeezing the glans penis whilst the examiner's finger is inserted into the patient's rectum. A positive response is shown by reflex contraction of the anal sphincter. It is observable in 70% of normal men (Bors & Blinn 1959) but false negatives are common.

When erectile or ejaculatory function is impaired, neurological assessment of the pelvis and lower limbs may be indicated. This is also an opportunity to check peripheral pulses in the lower limbs for evidence of peripheral vascular disease.

Involvement of the partner during physical examination

The same considerations apply for the man as for the woman (see p. 421).

Laboratory investigations

Checking urine for sugar is a simple procedure which can be done in the clinic and should be carried out for every man presenting with secondary erectile problems, and probably also those with late-onset ejaculatory disturbance.

Other tests should be based on appropriate clinical indications, derived either from the history or the physical examination. Indications for hormone measurement in men present the main difficulty. Any clinical evidence of hypogonadism (i.e. small testes, deficient body hair, gynaecomastia etc.) requires measurement of plasma testosterone, gonadotrophins and prolactin, preferably on more than one sample. Sex hormone-binding globulin measurement adds valuable information about total testosterone level (see p. 21). Loss of sexual interest in men above the age of 50 justifies hormonal assay, as in older men testicular function may decline without any obvious clinical signs of hypogonadism. In younger men, unexplained loss of sexual interest may warrant such investigations, though it is seldom that positive results will be obtained.

Prolactin also presents a problem in this respect. Hyperprolactinaemia in men is rare (see p. 99). It is usually (though not always) accompanied by lowered testosterone. It is therefore questionable whether prolactin should be measured unless the testosterone level is low.

Special investigations of sexual responses in men

Erectile dysfunction

If during interview or physical examination it has not been possible to exclude an organic factor contributing to the erectile dysfunction, there are a number of procedures which may throw further light on the aetiology.

Assessment of erectile function. The most direct procedures involve the measurement of erections which occur either physiologically or are pharmacologically induced. This can be done in three ways; by measuring erections during sleep (NPT), in response to erotic stimuli, and following intracavernosal injections of smooth muscle relaxants such as papaverine or phentolamine. With the first two, the occurrence of normal erections increases the likelihood of a predominantly psychogenic causation. The diagnostic significance of the intracavernosal injections remains unclear, but this procedure is now being used so widely that we will need to consider its value more closely. The evidence for the clinical value of all three of these procedures and their relation to each other will be considered in more detail below.

In terms of acceptability each has its advantages and disadvantages. Measurement of sleep erections is non-invasive, but to be done reliably does require spending two or three consecutive nights in a hospital bed or sleep laboratory, which is expensive. The main problem with the psychophysiological technique of eliciting erections in response to erotic stimuli is that stimuli such as erotic film or literary material have to be used. In my opinion, with appropriate selection of erotic material and careful explanation to the patient why the procedure is being used (and obviously his fully informed consent) offence can be avoided and useful information obtained. But there are some who object to such tests on moral grounds. Intracavernosal injections can be painful, albeit briefly. In a small percentage of cases they produce prolonged erections, which may require pharmacological reversal to avoid possible permanent damage to the erectile tissues, and there may be other potentially harmful long-term effects, such as intracavernosal fibrosis, which have not as yet been recognised. It is an interesting reflection on medical attitudes to sexuality that there are many surgeons who do not hesitate to elicit an erection by injecting a drug into the penis, but who would be very reluctant to elicit an erection with the use of erotic stimuli.

Assessment of the vascular supply to the penis. If an arterial factor is suspected (e.g. in older men, smokers, diabetics or those with hypertension or other evidence of cardiovascular or peripheral vascular disease) the following procedures can be used:

1. penile blood pressure index (PBPI; see below).
2. Doppler wave form analysis (see below).
3. Angiography.

Angiography

Arteriography of the internal pudendal artery and its branches is being used in a number of centres to investigate impotence thought to be associated with peripheral arterial disease (Ginestie & Romieu 1978; Michal & Pospichal 1978) (Figs 9.1, 9.2). These procedures are not without risk since they require a general anaesthetic and usually arterial catheterisation. The aetiological significance of these angiographic findings is still uncertain, and it may be that many men in the same age group as those patients studied would have such angiographic findings in the presence of normal erectile function. It also remains to be demonstrated that the presence of such lesions precludes a successful response to psychological treatment, or indicates a persisting erectile problem. Modern computer-assisted angiographic techniques allow investigation of the arterial tree following *intravenous* injection of radiopaque medium. The risks associated with such techniques are substantially less and, with further experience, our understanding of the relevance of arterial occlusion to erectile dysfunction should increase.

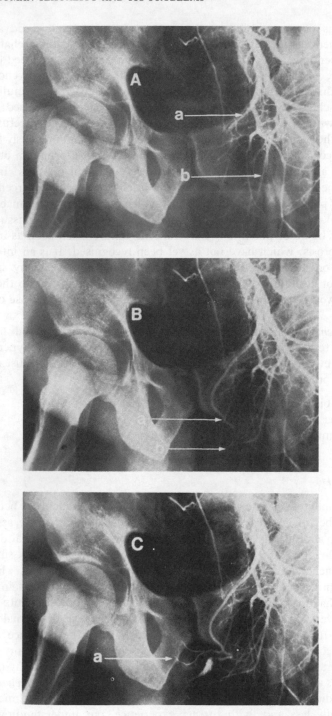

Fig. 9.1

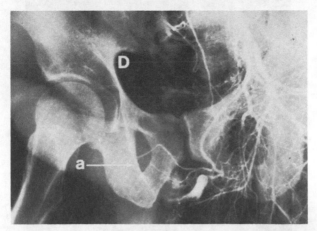

Fig. 9.1 Left-side selective internal iliac arteriography in a 24-year-old man with primary erectile dysfunction. The shadow of the penis is seen over the head of the right femur. **A** Early filling of (a) the accessory pudendal artery and (b) the internal pudendal artery of the left side. **B** Two seconds later. Further filling of (a); internal pudendal artery gives off perineal branches (b). **C** Two seconds later. Early filling of the three penile branches from the accessory pudendal artery (a). Bulbar shadow is clearly visible. **D** Two seconds later. Further filling of dorsal, deep and bulbar penile arteries (a). Although well calibrated, the filling from the accessory pudendal artery is delayed compared with that of the rest of the branches of the iliac artery. A similar pattern was observed on the right side. (Courtesy of Gorm Wagner & Richard Green)

Techniques of injecting radiopaque medium into the corpora cavernosa have been used to study the competence of the venous valves draining the erectile tissues (Fitzpatrick & Cooper 1975). Of particular therapeutic significance have been reports of abnormal venous drainage, usually involving arteriovenous anastomotic leaks through the tunica albuginea (Ebbehøj & Wagner 1979; see p. 377). Injections of radiopaque medium or the use of radioactive isotopes (e.g. xenon) have been used for this purpose (Wagner 1981). In some cases, correction of the erectile failure has been achieved by surgical closure of these anastomotic channels. At present it is not known how common such a condition is. Most of the reported cases have been in relatively young men whose arterial system should be otherwise normal.

Assessment of neurological function. Nerve damage can affect sexual response in three ways: via the neural control of erection, of ejaculation and via sensory pathways from the genitalia.

1. The neural control of erection. As discussed in Chapter 2, this supply is complex and probably involves autonomic fibres both from the sacral (nervi erigentes) and thoracic outflow (hypogastric nerve).
2. The neural control of ejaculation. This is more clearly dependent on the lumbar sympathetic outflow.
3. The sensory pathways from the genitalia. It has been shown in primates (Herbert 1973) and rodents (Larsson & Sodersten 1973) that section

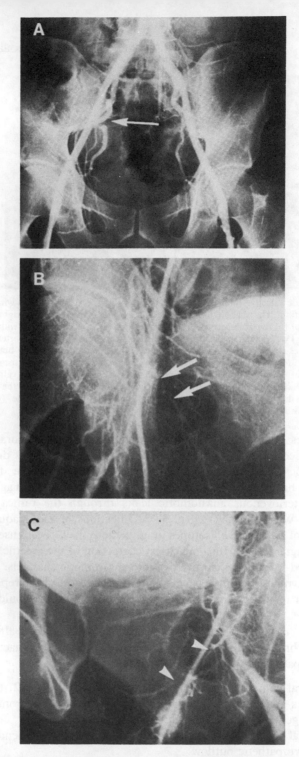

Fig. 9.2 Arteriography in a 47-year-old man with a 6-year history of erectile dysfunction.
A View of acute infarction and iliac region showing occlusion of proximal part of right
internal pudendal artery. **B** Right selective internal iliac arteriography. Between the arrows
can be seen the occlusion of the internal pudendal artery. **C** Left selective internal iliac
arteriography. The internal pudendal artery is occluded between the arrows. (Courtesy of
Gorm Wagner and Richard Green)

of the dorsal nerve of the penis severely disrupts mating behaviour. In humans, sensory input from tactile stimulation is clearly important for a normal sexual experience.

Tests of the integrity of these various neural pathways include:

1. Sacral-evoked responses (see below).
2. Tests of autonomic nerve function (see below).
3. Cystometrography and video cystometry. The neural supply of the erectile tissues is closely related to that of the bladder. Consequently, when pelvic nerve damage leads to erectile problems, bladder function is often affected as well. The cystometrogam is a systematic technique for assessing bladder function which can provide evidence of such neural damage. It is however relatively invasive, requiring catheterisation. It is usually only done when coexistent bladder symptoms warrant investigation, and is best combined with intravesical pressure recording in a full urodynamic study.
4. *Micturography*. This is a non-invasive technique in which the subject urinates into a special container for measuring the rate of urine flow. Flow rates have been found to be abnormal in some diabetic men with impotence, but also in some men with assumed psychogenic impotence, leading Buvat et al (1985) to suggest that flow rate may be affected by psychologically mediated mechanisms. More research on this simple procedure is required before its clinical value can be established.

Ejaculatory dysfunction

At the present time the only organic aetiology to account for absent or delayed ejaculation in men is either androgen deficiency (assessed by clinical examination and hormone assay) or neurological damage. Sacral-evoked responses can therefore be of value in investigating ejaculatory delay and have been found to be deficient in a number of such men (Brindley & Gillan 1982). Retrograde ejaculation can be established by microscopic examination of centrifuged freshly collected post-orgasmic urine, if the diagnosis is in doubt.

No organic cause of premature ejaculation has so far been identified which would lend itself to investigation.

Psychometric tests

A variety of pencil and paper tests to assess aspects of sexuality have been devised. Schiavi et al (1979) catalogued 50 of them. Some of the most widely used for sexual dysfunction include the Derogatis sexual function inventory (DSFI; Derogatis 1976), the sexual interaction inventory (LoPiccolo & Steger 1974) and the sexual experience scales (Frenken & Vennix 1981). A more recent brief questionnaire of sexual function is the

Golombok–Rust inventory of sexual satisfaction (GRISS; Rust & Golombok 1985).

In general such tests have not been shown to have diagnostic value (LoPiccolo 1985) and are mainly useful for research purposes. I will not attempt to consider them in detail in this book. For a review and critique of many of them see Conte (1983).

THE CURRENT STATUS OF SOME INVESTIGATIVE PROCEDURES FOR SEXUAL DYSFUNCTION

MEASURES OF ERECTILE FUNCTION

Nocturnal penile tumescence (NPT)

The normal occurrence of spontaneous erections during sleep, typically associated with rapid eye movement (REM) phases of sleep, was described in Chapter 2 (Fig. 9.3). The device most commonly used for continuous recording of such erections is the mercury-in-rubber strain gauge (see Fig. 9.4).

Karacan (1970) was the first to suggest that measurement of NPT might be useful in distinguishing between organic and psychogenic causes of erectile failure. If organic factors are involved, impairing the basic mechanisms of erection, then sleep erections should also be impaired. By contrast, psychogenic factors should have little or no influence during sleep.

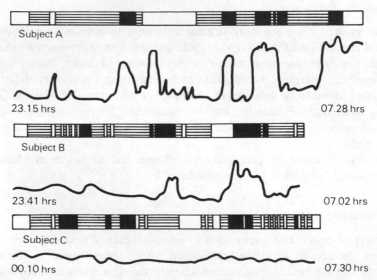

Fig. 9.3 Measurement of erections during sleep in three men. Subject A normal; subject B probable psychogenic erectile dysfunction; C diabetic dysfunction with severe autonomic neuropathy.
□ = awake ■ = REM ⊟ = non-REM

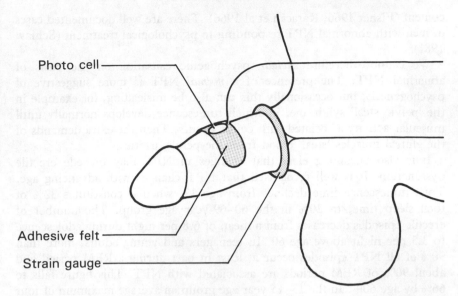

Photo cell

Adhesive felt

Strain gauge

Fig. 9.4 Measurement of penile erection, showing mercury-in-rubber strain gauge for measuring penile diameter and photocell for measuring pulse amplitude from the dorsal artery of the penis. (from Bancroft & Bell 1985)

Fisher et al (1975) and Karacan et al (1977) started publishing results of the use of NPT in the differential diagnosis of erectile dysfunction. Since then numerous comparable reports have appeared, though in very few have adequate attempts to validate the measure been involved. Nevertheless NPT has become a standard procedure in many sexological clinics, and often decisions whether to proceed with surgical implants are based largely on this test.

With time, the value of this test has received more critical appraisal, and whilst it continues to be of considerable interest, and can be of diagnostic value, it is now clear that its interpretation is much more complex than was at first thought.

In Chapter 2 we considered the chain of events leading to penile erection, pointing out that disruption of this chain can occur at various points (see Fig. 2.48, p. 126). In other words, impairment of NPT does not necessarily mean impairment of *peripheral* mechanisms of erection, such as vascular disease or damage to the peripheral nerves. NPT is impaired in hypogonadal states (see p. 93), during depressive illnesses (see p. 131) and in men with low sexual desire but not obvious evidence of organic disease. As suggested earlier, NPT can be seen as a 'window' into the neurophysiological substrate of central arousability, in which case, anything affecting that central system may be manifested as changes in the NPT. More direct psychological mechanisms also seem to be relevant. NPT is less marked during REM sleep when it is associated with dreams of high anxiety content (Fisher 1966; Karacan et al 1966). There are well documented cases of men with abnormal NPT responding to psychological treatment (Schiavi 1981).

We cannot therefore *exclude* psychogenic causation on the basis of abnormal NPT. The presence of a *normal* NPT is more suggestive of psychogenesis, but occasionally this can also be misleading, for example in the 'pelvic steal' syndrome, in which tumescence develops normally until muscular activity associated with coitus occurs. Then the extra demands of the gluteal muscles 'steal' blood from the penile arteries.

It is also becoming clear that changes in NPT may precede erectile dysfunction. It is well recognised that NPT changes with advancing age. Total tumescence time declines from age 13, when it constitutes 32% of total sleep time, to 20% in the 60–69-year age group. The number of erectile episodes decreases from a mean of 6.8 per night during adolescence to 3.5 per night above age 60. In teenagers and young adults, more than 90% of all NPT episodes occur at least in part during a REM period and about 90% of REM periods are associated with NPT. This figure falls to 66% by age 60+. In the 13–15 year age group an average maximum of four erections occur per night; three in the 30–39 age group; 2+ in the 40–67 group and 1.7 for the 70+ (Schiavi & Fisher 1982). It is not clear which mechanism is involved in this ageing process. Recently Schiavi (personal communication) found NPT to be impaired, to an extent often regarded as indicative of organic failure, in a group of older men who had no problems with erections during love-making. Presumably, in some way the capacity for spontaneous erection can decline whilst the ability to respond to tactile stimulation continues. This ageing trend could be reflecting the decline in sexual desire commonly associated with advancing age (see Chapter 5).

Schiavi et al (1985) have also found that whereas NPT is frequently impaired in diabetic men with erectile dysfunction, it can also be abnormal in some respects in diabetic men *without* erectile problems, raising the possibility that some subclinical change in central or peripheral responsiveness has already occurred. A similar finding was reported in a study comparing untreated hypertensive men with and without erectile dysfunction (Hirshkowitz & Karacan 1987).

Methodological issues

Somewhat surprisingly, NPT does not appear to be affected by previous sexual activity (Brissette et al 1985). Most authorities suggest that a minimum of two consecutive nights, preferably three, are required (Schiavi & Fisher 1982). Sleep is often poor during the first night, though it is not unusual to get a normal response on the first night.

Some workers recommend the simultaneous use of two strain gauges, one at the base, the other near the tip of the penis. In our experience the second gauge rarely provides additional information, though according to Schiavi

& Fisher (1982) it may identify abnormalities in the erection, such as Peyronie's disease.

Most experts also stress the importance of measuring sleep parameters as well as NPT, on the grounds that failure to recognise abnormal sleep patterns may result in misleading conclusions (Schiavi & Fisher 1982). Whilst this is undoubtedly true, polysomnography, as it is now called, which requires electroencephalogram, electro-oculogram and electromyogram as well as NPT measurement, is considerably more expensive and time-consuming than the simple recording of NPT. When cost is a factor, the costs and benefits have to be carefully weighed. Providing that NPT is seen as one of several methods of assessment, useful information can be obtained from NPT recordings without sleep data.

Attempts to measure NPT at home with simple devices such as the 'snap gauge' have not been convincing (Allen 1987), but the use of portable home monitoring does have potential (Procci et al 1983).

The most contentious issue in relation to NPT is the definition of a normal or adequate response. Most early reports relied simply on a measurement of circumference change. In one of the few attempts to validate the measure, Marshall et al (1981) found that a maximum circumference increase of more than 11.5 mm correctly identified psychogenic aetiology in 80% of cases. Other workers have used even smaller changes as criteria of response. But an 11.5 mm increase in circumference is usually a long way from full tumescence, not to mention a rigid erection.

Various other parameters can be measured, some of which are listed above in describing the changes with age.

In recent years, increasing attention has been paid to rigidity. Wein et al (1981) reported that 'normal' circumference increases can occur without sufficient rigidity for vaginal entry. It has also been shown that after a certain amount of tumescence, circumference change ceases to have a linear relationship with intracavernosal pressure (Godec & Cass 1981; Metz & Wagner 1981). Schiavi & Fisher (1982) assessed rigidity by waking the patient during a NPT episode, usually on the third night, and directly checking the rigidity of the erection. Various methods for quantifying the 'buckling force' have been devised. But waking the subject in mid-NPT is not without its problems. Various attempts to produce devices for continuously monitoring rigidity have been made. One such device, the Rigiscan, is commercially available but expensive. Though there have been some favourable reports about its validity (e.g. Bradley et al 1985), some workers have found it less useful, since it has a tendency to underestimate the degree of rigidity (e.g. Wooten & Fields 1987). Virag et al (1985) and Desai et al (1987b) have developed simpler devices based on the principles of tonometry and further evidence of their validity and clinical usefulness is awaited.

Although assessment of rigidity is clearly desirable, one should not be dismissive of the potential value of simple circumference measurement.

This may still have diagnostic significance, particularly in assessing other aspects of sexual responsiveness such as the disorders of sexual desire and the effects of drugs on sexual response.

Erectile response to erotic stimuli

Psychophysiological techniques for measuring responses to erotic stimuli have been used extensively for the past 20 years to assess sexual preferences and the outcome of modification of deviant sexual preferences (Bancroft 1974). Surprisingly little attention has been paid to the use of these techniques for the assessment of erectile dysfunction.

Kockott et al (1980) reported results of such an investigation in diabetic and non-diabetic dysfunctional men as well as normal controls. Two further comparable studies have been reported by Bancroft et al (1985) and Zuckerman et al (1985).

The most widely used method for measuring erection is the mercury-in-rubber strain gauge (Fig. 9.4). This is probably optimal for NPT measurement because of its relative immunity to movement artefact. But there are other methods, in particular those using solid-state semiconductor strain gauges (Bancroft 1974). The relative merits of these different procedures have been reviewed by Rosen & Keefe (1978). Changes are reported either in diameter or circumference (it is important to be clear which). Some studies have used percentage of full erection as their main variable. This is of doubtful value in studies of dysfunctional men in whom it is usually not possible to establish a full normal erection to provide the 100% change. As stressed in relation to NPT, diameter or circumference change does not indicate the degree of rigidity of an erection.

In our study (Bancroft et al 1985) we used erotic films and fantasies as stimuli and compared non-diabetic and diabetic dysfunctional men and

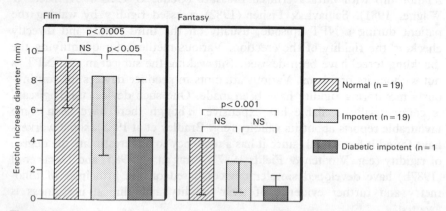

Fig. 9.5 Measurement of erectile response to erotic films and fantasies in three age-matched groups of men; normal controls, and non-diabetic and diabetic men with erectile dysfunction. (from Bancroft et al 1985)

age-matched normal controls. Response to erotic films was the best discriminator, with normal and non-diabetic dysfunctional groups producing significantly greater erections than the diabetics (Fig. 9.5). Interestingly, the non-diabetics did not differ significantly from the controls in this respect; some of them produced, usually to their surprise, good erections in the laboratory. Zuckerman et al (1985) reported somewhat different results. With three broadly similar groups, they found the non-diabetic and diabetic dysfunctional groups to be very similar in their response to erotic stimuli, and both significantly less responsive than the controls (though the non-diabetics produced significantly greater NPT than the diabetics — see below).

It is noteworthy that the mean level of response in these two studies was apparently different, with our study recording greater responses in all three groups. Thus the mean diameter change for the control groups was 9.3 mm in our study and 6.4 in Zuckerman et al's study. For the non-diabetic and diabetic dysfunctional groups the means were 8.3, 3.2, and 4.2, 3.2 respectively. Obviously, with relatively small size groups there is likely to be considerable variance from one study to another, perhaps particularly in the non-diabetic dysfunctional groups where the relevance of organic factors may be more obscure and hence psychogenesis more variable in importance. It is also important to consider methodological differences which could make quite a difference to the responsiveness of individuals in what is a rather strange laboratory setting. The erotic stimuli may have been more effective in one study than another. Certainly if such procedures are to be more widely used it is important that the methods should be reproducible and strictly adhered to.

We also divided our subjects into those with an without positive evidence of psychogenic factors from their history. In the non-diabetic group, the psychogenic subgroup produced significantly greater erections than the non-psychogenic. With the diabetics the difference was not significant, though the psychogenic diabetics did show a greater blood pressure response (Chapter 11, Fig. 11.2) and also a greater penile pulse amplitude response to erotic stimuli (see below).

A comparison of erectile response to erotic stimuli during the waking state and spontaneous erections during sleep in the same individuals is of obvious interest. Zuckerman et al (1985) found the two measures were positively correlated in their control and diabetic groups, but not in their non-diabetic dysfunctional group. We examined this relationship also (Bancroft 1984) and found that those men who produced an erectile response to erotic stimuli of greater than 5 mm increase in *diameter* almost always produced substantial NPT responses (see Fig. 9.6).

Obviously we would expect some association between these two measures, particularly at the most normal and abnormal ends of the spectrum. But it should not be assumed that they are assessing the same mechanisms. In Chapter 2 the variety of mechanisms which are or may be involved in

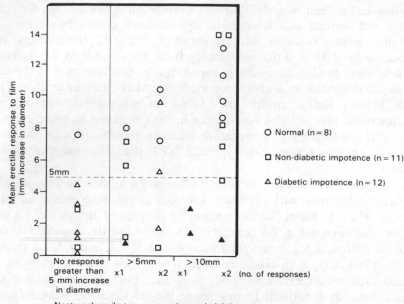

Fig. 9.6 Comparison of maximum erectile response to erotic films and maximum NPT in three groups of men. The NPT responses are categorised as (i) less than 5 mm increase (ii) greater than 5 mm increase or (iii) greater than 10 mm increase in *diameter*. All but one of the men with a response to film of more than 5 mm increase in diameter produced maximum NPT response of greater than 5 mm. (from Bancroft 1984)

erection were discussed. We do not yet know whether the sequence or combination of such mechanisms is the same during NPT as during response to erotic stimuli when awake. If it is not, the two measures may react differently to different types of pathology. Furthermore, evidence was also presented in Chapter 2 to suggest that different central pathways are involved for these two types of response, with NPT being androgen-dependent and response to visual erotic stimuli being androgen-independent.

Melman and his colleagues (1984) have been unusual in reporting their incorporation of measurement of response to visual erotic stimuli as part of the diagnostic 'package' in their sexual dysfunction clinic. They do not give details of their procedure but, in evaluating 70 men, they found 12 who produced greater responses to visual erotic stimuli than during sleep, with the converse applying in 10 men. In six patients a diagnosis of psychogenic dysfunction was made 'only by observing the response to visual sexual stimuli and would not have been possible with nocturnal penile tumescence alone'.

Hence we should regard these two procedures as being potentially different in their diagnostic application, and clearly we need more systematic studies of both procedures, but particularly the measurement of response to erotic stimuli, before we can properly evaluate their clinical relevance.

Penile blood flow during erection

Given the complexity of erectile physiology it would be valuable to have non-invasive procedures for measuring vascular changes in the penis during the development of physiological erection. With this objective, we explored the use of photometric measurement of pulse amplitude from the dorsum of the penis, using a photometer similar to that used widely for recording changes in vaginal blood flow (see below; Bancroft & Bell 1985). This device is attached to the dorsum of the penis with adhesive felt (see Fig. 9.4). The interpretation of this particular psychophysiological signal is not straight-forward, but it is reasonable to assume that changes in amplitude of the pulsatile signal reflect changes in pulsatile blood flow, in this case probably from the dorsal arteries of the penis.

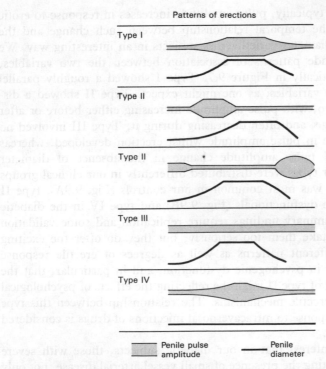

Fig. 9.7 Diagrammatic representation of four types of erectile response involving changes in penile diameter and penile pulse amplitude, showing the variable temporal relationship between the two parameters. (from Bancroft & Bell 1985)

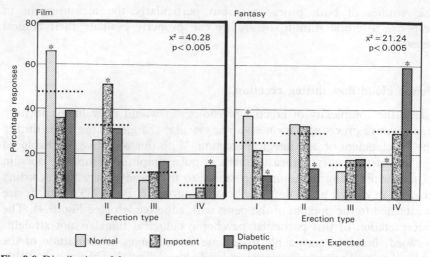

Fig. 9.8 Distribution of four types of erectile response to erotic films and fantasies in three groups of men, normal controls, non-diabetics and diabetics with erectile dysfunction. See Fig. 9.7 for description of response types. (from Bancroft et al 1985)

We found that, typically, pulse amplitude increases in response to erotic stimulation, but the temporal relationship between such change and the change in penile diameter varied across subjects in an interesting way. We identified four crude patterns of association between the two variables, shown diagrammatically in Figure 9.7. Type I showed a roughly parallel change of the two variables, as one might expect. Type II showed a dissociation of the two, with pulse amplitude increasing either before or after the diameter change, and often decreasing during it. Type III involved no appreciable change in pulse amplitude whilst erection developed, whereas Type IV involved pulse amplitude change in the absence of diameter change. These four types were distributed differently in our clinical groups (Fig. 9.8). Type I was most common in our controls (Fig. 9.9A), type II in the non-diabetic dysfunctionals (Fig. 9.9B) and type IV in the diabetic group. These preliminary findings require replication and some validation before we should take them too seriously, but they do offer the exciting possibility that different patterns as well as degrees of erectile response might be observed in psychogenic dysfunction, and in particular, that the dissociative pattern of type II might be reflecting the effects of psychological inhibition on the erectile mechanisms. The relationship between this type of response and response to intracavernosal injections of drugs is considered in the next section.

It was also of interest that in our diabetic subjects, those with severe retinopathy, indicating the presence of small vessel arterial disease, not only had significantly smaller baseline penile pulse amplitudes, but also smaller amplitude change in response to erotic stimulation (Bancroft et al 1985).

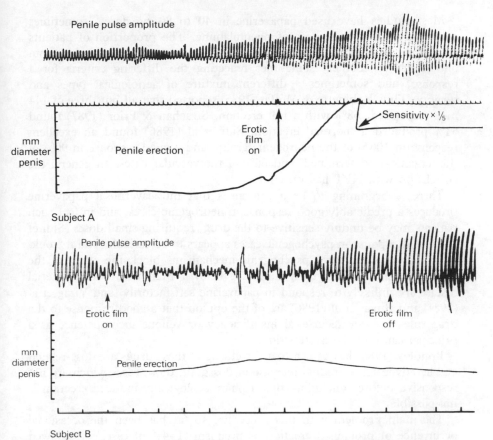

Fig. 9.9 Patterns of penile blood flow during erection. Subject A, a normal 26 year old man, produced a rapid erection associated with an increase of penile pulse amplitude indicating increased penile blood flow. The response starts before the erotic stimulus as he anticipates the film. Subject B is a 30 year old man with erectile problems. He shows a slight erection, accompanied by a *decrease* in penile pulse amplitude. This pattern is commonly found in impotent men, particularly those with likely psychogenic causation, and may prove to be of diagnostic significance.

Intracavernosal injections of smooth muscle relaxants

The discovery by Virag and Brindley of the erection-producing effect of intracavernosal injections of smooth muscle relaxing drugs was considered in Chapter 2. Since then the use of such injections for diagnostic purposes has increased substantially and they are now being used by urologists on a large scale (e.g. Williams et al 1987). Unfortunately, the enthusiasm for their use has not been matched by a preparedness to evaluate their effects with careful, systematic and well reported studies. There are a few such studies from which we can begin to piece together a picture of their diagnostic value.

Most studies have used papaverine in 40 to 80 mg doses, sometimes combined with a small dose of phentolamine. The proportion of patients responding to these injections with erection has varied considerably from one report to another, sometimes reflecting the differing criteria for a response, and sometimes a different mixture of aetiological types and severity. Thus Robinette & Moffat (1986) reported that all but three of 144 men responded, 68% with a full erection. Strachan & Prior (1987) found 51% produced a 'normal' erection. Sidi et al (1986) found an excellent response in 100% of the neurogenic group, and a good response in 90% of the 'organic–undetermined' and 66% of the vascular cases. In general the correlation with NPT has varied.

There is beginning to be a consensus that intracavernosal papaverine produces a predictably good response in neurogenic cases, and in fact such patients may be unduly sensitive to the drug, requiring small doses (Sidi et al 1986). Response in psychogenic cases appears to be variable, and it would seem that in some cases psychogenic mechanisms block the effect of the drug, though it is not clear how (see below). Men with severe arterial disease are unlikely to respond to papaverine satisfactorily, and Virag et al (1984) and Buvat et al (1986) are of the opnion that a good response to the drug rules out severe arterial insufficiency or venous incompetence as a principal cause of the dysfunction.

Brindley (1986) has shown that the effects of these drugs are dose-related and he advocates a gradual increase of dosage in those cases which are not responsive before concluding that a pharmacologically induced erection is not possible.

The main problem with this procedure so far has been the occasional occurrence of prolonged erection or priapism (1–4% of cases). If allowed to continue for too long this can lead to permanent damage to the erectile tissues, as happened in one case of psychogenic dysfunction reported by Buvat et al (1986). Guidelines vary from 6 to 8 to 12 hours before reversing the drug-induced erection with a counteracting drug (e.g. metaraminol; Brindley 1984). Such antidotes themselves have to be used with extreme caution because of potential hypertensive effects.

The combination of papaverine-induced erection with Doppler assessment of penile blood flow will be considered in the next section.

One aspect of this drug effect has received very little attention and yet may prove to be of fundamental importance. Zorgniotti & Lefleur (1985), in describing the self-administration of such injections as a method of treatment, pointed out that the injection 'can be followed by erection and coitus provided there is sexual stimulation'. Virag (1986) reported on the use of a very small dose of papaverine (8 mg) combined with visual erotic stimuli as a diagnostic procedure. These observations suggest that such drugs administered intracavernosally can facilitate the erectile response to sexual stimulation, even that which is mediated via the brain. This is of considerable clinical as well as theoretical interest.

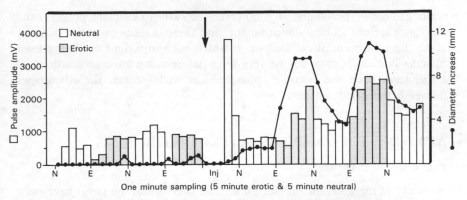

Fig. 9.10 Changes in penile diameter and penile pulse amplitude in response to erotic and neutral films before and after an intracavernosal injection of 30 mg papaverine. Both variables are sampled at one minute intervals. Neutral and erotic stimuli alternate, each of 5 minutes duration. This subject showed no erectile response prior to injection, but both penile diameter and pulse amplitude responses to erotic stimuli occurred after the injection. (Bancroft & Smith 1987)

We are currently investigating this possibility by combining the previously described technique for measuring response to erotic stimuli in which both erection and penile pulse amplitude are measured with intracavernosal injections of papaverine or phentolamine (Bancroft & Smith 1987). A typical response is shown in Fig. 9.10. Early results suggest not only that the erectile response to erotic stimuli is facilitated, but also that the penile pulse amplitude response in this combined test may have diagnostic value. A particularly striking case is shown in Figure 9.11.

There is little doubt that intracavernosal drug administration has provided us with a powerful technique for investigating (and possibly

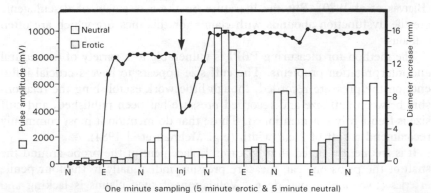

Fig. 9.11 A further example of erectile response before and after intracavernosal papaverine 30 mgm. This 20yr old man with psychogenic erectile dysfunction provides a striking example of the 'dissociative' Type II response described earlier. His penile pulse amplitude decreased sharply after the onset of each erotic stimulus, increasing dramatically after each offset. This pattern was amplified following papaverine in spite of a full erection being maintained throughout. (Bancroft & Smith 1987)

treating) erectile problems. It is however too early to evaluate properly the clinical value of this new development, and there is some cause for concern about the rather uncritical manner in which such injections are being used in some clinics. It may not be very long before some adverse reactions or longer-term problems become apparent. Let us hope that the advantages outweigh the disadvantages.

ASSESSING THE VASCULAR SUPPLY OF THE PENIS

Penile blood pressure.

A variety of methods for measuring arterial pressure in the penis have been reported. They usually combine a small inflatable cuff and manometer and detection of blood flow beyond the cuff by means of a 8–10 MHZ Doppler probe (Abelson 1975; Velcek et al 1980). (Other less frequently used methods include the use of a mercury-in-rubber strain gauge to detect pulsation (Britt et al 1971) and spectroscopy (Gaskell 1971).

The usual procedure is to place the inflatable cuff around the penis and to read the pressure in the cuff when the arterial pulse, distal to the cuff, and detected by the Doppler probe, disappears on inflation and returns after deflation. This is then compared with the brachial systolic pressure as the penile to brachial ratio (penile blood pressure index (PBPI), or penile brachial index (PBI)). The lower the index the greater the likelihood that arterial insufficiency is a contributory factor. Ratios of between 0.8 and 0.6 are regarded as suspicious, and below 0.6 is indicative of arterial insufficiency.

This measure has the virtue of being non-invasive and relatively easy to carry out. A certain amount of evidence validating this approach has been published, in particular comparison of dysfunctional and normal men (Blaivas et al 1980). But the literature on the assessment of vasculogenic erectile dysfunction abounds with claims for this measure which are often dubious.

The method for measuring PBPI is vulnerable to a variety of procedural and interpretation problems. The cuff size appears to have a crucial influence on the pressure recorded, though little work establishing the relationship between cuff size and recorded pressure has been published, and cuff size is frequently not mentioned. Those that do mention it most commonly recommend a cuff of 2 cm width (e.g. Melman et al 1984).

It is frequently stated that by careful placement of the probe around the shaft of the penis one can measure pressure individually in the four penile arteries (two dorsal, two deep). Validation of such claims is lacking and there is a growing belief that in the majority of patients it is only the dorsal arteries or their branches that are adequately assessed in this procedure. According to Sharlip (1986), digital pressure on the dorsal arteries at the base of the penis effectively obliterates all four arterial signals. There are also problems interpreting the functional significance of the ratio. It does decline with age in men who retain their capacity for erection (Kleinschmidt et al 1986), and has been shown to be equally impaired in diabetic men with and without erectile dysfunction (Buvat et al 1986; see p. 558).

Metz & Bengtsson (1981) have shown that PBPI values of less than 0.6 have some validity in the diagnosis of arteriopathy, but above that level the measure lacks specificity and is of uncertain diagnostic value.

Arterial wave form analysis

Doppler ultrasound technology is widely used for assessing abnormalities of flow in the arterial system. Spectral analysis of the ultrasound signal samples and digitalises frequencies relating to the velocity of blood in arteries. This allows various parameters to be identified and quantified. This technique has also been used in assessing flow in penile arteries. Once again we find too many reports in which very arbitrary criteria of somewhat doubtful reproducibility have been used, and there are similar methodological problems in discriminating between different penile arteries. However, this is a technique that can be applied systematically, and for which computer-based methods of data processing are available. Examples of normal and abnormal wave forms from penile arteries are shown in Figure 9.12. The height and slope of the 'up-stroke' reflect speed of flow, the dicrotic notch, which shows the signal changing in direction towards or even below the baseline, indicating reverse flow that may occur during diastole. Poor amplitude with no dicrotic notch indicates impaired flow, poor input or high peripheral resistance.

As we shall see below, interpretation of some of these parameters in vessels in the flaccid penis are probably subject to too much error and artefact to be of clinical value. We have used a method, the presence or absence of the dicrotic notch, as a simpler and reproducible qualitative sign of impaired flow (Smith et al 1987). This has correlated well with NPT. In 81% of men with a notch present, NPT was normal; most of the exceptions were men in whom a neurogenic cause was likely. A total of 88% of men *without* a notch had abnormal NPT.

Recent developments in measuring pulsatile flow

Two recent developments have improved the validity and reliability of wave form analysis and blood flow measurement. First is the use of intracavernosal injections of smooth muscle relaxant drugs such as papaverine to produce an erection so that blood flow can be assessed in the flaccid and the erect state. Second is a sophisticated form of ultrasound technology called the Duplex scanner; this makes use of ultrasound imaging of the penile tissues so that the penile arteries can be located. A second, linked Doppler probe is then focused on to the located vessel. With computer techniques such as fast Fourier transfer, blood flow in the arteries in the

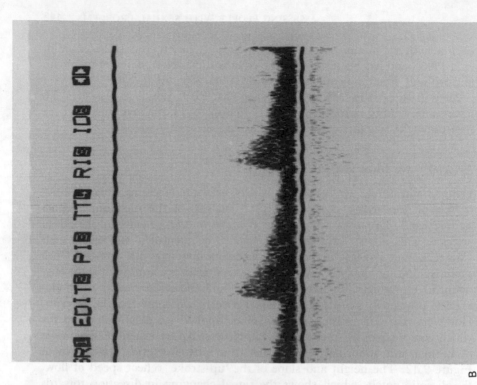

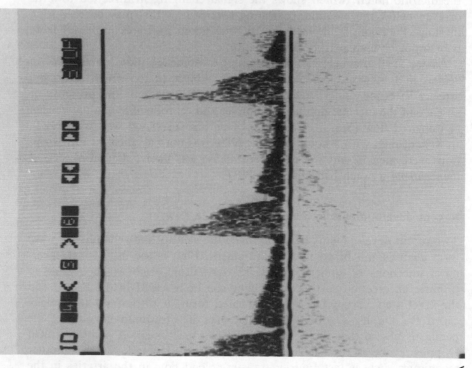

Fig. 9.12 Doppler wave form from the dorsal artery of the penis. **A** Normal, showing shoulder and clear dicrotic notch. **B** Abnormal, with poor amplitude, no shoulder etc.

flaccid and erect state can be assessed, and the diameter of the vessels measured by means of electronic calipers.

Lue et al (1985) used this technique in 23 subjects who were mainly sexually dysfunctional. In the flaccid state they found very variable size of the deep penile arteries, with little evidence of flow in them. Following papaverine, the diameter of the deep arteries and the blood flow within them increased to varying degrees. The authors concluded that the initial size of the artery is less clinically relevant than 'arterial compliance and dilatability'; also that assessment of the dorsal arteries is less informative than that of the deep arteries (they had some examples of good flow through the dorsal artery with poor tumescence).

Collins & Lewandowski (1987) applied the same technique to 47 men with suspected vasculogenic erectile dysfunction. In contrast to the first study (Lue et al 1985), they did detect flow in the flaccid deep arteries. They also found some association between increase in arterial diameter and the degree of erectile response after papaverine, but this relationship was not linear. Those with a poor erectile response to papaverine and little arterial dilatation were found to have disease of both deep and dorsal arteries on angiographic examination. There was also a small but interesting group showing arterial dilatation but poor erectile response. Four of these five men were found to have stenosis in the proximal pudendal artery, with relatively normal penile arteries angiographically. That is the type of vascular abnormality that might respond to revascularisation by surgery. The authors also suggested that the occurrence of a short-lived erectile response in association with normal arterial dilatation points to a possible venous leakage requiring cavernosography.

These methods show considerable promise, but the equipment required (e.g. the Duplex scanner) is very expensive and is unlikely to be available in many hospitals at the present time. The procedure is also very time-consuming. The results do, however, emphasise the need to assess vessels in the erect state. Desai et al (1987c) have reported on the use of the more conventional Doppler wave form analysis following intracavernosal injection of papaverine, with encouraging results.

TESTING THE NERVE SUPPLY TO THE GENITALIA

The bulbocavernosus reflex and sacral evoked responses

Brindley & Gillan (1982) have renamed the bulbocavernosus reflex the 'glandi-pudendal reflex', a name which they believe better describes the components of the reflex. Its receptive field is the glans of the penis or clitoris; the responding muscles lie in the pudendum and are enervated wholly (in the case of ichiocavernosus and bulbospongiosus muscles) and partly (in the case of the levator ani and external anal sphincter) by the pudendal nerve, with its roots from S2 to 4. Brindley & Gillan (1982) demonstrated that this reflex could be elicited in a sustained form by continuous vibratory stimulation of the glans, that it is not apparently influenced by psychological mechanisms, and is unilateral (i.e. it is elicited ipsilaterally by unilateral stimulation.

The method of eliciting this reflex during clinical examination was described on p. 425. This response can be measured in a much more precise and quantifiable way by means of *sacral evoked response testing*. This electrophysiological technique involves stimulation of the dorsal nerve of the penis by means of a skin electrode, and recording an electrical potential response with a receiving electrode on the perineum, as a needle electrode inserted into the perineal musculature (Ertekin et al 1985), by a surface electrode (Haldeman et al 1982) or by a surface electrode, mounted on a plastic plug, inserted into the anal sphincter (Galloway 1985). A normal latency of response in the perineum following stimulation of the dorsal nerve of the penis is in the order of 40 to 50 ms. Specialised electrophysiological equipment, capable of recording such time intervals, is therefore required. It is also necessary to average the responses from a rapid succession of repeated stimuli. In this way the signal can be amplified and the recurring evoked response distinguished from the background noise. This form of testing allows measurement of the threshold for stimuli to be perceived, and of the latency of the evoked response (see Fig. 9.13).

Abnormal responses in this test may reflect impairment of either the sensory afferent pathways or the motor efferent pathways supplying the perineal muscles. The role of the pudendal nerve fibres in sexual response is not clear. They are probably not involved in the neural control or erection, apart from the occasional contractions of the perineal muscles which produce transient increases in intracavernosal pressure and increased rigidity (see p. 59). Some hold the view that it is unlikely that pelvic autonomic neuropathy exists without the somatic nerves being affected (e.g. Herman et al 1986). On the other hand, damage to the peripheral nerves is likely to occur earliest in the longest fibres (Said et al 1983). If so, one can conclude that with a disease process such as diabetes, autonomic nerve damage may precede somatic nerve damage, at least in the pelvis, because of the longer fibres involved in the autonomic supply (see p. 18). Therefore, whilst an abnormal sacral evoked response probably indicates damage to the autonomic fibres as well, a normal response does not exclude the possibility of autonomic damage. (Desai et al 1987).

Direct attempts to test the integrity of the pelvic autonomic fibres have involved placement of an electrode, both for stimulation and response recording, on a catheter to be situated in the urethra at the level of the external sphincter (Desai et al 1987). The efferent autonomic supply to the corpora cavernosa is thought to run close to the urethra at this point in the neurovascular bundle (Lepor et al 1985).

A further extension of evoked response testing allows assessment of the neural pathways above the sacral cord. Thus evoked responses can be recorded from electrodes placed over the lumbar spine and on the scalp.

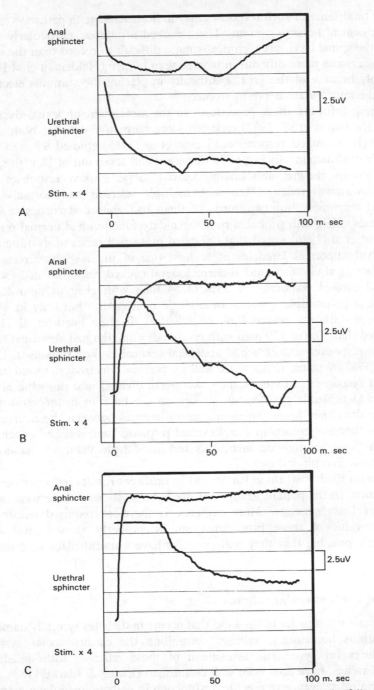

Fig. 9.13 Sacral evoked responses recorded from anal and urethral electrodes following stimulation of an electrode on the dorsum of the penis. **A** Normal response and latency; **B** delayed response; **C** absent response. (courtesy of Dr Angus McInnis)

Delay or absence of such responses may indicate damage to pathways higher in the central nervous system. These evoked responses, particularly those from the spinal level, are technically more difficult to record than the sacral responses, and more difficult in women than in men (Haldeman et al 1982), possibly because of the greater difficulty in placing the stimulus electrode over the appropriate nerve in women.

How helpful are these procedures in the assessment of sexual dysfunction? Haldeman et al (1982) reported some normative data for both sacral and cortical evoked responses. Ertekin et al (1985) studied 95 men with erectile dysfunction. Six out of 20 diabetics, and seven out of 18 with spinal cord lesions showed abnormally delayed sacral evoked responses (i.e. bulbocavernosus reflex). Men with multiple sclerosis had normal sacral evoked responses, but two-thirds of them had abnormal cortical evoked responses. Men with probable psychogenic dysfunction had normal results. Herman et al (1986) found that one-third of a small series of dysfunctional men had abnormal latencies in at least one of the responses recorded. Opsomer et al (1986) found abnormal sacral evoked responses in 24% and cortical evoked responses in 63% of 54 men with clearcut neurological disease (e.g. multiple sclerosis or diabetic neuropathy) but only in 4% of 183 men with no evidence of neurological disease. Porst et al (1987) reported that 50% of 130 men with erectile dysfunction had abnormal sacral evoked responses and 28% had abnormal cortical evoked responses. Desai et al (1987a), using urethral as well as perineal electrodes, tested sacral evoked responses in diabetic men, who were divided into probable neurogenic and probable psychogenic groups on the basis of history and other test results. They found no significant differences between the neurogenic and psychogenic groups in sacral evoked response latencies, and concluded that, at least in diabetic men, this test is of little value in diagnosing neurogenic erectile failure.

It seems likely that these varied and inconsistent results reflect important differences in the patient groups involved. In most cases these were aetiologically heterogeneous. More evidence is therefore required before the clinical value of these procedures can be properly asessed. But it is distinctly possible that they will prove to have a useful place in carefully selected cases.

Testing cardiovascular reflexes

Autonomic neuropathy of the kind that occurs in diabetes typically damages the various homeostatic reflexes controlling the cardiovascular system. Procedures for systematic assessment of these reflexes, with details of normal values, have now been well established (Ewing & Clarke 1982), and their clinical relevance to erectile dysfunction in diabetic men demonstrated (Ewing & Bancroft 1984; Bancroft et al 1985). Five procedures are involved:

1. heart rate response to the Valsava manoeuvre;
2. heart rate response to deep breathing;
3. heart rate response to standing up;
4. blood pressure response to standing up;
5. blood pressure response to sustained handgrip.

Abnormalities of the three heart rate tests are believed to reflect para-sympathetic damage; the two blood pressure tests reflect sympathetic damage. Parasympathetic damage typically precedes sympathetic damage in diabetes and therefore may be found on its own. It is rare to find evidence of sympathetic damage without parasympathetic damage.

The advantage of this procedure is that it is non-invasive and relatively easy to carry out. The disadvantage is that cardiovascular and not pelvic autonomic supply is being tested. Whilst it is unlikely that damage to one system would occur without damage to the other, it cannot be assumed that they always coexist, and they may develop at different rates. Nevertheless, evidence of sympathetic damage by this test in a diabetic with erectile dysfunction is strong evidence of a neurogenic component.

Peripheral nerve conduction tests

Measurement of nerve conduction velocity in peripheral nerves is a well established procedure in the assessment of peripheral neuropathy. Lin & Bradley (1985) have reported on the measurement of conduction velocity in the dorsal nerve of the penis in diabetic dysfunctional men and normal controls. They found significantly longer conduction times in the diabetic group, although the two groups did not differ in sacral evoked response latency. More evidence is required of this potentially interesting procedure.

Measurement of thermal thresholds

As mentioned earlier, peripheral neuropathy tends to appear first in the longer fibres. The unmyelinated fibres to the feet include the efferent auto-nomic and the afferent sensory fibres conveying pain and temperature sense. Tests of thermal sensation in the feet may therefore be a sensitive indicator of early neuropathy. Fowler et al (1987) compared two groups of men with erectile dysfunction. In one group of 15 (14 of them diabetic) a neurogenic cause was thought likely on the basis of history and other tests. The other group of 18 had various non-neurogenic aetiologies ascribed to them, including vascular and psychogenic. All of the neurogenic group had abnormal thermal threshold measurements, whereas the non-neurogenic group had results within the normal range. This is a potentially interesting method which deserves further study.

CONCLUSIONS

The clinical value of any of the diagnostic procedures reviewed in this chapter has not been clearly established. The procedure most extensively investigated, NPT, can be conclusive in some cases, at least in excluding significant organic aetiology, but more often the results are equivocal and have to be combined with the results from other procedures to build up a clinical picture. The presence of an abnormality on one of these tests may be relevant but it should not be assumed that it provides a sufficient explanation for the sexual dysfunction, and it is always important to consider the possible role of psychological factors. With further careful research the diagnostic power of each of these procedures should increase.

REFERENCES

Abelson D 1975 Diagnostic value of the penile pulse and blood pressure: a Doppler study of impotence in diabetics. Journal of Urology 113: 636–639

Allen R P 1987 Snap gauge compared to full nocturnal penile tumescence evaluation for evaluation of patients with erectile impotence. International Sleep Conference (in press)

Bancroft J 1974 Deviant sexual behaviour: modification and assessment. Clarendon, Oxford

Bancroft J 1984 Psychophysiological assessment of erectile dysfunction. In: Segraves R T, Haeberle H (eds) Emerging dimensions of sexology. Praeger, New York, pp 93–100

Bancroft J, Bell C 1985 Simultaneous recording of penile diameter and penile arterial pulse during laboratory based erotic stimulation in normal subjects. Journal of Psychosomatic Research 29: 303–313

Bancroft J, Smith G 1987 Penile diameter and pulse amplitude change before and after intracavernosal injection of smooth muscle relaxants in men with erectile dysfunction. Paper presented at 13th Annual meeting, International Academy Sex Research, Tutzing, W. Germany

Bancroft J, Bell C, Ewing D J, McCulloch D K, Warner P, Clarke B F 1985 Assessment of erectile function in diabetic and non-diabetic impotence by simultaneous recording of penile diameter and penile arterial pulse. Journal of Psychosomatic Research 29: 315–324

Blaivas T G, O'Donnell T F, Gottleb P, Labib K B 1980 Comprehensive laboratory evaluation of impotent men. Journal of Urology 124: 201–204

Bors E, Blinn K 1959 Bulbocavernosus reflex. Journal of Urology 82: 128

Bradley W E, Timm G W, Gallagher J M, Johnson B K 1985. New method for continuous measurement of nocturnal penile tumescence rigidity. Urology 26: 4–9

Brindley G S 1984 New treatment for priapism. Letter. Lancet: iii: 220

Brindley G S 1986 Maintenance treatment of erectile impotence by cavernosal unstriated muscle relaxant injection. British Journal of Psychiatry 149: 210–215

Brindley G S, Gillan P 1982 Men and women who do not have orgasms. British Journal of Psychiatry 140: 351–356

Brissette S, Montplaisir J, Godbout R, Lavoisier P 1985 Sexual activity and sleep in humans. Biological Psychiatry 20: 758–763

Britt D B, Kemmerer W T, Robison J R 1971 Penile blood flow determination by mercury strain gauge plethysmography. Investigative Urology 8: 673–678

Buvat J, Lemaire A, Buvat-Herbaut M, Guien J D, Bailleul J P, Fossati P 1985 Comparative investigation in 26 impotent and 26 non-impotent diabetic patients. Journal of Urology 133: 34–38

Buvat J, Buvat-Herbaut M, Dehaene J L, Lemaire A 1986 Is intracavernous injection of papaverine a reliable screening test for vascular impotence? Journal of Urology 135: 476–478

Collins J P, Lewandowski B J 1987 Experience with intracorporeal injection of papaverine and Duplex ultrasound scanning for assessment of arteriogenic impotence. British Journal of Urology 59: 84–88

Conte H R 1983 Developments and use of self-report techniques for assessing sexual functioning: a review and critique. Archives of Sexual Behavior 12: 555–576

Derogatis L R 1976 Psychological assessment of the sexual disabilities. In: The clinical management of sexual disorders. Williams & Wilkins, Baltimore

Desai K M, Dembrey K, Morgan H, Gingell J C, Prothero D 1987a The neurophysiological investigation of diabetic impotence: are sacral response studies of value? Paper presented at British Association of Urological Surgery Annual Meeting, Edinburgh

Desai K M, Floyd T J, Follett D H, Peake D R, Gingell J C 1987b The development of a new low cost penile rigidity indicator and new concepts in the quantification of rigidity. Poster presented at British Association of Urological Surgery Annual Conference, Edinburgh

Desai K M, Gingell J C, Skidmore R, Follett D H 1987c Application of computerised penile arterial waveform analysis in the diagnosis of arteriogenic impotence — an initial study in potent and impotent men.

Ebbehøj J, Wagner G 1979 Insufficient penile erection due to abnormal drainage of cavernous bodies. Urology 13: 507–510

Ertekin C, Akyurekli O, Gurses A N, Turgut H 1985 The value of somato-sensory evoked potentials and bulbocavernosus reflex in patients with impotence. Acta Neurologica Scandinavica 71: 48–53

Ewing D F, Bancroft J 1984 The evaluation of the autonomic nervous system in impotent males. International Angiology 3: 255–258

Ewing D J, Clarke B F 1982 Diagnosis and management of diabetic autonomic neuropathy. British Medical Journal 285: 916–918

Fisher C 1966 Dreaming and sexuality. In: Loewenstein R M, Newman L M, Schur M (eds) Psychoanalysis — a general psychology: essays in honor of Heinz Hartman. International University Press, New York pp 537–563

Fisher C, Schiavi R C, Lear H, Edwards A, Davis D M, Witkin A P 1975 The assessment of nocturnal REM erections in the differential diagnosis of sexual impotence. Journal of Sexual and Marital Therapy 1: 277–289

Fitzpatrick T J, Cooper J F 1975 A cavernosogram study of the valvular competence of the human deep dorsal vein. Journal of Urology 113: 497–499

Frenken J, Vennix P 1981 SES manual. Swets & Zeitunger, The Netherlands

Fowler C J, Ali Z, Kirby R S, Pryor J P 1987 The value of testing for unmyelinated fibre sensory neuropathy in diabetic impotence. Paper presented at British Association Urological Surgery annual conference, Edinburgh

Galloway N T M, Chisholm G D, McInnes A 1985 Patterns and significance of sacro-evoked response (the urologist's knee jerk). British Journal of Urology 57: 145–147

Gaskell P 1971 The importance of penile blood pressure in cases of impotence. Canadian Medical Association Journal 105: 1047–1050

Ginestie J-F, Romieu A 1978 Radiologic exploration of impotence Maritinus Nijhof, The Hague

Godec C J, Cass A S 1981 Quantification of erection. Journal of Urology 126: 345–347

Haldeman S, Bradley W E, Bhatia N N, Johnson B K 1982 Pudendal evoked responses. Archives of Neurology 39: 280–283

Herbert J 1973 The role of the dorsal nerve of the penis in the sexual behaviour of the male rhesus monkey. Physiology and Behaviour 10: 293–300

Herman C W, Weinberg H J, Brown J 1986 Testing for neurogenic impotence: a challenge. Urology 27: 318–321

Hirshkowitz M, Karacan I 1987 Nocturnal penile tumescence, hypertension and penile hemodynamics. International Sleep Conference (in press)

Karacan I 1970 Clinical value of nocturnal erection in the prognosis and diagnosis of impotence. Medical Aspects of Human Sexuality April: 27–34

Karacan I, Goodenough D R, Shapiro A, Starker S 1966 Erection cycle during sleep in relation to anxiety. Archives of General Psychiatry 15: 183–189

Karacan I, Scott F B, Dalis P T et al 1977 Nocturnal erections in differential diagnosis of impotence in diabetes. Biological Psychiatry 12: 373–380

Kleinschmidt K, Grohe C, Weisbach L 1986 Age related normal values for penile pressure index and penile temperature index in 123 urological patients. 2nd World Meeting on Impotence, Prague

Kockott G, Feil W, Ferstl R, Aldenhoff J, Besinger U 1980 Psychophysiological aspects of male sexual inadequacy: results of an experimental study. Archives of Sexual Behavior 9: 477–494

Kolodny R C, Masters W H, Johnson V E 1979 Textbook of sexual medicine, Little, Brown, Boston

Larsson K, Sodersten P 1973 Mating in male rats after section of the dorsal penile nerve. Physiology and Behaviour 10: 567

Lepor H, Grtegerman M, Crosby R, Mostofi F K, Walsh P C 1985 Precise localisation of the autonomic nerves from the pelvic plexus to the corpora cavernosa: a detailed anatomical study of the adult male pelvis. Journal of Urology 133: 207–212

Lin J T, Bradley W E 1985 Penile neuropathy in insulin dependent diabetes mellitus. Journal of Urology 133: 213–215

LoPiccolo J 1985 Diagnosis and treatment of male sexual dysfunction. Journal of Sexual and Marital Therapy 11: 215–232

LoPiccolo J, Steger J G 1974 The sexual interaction inventory: a new instrument for assessment of sexual dysfunction. Archives of Sexual Behavior 3: 585–595

Lue T F, Hricak H, Marich K W, Tanagho E A 1985 Vasculogenic impotence evaluation by high-resolution ultrasonography and pulsed Doppler spectrum analysis. Radiology 155: 777–781

Marshall P, Surridge D M, Delva N 1981 The role of nocturnal penile tumescence in differentiating between organic and psychogenic impotence: the first stage of validation. Archives of Sexual Behavior 10: 1–10

Melman A S, Kaplan D, Redfield J 1984 Evaluation of the first 70 patients in the center for male sexual dysfunction of Beth Israel Medical Center. Journal of Urology 131: 53–55

Metz P, Bengtsson J 1981 Penile blood pressure. Scandinavian Journal of Urology and Nephrology 15: 161–164

Metz P, Wagner G 1981 Penile circumference and erection. Urology 18: 268

Michal V 1982 Arterial disease as a cause of impotence. Clinics in Endocrinology and Metabolism 11(13): 725–748

Michal V, Pospichal J 1978 Phalloarteriography in the diagnosis of erectile impotence. World Journal of Surgery 2: 239–248

Morokoff P, Heiman J 1980 Effects of erotic stimuli on sexually functional and dysfunctional women: multiple measures before and after sex therapy. Behaviour Research and Therapy 18: 127–137

Opsomer R J, Guerit J M, Wese F X, van Caugh P J 1986 Pudendal cortical somatosensory evoked potentials. Journal of Urology 135: 1216–1218

Porst H, Tackmann W, van Ahlen H 1987 Neurophysiological investigation in potent and and impotent men — results of BCR-latencies and somatosensory evoked potentials (SSEP)?

Procci W R, Moss H B, Boyd J L, Baron D A S 1983 Consecutive-night reliability of portable penile tumescence monitor. Archives of Sexual Behavior 12: 307–316

Robinette M A, Moffat M J 1986 Intracorporal injection of papaverine and phentolamine in the management of impotence. British Journal of Urology 58: 692–695

Rosen R C, Keefe F J 1978 The measurement of human penile tumescence. Psychophysiology 15: 366–376

Rust J, Golombok S 1985 The validation of the Golombok–Rust inventory of sexual satisfaction. British Journal of Clinical Psychology 24: 63–64

Said G, Stama G, Salva J 1983 Progressive centripetal degeneration of axons in small fibre type diabetic polyneuropathy: a clinical and pathological study. Brain 106: 791–807

Schiavi R C 1981 The diagnosis of erectile disorders. In: Hock Z, Lief H E Proceedings of the 5th World Congress of Sexology. Excerpta Medica, Amsterdam

Schiavi R C, Fisher C 1982 Assessment of diabetic impotence: measurement of nocturnal erections. Clinics in Endocrinology and Metabolism 11(3): 769–784

Schiavi R C, Derogatis L R, Kurianski J, O'Connor D, Sharpe L 1979 The assessment of sexual function and marital interaction. Journal of Sexual and Marital Therapy 5: 169–223

Schiavi R C, Fisher C, Quadland M, Glover A 1985 Nocturnal penile tumescent evaluation of erectile function in insulin dependent diabetic men. Diabetologia 28: 90–94

Segraves K A, Segraves R T, Schoenberg H W 1987 Use of sexual history to differentiate organic from psychogenic impotence. Archives of Sexual Behavior 16: 125–138

Sharlip I D 1986 The case against using Doppler auscultation of the penis to diagnose arteriogenic impotence. 2nd World Meeting on Impotence, Prague

Sidi A A, Cameron J S, Duffy L M, Lange P H 1986 Intracavernous drug-induced erection in the management of male erectile dysfunction; experience with 100 patients. Journal of Urology 135: 704–706

Smith G, Chisholm G D, Pye F, Bancroft J 1987 Doppler penile pulse wave forms and nocturnal tumescence testing in erectile impotence. Paper presented at BAUS, Edinburgh

Strachan J R, Prior J P 1987 Diagnostic intracorporeal papaverine and erectile dysfunction. British Journal of Urology 59: 264–266

Velcek D, Sniderman K W, Vaughan E D, Sos T A, Muecke E C 1980 Penile flow index utilising a Doppler pulse wave analysis to identify vascular insufficiency. Journal of Urology 123: 669–673

Virag R 1986 The screening of impotence by the use of visual sexual stimulation after intracavernous injection of a small (8 mgm) dose of papaverine. 2nd World Meeting on Impotence, Prague

Virag R, Frydman D, Legman M, Virag H 1984 Intracavernous injection of papaverine as a diagnostic and therapeutic method in erectile failure. Angiology 35: 79–87

Virag R, Virag H, Lajujie J 1985 A new device for measuring penile rigidity. Urology 25: 80–81

Wagner G 1981 The diagnostic value of blood flow determination of corpus cavernosum in the flaccid and erect states. In: Hoch Z, Lief H E (eds) Proceedings of the 5th World Congress of Sexology. Excerpta Medica, Amsterdam

Wein A J, Fishkin R, Carpiniello V L, Malloy T R 1981 Expansion without significant rigidity during nocturnal penile tumescence testing; a potential source of misinterpretation. Urology 126: 343–344

Williams G 1987 Erectile dysfunction: diagnosis and treatment. British Journal of Urology 60: 1–5

Wincze J, Hoon E, Hoon P 1976 Physiological responsibility of normal and sexually dysfunctional women during erotic stimulus exposure. Journal of Psychosomatic Research 20: 445–451

Wincze J, Hoon E, Hoon P 1978 Multiple measure analysis of women experiencing low sexual arousal. Behaviour Research and Therapy 16: 43–49

Wooten V, Fields T J 1987 Evaluation of the Dacomed Rigiscan device. International Sleep Conference

Zorgniotti A W, Lefleur R S 1985 Autoinjection of the corpora cavernosa with a vasoactive drug combination for vasculogenic impotence. Journal of Urology 133: 39–41

Zuckerman M, Neeb M, Ficher M et al 1985 Nocturnal penile tumescence and penile response in the resting state in diabetic and non-diabetic sexual dysfunctionals. Archives of Sexual Behavior 15: 366–376

10

Helping people with sexual problems

THE HISTORICAL BACKGROUND

It should now be clear that the variety of problems relating to human sexuality requires a broad spectrum of help and treatment. Not only do we have to consider physical or medical factors, but also individual problems in the acceptance of sexual feelings as well as conflict within sexual relationships. Such problems may arise in the context of conventional sexual relationships, or relate to homosexuality or to other unconventional, stigmatised or deviant manifestations of sexuality.

Over the past 50 years there have been major changes in social and professional attitudes to the treatment of such problems. These stem from influences which are mostly emotive or ideological rather than rational. The situation is still in a state of flux but there is reason to think that progress towards a rational approach is being achieved.

Of importance have been theoretical and often ideological differences about the causation and appropriate treatment of sexual problems. Probably the most dominating influence in the first half of the 20th century was psychoanalysis. Sexual problems, whether experienced as dysfunction or deviance, were regarded as symptoms of disorders of personality development, hence their effective treatment was seen to require psychoanalytic therapy, usually of a fairly prolonged kind. The essence of this approach is described by Rosen (1977). 'Full analysis is usually four or five times weekly, and extends for many years because of the time necessary to effect structural changes in the personality concerning events in earliest childhood which are totally unconscious'. Much reliance is placed on analysing the 'transference' which is a process 'whereby the patient, following the basic rule of free association, relives within the therapeutic situation past psychic events in their fullest recall . . . The therapist is regarded as being the other person or persons in that past relationship or experience . . . The process of verbalising such reliving, which partakes of abreaction in its emotional expression . . . is known as working through'. In this way the defences against these early stresses are gradually relinquished and conflicts resolved. However, 'because one is dealing in the sexual disorders with pleasurable aspects which the patient does not wish to give up, and painful guilts, anxieties and losses the patient does not wish to encounter, progress is slow and proceeds against constant resistance' (Rosen 1977).

The restriction of this kind of prolonged treatment to those who were able to pay, or were seen to be likely to respond, and the very uncertain efficacy of such methods has meant that for the large majority of people with sexual problems, help has appeared to be inaccessible and the prospects for change slim.

This psychoanalytic view, more predominant in the USA than in Europe, has always been countered to some extent by a more pragmatic and directive view of psychological treatment, in which learning or re-learning or the acquisition of healthy habits has been the basic theme. In an early crude form this was shown in the various attempts to discourage masturbation, believed to lead to all types of problems, sexual and otherwise. Towards the end of the 19th and in the early parts of the 20th century hypnosis enjoyed a vogue, and is still in evidence to a limited extent today. Von Schrenck-Notzing (1895) wrote a monograph on the use of hypnotherapy in the treatment of various sexual problems. He derived the principles of treatment from the more general ones of education, the aim of which was 'to create a series of habits by means of direct persuasion, acts, imitation and admiration'. Using 'suggestion' in its widest sense, he regarded all education as a combination of co-ordinated and well considered suggestions. He believed sexual problems stemmed from 'faulty habits' and in his view, if such habits could have been prevented by correct education, then they should be to some extent reversible by re-education. Hypnotic suggestion was thus used to facilitate this process, in which patients were encouraged to try out and persevere with normal sexual activity, often using prostitutes as a source of experience.

Other authorities, such as Moll & Charcot, at this time advocated direct behavioural intervention (see Bancroft 1974). Whilst such approaches seem crude today, they contain much of the essence of more modern behavioural methods.

One therapeutic factor which has a long history is the imposition of a ban on full intercourse whilst encouraging more limited sexual contact. John Hunter wrote in 1786 (see Hunter & MacAlpine 1963) how he had helped a man who was troubled by erectile impotence by advising him 'to go to bed to this woman, but first promise to himself that he would not have any connection with her, for six nights, let his inclinations and powers be what they would; which he engaged to do; and also to let me know the result. About a fortnight after he told me that his resolution had produced such a total alteration in the state of his mind, that the powers soon took place, for instead of going to bed with the fear of inability, he went with fears that he should be possessed with too much desire, too much power, so as to become uneasy to him, which really happened'. This commonsense principle features in many more modern directive approaches.

Others in more recent years have advocated practical steps such as progressive relaxation (Schultz 1951), a 'stop–start' method for controlling premature ejaculation (Semans 1956), the use of graded dilators for vaginismus and self-stimulation techniques for unresponsive women (Hastings 1967). These were essentially empirical approaches and were not based on any particular theoretical assumptions.

Modern behaviour therapy became established in the 1950s and 60s. Practical behavioural approaches were based on the theoretical principles of learning derived from laboratory experiments. This basis claimed to endow such treatment with a scientific respectability, in contrast to the more mundane commonsense basis of earlier practical approaches. This scientific respectability has proved to be an illusion, as the early theoretical assumptions have failed to be justified, but it did motivate many scientifically minded clinicians to explore these treatment approaches. And whilst the early theoretical assumptions have largely given way to a more empirical approach, a tradition of careful measurement and evaluation of treatment has been established which has always been notably lacking in the psychoanalytic arena. As we shall see in this chapter the behaviourist's enthusiasm for evaluation has sometimes obscured the realities of what can be evaluated, betraying a form of naivety which has not troubled psychoanalysts. Much of this 'scientism' of early behaviour therapy was a reaction against the ascientific nature of psychoanalysis and hence ideological polemic influenced behaviour therapists as much if not more than psychoanalysts. As a consequence of these early theoretical constraints, treatment of sexual problems was mainly confined to those conditions which fitted an appropriate experimental learning model, hence the early emphasis on aversive conditioning and the modification of 'undesirable' sexual behaviours, such as homosexuality. These aversive procedures, which evoked considerable ingenuity amongst their innovators, seem of very limited relevance nowadays, not simply because of their doubtful efficacy. Now there is much more emphasis on positive approaches — learning new behaviours rather than actively discouraging old ones (Bancroft 1974). Behaviour therapy for the much more widespread problems of sexual dysfunction received very little attention. Occasional case reports of the use of systematic desensitisation (Lazarus 1963; Brady 1966; Friedman 1966; Wolpe 1969) appeared but were few compared to the literature of the treatment of deviant sexuality.

Alongside the psychoanalytically and behaviourally oriented therapists have been those advocating surgical, pharmacological or mechanical methods of treatment. In the 1930s there was a brief interest in a variety of surgical procedures for impotence, such as cautery and the passage of cold sounds, tightening of the perineal musculature, the application of testicular diathermy or galvanic stimulation of the perineal musculature (Johnson 1968). Not surprisingly, in view of the lack of any sensible rationale, such methods did not survive for long. The main surgical procedure to have been used for treating female dysfunction is Fenton's operation for vaginismus. Posterior wall vaginal repairs are sometimes carried out to increase vaginal tightness. There a few proper grounds for such procedures nowadays.

Surgical treatment of erectile failure has however entered a new and important phase. The 1940s saw the first attempts at inserting penile splints. In the past 15 years there has been a dramatic increase in the use of such surgically implanted prostheses, accompanied by considerable technical ingenuity. Vascular surgery for erectile problems attributed to vascular pathology is also being explored. We will consider these surgical developments later in this chapter. Of particular importance however has been the increased interest in methods of investigation and diagnosis (considered in Chapter 9); these methods have developed alongside the surgery, ostensibly to identify those cases where organic aetiology justifies surgical treatment. The tendency to see sexual dysfunction as *either* organic *or* psychogenic is not being relinquished easily, in spite of unremitting evidence that both types of factor are more often than not involved. Nevertheless this era of objective assessment is substantially advancing our understanding of the pathophysiology of sexual function.

Non-surgical mechanical devices have usually been in evidence. The coital training apparatus of Loewenstein (1947) was an early example. More recently we have seen penile rings and suction apparatus. We will consider these under sexual aids, below.

Not surprisingly with the identification of sex hormones, and in particular testosterone, attempts to use these hormones to treat sexual problems were made. Whilst there were some early successes (e.g. Hamilton 1937) most reports were negative. Heller & Myers (1944) claimed a good response in impotent men who had raised urinary gonadotrophins, indicating testicular failure. They called this the 'male climacteric syndrome'. Testosterone was also reported to be effective in increasing libido in women (Salmon & Geist 1943). These reports were anecdotal and somewhat impressionistic. After a phase of interest during the 1940s, disillusion set in, apart from the occasional enthusiast (e.g. Tuthill 1955). Little interest in hormone therapy was then shown until recently, with the major improvements in hormone assay and the resultant spate of clinical research into endocrinological mechanisms (see Chapter 2).

In an era when we seek drugs to solve most problems there has been a notable lack of pharmacological agents to help sexual difficulties. Of course the search for the effective aphrodisiac is older than alchemy (Taberner 1985). There have been some interesting developments in the last few years, with the introduction of intracavernosal injections and the evaluation of systemic drugs such as yohimbine. We considered some of the evidence in

Chapter 2 and will review the therapeutic implications in this chapter. But the significant pharmacological breakthrough still eludes us.

Also to be taken into account is a substantial increase in our basic understanding of sexual physiology. It is now possible for sex therapists to employ a fairly thorough knowledge of the anatomy and physiology of sexual response in their treatment methods. Such a basic factor was notably lacking in most sex therapy prior to 1960. To some extent this physiological trend has 'overswung'. We are once again in a phase of undue emphasis on physical factors and over-enthusiastic application of physical methods of treatment.

Whilst there have been these substantial developments in both psychological and physical methods, the amount of dialogue between the exponents of these contrasting approaches has until recently been minimal. In fact ideological barriers have existed. Until recently there has been little attempt to place these contrasting approaches into a common perspective, or to explore factors that might in particular cases indicate one approach rather than another, or favour a combination of approaches. In the past 5 years this situation has started to improve, with growing collaboration between surgical, physiological and psychological researchers.

Of importance in the UK was the development of sexual counselling techniques within the Family Planning Association. This was mainly under the influence of Michael Balint, who had applied his psychoanalytic training to devise ways for general practitioners to achieve more limited aims in a short time with a wide range of problems (Balint 1957). In 1958, Balint, together with a group of family planning doctors, started to apply these principles to the sexual problems that presented in family planning clinics. A central feature was the vaginal examination which was not only used for diagnostic and educational purposes, but also as a powerful method of eliciting emotional reactions relating to the genitalia and their functioning. In addition, doctors developing this approach focused on their own emotional reactions to the patient as another important source of information. Over the next few years, a treatment approach and method of training was devised and these are now being learnt by many doctors in the UK (Tunnadine et al 1981). Because of this focus on the vaginal examination, the emphasis has been on female problems, in particular those involving non-consummation, and also on working with the individual woman rather than the couple. This group has claimed good results (e.g. Bramley et al 1983). Unfortunately their attempts to evaluate their results have been limited or seriously biased in various ways. They have also shown a tendency to draw spurious comparision with the results from other approaches, claiming superiority for their method which the evidence certainly does not justify (Bancroft 1985). Also, as is characteristic of other psychoanalytically oriented methods, it is difficult for the uninitiated to grasp what it is that the therapist actually does to bring about therapeutic change. Relatively little has been written, though the reader will obtain some idea of this approach from Courtenay (1968), Tunnadine (1970, 1980) and Draper

(1983). One obtains a cleared idea of the nature of the underlying problems than of the method of resolving them, and the impression obtained is that these workers typically deal with a narrower range of problems than would normally be encountered in a general sexual problems clinic. Nevertheless, this approach, now well established, is of interest and presents one of the first attempts to bridge the psychosomatic gap in treatment. It is to be hoped that in the future the proponents of this approach will be less doctrinaire and more prepared to share their methods and experiences with those from other treatment backgrounds.

In the development of sexual therapy 1970 proved to be a crucial year. Masters & Johnson published their book Human Sexual Inadequacy claiming impressive results in a large number of couples with sexual dysfunction, using an intensive but very brief treatment method which lasted only 2 weeks. They also presented follow-up data for at least 5 years.

The impact of this book, for all its unreadable prose, has been enormous and the repercussions are still continuing. This was no mere case report which could be ignored, but involved large numbers by any standard of treatment outcome research. There was no difficulty in criticising Masters & Johnson's results — their patients were obviously highly selected, treated in special, and for most patients, inaccessible circumstances, and their methods of assessing change left a great deal to be desired. They presented their results in terms of 'failure', meaning the failure 'to initiate reversal of the basis symptomalogy of sexual dysfunction for which the unit (i.e. couple) was referred'. Such vagueness prevailed but was accompained by such apparently conservative and over-cautious methods of reporting that its shortcomings were often overlooked. Failure was often interpreted by others as the reciprocal of success. In other words, 20% failure was taken to mean 80% success (Zilbergeld & Evans 1980; see p. 493 for fuller discussion).

But in spite of such valid criticism, there was no escaping the conclusion that a lot of people with sexual dysfunction had benefited substantially from a very brief, directive method of treatment. This has led to some revision of views by the less entrenched of the psychoanalytic camp. Thus Rosen (1977) listed four types of psychoanalytically oriented help which is needed for sexual problems.

1. Counselling, which aims to educate as well as challenge guilty attitudes and hence to 'give permission'.
2. Supportive psychotherapy when 'patients who present with sexual inhibitions or simple regressions such as uncomplicated secondary impotence or loss of libido, are best treated with short courses of individual or group therapy'. This does not make use of transference analysis but offers some interpretation of underlying motivations or resistance and facilitates expression of associated affects.
3. Intensive analytical insight psychotherapy.
4. Full psychoanalysis.

Rosen, in other words, is acknowledging that there are problems which will benefit from simple short-term approaches, though he is somewhat vague about how to recognise them.

Masters & Johnson also emphasised the couple rather than the individual, though this must be seen as part of a more general tendency away from the individual and towards couple, group and family techniques. To some extent, this swing has passed its peak and for sexual problems attention to individual treatment, even when a couple exists, is once again receiving attention.

Many behaviourally oriented therapists accepted Masters & Johnson's ideas enthusiastically. For those who had been working with more conventional behavioural therapy techniques prior to 1970, this new approach provided a more comprehensive package which made sense. More 'hard-line' behaviourists have looked at Masters & Johnson's very empirical atheoretical approach with suspicion, either accusing them of plagiarising behaviour therapy techniques without appropriate acknowledgement (Dengrove 1971) or regarding the method as no different to systematic desensitisation (Laughren & Kass 1975). Others have stated that Masters & Johnson's method would be even more effective if it was based on proper principles of behaviour modification (Murphy & Mikulas 1974).

Many modifications and additional innovations followed Masters & Johnson's report, usually accompanied, at least in the USA, with considerable optimism about efficacy and striking claims of success. Reactions in the UK and Europe have been somewhat more guarded, helped by an early recourse to controlled outcome studies and the sobering results produced.

It has become clear, even to those working in the USA, that the extreme optimism of the early 1970s was deceptive. A more realistic and less simplistic view is beginning to emerge which recognises the considerable heterogeneity of problems that present for sex therapy, with their widely differing therapeutic needs and prognoses.

The eclecticism associated with modern sex therapy has been refreshing, particularly compared with the polemic that has prevailed between psychodynamic and behaviourally oriented therapists working in other fields. Helen Kaplan (1974) set an example in her attempts to combine behavioural and psychoanalytic principles. Whereas the behavioural approach in its traditional form has value when modifying specific aspects of behaviour (e.g. phobic anxiety, obsessional rituals, smoking), sex therapy more often than not has to deal with the complexities of the relationship; whereas specific behavioural techniques may be helpful, their effects are usually mediated by highly complex inter- and intrapersonal processes. It is thus not surprising that sex therapists developed their eclecticism at a relatively early stage.

MARITAL THERAPY OR SEX THERAPY?

An issue of growing importance is the extent to which sex therapy needs to focus on non-sexual aspects of the relationship. This practical aspect of treatment will be discussed in more detail later. But we are increasingly seeing a combination of sex therapy and marital therapy.

Marital therapy has been through interesting phases of development in the past 25 years or so. On the psychoanalytic side we have seen innovation in working with couples rather than individuals, often with two therapists, whilst taking into account the unconscious processes which influence an individual's choice of partner and the type of interaction with him or her. Developments at the Institute of Marital Studies in Britain were documented by Pincus (1960). Dicks (1967), in his classic text Marital Tensions, described how he treated marital disturbance within a National Health Service clinic.

Family therapy has been in the ascendancy (Skinner 1976). With its background in psychoanalytic theory it has been much influenced by general systems theory, which emphasises the extent to which actors or components in a complex system interact with one another. A simple example is a central heating system in which, by means of a thermostat, the boiler switches on and off according to the temperature, showing homeostasis. In Chapter 2 we considered far more complex systems such as the hypothalamo-pituitary-gonadal axis, where both positive and negative feedback loops contribute to homeostasis. Systems theory is highly relevant in such a case, though the degree of predictability of the system is limited because of its variety of inter-relationships with other systems. Applying systems theory to the couple and family is in my view based on crude analogy at best. Homeostasis assumes a degree of stability of the system which is of doubtful relevance to human relationships. Systems theorists have tried to get round this by adding the concept of 'morphogenesis' to homeostasis, leaving us with a system sufficiently fluid and dynamic to account for any development in retrospect but defying prediction — a hall-mark of psychoanalytic theory. However this systems approach does have the virtue of focusing our attention on the interaction as at least a two-way process. Following such principles many family therapists doubt the effec-tiveness of marital therapy which does not take the children into account. According to Whitaker (1975), marital therapy without the children should be redefined as family therapy for a subgroup. Treacher (1985) has provided a useful discussion of the application of systems theory to marital counselling.

In the development of behavioural marital therapy we find a microcosm of the evolution of behavioural psychotherapy in general. Early efforts of conventional behaviourists such as Stuart (1969) saw the application of operant principles and token economies. Agreement was reached by the couple about which behaviours deserved reward or positive reinforcement.

In order to elicit or request such a behaviour from one's partner it was necessary to hand over a token or reward. As a closed economy was involved (i.e. there were a limited number of tokens in circulation), each partner would have to behave positively sufficiently often in order to earn enough tokens to purchase behaviours from the other. Other less extreme versions of this approach involved contingency contracting when an explicit and often written agreement was reached about what behaviour should get what kind of reward, e.g. if the husband talks to his wife for 30 minutes she will have sexual intercourse with him. The extent to which behaviour therapists were prepared to reduce marital interaction to this bartering level was an indication of their reluctance to consider anything except overt behaviour. In so far as such approaches succeeded, they probably did so by improving communication; negotiation of a specific behavioural contract is an effective way of finding out about one's partner's likes and dislikes. But there are alternative ways of attaining that goal which are more compatible with the principles of mutual trust and caring that one is striving for in any close relationship. After this naive beginning, behaviour therapists became less prepared to believe that they were shaping the behaviour of their couples in the way that Skinner shaped his pigeons. Instead they became more directly concerned with improving communication, dealing more appropriately with feelings, avoiding coercive and destructive patterns of interacting and using more effective problem-solving tactics (Patterson & Reid 1970; Jacobson & Margolin 1979; Stuart 1980; Hahlweg & Jacobson 1984). Their theoretical basis is now less to do with operant conditioning and more with social exchange theory (Kelly & Thibaut 1978) and social learning theory (Bandura 1977).

Part of the process of behaviour therapists becoming more interested in human beings and less in pigeons has been their recognition, a reluctant one for many, that one has to look further than overt behaviour and consider the thought processes accompanying it. In the early days of behaviour therapy this was seen by the purists as an abandonment of the scientific objectivity on which the new approach was based and a regression to discredited introspective techniques. However, those clinicians who were using the behavioural techniques found it increasingly difficult to ignore these more subjective aspects. If one stands back and views the development of these behavioural methods over the past 20 years, it is difficult to avoid the conclusion that individual therapists choose a treatment method and a theoretical perspective that best suit their personality and cognitive style. There are some, and I include myself in this category, as I shall reveal in this chapter, who are prepared to be eclectic and combine fragments of methods or tactics if they seem to be useful. It is helpful to have a framework in which to order such fragments but this is not the same as a theoretical system (see Bancroft 1974 for comparison of a treatment procedure and a theoretical model). There are others who need to identify clearly with a specific school of thought and for whom eclecticism is some sort of threat to their professional identity. Thus, when cognitive processes became the focus of attention in the late 1970s, we found some traditional behaviourists retreating into their entrenched purist positions and rejecting 'the soft tendency', whilst others produced a 'new doctrine' called cognitive therapy, endowed with its own special jargon (an inevitable feature in the separation of professional groups), its own journal and conferences. Thus to some extent we have seen a split in the behaviour therapy movement comparable to the ideological divides that have riven the psychoanalytic movement. I therefore have mixed feelings about the recent developments in cognitive therapy. The commitment to precise definition carried forward from traditional behaviour therapy has been useful in clarifying certain concepts and tactics. But the mystification, by means of special terminology and training methods, of a therapeutic process which in my view is the concerted application of commonsense, reveals an unwelcome tendency to professionalism. We will consider the use of cognitive methods of various points in this chapter. But they will form parts of a multi-faceted therapeutic approach rather than constituting specific treatments in their own right (e.g. Beck 1976; Meichenbaum 1977). It helps to put these new ideas into perspective by comparing them with rational emotive therapy (RET), pioneered some time ago by Albert Ellis (1962); although it involves many Ellis idiosyncrasies, RET shares much common ground with cognitive and behavioural programes. (Dryden (1985) has considered the application of RET to marital problems.)

In marital therapy as well as sex therapy we see a refreshing readiness for therapists from differing backgrounds to exchange ideas and borrow from each other. In Dryden's book Marital Therapy in Britain (1985) there is an interesting discussion of the similarities and differences of several approaches to marital therapy. In the National Marriage Guidance movement in Britain we have seen an approach rooted in Rogerian principles (Rogers 1951) with a reliance on psychoanalytic concepts to gain understanding of the dynamics of marriages, but with an increasing tendency in recent years to employ more directive task-oriented, problem-solving methods (e.g. Egan 1975). It has also been of interest to see how the Marriage Guidance movement has incorporated sex therapy into its scheme of things. In the mid 1970s, Paul Brown, a clinical psychologist, taught marriage guidance counsellors a modification of Masters & Johnson's approach (Tyndall 1985). This was seen as a radically different technique to the traditional counselling for non-sexual marital problems and hence it was allowed to develop as a separate subspeciality with its own training programme. Clearly in the early days this degree of separation was necessary to avoid confusing the aims and principles of their traditional approach. But now that marital counselling is becoming more directive and task-oriented we are beginning to see an integration of these previously distinct methods.

The approach to sex therapy described in this chapter will demonstrate this eclecticism, as well as a readiness to work with both sexual and non-sexual problems in the same counselling relationship.

SOCIAL INFLUENCES

Apart from the theoretical and ideological influences already discussed, recent changes in sex therapy have also been affected by changes in social attitudes to sex. These were marked during the 1960s, and we have already discussed the major changes that became evident during that decade and the various societal factors which may have contributed to them. Changing expectations of sex, particularly for the increasingly liberated woman, and the fostering of these expectations by the media led to increased demands for professional help. During the 1980s some commentators have had the impression of a move back towards more traditional or at least less liberated attitudes towards sexual relationships. This swing of the pendulum is in the process of receiving an almighty shove from the AIDS scare, though it is too soon to judge the effects this will have. Certainly there are likely to be changes in attitudes to unconventional and casual sex, not all of them for the better.

Another issue has to be faced if modern sex therapy is to realise its potential on a worldwise basis. In its origins, and the basic sexual values underlying it, sex therapy is clearly middle-class. It is true, as discussed in Chapter 4, that many of the social class differences in sexual attitudes and behaviour are diminishing, at least in the USA and western Europe. But there are many parts of the world where a concern about sexual problems is growing and where several of the basic assumptions of sex therapy, concerning the good sexual relationship and the need for an egalitarian, reciprocal relationship between man and woman, have almost revolutionary significance. Even within our own society we must exercise caution to avoid provoking conflict with the subcultures of our patients, creating more problems than our therapy solves (Bancroft 1981).

Sex therapy gets caught up in other social processes which should make us, as therapists, cautious. Thus, in the USA, we have seen an increase in the request for help with orgasmic difficulties which now seem to have passed its peak. Did sex therapy, through the media, alter at least temporarily the expectations of women? Now we are seeing a rather dramatic change of emphasis towards disorders of sexual desire. As indicated earlier (see Chapter 8) it is commonplace for women to report virtually no spontaneous sexual desire and this does not necessarily lead to problems. Is there now a danger that such women will be encouraged to see themselves as pathological or needing treatment? How often are we 'medicalising' what is in fact a relationship problem?

Sex therapy therefore requires us to take a broad multidisciplinary grasp of human sexuality, with psychological, physiological and sociological factors viewed in their proper relationship to one another and with due consideration of the ethical implications. There is a long way to go before we can hope to reach that happy state of affairs.

AN APPROACH TO TREATMENT — COUPLE THERAPY

Psychological methods of treatment are used in a variety of contexts:

1. simple counselling for the individual or couple;
2. couple therapy;
3. individual therapy;
4. group therapy.

In addition there is scope for using:

1. hormone or drug therapy;
2. sexual aids;
3. surgical treatment.

These last three treatments should be, but often are not used in combination with one of the above psychological approaches. Obviously couple therapy is most suited for dealing with sexual problems within existing relationships, individual therapy is best for individual problems and group therapy for either.

Each of these treatment approaches will now be considered in more detail. It is assumed that appropriate assessment of the problem, as described in Chapter 9, has already taken place and an offer of counselling or therapy has been made and accepted. The approach used by the author in each case will be described in some depth and will be followed by a discussion of the main points of contrast with the methods of other sex therapists and a brief review of the available and relevant research evidence. As couple therapy in the most widely used at present it will be dealt with most fully. Most of the basic principles relevant to individual and group treatment will be covered under that heading to avoid repetition.

SIMPLE COUNSELLING

Many people have difficulties in adjusting to a rewarding sexual relationship because of relatively simple problems such as ignorance or misunderstanding of what to expect, or some degree of unjustified guilt or anxiety. They may benefit from very limited counselling. Many professionals are able to offer such counselling without having either the time or expertise to embark on the more specialised forms of treatment described below. If such counselling helps, all well and good. If it does not, more substantial help can be offered or arranged. One can confidently conclude that no harm is likely to result from such a policy.

The basic elements of such simple counselling have been well described by Annon (1974). The counsellor's contributions can be listed under the following headings:

1. Limited information: the provision of basic facts about normal sexual response and the countering of myths about norms of behaviour. Such

information may not need to be comprehensive but limited to the specific problem area (e.g. the majority of women need some clitoral stimulation to achieve orgasm during intercourse. A woman may get more pleasurable sensation from intercourse in the male superior position if she fully flexes her hips etc.).

2. Specific suggestions. These may involve techniques of self-stimulation and masturbation, the use of vibrators, trying different positions during love-making, increasing the level of communication and so on.

3. Permission and reassurance. Often in providing information and making specific suggestions to try out new and previously unacceptable behaviours, one is giving permission. This is often as important or more so than the suggestions themselves. The effectiveness of such permission depends on the patient having a positive opinion of the counsellor.

4. Facilitate communication. Establish with the individual or couple an appropriate and comfortable vocabulary for talking about sexual matters and provide a model for such comfortable communication. With a couple this experience may make it easier for them to discuss the issues with each other, a very important need in many cases.

Such counselling is largely based on commonsense and need only occupy one or two half-hour sessions. A follow-up appointment is useful as it keeps open the channels of communication with the counsellor and provides an opportunity to consider more systematic help if needed. As yet there is no research evidence of the efficacy of or indications for such an approach.

Although simple, this form of counselling does have certain requirements, the importance of which should not be underestimated. The counsellor should *feel* relaxed and comfortable with sexual issues, whilst making it easier for other people to talk comfortably about sex. In addition to having sufficient knowledge about human sexuality to permit him or her to be confidently informative, it is also desirable to be adept at recognising poor communication and teaching basic communication skills.

COUPLE THERAPY

There are many factors contributing to sexual problems that need to be dealt with in therapy: anxiety, anger, insecurity, guilt and low self-esteem are particularly important. The advantage of the treatment approach described in this section is that it is designed to deal with all of these if and when they arise. This method is based on that of Masters & Johnson (1970) though, as will be discussed later, there are some important differences and behavioural and cognitive methods of dealing with the non-sexual aspects of the relationship will be described when appropriate.

The objective of couple therapy is the establishment of an emotionally secure relationship that allows normal sexual responses to occur and be enjoyed. It is important not to make aims too specific. Half the battle is to distract the couple from being goal-oriented in their love-making, as this leads to performance anxiety and the tendency to become a spectator rather than a participant. There are certain types of sexual dysfunction that require particular attention (e.g. vaginismus and premature ejaculation), but for most sexual problems, including erectile failure and orgasmic difficulty, the main emphasis is on the nature of the sexual interaction and away from the specific sexual response. Even with vaginismus and premature ejaculation it is usually necessary to check that the couple are relating and communicating comfortably and appropriately before the specific problem can be dealt with properly.

The couple are asked to carry out certain sexual assignments whilst agreeing to keep within certain limits. The assignments involve mutual touching, called by Masters & Johnson 'sensate focus'. The initial limits exclude genital touching or intercourse. This combination of specified tasks and agreed limits can have a variety of effects. It may certainly reduce performance anxiety and hence improve natural sexual responsiveness. It may help to identify the threat of being trapped in a situation from which one cannot escape. A woman may be reluctant to attempt these first assignments for fear that her partner will become aroused and then demand or expect intercourse. This in turn reveals a lack of trust in the partner, doubts that he will keep to the agreed limits. The partner's reaction to this may reveal highly relevant attitudes about male sexuality. He may not trust himself either, on the grounds that a male who is sexually aroused cannot be expected to be responsible for his behaviour, and so on. Each of these reactions may be important for understanding the problem. Resentment is commonly revealed at this early stage; to touch one another in this mutually caring way is very difficult if each is feeling angry with the other. Resentment may be expressed that your partner is getting more pleasure than you are. A host of problems may be revealed by setting these sensate focus and subsequent assignments.

The therapist then has to use his psychotherapeutic skills to resolve these problems as they arise. He must be prepared to encounter a complex of inter- and intrapersonal processes, requiring a flexible approach.

The treatment technique

Now let us look at this treatment method in considerably more detail. The style can best be described as behavioural psychotherapy, the essence of which is a combination of doing and understanding, i.e. getting patients to try things and helping them to understand the difficulties they have in carrying them out. The framework of therapy and the structure of the therapy session can therefore be summarised as follows:

1. Set appropriate behavioural assignments (homework; the behavioural component).

2. Examine the patient's attempts to carry out those assignments.
3. As a result, identify those obstacles (attitudes, fears, or other feelings) underlying the difficulties encountered.
4. Help the patient to modify or reduce those obstacles so that the behaviours can be carried out successfully (the educational and psychotherapeutic components).
5. Set the next appropriate behavioural assignments.

The particular strength of this combination is that the setting of relevant target behaviours is a rapidly effective way of uncovering the crucial inter- or intrapersonal problems behind these obstacles which must be dealt with. Such an approach is a combination of behavioural change and discovery. The therapist can reasonably assume that relevant material will emerge during the course of treatment. This is an important point because it means that the information necessary for treatment does not have to be obtained in the initial assessment, which can then focus more appropriately on establishing whether treatment is indicated and which type of approach is most likely to be beneficial, as well as establishing a 'contract' for that treatment. This means there need be no delay in getting the couple actively involved and started on a behavioural programme, provided that appropriate assignments suggest themselves. Let us look more closely at the components of treatment.

The behavioural component

Regardless of the precise nature of the sexual dysfunction it is considered appropriate at the outset to focus on basic elements of the relationship, on the assumption that unless the relationship works well with good communication and both partners feeling secure, it will be difficult to alter the specific sexual problem. Often by simply improving these basic aspects of the relationship, the specific sexual dysfunction recedes without special attention.

The first assignments concern the couple's method of communication during love-making, both verbal and physical, and their ability to make each other feel secure. The early sensate focus stages advocated by Masters & Johnson (1970) are particularly effective in this respect and are of universal relevance because they check the interpersonal processes which are fundamental to any sexual relationship. We can therefore ask any couple to embark on these assignments at an early stage in counselling, knowing that they will be relevant. Thus these initial stages are sufficiently standardised to warrant the use of written instructions. The couple are given a booklet at the outset which, in addition to containing some basic principles of sexual interaction, describes in detail the first few behavioural steps or stages of the programme. The partners are asked to read through the booklet and discuss their reactions with the counsellor before going over the first behavioural assignments again. The couple then take the booklet home with them. A copy of the booklet with details of how we use it is given in the Appendix (p. 535).

Basic communication skills

The golden rule of communication within close relationships is to self-assert and self-protect; that is, to tell one's partner what one wants as well as what one finds hurtful or unpleasant. What at first sounds like self-centredness works well provided that both partners follow the same principle. At the beginning of counselling the couple are asked to practise this golden rule in some relatively trivial, non-sexual situation, emphasising the use of 'I' language, or the use of the personal pronoun. Thus the typical question: 'Shall we go to the cinema tonight?' becomes: 'I would like to go to the cinema. Do you want to come too?' The answer might be: 'Yes, I would like to come' or 'I'm easy, but if you would like company I'll happily go along with you' or 'No, I would much rather stay in tonight, but you go on your own if you would like to' or 'No, I was hoping that we could both stay at home — there are a number of things I would like to discuss with you'. Such exchanges are direct and clear. When there are differences in needs or wishes these are not removed but they are clearly identified so that their resolution is much easier.

Throughout counselling, attention should be paid to this aspect of the relationship, concentrating not only on correct communication of meaning but also of feeling. We will consider problems of anger and resentment more closely later.

Sensate focus

Stage one

Self-protection and self-assertion are central to these early stages of the behavioural programme.

The couple are asked to take it in turns to touch each other when both are unclothed, comfortable and securely private. An agreement is made before starting that no attempt at genital touching or intercourse will be made by either partner, but that other parts of the body should be explored. The person doing the touching should be doing it for his or her own sake — to enjoy the touching (i.e. self-asserting). The person being touched has only one task: to indicate if he or she is finding anything unpleasant, however slight (i.e. self-protecting); the person doing the touching will then stop or change what is being done (Fig. 10.1). When either person has had enough (however long or short a period of time) the partners change place and the other one becomes the active toucher. This alternating pattern applies also to the initiating process; the couple are asked to take it in turns

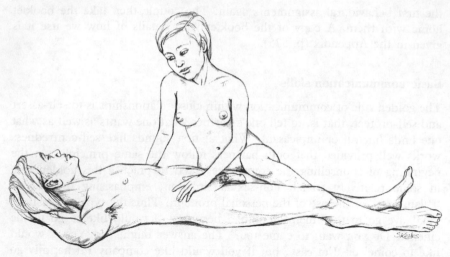

Fig. 10.1 Sensate focus.

to invite the other to have a touching session with the understanding that the invitation can be declined without offence.

A general principle of this kind of counselling is that the reasons for each assignment are explained to the couple. There is no magic involved — we are encouraging them to use commonsense principles of relating and it is important for them to understand those principles so that they can make use of them in the future should the need arise. There are two particular aspects of this first stage which need careful explanation:

Setting limits. This has two principal purposes:

1. to eliminate performance anxiety. As there is no need for any sexual response, both partners will be able to relax and enjoy the physical intimacy. It is not unusual for couples to experience considerable relaxation and enhanced enjoyment at this first stage and this is a useful indicator of the importance of performance anxiety.

2. to check feelings of trust; will the partner agree to stick to the limits? Often in a sexually troubled relationship, one partner reaches the conclusion that the other (most often the male) is not to be trusted, hence if any form of intimacy is permitted, full sexual intercourse will be expected or demanded. Hence even minimal physical expression of affection is avoided. If such lack of trust is important it will quickly become evident at this stage.

Touching for your own pleasure. This instruction has three principal purposes:

1. to check that each person feels comfortable being sexually assertive and does not have to give pleasure first before being able to experience it.

2. to allow each person to discover (or rediscover) that touching can be pleasurable in itself. If the toucher is preoccupied with the effect being produced on the partner, this subjective response is often lost or blunted.
3. to remove a sense of obligation to respond on the part of the recipient — 'he is trying to turn me one, why aren't I feeling anything?'. This relief from performance pressure often allows the person being touched to enjoy the experience more, even though this is not the primary intention.

Couples often have difficulty grasping this notion of 'touching for your own pleasure' and careful questioning is required to establish that they have understood. When both partners are comfortable with this stage, they progress to stage two.

Stage two

This differs from stage one only in that the person being touched is asked to give positive as well as negative feedback; in other words to indicate what is enjoyable as well as what is unpleasant. The touching partner can then act accordingly.

These first two stages typically reveal problems of mistrust, unresolved resentment or poor communication. 'Breaking the ban' (i.e. going on to intercourse) may occur and this is usually informative if discussed is sufficient detail. Typical explanations include:

1. not understanding the instructions or not seeing the point of them;
2. the underlying attitude that once sexually aroused a man does not normally act in a responsible fashion — responsibility is left to the woman, often an attitude shared by both partners which fosters the woman's resentment and loss of sexual responsiveness;
3. a subtle form of sabotage of the counselling if there is concern by one or other partner that the key issues are not being dealt with.

Stage three

The same basic principles apply, including the alternation of who initiates and who is active. Now genital touching can be included. (see Fig. 10.2) Orgasm should not be the aim, but may be allowed to occur. The main objective is simply to enjoy the experience of touching and being touched. If premature ejaculation is a problem, specific instructions about the 'stop–start' technique are given at this stage (see p. 544).

Fear of loss of control, sexual guilt or other unresolved sexual anxieties often become apparent at this time. Men with erectile problems may now realise the extent to which they have become spectators of their erectile response. Paradoxical instruction to get rid of any erection as soon as it

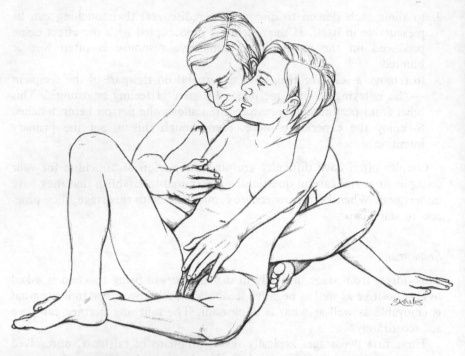

Fig. 10.2 Armchair position. This allows the man to stimulate the breasts and vulva of the woman in a non-threatening position. The woman can clearly guide her partner's hand.

occurs is sometimes useful. Generally each partner should learn to recognise when he or she is becoming a spectator and practise ways of stopping this. This may involve 'switching on' some pleasant distracting image, or if necessary stopping temporarily to disrupt the process.

When a couple are able to deal with a particular behavioural stage without difficulty, they move on to the next stage. However, behavioural progress may be halted for some time whilst crucial inter- or intrapersonal conflicts are resolved.

Subsequent stages are tailor-made to suit the needs of the particular couple, but usually involve a gradual progression, with short periods of vaginal entry, exploring different positions, and so on (see p. 543). Specific techniques dealing with premature ejaculation, vaginismus or other specific dysfunctions are incorporated into the programme (see below). The same basic principles continue to apply, with either partner being able to say 'stop' at any stage if he or she is aware of anxiety or other negative feelings. If necessary they should go back to an earlier stage which is less difficult.

The educational component

Overcoming ignorance and countering false expectations about what is normal or socially acceptable is as important in this context as in the simple counselling approach. Factual information should be provided, when relevant, throughout treatment. A didactic teaching session about normal male and female anatomy and sexual physiology is included, usually before the behavioural programme reaches the stage of genital touching. In this way the therapist can ensure that an appropriate shared vocabulary has been established before getting on to that stage. Films, pictures, models or rough sketches by the therapist can be all be used to aid this educational process. In particular the couple's attention is focused on to those aspects of anatomy and physiology which are especially relevant to their problems, e.g. the pelvic floor muscles for the woman with vaginismus or normal ejaculatory physiology for the premature ejaculator. The physical examination, as discussed in Chapter 9, is a further opportunity for providing information.

Another aspect of the educational component is ensuring that the couple understand why progress has been made so that they can apply the same principles in future when the need arises.

The psychotherapeutic component

In some cases the setting of appropriate behavioural tasks is all that is required of the therapist for improvement to occur. The reasons for this are often not clear but the reduction of performance anxiety, the increased sense of security with a partner that follows the setting of defined limits, the information and education that inevitably accompanies such behavioural analysis and goal-setting, the enhanced sexual response that may follow a novel approach and the permission of the therapist that explicitly or implicity accompanies the instructions may all play a part.

In the majority of cases, however, difficulties in carrying out a specific behavioural task will be experienced at some stage. The psychotherapeutic skills of the therapist then become important. It is at this point that the inexperienced therapist is likely to flounder. Whereas there are various theoretical models which could guide the therapist at this point, the following description is broadly eclectic.

Facilitating understanding

Reaching understanding of why one has difficulty carrying out a particular task is often followed by a reduction of that difficulty. A female patient was finding that during her love-making sessions she would start to become aroused and then suddenly 'switch off' and be unable to respond further. After several experiences of this kind and repeated consideration of why this might be so she eventually recalled that during her childhood she had the habit of masturbating to orgasm whenever she had been naughty and received punishment or criticism. She realised that the link between the sexual excitement and naughtiness had made it difficult for her to incorporate her sexual response into the good and loving relationship she had with her husband. Following this insight, the switching-off process ceased and she was able to experience orgasm during intercourse. Not infrequently, gaining understanding in this way is followed by behavioural change. What presumably happens is that the patient, having identified the most likely cause of the difficulty, now looks at the behaviour in a new light. If the original source of threat was during childhood, it is now looked at through adult eyes. The threat is reappraised and often found to be no longer threatening. Nowadays this is called 'cognitive restructuring'. Such reappraisal may continue between treatment sessions. What can the therapist do to facilitate it?

1. Attempting further appropriate behavioural tasks may help to focus on the specific problem. It may be particularly helpful to identify the difference between a person's reactions to two subtly different tasks. Why is it more difficult for a woman to become aroused when she takes the initiative than when her partner starts love-making? Why is it easier to indicate to one's partner what is unpleasant than what is pleasant?
2. Encourage the correct identification of feelings that accompany a particular difficulty. Is it anger, fear, anxiety etc.? Are particular thoughts evoked each time the difficult behaviour is attempted (eg. 'Do you find yourself thinking about your partner's past infidelity or some traumatic experience you had during childhood?')?
3. Encourage patients to find their own explanation. The therapist should start to produce in his or her mind a list of possibilities as soon as the difficulty is encountered and look for evidence to support or reject each one. But it is probably more effective if patients can produce the best explanation themselves rather than having it provided for them. They should be encouraged to produce their own list of possible explanations and to test them out. If this is not successful, the therapist can adopt a Socratic approach, when, with a particular explanation in mind, a patient is questioned in such a way as to increase the likelihood that he or she will consider that possibility. As a last resort, explanation can be offered by the therapist, preferably giving more than one alternative so that the patient can still choose which is the most appropriate.

The problem may nevertheless remain unchanged or incompletely resolved after such insight. Further steps then need to be taken.

Helping to resolve the difficulty

The active steps the therapist can take at this stage are considered under four headings:

1. Making explicit the patient's commitment to specific changes. At the start of treatment, the ultimate goals are deliberately vague, with the emphasis on improving the quality of the sexual relationship rather than

the efficiency of the sexual performance. But as treatment proceeds and specific obstacles are encountered, it becomes necessary to establish whether or not the patient or couple want to overcome a particular obstacle or problem. Thus if a woman has difficulty in touching her partner's penis, is this something she wishes to overcome? Is this resistance regarded by her as a nuisance (i.e. 'ego-alien') or is it consistent with her value system (i.e. 'ego-syntonic') and not something which ought to be changed? Phobic anxiety is a good example of an ego-alien resistance. The patient acknowledges that the anxiety is unreasonable or undesirable and wishes to be rid of it. If this is made clear then various steps can be recommended to overcome it. Obtaining explicit commitment of this kind is the next appropriate step in counselling.

2. In such circumstances one can set further appropriate behavioural steps specifically designed to overcome the resistance. Recommending a graded or hierarchical approach may be useful. Thus the woman who is reluctant to touch her partner's penis is encouraged to do so initially for a very short time. A woman who fears anything entering her vagina may be encouraged to insert her finger a short distance and for just 1 or 2 seconds. In general this approach involves the use of small steps which do not overwhelm the patient with anxiety, and encouragement to 'stay with' the anxious feelings, rather than avoid them, until they start to decline.

3. Alternatively such anxious feelings can be challenged at a cognitive level. Such reality confrontation may be applicable to either the ego-alien or ego-syntonic block. In the latter case, when the patient indicates no wish to overcome a particular resistance, the therapist has to judge the extent to which this is genuinely in conflict with the goals of treatment. This is often an issue in relation to masturbation. The therapist may recommend self-stimulation or individual sensate focus as an appropriate behavioural assignment and not infrequently the patient refuses on the grounds that such behaviour is unacceptable. Patients may assert that they came for help with the sexual relationship with their partners and not for their individual sexual feelings. It is then sensible to consider whether there are alternative routes to reach that goal, rather than insisting on following the prescribed path. A woman who is reluctant to touch her partner's penis can be confronted with the fact that such touching is particularly enjoyable for him. Is it that she is reluctant to give him pleasure? If she regards genital touching of any kind as unacceptable, the therapist can justifiably point out that such a view is incompatible with the patient's stated objectives. Knowing whether to accept a patient's values or challenge them presents one of the ethical problems in sex therapy (Bancroft 1981).

Often there is a need to confront patients with the inconsistencies between their beliefs or expectations and their actions. Such reality testing may involve providing factual information to challenge their beliefs (e.g.

the common belief that 'normal' women experience orgasm from vaginal intercourse alone, which may make it difficult for a woman to accept or enjoy direct clitoral stimulation). The permission-giving role of the therapist involves confronting the patients with inconsistencies between their values and those of the therapist: 'You may regard that as wrong but as far as I am concerned it is a perfectly acceptable thing to do'.

Facilitating the expression and communication of affect

As indicated in Chapter 8 there is commonly a link between sexual dysfunction and negative emotional reactions. The correct labelling of these associated affects is part of the process of understanding the difficulty. Often the affect stems from interpersonal problems, such as insecurity or resentment towards the partner. It is a basic assumption that such feelings, when unexpressed or misunderstood by the partner, serve to keep the problem going. Thus an important role for the therapist is to facilitate their expression in addition to helping their partner understand them. Often the difficulties in doing so reflect lifelong attitudes to dealing with anger or feelings in general which the individuals have brought with them into their relationship, such as the belief that it is wrong to show anger or fear, or concern that the relationship may not survive their expression. The therapist therefore has three tasks: firstly, to educate the couple about the adverse effects unexpressed or misunderstood feelings produce in intimate relationships and in the healthy use of appropriate methods of expressing them. Secondly, to help the couple to recognise particular instances when such feelings arise and are dealt with inappropriately or misunderstood, i.e. give feedback. Thirdly, to help them to work out more satisfactory ways of expressing and communicating their feelings, giving them behavioural tasks in trying out these new tactics, much as other behavioural assignments are used.

Identifying negative patterns of marital interaction

It is commonplace when working with sexual problems to become confronted with the non-sexual aspects of the relationship, as I stressed earlier. Unresolved anger may cause havoc in the sexual relationship but originate from non-sexual exchanges. Patterns of miscommunication may interfere with sexual intimacy but be reinforced in other contexts. An analysis of these non-sexual interactions is often necessary if these various non-sexual obstacles are to be dealt with and if progress in the sexual relationship is to be permitted.

We have already considered communication skills. Mackay (1985) has summarised the other common obstacles as follows:

1. *low levels of rewarding interactions*;
2. *coercive patterns of relating*, e.g. passive aggression, when positive rein-

forcement is deliberately or unconsciously withheld (e.g. a wife may refuse to have sex because she feels her husband has failed to give her appropriate support in dealing with the children) or aversive control, when compliance is obtained under threat (e.g. 'If the house isn't tidy when I get home I'm going to the pub'. If in such a situation the house is tidied it will be the result of appeasement and not a positive gesture of affection).
3. *poor problem-solving skills.* Many conflicts result from or are at least aggravated by the couple's inability to deal appropriately with otherwise ordinary problems confronting their marriage or their parenting.

The therapist can guide the couple in developing better problem-solving skills (for a description of the problem-solving approach see Greenwood & Bancroft 1988; and, as applied to marital therapy, Jacobson & Margolin 1979). Coercive behaviour should be pointed out and its destructive effects emphasised. The therapist has a vital feedback role in this respect. If such behaviour is motivated by unresolved anger, attention will need to be focused on dealing with that anger in more appropriate ways. Sometimes these coercive forms of interacting become like ingrained habits and need to be checked repeatedly. At the same time the couple are encouraged to increase the frequency of positive behaviours. Liberman et al (1980) describe a simple exercise called 'catch your spouse doing something nice'. Both partners are asked to record separately all such positive behaviours and to exchange their lists with each other at the end of each day, explaining clearly why each incident was rewarding. The emphasis, in other words, is on positive rather than negative exchanges. I tell couples that a healthy relationship does not require frequent gestures of spontaneous goodwill to keep it content. Many of the behaviours in a marriage — preparing meals, taking the dog for a walk, getting the shopping — are routine tasks which, whilst contributing to the running of the marital unit, do not involve spontaneous gestures of goodwill. But every now and then, when feeling positively towards one's partner, an otherwise unexpected spontaneous gesture is beneficial. In an unhappy marriage I draw the analogy of the sun occasionally breaking through the clouds and temporarily warming the day. Whilst the clouds may remain very much in evidence, as long as these sunny spells occur occasionally and with increasing rather than decreasing frequency then progress is being made.

Often apparently spontaneous gestures need careful scrutiny; they may conceal subtle forms of coercion. For example, a wife may cook her husband his favourite meal — it seems like a positive act, but she chooses to do it at a time when she knows he is going to be late home so that she can criticise him for spurning her warm gesture. Once again sensitive feedback is needed in such cases.

Dryden (1985), in describing the rational–emotive approach, points out certain styles of unhelpful thinking that can aggravate these negative marital patterns. He draws the distinction between expressing desire for certain responses from the spouse, and *insisting* that they occur. The first can be constructive, the second destructive. He describes 'awfulising' when something undesirable is exaggerated as 'awful' (i.e. 100% bad) rather than just 'not good'. A variant of this is to jump to the conclusion that a situation is 'intolerable' rather than 'undesirable but capable of being tolerated'. These are examples of how rational–emotive (and cognitive) therapists encourage less irrational and hence less destructive styles of thinking. These can all be seen as variants of the principal of reality confrontation, described earlier.

The patient–therapist relationship

In terms of the transactional analyst, this type of counselling requires an adult–adult relationship, not that of a parent–child or doctor–sick patient. The patient, or in this case both patients, need to accept responsibility for the work that has to be done. The therapist can help by offering specific suggestions and in other ways, but it is up to the couple to make use of that help. For the same reason, as I indicated earlier, the therapist needs to explain why each suggestion is being made — the emphasis should be on education and re-learning rather than cure* The quality of the relationship between therapist and patient is crucially important. Some psychotherapists talk of the therapeutic alliance (Dryden & Hunt 1985). This involves being explicit about the goals of counselling, the need for commitment and probable duration and timing of counselling sessions and so on. Certainly one needs to establish a basis of trust and mutual respect before the couple can be expected to make constructive use of this type of treatment programme.

Unfortunately one cannot relate to a couple — so two therapeutic alliances have to be established. For this purpose the first treatment session (i.e. after the treatment contract has been agreed) is spent largely with each partner on their own. It is at this stage that I give the couselling notes for one partner to read whilst I talk individually to the other (see p. 535). One of the most important objectives in these individual sessions is to establish a rapport with each partner. Often the best way to achieve this is to get each to describe some crucial sexual experience which conveys how he or she feels about sex and sexuality. It is often more fruitful to spend time dealing with one such incident in depth than to cover a variety of experiences superficially. If, by focusing on that key experience the therapist begins to understand how that person feels about sex, and if in return the patient realises that he or she is understood, then the therapeutic alliance is off to a good start.

However, it is unusual for a couple to seek counselling with both partners

---

* There is a dilemma whether some people gain more from being cured than educated, and whether the therapist should collude with this. See Bancroft (1986).

equally identified with the problem. More often than not it is easier to empathise with the person who 'has the problem'. He or she is less likely to be defensive; by seeking help they have explicitly acknowledged that they have a problem. For the partner it may be much harder. To what extent do they have a problem themselves? To what extent have they realised they have a problem, let alone admit it to others? The therapeutic alliance may therefore be more difficult to establish with the non-presenting partner — unless it is the wrong sort of alliance when the non-presenting partner joins forces with the therapist to treat 'the one with the problem'. Not infrequently, reluctance of the partner to participate or even attend for the initial consultation reflects an anxiety that their own often ill-defined problems may come to the surface. Such a partner may need very sensitive handling before he or she is sufficiently unthreatened to participate constructively in the programme.

The behavioural assignments are not only powerful tools for revealing the underlying problems, they are also sensitive indicators of the couple's acceptance of the therapist. This is one of the most important questions the therapist should be asking in the first three or four sessions of treatment: do the couple accept that the treatment programme is appropriate? Their initial reaction to reading the counselling notes can be helpful in this respect, and their reactions to the early homework assignments are usually highly informative. Politeness may make it difficult for some couples to express their doubts, and if there appears to be ambivalence in carrying out the early assignments or less subtle evidence of a weakening commitment to making or keeping appointments, the therapist should make it easy for them to admit that they do not see the point of what they are being asked to do. I have already stressed that it is the responsibility of the therapist to explain the rationale of each step in treatment, and that often has to be done more than once.

Common doubts expressed by patients in early stages include feelings that the behavioural programme is too clinical or too standardised. This reaction deserves respect and should be dealt with properly. It should be explained that basic or relatively standardised steps are advised because they are believed to be fundamental to any good relationship. It is worth pointing out that *any* couple may benefit from going through these early stages, regardless of whether they have problems. A periodic refresher course in communication and self-assertion could be widely recommended if couples were prepared to take the time and make the effort. But whilst the initial steps are relatively standardised, how the couple react to them will be unique and may reveal important information about their problems. If the steps are carried out properly and without difficulty, they can move on to the next stage without delay. As time goes on assignments will become more tailor-made to suit their needs. This type of explanation is usually effective in allaying such doubts.

Sometimes inexperienced therapists lose the confidence of the couple because they stick too rigidly to the prescribed behavioural programme and fail to respond appropriately to their particular needs or difficulties.

The therapist should aim to keep in touch with how the couple feel about the treatment *throughout*, though this is usually easier after the first few sessions. Similarly, a continuing effort is required to maintain a balanced relationship with both partners. It is all too easy to concentrate on one, or give the impression of 'ganging up' on the other, or alternatively leading the other to feel neglected. The partner may collude with this neglect so that he or she can maintain the role of being uninvolved. It is not unusual during treatment to get stuck and to feel that some time spent with the partners individually might help. This can be useful, but it is important to use this 'splitting' up in a balanced way and whenever possible, to bring back into the couple-sessions the main points that emerge, if the individuals agree.

The basic theme of security in the sexual relationship is emphasised in the early stages by the authoritative setting of limits by the therapist. But this externalisation of control on to the therapist has to be gradually reversed so that by the end of treatment the couple have taken back responsibility and demonstrated to each other and to the therapist that they are capable of setting and keeping to limits when necessary. Only then will their feelings of safety continue into the future.

In a similar way, the therapist must of necessity invade the private world of the couple in the early stages with detailed questions and limit-setting. But by the end of treatment they should hve regained their privacy. It is reassuring at this stage when the couple becomes reluctant to give all the details of their love-making session. By then the therapist should have established enough confidence in the therapeutic relationship to know when to accept assurances that all is well without going into detail, something that is not possible at the outset of treatment.

It is important not to underestimate the motivating effect of frequent visits to the therapist. If after such frequent and regular visits treatment suddenly stops there is likely to be a loss of momentum in the sexual relationship and the couple's progress may go into reverse. As a general rule it is sensible gradually to extend the intervals between visits in the latter part of treatment so that the couple's own motivation can be seen to be working.

One aspect of sex therapy which has received a lot of attention is whether to work with one or two therapists. Masters & Johnson (1970) based their approach on a dual-sex therapy team. Clearly this has some advantages. Both the male and female point of view are represented. There is less likelihood of one partner feeling in the minority (though it is not difficult to end up with three against one!), and it is an advantage to have one therapist taking a back seat, observing whilst the other is locked in therapeutic interaction. However, co-therapy is not easy. It is important to feel comfortable with one's co-therapist and it can take time for that comfort to develop, even when the two therapists have complementary attitudes, values and styles of working. When it is not comfortable the co-therapists can present to the patients a bad model of a relationship. Possibly most important, two therapists are twice as expensive as one, and as we shall see later in this chapter, there has been a consistent failure to demonstrate a superiority of outcome with two therapists. Co-therapy is often used as a training model, but even this has serious limitations. If one co-therapist is experienced and the other a novice this inequality can make both feel awkward and they may function below their best. Whilst it may be informative for the trainee, it is unlikely to be in the best interests of the couple. Observing an experienced therapist, either by sitting in as a non-participating observer, or watching through a one-way screen, is probably a superior training model.

Specific techniques for particular forms of dysfunction

The approach described above forms the basis of sex therapy which focuses on the relationship. No other special procedures may be needed; the reduction of anxiety, the lessening of resentment, increased feelings of security or generally better communication and understanding combined with the 'permission-giving' role of the therapist may suffice. However a variety of techniques dealing with specific problems can be added to this general programme. Some of these will be described here. Further detail and suggestions can be obtained from Masters and Johnson (1970), Kaplan (1974), LoPiccolo (1977), Arentewicz & Schmidt (1983) and Hawton (1985).

Erectile failure

Once erections are starting to occur during genital touching, a form of paradoxical intent may be used. The couple are told to get rid of the erection as soon as it develops, by whatever means are effective, and then resume the touching and caressing. The purpose is both to demonstrate that erections can go and return and to counter the tendency to feel that they should be used as soon as they arise.

It is also important to avoid making a major change from foreplay to intercourse, as this is often the point at which performance anxiety returns. Thus a gradual approach involving genital contact and partial and very brief penile insertion is indicated (see Appendix, p. 543). This is best achieved with the woman in the female superior position (see Fig. 10.3) so that she is taking responsibility for vaginal entry and can control entry in a graduated fashion.

Premature ejaculation

Once the stage of genital touching has been reached the couple should be

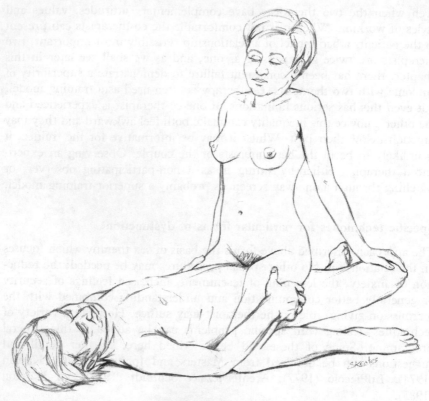

Fig. 10.3 The female superior position, in which the woman is above to control entry of the penis into her vagina. It also allows her to feel safe and not trapped under her partner's body, whilst at the same time permitting the man to relax without the responsibility for vaginal entry.

instructed to spend part of the time each session practising the 'stop–start' technique. Initially this involves manual stimulation of the man's penis by his partner. This should continue until he feels close to the point of ejaculatory inevitability (see p. 78). He then signals to his partner to stop. Stimulation is then resumed after a few minutes and the whole process is repeated many times. Usually, providing the relationship between the couple is free from tension and insecurity, this approach will lead to a gradual increase in ejaculatory control. When confidence at delaying ejaculation from manual stimulation is established, the couple move on to using short periods of vaginal entry (with the woman in the female superior position). Often the switch from manual to vaginal stimulation is the most difficult; the sensation of being inside the vagina may have a 'triggering' effect on ejaculation. In such cases the initial vaginal entry, or even only genital apposition, may have to be very brief until control starts to develop.

If necessary, stimulation can be stopped well in advance of likely ejaculation to create confidence that control is possible. Occasionally merely stop-

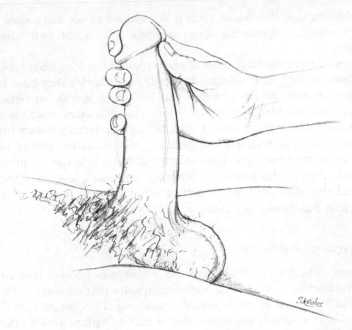

Fig. 10.4 Squeeze technique in the management of premature ejaculation. If the 'stop-start' technique fails to control ejaculation, squeezing the penis in the manner shown can be used by the partner to delay ejaculation when the man indicates that ejaculation is imminent.

ping and starting is ineffective and the additional use of the squeeze technique (Masters & Johnson 1970) may be used, in which the female firmly squeezes the penis between her thumb and forefinger at the level of the frenulum. This slightly painful procedure should inhibit ejaculation (Fig. 10.4). As with the 'stop–start' method, the procedure needs to be repeated many times.

Ejaculatory failure

The first objective in these cases is to help the patient to ejaculate easily and comfortably in the presence of his partner but *outside* the vagina. This may in itself be the main hurdle, as inhibition about letting ejaculation escape or becoming uncontrolled may be fundamental to the problem. Because of the high level of central inhibition of ejaculation that is assumed to exist in such cases, vigorous stimulation using a lubricating jelly or cream may be needed to overcome the block. This superstimulation should be used for relatively short periods initially, gradually lengthening the time as the individual finds himself enjoying the process and becomes less goal- (i.e. ejaculation) oriented. Often the female partner will need to be encouraged to stimulate the penis with sufficient vigour. Once ejaculation occurs predictably outside the vagina then it is induced closer and closer to the vaginal opening, introducing short periods of vaginal entry into the procedure.

In many of these men a pattern of masturbation has long been established which involves very vigorous stimulation. It is as though they have become dependent on this strong stimulus and are quite unable to obtain sufficiently strong stimulation from the vagina. In such cases, once ejaculation occurs predictably in the partner's presence and preferably induced by her, a gradual process of reducing the intensity of stimulation should be used so that the contrast between vigorous manual and gentle vaginal stimulation is reduced. Part of the process is lowering the man's level of active inhibition and this may arise as a result of other psychological or attitudinal changes that accompany sex therapy.

Female orgasmic dysfunction

If orgasmic difficulty is a consequence of a failure to become aroused, then the general improvement and increased enjoyment that accompany the basic programme may well result in orgasm occurring. In some women there is particular anxiety about orgasm, either a fear of failure which effectively inhibits the response, or a fear of loss of control or some other consequence of letting oneself go (see Chapter 8).

During the basic part of the programme it is desirable to avoid becoming too goal-oriented in this respect, as this is likely to defeat the purpose. However, it may be appropriate to encourage the woman, *in addition* to following the programme with her partner, to carry out some individual sessions in which a gradual programme of relaxed self-touching is followed. Vibrators are sometimes useful in producing the first orgasm. Women may find it easier to experience this on their own and then to introduce the appropriate stimulation technique into their sessions with the partner. Role playing may also be helpful. The woman is asked to pretend that she is losing control and having an orgasm. This may then help her to resolve fears of what it would be like in reality (Heiman et al 1976).

Vaginismus

With this problem it is especially important to help the woman become comfortable at exploring her own genitalia and inserting her finger. Finger insertion first by the therapist, then by the woman herself on her own and subsequently by the male partner, may be all that is needed, combined with the basic programme. Often, however, additional dilatation is useful and graded dilators can be used. The woman should be shown how to insert these, asked to practise inserting them on her own and, when sufficiently confident, show her partner how to insert them.

Low sexual desire

This problem, which is often extremely difficult to treat, requires a more careful initial analysis than is necessary for other types of dysfunction. This is because of the very heterogeneous nature of this category and the different types of approach that may be needed. These issues are therefore considered in more detail in Chapter 8. Helping the individual with low sexual interest is considered on p. 503.

Illustrative case

The following case illustrates various aspects of the counselling process.

> Morag, aged 32, and Ian, aged 35, had been married for 6 years. It was the second marriage for both. Morag presented with loss of sexual interest since the birth of her child 4 years previously. There had been little sexual activity since that time. Sex had never been satisfactory for her and the birth of her child was an opportunity to opt out of active sex. In the past she had not found sexual intercourse unpleasant but was rarely orgasmic. Ian had gradually been exerting pressure on her to respond.
>
> Morag had a very negative relationship with her mother who had always undermined her self-confidence whilst being emotionally demanding. Her father had interfered with her sexually when she was a child and her parents separated when she was 9. She first married when 18, very much to escape from her unhappy family background. Sex was not particularly satisfactory at that stage and they separated after 3 years.
>
> Ian's first marriage had been a disaster sexually and had lasted only a short time. Following that he had experienced a sexually satisfactory relationship with an older woman before meeting Morag.
>
> When given the instructions for stage one of therapy, Morag expressed uncertainty whether she would be able to cope. At the next session Ian reported difficulty in keeping to the limits and Morag had lain on her tummy to make sure he did not touch her genitalia. She described a fear of entrapment, partly because she believed it to be unfair to start something and not be prepared to see it through. This attitude was comparable to that of Ian who did not expect to be held responsible for controlling himself once sexually aroused.
>
> At the third treatment session, Morag reported no attempts at sensate focus. She had avoided it. She described feeling unfeminine, with low self-esteem, especially about her body. She was asked to spend time examining and exploring her body and to identify its good and less good features. At the next session she said that she was unable to think of her body in sexual terms and she linked this to feelings of rejection as a child, particularly stemming from her mother's behaviour. She denied any sexual awareness or interest until her marriage at 18, which she entered into for non-sexual reasons. At this session it was pointed out to her that she would need to take at least limited action in attempting stage one if she was to benefit from the therapy. By the end of that session she was feeling under some pressure from the therapist.
>
> On the next visit they confessed to breaking the ban. They had had sexual intercourse on three occasions and she was orgasmic on one, the first time

for 3 years. Morag had suggesting breaking the ban and Ian had agreed. In spite of her improved response she described her continuing difficulty in relaxing during love-making. They were told that the improvement that had occurred was reassuring since it demonstrated that her capacity for sexual response was still there. However, the fact that she was unable to relax, and that she had found it necessary to make this jump from doing nothing to having intercourse, made it likely that the crucial underlying problem had not yet been identified or resolved. Morag was told that it was important for her to be able to say 'stop' without feeling guilty or apprehensive. They were asked to go back to stage two, progressing to stage three (i.e. genital touching) before the next visit if all went well.

During the next 2 weeks, Ian wanted to go further and Morag was able to say 'stop' without any difficulty. This was important for her as she was still feeling tense. Ian therefore suggested that they stayed at stage two. He was beginning to realise the importance of not putting pressure on Morag. However, following the sixth treatment session, Ian refused Morag's invitation for a session on four successive occasions. He said he was feeling at the bottom of the pile of Morag's priorities and was able to express his resentment at the next visit. Following this the homework sessions almost came to a stop. On the eighth visit the therapist re-established a commitment to at least one session per week, progressing on to vaginal containment when they felt ready.

At the ninth visit, Morag reported that she had been unable to start any session. On close questioning she revealed that it was the thought of vaginal entry that seemed to put her off. She was asked to suggest possible reasons for this. She gave a list which included: 'sex is not nice'; her early experiences with her father; fear of loss of control; not making a noise; 'messy' and 'I just don't fancy it'. She was then asked which of these seemed most important. Rather tentatively she chose the early experiences with her father. She was then encouraged to talk about this and produced a rather different story to her initial account. The experiences occurred rather later (aged 11 to 12) when she was visiting her father and his second wife, and continued over a period of 1 year. Her father would insert a finger into her vagina and ask her to touch his penis. She described feeling a mixture of guilt and fear and had been unable to talk to anyone about it. Morag looked emotionally drained by the end of that session and that evening phoned the therapist asking for an appointment on her own. She was seen the next day and went on to recount a later phase, involving mutual masturbation with a girl at school when aged 13. This continued for about 2 years. She was reluctant to talk about this in front of Ian, not being sure how he would react. She was encouraged to do so and by the next joint session had been able to tell him all the details. This was discussed at the session with Ian, who accepted it all without difficulty.

Following this, progress continued. For a short time Morag became somewhat demanding sexually, leaving Ian feeling slightly overwhelmed. But thereafter they settled into a comfortable and mutually enjoyable sexual relationship. At the last visit to the therapist (the 12th) Morag described feeling quite different about herself and no longer under pressure. Ian felt much closer to her and realised the importance of not putting her under pressure. They both agreed that, should they have further difficulties, they would go back to an earlier stage of the programme and rebuild their confidence.

This course of treatment illustrates well how the early stages of the programme deal principally with interpersonal issues — in this case the need to establish trust and reduce pressure, to allow Morag to say 'no' and to get Ian to see that he was being irresponsible in his sexual demands, and not just 'a normal male'.

By the time genital stages were being dealt with, trust was being established, making it easier to reveal and work through highly sensitive and unresolved feelings from childhood experiences. It was noteworthy in this case how informative the various blocks in treatment proved to be. Morag had reacted to pressure from the therapist by breaking the ban. This may have allowed her to avoid what would have been the next more difficult stage in the graduated behavioural programme. But it was also useful in revealing Ian's tendency to be irresponsible with his ready acceptance of her suggestion. This helped him to realise the part he was playing. It also demonstrated that simply having sexual intercourse, even with orgasm, was not sufficient, as she was still feeling tense. As is often the case, following this act of apparent sabotage, some important information was revealed. In this instance it was Morag's anxiety about her sexual identity stemming from her incestuous and her adolescent homosexual experiences.

Some therapists may have chosen to deal with the incest experience at the outset — on the basis of her initial history. In my view she would have found it more difficult to talk more openly at that stage, not having established trust with either her husband or the therapist, and it is unlikely that she would have revealed her anxieties about her lesbian experiences. The vaginal entry phase of the programme acted as a cue for these sensitive issues — clearly linked in her mind with her father's finger insertions. Sensitive material can be expected to arise at the appropriate part of the behavioural programme, providing that the therapeutic relationship and a safe relationship with the partner have been established. Initial history-taking, however detailed and prolonged, cannot be relied on to uncover such material if the patient is not ready to reveal it.

Morag was able to ask for individual sessions when she had uncertainties about how her husband would react. Many patients are not assertive enough to do so, and the therapist should be alert to this need. Couple therapy can get blocked by the difficulty of one partner revealing crucial information in front of the other. In this case the therapist made the error of not seeing Ian on his own. Often when one partner, particularly the presenting partner, shows some fundamental change, the other partner may feel under threat or confused. This is usually a transient reaction if dealt with appropriately.

Sex therapy in patients with organic impairment

In many couples who present with sexual problems, physical disability either directly affects the sexual response (e.g. in erectile dysfunction) or makes normal love-making difficult because of pain or immobility, or embarrassing because of disfigurement or problems such as ileostomies. Whilst it is clearly important to treat such physical factors whenever possible, it is unfortunately true that in most cases there is little more that can be done to reduce the physical problem. As emphasised in Chapter 8, the involvement of physical processes does not mean that psychological factors are unimportant. They are always important in some sense. Nor does it mean that sex therapy or counselling has nothing to offer. Often the only way to assess the relative importance of psychological factors in the presence of physical aetiology is to see what improvement can result from sexual counselling. Thus in the majority of cases a trial of counselling is justified and may lead to substantial improvements. But even in those cases where sexual dysfunction is largely due to physical factors, counselling can make a substantial difference in helping the couple to get the best out of their sexual relationship within the limits imposed by the physical disability. In particular it is important to 'give permission' and reduce the psychological barriers to exploring alternative methods of love-making.

The principles of counselling in such cases are basically the same as those described previously. The main difference is that it may be necessary to work on the assumption that full genital responses will not occur. This is why it is important to have the opportunities for satisfactory diagnostic investigation before embarking on counselling. It is demoralising to persevere with sex therapy in the belief that the problem is psychological when in fact physical impairment makes normal response impossible. It is much better to begin counselling with a reasonable idea of the likelihood of physical impairment being involved, even if the contribution of psychological factors is not yet clear.

With surgical methods of treatment, particularly penile prostheses, counselling is particularly valuable, firstly in helping the couple to decide whether this form of help will be appropriate for them. Some couples, when they are able to discuss the implications fully and explore other approaches to love-making, decide that an erect penis is not *essential* for enjoyable sex. For those who choose this form of treatment, the improved communication that results from counselling will have made it easy for them to incorporate the 'post-surgical penis' into their love-making. I would advise any couple contemplating an implant to have counselling first. Unfortunately some couples are not prepared to do so, preferring to see the problem in physical terms.

Couple therapy for homosexuals

Homosexual couples also have sexual difficulties and need help. The similarities and differences in their problems are discussed in Chapter 8. Until recently help was hard to find, or at least concealed within the homosexual underworld. Masters & Johnson (1979) presented a unique report of a series of 84 homosexual couples, 25 of them lesbian. They reported good results using essentially the same approach as they use with heterosexual couples. They do state that homosexuals are less likely than heterosexuals to offer the level of co-operation needed for optimal treatment. This may be a result of the therapists not being gay themselves.

Since that report a number of gay therapists have described their treatment methods when working with gay couples. McWhirter & Mattison (1980) reported their results with 22 gay male couples and in a later paper (McWhirter & Mattison 1982) proposed that the single most important factor in the treatment of gay couples was the total absence of unresolved homophobia in the therapist. Gordon (1986), in reviewing the recent literature of the treatment of gay couples, concluded that a combination of a Masters & Johnson-type approach combined with clear gay affirmation is appropriate for gay couples. The evidence for lesbian couples is more limited, but presumably a similar conclusion would be appropriate.

Couple therapy for different ethnic groups

The Masters & Johnson approach to couple therapy has been described as white, middle-class and Anglo-Saxon in its implied values. Certainly we have to be cautious when using this approach with couples from different ethnic or religious backgrounds to that of the therapist. Wyatt et al (1978) discussed some of the problems arising when white therapists work with black Afroamerican couples, including the particular myths of black sexuality and the resentment that may be felt by some black patients towards white therapists. D'Ardenne (1986) discussed the problems of sex therapy with Asian couples in Britain and stressed the importance of adapting the treatment approach to the needs and expectations of a particular cultural group. Fortunately, this form of behavioural psychotherapy is adaptable in this way. But a tendency to impose our hallowed values on to others sometimes creates more problems than it solves, and behoves us to compare ourselves with the Christian missionaries. Certainly the conflict of values that sex therapy can provoke poses one of the main ethical issues in sex therapy (Bancroft 1981).

Comparison with other approaches to couple therapy

The method outlined above has much in common with that described by Masters & Johnson (1970). There are apparent differences, with much more emphasis in the above account on the psychotherapeutic component and more in Masters & Johnson's account on the behavioural component. On the basis of further writing by Masters & Johnson (1976) and their associates, and discussions with therapists who have been trained by them*, it is clear that their original book underemphasised the importance they attach to psychotherapy and the non-sexual aspects of the relationship. Tullman et al (1981) reported evidence from the Masters & Johnson Institute of

---

* I am particularly indebted in this respect to Philip and Lorna Sarrel.

substantial changes in communication skills in couples undergoing sex therapy there. Nevertheless, their early account has led to considerable misunderstanding. Many psychoanalytically oriented therapists have assumed that their method is behavioural to the point of being mechanical, whilst many behaviour therapists have assumed that they can apply their method without tangling with the complexities of such cognitive and emotive aspects. I have reached the conclusion that Masters & Johnson are skilled psychotherapists who until recently have been unwilling or unable to describe their psychotherapeutic technique.

There are however some important real differences. Working in a busy outpatient clinic, with limited time, I do not place so much emphasis on an intensive initial assessment and relatively prolonged history-taking. This issue was discussed more fully in Chapter 9. As mentioned earlier, we usually work with single therapists and see patients on a weekly or fort-nightly basis for an average of about 12 sessions, seldom more than 15. Masters & Johnson see their couples daily for 2 weeks, usually with them living away from their normal environment. Some research evidence on these aspects will be discussed later.

Arentewicz & Schmidt (1983) have given a detailed description of the method they and their colleagues have used in the treatment of a large number of couples. Their method is also closely derived from Masters & Johnson, but they focus predominantly on behaviour. Their behavioural tasks are similar to those I have already described, except that they are much more directive in telling the couple what to do. Thus they specify how long each session and part of a session should last, whereas I encourage the couple to set their own pace and timing. What is most noticeably different, judging by their admirably detailed description of their treatment procedure, is the little attention they pay to what I have called 'the psychotherapeutic component' — in particular the use of behavioural assignments as a method of uncovering the underlying problem. They refer to these aspects in passing. In talking about avoidance behaviour, by which they mean reluctance to carry out certain aspects of the behavioural programme, they advise as follows:

> These problems can often be solved by discussing them in detail in sessions, by repeating the exercises, by recapitulating the rules and the purpose of caress, or where necessary by adding behavioural instructions, for example for desensitisation of specific reactions of aversion . . . . If avoidance behav-iour persists the therapist should insist on compliance with the rules and comfront the partner with their avoidance behaviour and the underlying problem. Most difficulties can be solved by these methods. However there are couples who put up strong resistance; *the basic problems then have to be discussed and worked through as best the therapist can with his specific training and therapeutic orientation* (my italics).

Further important differences arise when we consider Kaplan's approach (1979). She divides her causes of sexual problems into different levels, using a physical analogy which is typical of psychoanalytic theory. She deals with the more superficial or immediate causes, using simple behavioural techniques. If, in spite of that, problems remain, she looks for deeper or more remote causes and switches into a more psychoanalytic mode. Although she sees these approaches as being capable of integration, one consequence of her model is that attention is first paid to the sexual dysfunction. With the Masters & Johnson model, attention is first paid to the relationship. This represents an important divide in modern sex therapy. I place myself firmly in the latter category.

The approach I have described here clearly borrows tactics from a variety of theoretical models and is in that sense eclectic. I am also prepared to combine sexual counselling with drug or hormonal treatment (see below). In drawing these contrasts with other approaches I am not commenting on their relative efficacy. It is extraordinarily difficult to demonstrate superiority of one method over another, as we shall see later. What is important is to adopt an approach which suits the temperament and style of the therapist. To some extent the couple, in accepting or rejecting offers of help, will then select the therapist who best suits them.

THE OUTCOME OF SEX THERAPY FOR COUPLES

The largest series of treated cases for which outcome has been reported is that of Masters & Johnson (1970). As described on p. 46, they have used an unusual method of reporting outcome — by giving the failure rate rather than the success rate. This has led to considerable confusion, as many have interpreted a 20% failure rate to mean a 80% success rate. Masters & Johnson have been fiercely criticised for this, most notably by Zilbergeld & Evans (1980). Masters & Johnson defended their position at the World Congress of Sexology in Washington in 1983 (Masters et al 1983) and in view of the controversy surrounding this issue it is worth dwelling a little on what they said.

They first admitted that their method was less than satisfactory, but that it reflected the state of the art at the time. They quoted Bergin, an authority on psychotherapy outcome studies, as saying in 1971: 'It is impossible to conclude very much from gross studies of therapeutic effects'. They justified their use of failure rates as follows: 'When symptoms were not reversed, it was quite obvious; whereas when symptoms were reversed little was known about whether that actually constituted sexual health'. After comments that they were reluctant to ask questions about the frequency and effectiveness of specific sexual responses, as it would encourage the goal-oriented attitude which they aimed to avoid, they went on to describe the criteria that were in fact used for each type of dysfunction. For erectile impotence, failure was adjudged if erection sufficient for coitus was not maintained in at least 75% of opportunities. They pointed out however that at their end of treatment assessment, this would probably be based on only three or four such opportunities. With premature ejaculation, failure was the inability to maintain coital thrusting long enough for the partner to be orgasmic in the majority of opportunities, or if the partner had difficulty with orgasm herself, the inability to delay ejaculation 'for the length of time he wished'. Women with orgasmic dysfunction were failures if they 'did not reach orgasm in a consistent fashion during sexual opportunities . . . 50% being a general guide'.

They went on to describe in detail the outcome criteria they are currently using (Masters et al 1983), although as far as I know they have not as yet reported results with these criteria, and we must await such evidence before we can evaluate them.

Masters & Johnson's defence contains some special pleading, but they do make an important point — the difficulties of defining success when evaluating sex therapy. As we shall see from other studies, no one has satisfactorily resolved that problem. This is an important issue because more often than not the specific dysfunction is only one aspect of the sexual relationship and therapy can achieve substantial improvement in the quality of the relationship whilst leaving the dysfunction largely unaltered, as, for example, in some cases of erectile failure of organic origin.

At this stage in the outcome controversy it is still difficult to escape the conclusion that Masters & Johnson have been unusually successful with their treatment, probably as a result of a combination of effective selection (both explicitly and implicitly) and powerful psychotherapeutic skills. Certainly much of Zilbergeld & Evans' critique is not only distorted but unhelpfully destructive. With these considerations in mind, we can look at the results reported by Masters & Johnson (1970) in more than 500 couples (Table 10.1).

They also reported a 5-year follow-up of 313 couples who were non-failures at the end of treatment and found a relapse rate of only 5.1% — most commonly with secondary erectile dysfunction (11.1%).

Table 10.1 Failure rates reported by Masters & Johnson

Sexual problem	Percentage failure
Orgasmic dysfunction	
Primary	16.6%
Secondary	22.8%
Vaginismus	0%
Erectile dysfunction	
Primary	40.6%
Secondary	26.3%
Premature ejaculation	2.2%
Ejaculatory incompetence	17.6%

The next most substantial follow-up study was from Arentewicz & Schmidt (1983) reporting on 262 treated couples. They were followed-up by questionnaire at 1 year and from $2\frac{1}{2}$ to $4\frac{1}{2}$ years after the end of treatment. However they obtained information from only 50% at 1 year and 42% at the later follow-up. The authors concluded that those followed-up were representative of all who had completed treatment as they did not differ in their amount of change at the end of treatment from those they could not contact. This however is a suspect conclusion and we must be cautious in generalising from their follow-up data, presented in Table 10.2. As we shall see, failure to gain the co-operation of couples for follow-up has plagued most of the studies so far.

A number of reports have give a crude global assessment of outcome at the end of therapy. Thus Bancroft & Coles (1976) reported on 78 couples who entered therapy in Oxford: 32% showed a successful outcome, 31% worthwhile improvement and 32% no change or dropped out. These were similar to results reported elsewhere in the UK at that time (Duddle 1975; Milne 1976). Hawton (1982) later reported a further 100 couples treated at Oxford. At the end of treatment the problem was rated as resolved or largely resolved in 66%, slightly improved in 12% and unchanged in 21%. The best outcome was for vaginismus and erectile dysfunction.

Table 10.2 Changes in sexual functioning classified by type of sexual problem at end of treatment and at follow-up (Arentewicz & Schmidt 1983)

	Orgasmic dysfunction	Vaginismus	Erectile dysfunction	Premature ejaculation	Total
At end of treatment					
n	108	27	57	31	223
Dropped out	24%	11%	13%	13%	17%
No change	2%	0%	4%	0%	2%
Slightly improved	4%	11%	4%	3%	5%
Improved	50%	11%	30%	43%	40%
'Cured'	19%	67%	49%	40%	35%
After 1 year (compared with end of treatment)					
n	51	16	29	15	111
The same	39%	56%	48%	33%	43%
Better	25%	19%	14%	13%	29%
Worse	24%	12.5%	24%	47%	25%
Separated	12%	12.5%	14%	7%	12%
After 2–4 years (compared with 1 year follow-up)					
n	44	14	23	13	94
The same	50%	64%	48%	15%	47%
Better	18%	7%	9%	46%	18%
Worse	18%	14%	26%	31%	21%
Separated	14%	14%	17%	8%	14%

Heisler (1983) reported outcome in 998 couples assessed for sexual problems by marriage guidance counsellors with special training in sex therapy. 25% were deemed not suitable for such treatment and 28% failed to complete treatment once started. This left 47% who completed treatment. Of those, 70% showed a marked improvement. Warner et al (1987) reported on 1194 referrals to sexual problem clinics in Edinburgh during a 3-year period. Of these, 478 (51% of those with a current partner) were offered couple therapy. At the time of the report 40% of these couples had completed treatment and 35% had dropped out of treatment. For those who completed or dropped out, the outcome was reported to be good in 35%, and moderate in 25%. The best outcome was for vaginismus.

Vansteenwegen et al (1983), from Belgium, reported on 192 patients; 177 of these were treated with their partner and 15 were treated individually. Treatment was successful in 46%, caused improvement in 17.5% and showed no change or worsened in 37%.

A number of long-term follow-up studies have now been reported. Dekker & Everaerd (1983) attempted to follow-up 140 couples from 5 to 8 years after treatment, using postal questionnaires. Only 46% responded appropriately. Of those for whom information was available, 21% had separated or divorced. It is difficult to draw conclusions from this report. A number of different treatment methods had been used and their methods of assessment were difficult to follow. The authors concluded that improvement obtained during treatment was fairly stable during the follow-up period in those couples who had stayed together.

DeAmicis et al (1985) successfully followed-up 38 couples after 3 years, (47% contact). They found some evidence of treatment gains being maintained, but there was a fair amount of relapse. They also reported in a separate paper (DeAmicis et al 1984) on the follow-up of 49 couples who had been assessed but not treated 3 years previously. In general they had not shown much change in their sexual behaviour during that time, although approximately 50% had sought treatment elsewhere in the interval.

Watson & Brockman (1982) followed-up 116 couples but were only able to obtain information from 53% of them, with follow-up periods averaging 13 months. Of 29 couples who had improved at the end of treatment and who were followed-up, 16 (55%) had maintained their improvement. A total of 35% of couples had separated, though these were significantly more likely to be amongst those who had not responded to treatment or had not been treated. This figure seems high and may reflect a tendency for couples with more severe marital problems to be treated than would be typical in many sexual problem clinics.

Heisler (1983) attempted to follow-up couples who had been treated by marriage guidance counsellors but succeeded in only 36% of cases. Within that subgroup 41% had maintained their improvement, 41% had shown some return of problems, whereas the remainder reported further improvement since the end of treatment.

Hawton et al (1986) proved somewhat more successful in contacting their ex-patients. Of 140 couples who had entered therapy 1 to 6 years earlier, in 75% of cases at least one partner was contacted and usually interviewed. Recurrence of or continuation of the presenting problem was experienced at some stage during the follow-up period by 75% of couples, though in a third of them this did not cause concern. Almost a half of those who had experienced these recurrences were able to deal with them effectively, often by adopting strategies learnt during therapy. In all, 17% of the relapsing couples had sought further help; 13% of the original group had separated.

The outcome for different types of sexual dysfunction also presents a confused picture. The most consistent findings are for good results with vaginismus (Masters & Johnson 1970; Arentewicz & Schmidt 1983; Bramley et al 1983; Hawton et al 1986) and poor results for low sexual desire (DeAmicis et al 1985; Hawton et al 1986). The evidence of prognosis for orgasmic dysfunction and erectile failure is much more variable, and in the latter case may reflect varying degrees of selection of cases without organic impairment. Premature ejaculation, whilst often helped initially, appears to relapse much more often than Masters & Johnson's figures would indicate. Arentewicz & Schmidt (1983) made this interesting comment: 'Maybe therapists too readily considered premature ejaculation a purely technical problem and so were distracted from dealing with deeper rooted problems between the partners or in the patient'.

In conclusion, the picture presented by follow-up studies of outcome is confused (several of the papers are difficult to follow) and somewhat discouraging. In my view this is in part because we have not as yet defined satisfactorily what we mean by a successful outcome in such a complex entity as a sexual relationship. For all the scorn that has been poured on Masters & Johnson for their lack of rigour and definition, there has been a notable absence of any better model of how it should be done, reflecting I believe the inherent difficulty of the task. Arentewicz & Schmidt (1983) should perhaps take the greatest credit for the care they have taken, but the very complexity of their analysis precludes making any summary assessment of success. It may be that there is no alternative to defining various aspects of the sexual relationship, e.g. sexual response, communication, enjoyment etc. and assessing each separately. As far as erectile dysfunction is concerned, it is now abundantly clear that careful evaluation of possible physical factors is required, something that has been lacking from most treatment studies hitherto. With low sexual desire we have a good example of a label covering a heterogeneous mixture of problems with very different prognoses. Much more thought and debate will be required before we can begin to talk about the effectiveness of sex therapy with any statistical confidence.

Controlled treatment outcome studies

Modern sex therapy, particularly that derived from Masters & Johnson's approach, has been popular amongst behaviour therapists. The early days of behaviour therapy were characterised by a striving for scientific respectability, mainly through the application of modern learning theory to the modification of behaviour (e.g. Eysenck 1964). This was in part a reaction to the ascientific nature of psychoanalysis. As clinical experience accumulated, the relevance of learning theory became increasingly suspect, particularly as behaviour therapy started to tackle increasingly complex behavioural problems (such as sexual or marital problems). Yates (1970) suggested that the essence of behaviour therapy was in the application of experimental method to the single case study. Most other behaviour therapists, however, applied their scientific rigour in controlled evaluation of treatment using group designs. There have now been a number of such studies in the field of sex therapy. For much of my earlier career I was involved in such treatment outcome research. At that stage I never doubted that it was the right thing to do, though it became necessary to live with results that were predominantly negative. In the first edition of this book I wrote:

> It is surprisingly difficult to demonstrate superiority of one psychological treatment method over another. The cynic might conclude that none of the methods are therefore of any particular value. But there are other explanations to be considered. Properly controlled treatment studies involve careful evaluation and measurement which in itself may alter behaviour in a positive way, thereby reducing observed treatment effects. The restraints of a controlled research design often impose restrictions on therapists' functioning which may impair their therapeutic efficacy, whatever method they may be using. And, perhaps most important, problems being treated are usually regarded as relatively homogeneous. Given the considerable individual variance in factors which may affect response to treatment, and the usual failure to balance for these in the design, we should expect treatment effects to be obscured.

Subsequent and somewhat painful experience has led me to attach overriding importance to the last of these explanations.

When in Oxford I had the unusual experience of participating in a controlled treatment outcome study which demonstrated the substantial superiority of one method over another. The patients were women with sexual unresponsiveness, and the effective method was hormonal (i.e. testosterone) not psychological; the hormonal method was superior to the tranquilliser, diazepam. Both groups of women, together with their partners, also received sex therapy of Masters & Johnson-type (Carney et al 1978). It was particularly salutary that two attempts to replicate this finding failed. In each case testosterone was compared not with diazepam but with placebo. Placebo was as effective if not more so than testosterone (Dow 1983; Mathews et al 1983). One possible explanation for this failure to replicate was that in the original study diazepam was having an adverse effect, possibly by reducing the effectiveness of counselling, whereas testosterone was having no effect.

In Edinburgh we carried out a comparable study with male sexual dysfunction, comparing testosterone with placebo, both in combination with sex therapy. We found trends in favour of placebo; but there is no reason why testosterone should be *less* beneficial than placebo in men. We also found that in spite of randomisation there were differences in the two treatment groups (i.e. testosterone and placebo) *before* treatment in variables which were found to have prognostic significance. In some cases these pretreatment differences reached statistical significance. It was apparent that they could have accounted for the post-treatment differences, making the results *uninterpretable*. We had been unlucky in our randomisation. But this experience emphasised the importance of balancing for pretreatment variables of prognostic significance. In our case we had imbalance of statistically significant proportions. But such significance levels are arbitrary and their biasing effect on the results depend on the *degree* of the difference, not on whether it is statistically significant.

In other controlled treatment studies to date, virtually no attempt has been made to balance prognostic variables, partly because we have so little evidence of what the important variables might be. It is generally assumed that by using random allocation of subjects to treatment groups, the important variables will be evenly distributed. If large numbers are involved this is a realistic expectation. But such studies are difficult and time-consuming and numbers are usually small.

If prognostic variability is not controlled there are two important adverse effects. If one treatment group has a better prognosis than the other, bias will be introduced, inflating or cancelling out real treatment effects or producing spurious effects where none exist (as probably happened in our ill-fated study). Secondly, if prognostic variability is not taken into account in the analysis it will add to the experimental error. Since the statistical significance of a treatment effect is measured in relation to this residual error, moderate treatment effects will remain undetected, unless the sample size is increased substantially. When we look at the various studies in the literature we find in the majority of cases no significant differences between treatments, and in a few, weak effects which usually are not consistent across studies. Anyone who has clinical experience of sex therapy will know how variable couples are in their response to treatment. Some improve with apparent ease and little therapeutic effort; others are notably resistant to change. This variability in outcome is likely to be at least as great if not greater than the differences between a 'good' and a 'bad' treatment method. Thus the predominance of negative findings may simply mean that genuine and worthwhile treatment effects have been obscured by the variance attributable to prognostic variability. We reported our ill-fated study as a cautionary tale (Bancroft et al 1986) and in the second part of the paper examined in detail the methodological issues involved (Warner & Bancroft

1986). We realised that if, as is usually the case, modest numbers are involved in controlled treatment outcome studies, it is of crucial importance to identify and control for the key prognostic variables. As this has seldom been done we must reluctantly conclude that the substantial amount of work that has gone into these various studies up to now has been of very limited value. If a reasonable proportion of the research effort that has been expended in such studies had been directed at identifying and measuring prognostic variables, we would be in a much stronger position to carry out worthwhile outcome studies in the future. There is nothing new about these conclusions; statisticians and methodologists have been making these points for long enough. But for some reason, those involved in such treatment outcome research, myself included, have preferred to turn a blind eye to this aspect.

I will therefore not dwell on these various studies expect to mention them briefly as readers may wish to reach their own conclusions on this rather fundamental point. I will then consider the limited information we do have about prognostic indicators.

A number of studies have investigated practical aspects of the treatment format. Thus, a comparison of the use of one and two therapists was carried out by Arentewicz & Schmidt (1983), Crowe et al (1981), Heiman et al (1985) and Mathews et al (1976). Apart from the last study, which found a weak superiority of two therapists over one when using the Masters & Johnson approach, no significant differences in outcome have been observed. Comparisons of daily and weekly treatment sessions (Arentewicz & Schmidt 1983; Heiman & LoPiccolo 1983) or between weekly and monthly sessions (Carney et al 1978) have also found little difference. These negative results have been taken to justify the use of firstly, one therapist rather than two, as it is cheaper and secondly, weekly sessions rather than daily as they are more convenient. But the replication of negative findings does not have the same significance as replication of positive findings. At best we can conclude from these studies that the differential effects of these procedural variations are small in comparison with the variability of outcome which occurs in any case. It remains distinctly possible that in *certain types of case* two therapists may be superior to one, or daily sessions more effective than weekly. At the moment we can go no further than that.

The following studies have compared variations in the treatment process for couple therapy, e.g. comparing the Masters & Johnson approach, systematic desensitisation, communication training, marital therapy, sex aids or self-help methods: Kockott et al 1975; Ansari 1976; Mathews et al 1976; Everaerd 1977; Riley & Riley 1978; Crowe et al 1981; Everaerd & Dekker 1982; Dow 1983; Libman et al 1984; Kilmann et al 1986. Attempts to evaluate combinations of drug or hormone treatment with couple therapy include studies by Carney et al 1978; Mathews et al 1983 and Dow 1983. Munjack et al (1984) reported an evaluation of rational–emotive therapy in the treatment of erectile dysfunction. Other studies more relevant to individual or group therapy will be cited later in this chapter.

Prognostic indicators

Most available evidence of variables which predict outcome in couple therapy have been derived as by-products of controlled treatment outcome studies which were not designed primarily for this purpose (e.g. Mathews et al 1976; Whitehead & Mathews 1977, 1987), or from retrospective case note studies (e.g. Glover 1983). One systematic prospective study aimed primarily at prognosis has been reported by Hawton & Catalan (1986). A series of 154 couples, receiving Masters & Johnson-type therapy, were assessed before treatment for levels of sexual knowledge, motivation for treatment, how much the therapist liked the couple, global ratings of the quality of both general and sexual relationship, and psychiatric status. The initial response to treatment was assessed after the third treatment session. Outcome was assessed by the therapist after the last treatment session, whether or not treatment had been completed. Failure to complete treatment was significantly associated with lower social class and lower motivation on the part of the male partner, poorer general relationship and poorer progress by the third treatment session. Outcome of the whole group was related to the quality of the general relationship as rated by the therapist and female partner (though not by the male), and to motivation of the male partner. The extent to which couples were carrying out their homework assignments by the third session was also highly predictive of outcome. The prognostic importance of the general relationship has been found in a number of studies (e.g. Cooper 1969; Lansky & Davenport 1975; Mathews et al 1976; Leiblum et al 1976; Snyder & Berg 1983; Whitehead & Mathews 1987). It is clearly highly desirable that this aspect is appropriately measured and balanced by means of blocking in future treatment studies.

Other variables may also be shown to be important, particularly with certain types of problem. The more prognostic variables that are identified, the more complex (and impracticable) a balanced design becomes. Elsewhere (Warner & Bancroft 1986) we have discussed the possibility of using a single composite prognostic variable by such means as discriminant function.

There is also a need to identify prognostic factors which relate to the specific method of treatment in use. When we compare two forms of treatment, we are assuming crucial differences in the treatment process (e.g. one method may focus on communication skills, the other on anxiety management). In such circumstances we need measures of the relevant pretreatment status (i.e. communication skill or anxiety) which will indicate prognosis. We then require our two treatment groups to be adequately matched on both these variables. For this purpose what is required is a conceptual analysis of the treatment process which is typical of sex therapy. Treatment process research of this kind has been attempted with little success in the non-directive field, though with somewhat more interest in a comparison of behavioural and non-behavioural psychotherapy (Sloane et al 1975). But as yet it has not been seriously attempted in the sex therapy field.

More research is certainly required in this respect if we are to expect worthwhile benefits from treatment outcome studies in the future. The immediate research needs are of three types: the study of commonsense prognostic indicators, such as general relationship and motivation, along the lines of Hawton & Catalan's (1986) study; the development of appropriate methods of measuring these variables and producing composite prognostic scores (e.g. discriminant function scores), and the analysis of treatment process that will allow the identification and measurement of patient characteristics relevant to that process.

INDIVIDUAL THERAPY

A proportion of patients presenting with sexual problems have no current sexual partner. Obviously couple therapy is not a possibility for them. Others do have partners but either they will not participate in treatment or the patients do not want to involve them. Individual or group therapy may be the only available option. For many the problem is in any case an individual one, e.g. long-standing sexual inhibitions or a primary lack of any sexual interest, inappropriate sexual preferences that are incompatible with stable sexual relationships, or problems of self-control which may bring the individual into conflict with the law.

THE PATIENT–THERAPIST RELATIONSHIP

In individual therapy the nature of the patient–therapist relationship requires special attention. It is easier in these circumstances for the patient to develop a dependent child–parent relationship with the therapist than it is for the couple. It is therefore particularly important to spell out the limits of the therapeutic relationship. The onus for change lies with the patient, not with the therapist. The relationship is primarily an educational one between two adults, one providing expertise, the other making use of that expertise in an active way. There are occasions when it is appropriate to allow a more dependent doctor–sick patient type of relationship to develop but we are then talking about relatively long-term psychotherapy. The patient may then be allowed to regress to this less adult-like role, whereas in modern sex therapy such regression is resisted. In individual therapy, the sex of the therapist has an added importance. The vicarious sexuality of a psychotherapeutic relationship should never be denied. When the focus of therapy is the patient's sexual life, this is even more important. In some cases this may be a therapeutic advantage. A shy inhibited male, lacking self-confidence and fearing rejection by all women, may find the vicarious sexuality of the relationship with a female therapist reassuring. That is not to advocate sexual contact between therapist and patient. In my view the advantages of the sexuality of the therapeutic relationship rely on the taboo against therapist–patient sex being firmly upheld (Bancroft 1981). For others a good relationship with a therapist of the same sex may be more important, not only reinforcing the patient's gender-related self-esteem but also providing a model of certain behaviours.

The contract for individual therapy

With couples it is possible to negotiate objectives of treatment which affect and are accepted by both partners. With the individual the goals of treatment should not be dependent on others who are not directly involved; they should be relevant to the individual alone. If improvement occurs in the individual's sexuality and self-esteem then benefits may well extend to his or her relationships with others, but that should not be the primary objective of treatment. It is no use relying on homework assignments for a couple when only one has agreed to do them.

THE BASIC PRINCIPLES OF TREATMENT

The principles of behavioural psychotherapy, already described for couple therapy, are just as applicable to the individual, with a combination of behavioural, educational and psychotherapeutic components. The main difference is that as a relationship is not directly involved in treatment, a more idiosyncratic, tailor-made set of assignments is necessary from the start. For this reason more time is usually needed in the initial assessment and behavioural analysis before appropriate assignments are identified.

Let us consider some particular types of treatment objective when working with the individual.

Marked sexual inhibition or absence of sexual desire

A person with such a problem may complain that his or her rather negative approach to sex is a barrier to establishing a rewarding sexual relationship. A normal relationship may be desired or children wanted.

Many such people have difficulty in accepting with comfort their sexual feelings and bodily responses. This may be an aspect of their general personality which avoids any form of undue hedonism or loss of control in particular, or it may be more specifically linked to avoidance of or discomfort with sexual pleasures.

The sensate focus approach, which is described above for the couple, may be relevant to such a person, carried out on an individual basis. The patient is asked to agree to limits — no genital touching initially — but to spend time exploring the feel of the body, the effects of different types of touch or stimulation, perhaps experimenting with a variety of stimuli such as creams, lotions, water baths, vibrators etc. Patients are encouraged to make time and space just for themselves, to pamper themselves, to listen to good music, read interesting erotic literature, look at pictures, enjoy nice smells and so on.

Advocating such an approach may quickly uncover negative attitudes about body pleasure and sexuality. It may also reveal discomfort with body image. As described in Chapter 8, feeling bad about one's body does not enhance sexuality. There may be rational grounds for such negative feelings, e.g. being overweight, too thin or unfit. If so, there may be good reasons for suggesting specific goals to improve self-image, e.g. dieting, exercise, yoga etc.

Step by step, individuals are encouraged to explore their genitalia in privacy, and with the use of a good mirror. This should eventually lead to gentle genital caressing whilst continuing the earlier body caressing. Negative attitudes about masturbation may be crucial at this stage. The beginnings of sexual excitement in response to such self-caressing may lead the patient to stop suddenly, fearing where the arousal may lead. Fears of loss of control may have to be resolved before further progress can be made.

Relaxation exercises may be usefully incorporated into this sort of programme, mainly to allow the individual to reduce tension before embarking on the pleasuring exercises and also to enhance body awareness. Much of the loss of erotic sensitivity that people experience is because they dissociate themselves from their bodily and tactile sensations by focusing their minds on other matters. An important objective is to 'tune in' to the sensations they are experiencing, either in the part of the body that is being touched or the part that is doing the touching. Avoidance of the spectator role in particularly important at this stage. Kegel's exercises for increasing tone and control over the pelvic floor muscles may be useful for some women, giving them an increased sense of awareness and control over their own bodies.

As in couple therapy, each new behavioural step may encounter some emotional block which then has to be identified and worked through. The principle of desensitisation, as described above, may be useful. Pictures of certain types of sexual activity may arouse anxiety and gradual repeated exposure to such pictures, accompanied by the reassurance and 'permission' of the therapist, who looks at the pictures with the patient, may serve to desensitise this anxiety. Taboo words or ideas may lose their threat by their repeated use or discussion during therapy. The therapist is therefore using a combination of education, permission-giving, desensitisation and the psychotherapeutic resolution of emotional blocks and conflicts when appropriate.

Lack of sexual interest which results from active psychological inhibition may respond to this approach. But as discussed earlier (see p. 402), there are other explanations needing different approaches. It is important to point out that although an individual may lack any spontaneous sexual interest or desire, this does not preclude him or her from responding to appropriate stimulation with sexual arousal and pleasure. As we discussed in Chapter 2, there are many women who seldom if ever experience spontaneous sexual desire and yet are able to respond with pleasure to their partner's advances. Lack of desire of this kind may be more problematic in a man, particularly if both he and his partner expect him to take the initiative.

Those individuals with lack of sexual desire may find it helpful to use erotic films or literature as well as novel forms of tactile stimulation, such as vibrators (Gillan 1977).

Specific sexual dysfunctions

A proportion of specific sexual dysfunctions can be usefully treated by individual therapy. Vaginismus is a good example. Self-exploration and the use of dilators, as described on p. 486, may be effective without having to involve the partner directly. In many cases this approach leads to consummation of a previously unconsummated marriage (Ellison 1968). Vaginismus is often one of the easiest sexual problems to treat, hence the frequent success with individual as well as with couple therapy. However some women are particularly resistant to treatment and may require either skilful couple therapy or long-term individual therapy.

Orgasmic difficulty in women may also respond to a masturbation programme as described above (LoPiccolo & Lobitz 1972). The capacity for orgasm acquired during such an individual approach does not necessarily generalise to sexual involvement with a partner, but it will do in a proportion of cases.

Males who are unable to ejaculate, even during masturbation on their own, may be helped to overcome this by following the individual sensate focus and masturbation programmes described above. Fear of losing control or discomfort at 'making a mess' are often important obstacles to be overcome. Vibrators may also be useful for this purpose (Schellen 1968; Geboes et al 1975).

Premature ejaculation may be helped by an individual 'stop–start' technique, as originally advocated by Semans (1956). Often control is only a problem when with a partner, but if ejaculation does occur very quickly during masturbation then this individual approach may help to increase self-confidence when with a partner.

Problems with erection are more difficult to treat on an individual basis, particularly when performance anxiety is a major factor. It is often assumed in such cases that erections during masturbation will be unaffected and that if they are, some organic factor is involved. This is not however the case, as masturbation may become an important test of erection and also suffer the effects of performance anxiety. If that is so, individual sensate focus may help the individual regain his erections during masturbation and increase his self-confidence to some extent. How best to tackle sexual encounters with a partner can be usefully discussed. Usually performance anxiety is much more troublesome if the man has to conceal it from his partner. Being able to share one's concern and obtaining a sympathetic and caring response is half the battle. He should therefore avoid sexual encounters where the reaction of his partner to sexual failure will be unpredictable. He should be encouraged to see himself as someone needing a relatively stable and secure relationship for his sexuality to be properly expressed, rather than as a potential sexual athlete. When he does find a partner he can trust he should prepare himself with some convincing reason for not engaging in sexual intercourse too quickly. If he has chosen his partner sensibly this will not be a problem, as she may also be happier to take things slowly. Engaging in mutual caressing with a clear commitment not to attempt intercourse (as in the early stages of couple therapy) may well allow him to experience full erection and increase his self-confidence. During the counselling sessions, his experiences during such encounters can be discussed and the appropriate lessons learnt from them.

In some men with erectile problems, their histories suggest a more basic difficulty in incorporating sex into a loving relationship, or of tolerating sexual intimacy. In such cases more long-term individual psychotherapy should be considered.

Psychophysiological techniques

Behaviourally oriented therapists have not been slow to exploit modern electronic technology in treatment. Biofeedback as a method of treatment is now fashionable. Some indication of a physiological response, whether it be heart rate, blood pressure, electromyogram or electrodermal activity, is fed back to the subject as a visual or auditory signal. He is then asked to control the response by whatever means possible. Whilst this approach is of considerable theoretical interest, particularly in increasing our understanding of autonomic control and conditioning, the therapeutic usefulness of such techniques is far from established. Unfortunately, the commercial potential of selling 'scientific' instruments for treatment purposes has been quickly recognised and there is no shortage of therapists who engage their patients in these procedures, impressing them with the flashing lights and digital dials of modern technology. The scope for the effects of suggestion is considerable.

There have been one or two attempts to use such feedback therapeutically, but as yet there is no evidence that it has therapeutic value for erectile problems. However one should not overlook the therapeutic potential of simply measuring genital responses. Csillag (1976) compared the effects of feedback on erection in two groups of normal and impotent men. Whereas the results were inconclusive about the effects of feedback per se, it was noteworthy that the erectile responses of the impotent men, elicited by erotic stimuli in the laboratory, increased with repeated testing. In a few cases this improvement appeared to generalise to their sexual encounters outside the laboratory.

In Chapter 9 I described the psychophysiological techniques for assessing erectile response to erotic stimuli as a method of investigation. Not infrequently a man who is complaining of impotence will be surprised by the strength of his response to an erotic film in the laboratory. Its degree and comparability with the responses of normal men can be pointed out to him and this may, by increasing his self-confidence, have a therapeutic effect. At the present time this cannot be regarded as a method of treatment, but rather a therapeutic side-effect of a diagnostic procedure. It may be counterproductive if the patient views this procedure as a form of therapy, as this would alter his expectations, increase his performance anxiety and, in the event of no response, further undermine his confidence.

Modifying sexual preferences and related problems of sexual identity

An individual's sexual preference may create problems because it is incompatible with a stable loving sexual relationship (e.g. fetishism or sadomasochism), or because it precludes a conventional sexual relationship (e.g. homosexuality) or because it cannot be expressed without incurring the risk of severe penalties (e.g. paedophilia). The individual who is concerned about his or her homosexuality and who seeks help to become heterosexual presents for treatment much less often now than was the case 20 years ago. It is more likely to be a male than a female who presents in this way and in the discussion that follows the patient will be assumed to be male. The same general principles apply however to a female with such a request.

Ethical implications

On several occasions in this book I have referred to the ethical controversy surrounding the treatment of homosexuality. Before proceeding any further it is therefore necessary to place these ethical issues into perspective.

Ever since people have actively defended the homosexual in society from social repression, there has been criticism of any attempt to alter homosexual preferences (see p. 311). This criticism is usually based on three main points. First, any attempt to alter homosexual preferences is reinforcing or colluding with negative social attitudes towards homosexuality. Secondly, individuals who ask for such help are not really doing so from free will but because they are under social pressures to confrom. Thirdly, such treatment is undesirable because it is unnatural; the natural sexual preference for the homosexual is someone of the same sex. To attempt to make it otherwise is to impose an unnatural status. My reactions to these points have been discussed more fully elsewhere (Bancroft 1981) but they will be briefly summarised here. Two issues face the therapist: his or her role in influencing social attitudes and his or her responsibility to the patient. Placing the needs of society before those of the patient threatens the most basic principles of the caring professions. But it does not have to be an either–or situation. If all the therapist does in this respect is engage in treatment aimed at altering homosexual preferences to heterosexual, he cannot escape the charge that, however unwittingly, he is reinforcing negative attitudes to homosexuality. If on the other hand he not only takes what steps he can to oppose negative and repressive social attitudes and policies towards homosexuality, but also makes genuinely clear to his patients his acceptance of homosexuality as an alternative lifestyle, then he can properly help an individual who is concerned about his sexual orientation explore the alternatives open to him. This issue has taken on an added dimension with the AIDS epidemic. On the one hand the likelihood that homosexuality will be stigmatised in society has been increased; on the other hand the fear of AIDS may well discourage some who until recently would have explored their sexual feelings in the gay community. The ethical dilemma has therefore become sharpened, but the principles in resolving it have not changed.

One of the alternatives open to a person who is unhappy about his homosexual feelings is to explore heterosexual relationships and to make use of appropriate counselling in the process. It is sometimes said that as soon as you talk of therapy in this context you are implying illness, and homosexuality should not be seen as an illness. But this is a specious play on words. Much of what a therapist does, not only in the field of sexual problems but in many other situations, is not treating illness but helping people tackle problems of living. It is often important to make this distinction explicit (Greenwood & Bancroft 1987). The term 'counselling' may be used to avoid the implication of illness, but in reality the boundaries between psychotherapy, behavioural or otherwise, and counselling are impossible to define. If they exist at all they are in terms of degree or emphasis.

As far as free choice is concerned, there is no doubt that many people who seek to change their homosexual orientation are ashamed of it and are responding to the social stigma. They may well expect the therapist to share the usual negative social attitudes, a further reason for the therapist to dissociate himself explicitly from this point of view (if in fact that is what he believes). But in my view it is arrogant to deny a person the right to choose to conform. To imply that such a choice is never 'free' is to throw doubt on the 'free choice' of most forms of psychological help. The therapist is entitled to decline to help a person who wishes to change his sexual orientation. But that does not mean that he is justified in attacking or criticising those who *are* prepared to offer such help.

It nevertheless is important that the therapist should encourage the individual to consider the alternatives as clearly as possible, and to identify the various pressures, internal and external, that are pushing him in one direction or another. This should precede any decision about treatment goals. Clearly it is difficult for a therapist to adopt this role in an unbiased way if he or she harbours any negative feelings about homosexuality. It is also difficult for a therapist who believes 'you are either one thing or the other' — the presence of any homosexual feeling may be seen as clear evidence that one is gay. This has been a characteristic of some gay counsellors, at least in the past.

The third point, the 'naturalness' of the homosexual state, implies a knowledge and understanding of homosexuality that we do not possess. It is possible, and indeed likely, that for some homosexuals their preferences reflect an innate characteristic. Any struggle to establish heterosexual preferences may well be 'unnatural' for such a person. But not only are we uncertain as to whether such an innate propensity exists, we are even less able to recognise those to whom it applies. It has often been said that if the homosexual responds to treatment by becoming heterosexual, then he was not a 'proper' homosexual in the first place. Havelock Ellis (1915) said this of the early therapeutic attempts of the hypnotherapists, and it has been said more recently of the 'conversion' successes reported by Masters & Johnson (1979); e.g. Zilbergeld & Evans (1980). The circularity of such reasoning is obvious. Those who responded to Masters & Johnson's treatment may not have been representative of the homosexual population. But the fact is that they presented themselves for help and had experienced homosexual feelings. As discussed in Chapter 3, the determinants of both homosexual and heterosexual preferences are likely to be many and varied. Whilst there may be some people whose homosexual preferences are not only established early but are stable and immutable, there may be others whose preferences are likely to change in suitable circumstances. They are entitled to seek help to explore such a change.

Homosexual preferences

Let us now consider what approach the therapist can take with someone concerned about his homosexual feelings. It should now be clear that there is a fair amount of groundwork to be done before arriving at any agreed treatment goals.

First, consider the alternatives. Often the patient will present a very negative view of his homosexuality, stressing that he wants to be rid of it. The therapist should encourage the patient to talk about these feelings. There is a tendency for therapists to fall over themselves in declaring their acceptance of homosexuality, and in the process fail to listen to the patient's real concerns. After inviting a full account of the patient's sexual feelings and his attitudes towards them, the therapist can then start to reveal his own point of view. Apart from the obvious issue of social acceptability, the therapist can ask what ways heterosexual relationships are more advantageous than homosexual ones. In answering this, the patient may reveal that he sees (or has experienced) homosexuality as an exciting but impersonal affair, usually followed by feelings of disgust or shame. In contrast, he may see heterosexuality as involving love and a more consistent and stable intimate relationship. If so, it should be explained to him that the impersonal quality of homosexuality, whilst quite common, is by no means inevitable. Much of it reflects the negative view the homosexual often has of his own sexuality, making it more difficult for him to see his sexual feelings as good or loving. It should be stressed that homosexual relationships can be as good and loving as any, and that there is no shortage of heterosexual relationships that are seriously deficient in these respects. Taking this line, the therapist is reinforcing the view that sex is at its most valuable when it is used to enhance a relationship, reflecting the particular set of values espoused in Chapter 1. Some therapists will reinforce the idea that sexual pleasure, whether homo- or heterosexual, is a worthwhile goal in its own right. I would prefer to recognise its value in the context of a personal relationship, emphasising that it is the quality of the relationship rather than the gender of the participants that is of importance.

A patient can then be asked what he sees as the main obstacles to achieving a rewarding sexual relationship, whether homosexual or heterosexual. Often he will believe that in order to succeed in a heterosexual relationship he will have to get rid of his homosexual feelings. In the past many therapists would have agreed with him. It is now more appropriate to introduce the concept of bisexuality, pointing out that it is possible, at least for some individuals, to enjoy sexual relationships with either male or female partners, though not necessarily at the same time. The therapist will be interested to know whether any heterosexual attraction or interest has been experienced recently or in the past; also whether heterosexual experiences in reality or in imagination have caused anxiety. If so, in either case, the prospects of change in the heterosexual direction are probably more substantial than if an unremiting sexual indifference to the opposite sex has prevailed.

By this stage, and it may have taken more than one session to get there, the patient can be asked more specifically what help he would like. Not infrequently, after this process of exploration of feelings and values he prefers to go away and try things out for himself. Perhaps he was looking for reassurance, or permission, or just needed a chance to clarify his own thoughts. He may now feel more comfortable about entering into a homosexual relationship. Putting him in touch with a homosexual counselling service may be helpful, giving him a chance to discuss these issues with other homosexual people. He should in any case be encouraged to allow himself time. He does not have to decide on his sexual orientation in a hurry — he may need to try a number of different relationships before he is clear about the sexual identity and type of relationship that suits him best. He should be warned against pressures to make premature decisions that may come from either heterosexual or homosexual directions.

If on the other hand he still seeks help from the therapist he can be offered two broad alternatives: improving or establishing a rewarding homosexual relationship, or exploring heterosexual relationships, extending his range of possibilities. The patient may still specifically request treatment to get rid of his homosexual feelings. I would then make it clear that I am *not* prepared to help with that particular goal

If he decides to accept his homosexual feelings but still welcomes help, a commonsense counselling approach can be used. There is first the need to identify specific problems and their associated feelings. Problems likely to be encountered can be considered under four headings:

1. guilt about homosexual feelings and being unable to accept homosexual expression of love;
2. problems in forming or maintaining a close intimate relationship with a person of the same sex;
3. sexual difficulties in a homosexual relationship;
4. coping with the social stigma that a homosexual encounters in our society.

For the second and third of these headings, the counselling approach is not fundamentally different to that used for a heterosexual person with similar problems. In some instances, as with heterosexual patients, more profound conflicts or personality problems may warrant longer-term individual psychotherapy.

If the patient decides that he would like to explore a heterosexual relationship, a realistic contract should be agreed. He should be encouraged to see subsequent attempts as an experiment and keep his homosexual feelings in reserve as an option to fall back on if his heterosexual encounters do not succeed. It is important not to foster over-optimistic expectations but rather to see success as a possibility that will not be realised unless such attempts are made.

Having agreed on such a contract, the programme to be followed will focus on two broad aspects: firstly, fantasy and secondly, real interactions with a potential partner. Usually the fantasy approach offers the most immediate scope. Attention is paid to the patient's usual masturbation pattern, with particular emphasis on the fantasies normally used. As an assignment he is asked to try out different fantasies involving some hetero-sexual component and to report back to the therapist his reactions to them and to what extent they were compatible with sexual arousal. The purpose of this is twofold: first, it helps him to find the best approach to an effective heterosexual fantasy world and secondly, by examining his reactions to different fantasies, possible sources of anxiety may be identified. These may include, for example, fear of being sexually inadequate, of being rejected, having to take a dominant role or having to be ultramasculine, or unease or disgust with female genitalia. Such fears or negative feelings can then be discussed and placed in a more realistic perspective. Heterosexual fantasies may need to be voyeuristic initially, e.g. watching another man making love to a woman. This, whilst clearly heterosexual, allows a homosexual component as the patient may focus as much on the man in the image as on the woman. By shaping the fantasy the subject's involvement may gradually increase.

There are two approaches to the use of fantasy in this situation. Some therapists advocate the use of the subject's favourite homosexual fantasy during masturbation, with instructions to switch to a heterosexual fantasy just before orgasm occurs. On subsequent occasions the heterosexual fantasy is introduced earlier and earlier in the sequence (Marquis 1970). This so-called 'orgasmic reconditioning' has been attributed to a conditioning procedure, although in fact it is closer to backward conditioning (i.e. with the unconditioned stimulus preceding the conditioned stimulus), which is known to be ineffective in laboratory learning experiments. In practice I have not found this procedure particularly helpful and prefer the fantasy shaping approach whereby a heterosexual component is added to the fantasy, sufficiently limited not to interfere with the sexual response and then, with practice, gradually extended (Bancroft 1971). If a phobic response to heterosexual contact is revealed, a desensitisation approach may be helpful (Bancroft 1974). Most commonly the anxiety that does arise stems from a fear of failure or rejection, but it may involve a phobia of female genitalia. With this approach, response to fantasy may progress, whilst at the same time important sources of anxiety or ignorance about heterosexual relationships are revealed and dealt with using the educational and psychotherapeutic components of treatment. At an appropriate stage the patient is encouraged to seek out some limited contact with a woman he finds attractive. If necessary the basic steps of sociosexual behaviour are discussed. How do you first show that you are interested? How do you ask for a date and so on? Limited goals of this kind are agreed with the therapist and the consequences reported back at the next session.

Some patients may already have established a relationship with a woman. Appropriate gradual steps to love-making can then be discussed and tried out. Probably the situation providing the greatest therapeutic potential is when such a heterosexual partner is prepared to come into couple therapy. This is the approach used successfully by Masters & Johnson (1979). Couples were taken through a similar behavioural programme to that undertaken by heterosexual couples presenting with sexual dysfunction. Unfortunately opportunities to do this are few, and the most unusual aspect of Masters & Johnson's 'conversion' treatment for homosexuals was that they were able to get so many people to come into therapy with a co-operative sexual partner.

So far we have considered the usual model of behavioural psychotherapy, with the emphasis on behavioural assignments to be carried out between treatment sessions. In the 1960s and early 1970s, when behaviour therapists were paying more attention to altering homosexual preferences, a variety of ingenious treatment techniques were used within the treatment session. Initially these were of a negative kind and comparised various aversive procedures for suppressing homosexual responses. As stated earlier, these are no longer considered appropriate, not only because of their negative connotations but also because they were less effective than more positive approaches in achieving their goals. Later, various methods for conditioning or enhancing sexual responses to heterosexual stimuli were introduced, usually to be applied in a laboratory setting. (For a detailed review see Bancroft (1974)). Few of these have much relevance today. The emphasis now is more on the behaviours that can be carried out in the patient's own time, with treatment sessions used to deal with the problems arising and to decide on the next appropriate assignments.

The measurement of erections to different types of stimuli may however be useful in some cases. By monitoring erections whilst the patient tries out different fantasies, much may be learnt about the sexually arousing or sexually inhibiting elements in a specific fantasy. With this information a more effective programme of fantasy shaping may be devised (Bancroft 1971).

Other types of sexual preference

Problems associated with fetishism, sadomasochism or other preferences which are not necessarily illegal, arise only occasionally in the clinic. This may be because people with such preferences have no particular wish to alter them. They are not subjected to the same degree of social stigma as the homosexual. Nevertheless their reasons for seeking help may need to be explored. Often a married man seeks treatment because of pressure from his wife, whereas he himself may be very ambivalent about change. These patterns of sexual activity often have a divisive effect on the sexual relationship. Some partners accept them and may even enjoy them, but for the majority this is not the case.

When a partner is involved, it is important to consider carefully whether individual or couple therapy is indicated. Often a fetishistic or sadomaso-chistic pattern becomes accentuated because of difficulties in the sexual relationship. When the relationship is going well these sexual tendencies often lose their importance. Thus, when possible, it is preferable to take the couple into therapy, focusing on their basic sexual relationship and not on the deviant preference per se.

When this is not possible or appropriate a similar use of masturbation training and shaping of fantasies, as described above, may sometimes be helpful.

Problems of sexual self-control

When an individual expresses concern about his ability to control unwanted sexual urges, he is often more likely to benefit from help which aims to strengthen more positive and acceptable aspects of his sexuality. Increasing confidence in one's ability to enjoy and cope with a normal sexual relationship (either hetero- or homosexual) is likely to reduce the urge to behave in unacceptable ways. Often the drive to such acts has a neurotic quality, stemming from anxiety about one's sexual identity or status.

In some cases, however, such positive approaches will either not be relevant or not sufficiently effective to avoid the possibility of trouble with the law or marital crises. Direct help in increasing self-control may then be needed. The principles of this are discussed in Chapter 13 in relation to sexual offenders and will not be repeated here.

THEORETICAL CONSIDERATIONS AND RESEARCH EVIDENCE

The approach to individual therapy described here is based on the same eclectic model of psychotherapy described for couple therapy. We are faced with similar problems when we turn to the literature on individual treatment outcome research. One controlled study deserves closer attention, however, as it has partly avoided the pitfalls described earlier. Obler (1973) compared systematic desensitisation with group therapy and no treatment in individuals with sexual anxiety of various kinds. The unique characteristic of this study is that subjects were chosen whose problems were appropriate for the method of treatment being used. Systematic desensitisation is specifically designed to reduce or improve the management of anxiety. Sixty-four subjects were selected from a group of 225 volunteers on the basis of their Taylor manifest anxiety scale scores. A degree of homogeneity was thus obtained in a variable which was relevant to one of the treatment methods, and a convincing superiority of systematic desensitisation was demonstrated. The weakness of this study is that this selection was relevant to only one of the treatment methods. Ideally the authors should have selected a second group with characteristics which were favourable to group therapy (if such characteristics were known) and then ensured that both patient groups were equally represented in each treatment group. This early study, which is of limited clinical relevance, does nevertheless underline the importance of selecting the patient to suit the treatment and vice versa. Other studies of systematic desensitisation for a variety of sexual problems are reviewed by Laughren & Kass (1975). Additional controlled studies of individual therapy for various kinds of female sexual dysfunction include Munjack et al (1976); McMullen & Rosen (1979); Roughan & Kunst (1981); Nairne & Hemsley (1983); Trudel & Saint-Laurent (1983).

For the modification of sexual preferences, a much more extensive literature exists. This is mainly concerned with evaluating specific techniques, such as aversive methods, positive conditioning or imaginal systematic desensitisation of heterosexual anxiety. In my view not only do most of these techniques have limited relevance to current treatment but their original theoretical basis is now very doubtful. There are some behaviour therapists who continue to view these methods as the mainstay of their treatment programmes. I see them as being of occasional use as ancillary procedures incorporated into a more comprehensive behavioural psychotherapy programme. (For a full review of this literature and theoretical critique see Bancroft 1974.)

GROUP THERAPY

Treating people in groups rather than as individuals has been popular for many years. Until recently most group therapy has been psychoanalytically oriented, but in the past 15 years or so most theoretical approaches to treatment have been applied in a group setting.

The use of groups has certain advantages, which tend to apply whatever the theoretical orientation of the group leader. The relationship between the patient and the therapist is much less crucial; the important relationship is between the patient and the group. Though this can lead to dependence on the group, this is usually less problematic than the dependency which may develop in individual therapy. The sexuality of the patient–therapist relationship is also easier to handle in a group.

One of the advantages of couple therapy over individual therapy is that the couple brings the most relevant relationship into therapy, allowing the therapist much more direct access to the relationship problem. In a group, relationships emerge between group members which can also be used in the treatment process. This is particularly valuable for the socially isolated individual whose problems may be related to interpersonal difficulties, or for the institutionalised patient (e.g. in prison) who is denied the opportunity of normal relationships which would provide not only the practice ground but also the evidence of progress.

A number of other advantages stem from being part of such a group. Once it is cohesive, its members may be less likely to drop out of treatment than if they are participating in individual or couple therapy (O'Gorman 1978; Duddle & Ingram 1980); there is a loyalty to the group, or alternatively a fear of loss of face, that keeps them going. The group may well have shared objectives. Group cohesiveness enhances the individual's motivation to try out new behaviours. Explanations or interpretations of resistances or blocks are provided by the group. The individual receiving such a group interpretation is likely to be influenced by it because he or she has also participated in providing such interpretations to others in the group. The group gives permission for new behaviours or values which may be more effective than permission from one therapist. Progress of any individual member acts as encouragement for the others, whereas conversely group members experiencing setbacks may gain support from the group.

There are also more practical advantages. In most cases more patients can be treated for a unit of therapist's time than with individual or couple therapy. Information or educational material can be provided more economically (e.g. showing the group a film).

There are also disadvantages. Many people are reluctant to join a group, fearing exposure and loss of confidentiality. This may be less of a problem in the USA, where at least the articulate middle classes appear to be more accepting of self-disclosure in groups than are typical Europeans. It may also be more of a problem when dealing with sexual difficulties. Several workers in the UK have had difficulty getting treatment groups started for lack of enough suitable people (e.g. Duddle & Ingram 1980). In mixed-sex groups (unusual for sexual problems unless couples are involved) or groups of homosexuals, pairing off outside the group can have a destructive effect on the group process. For those in group therapy, the attachment to the group may be threatening to their partners or other family members not involved. (This of course also applies to individual therapy.)

Some of the earliest use of groups for sexual problems was reported by Stone & Levine (1952). In the 1960s group therapy for homosexuals was being used, though the treatment goals were usually assumed to be heterosexual adjustment (e.g. Birk & Miller 1970). The use of groups for sexual dysfunction has increased noticeably since the early 1970s. This has reflected the general interest in sex therapy, and has usually involved the basic principles of behavioural psychotherapy that have already been described in relation to couple and individual treatment.

More traditional methods of behavioural therapy have been used in groups. O'Gorman (1978) used systematic desensitisation as a group process for women with sexual unresponsiveness. In most recent groups however the same sort of behavioural assignments that would be used in couple or individual therapy are agreed to by the group, with members going home to try them out. Assignments may vary from person to person but are discussed by the group as a whole. In this case each individual reports back on his or her progress or lack of it to the group rather than to the therapist, and the group helps to resolve the resistances or shift the attitudes that arise (e.g. Barbach 1974; Leiblum et al 1976; Kaplan et al 1974).

Others have emphasised the educational rather than the psychotherapeutic component. Thus Gillan et al (1980) used a very structured programme with emphasis on didactic material, watching films etc. and with the group carrying out the same homework assignments at each stage. An educational emphasis has been used in intensive weekend workshops for groups of individuals or couples (Leiblum & Rosen 1979). Others have used short intensive periods to combine group and couple processes. Blakeney et al (1976) treated couples for 2½ days with a combination of group and individual counselling sessions. Csillag et al (1981) used a combination of groups, relaxation training, role-playing, films and individual counselling sessions during a 5-day inpatient period in hospital, which also allowed the couples time and privacy to try out their newly learnt ideas.

The most popular format is to use groups of the same sex. Varied sexual dysfunctions may be involved (Zilbergeld 1975; Leiblum & Ersner-Hershfield 1977) but usually the members of the group have similar problems, e.g. orgasmic difficulty (Barbach 1974; Gillan et al 1980), vaginismus (Becker, personal communication) or erectile impotence (Lobitz & Baker 1979).

Others have used groups of couples, either with varied problems (e.g. Leiblum et al 1976) or specific problems such as premature ejaculation (Kaplan et al 1874). O'Gorman (1978) ran two parallel groups, one for dysfunctional women, the other for their male partners.

Whether to use groups of individuals or couples remains debatable. Obviously for people without sexual partners, group treatment has advantages. Also for people whose partners refuse to participate in couple therapy a group may provide the best option, although if, for example, all had unco-operative husbands, improvement in marital harmony should not necessarily be expected! The effect of group cohesiveness may be to alienate the women even more from their spouses. This can also be a problem, even when the sexual partner is not unco-operative. Schneidman & McGuire (1976) and Leiblum & Ersner-Hershfield (1977) gave examples of women whose partners reacted to their increased sexual esteem and assertiveness with resentment or hostility. Involvement of those partners in treatment may have avoided that. A further crucial issue is the extent to which behavioural change on an individual basis generalises to the sexual relationship. In the treatment of orgasmic difficulty in women, several studies have reported substantial success in helping women to become orgasmic during masturbation on their own, but the extent to which they become orgasmic with their partners is much less certain (Leiblum & Ersner-Hershfield 1977). On the other hand, Ersner-Hershfield & Kopel (1979) found no difference in this aspect between women who were treated individually and those treated with their partners in couple groups. At first sight this is surprising though we have ceased to be surprised by negative results in small comparative outcome studies.

There are also problems with couple groups. The ability for a particular couple to sabotage a group is probably greater than for an individual. Selection of suitable couples is important, and severe marital discord may prove to be a contraindication (Leiblum et al 1976).

Research evidence

So far the evidence of the efficacy of group treatment is mainly from uncontrolled studies (Mills & Kilman 1982). Controlled outcome studies include those by O'Gorman (1978); Golden et al (1978); Gillan et al (1980); Price et al (1981); Cotten-Huston & Wheeler (1983). One study worthy of special comment was reported by Hartman (1983). He used couple group therapy but crossed over between sex therapy and marital therapy, i.e. half the couples started with sex therapy and moved on to marital therapy and half in the reverse order. The use of a cross-over design does reduce the problem of prognostic variability, as each couple acts as their own control. The problem with cross-over studies is the possibility of carry-over effects, when behavioural change becomes self-sustaining. This is particularly likely when working with couples. Nevertheless, Hartman was able to describe some effects. Sex therapy produced more change than marital therapy for both partners in the dissatisfaction with frequency of sexual activity. For women, sex therapy produced more improvement in sexual enjoyment, though men tended to show more change with marital therapy in this respect.

As with most other forms of sex therapy, we will need much more sound evidence before group therapy finds its proper place.

THE USE OF SURROGATE PARTNERS

The sexually dysfunctional individual without a partner has, for reasons already discussed, few opportunities for effective help. Surrogate partners have been used by some therapists to overcome this problem, i.e. the therapist provides someone other than himself to become sexually involved with the patient for therapeutic purposes. The unacceptability of sexual involvement by the therapist is assumed by all but a very few (Bancroft 1981). The surrogate partner, who is concerned and sympathetic as well as knowledgeable about sexual problems, can be seen to provide the advantages of having sex with one's therapist without the disadvantages. Masters & Johnson (1970) treated 41 of their 448 male patients using surrogates. They did not use male surrogates for female patients however and have now stopped using surrogates altogether. Cole (1985) uses both male and female surrogate partners.

The ethical issues are complex. Surrogate therapists have been likened to prostitutes. The comparison is debatable, but in any case the ethical status of prostitution is far from clearcut. Usually women involved as surrogates in no way regard themselves as prostitutes. Their real motives are a matter of interest but are not readily apparent (Cole 1985).

Concern has been expressed about confidentiality as well as the legal complexities of such relationships. Masters & Johnson abandoned the use of surrogates, concerned that they were becoming too much like therapists, and hence raising all the ethical problems of sexual contact between the patient and the therapist (Masters et al 1977). Cole (1985) described his surrogates as 'therapists'. Sommers (1980) referred to his surrogates as 'sexual therapy practitioners'. In California, where surrogates are relatively numerous, they have formed their own professional organisation together with a professional code of practice (Jacobs et al 1975). There is therefore no doubt that the distinction between therapist and surrogate is now blurred.

Judging the efficacy of such treatment also has ethical implications. Is such judgement based on the quality of sexual performance or on the nature of the sexual relationship established with the surrogate? For those who regard the relationship as the main concern, this will seem of crucial significance.

Nevertheless, too hasty a rejection of surrogate therapy may be unjustified. There may be some individuals whose sexual lives will be genuinely enhanced by such experience and who may be difficult to help in other ways. An open mind is appropriate, but the ethical problems cannot be dismissed easily.

THE THERAPEUTIC USE OF DRUGS AND HORMONES

In Chapter 2 we considered the effects of pharmacological agents on the sexual response system. In the last few years there has been increasing interest in this field, and it remains possible that before long some important breakthrough in pharmacological treatment will occur. But as yet that is still some time away and the role of drugs in the management of sexual dysfunction remains very limited.

Intracavernosal injections

One of the most remarkable developments has been the use of intracavernosal injections of smooth muscle relaxants, such as papaverine and phenoxybenzamine. These drugs are being used widely for diagnostic purposes (see p. 441), and now their therapeutic possibilities are being increasingly explored. Brindley (1986) reported on 127 men with erectile dysfunction who received intracavernosal injections of either phenoxybenzamine or papaverine. Erections resulted in 113 cases. Dosage may be important and Brindley recommends increasing the dosage on three occasions before deeming the drug to be ineffective. Seventy-three men have injected themselves at home in order to have sexual intercourse and at the time of Brindley's report 54 were still doing so. He restricts the use of these injections to a maximum of one per fortnight. Therapeutic use of self-injection has also been reported by Virag et al (1984) and Zorgniotti & LeFleur (1985).

In a more systematic study, Keogh et al (1986) compared papaverine (60 mg), phenoxybenzamine (6 mg) and placebo (saline) in a double-blind cross-over design involving monthly injections in 34 men with assumed organic dysfunction. Twelve men (35%) developed full erections following papaverine, seven (20%) did following phenoxybenzamine and none did after placebo. Twenty-one (62%) developed partial erections after each of the active drugs and four (12%) did after placebo.

Phenoxybenzamine should probably not be used now. It has been shown to be carcinogenic in some animals (Brindley 1986) and repeated injections into the corpora cavernosa of rabbits produced an acute inflammatory reaction (Stackl et al 1986).

One of the unsatisfactory aspects of this burgeoning literature is the lack of attention to detail of the response to these injections, in particular the extent to which responses continue to occur in the short term. The implication of several reports is that erections not only occur within a few minutes of the injection (in a proportion of cases) but may also recur during the next day or two. In Chapter 9 we showed evidence of how these injections can enhance the erectile response to visual erotic stimuli. This effect, if it persisted for any length of time, would be preferable to a sustained erection as well as being of considerable theoretical interest. Keogh et al (1986) reported that erectile response was enhanced over the ensuing month in 41% of papaverine cases, 29% of phenoxybenzamine and also in 29% of placebo cases. We need more systematic evidence of these crucial effects before we can assess the therapeutic potential of this new approach.

Injections are not an attractive method of administration for many people, though they seem to be acceptable to some. They may be of particular relevance to insulin-dependent diabetic men who are used to injecting themselves in any case. The long-term consequences of repeated intracavernosal injections are not known — though Brindley has been on the look-out for fibrosis at the injection site. Persistent erection occurs in approximately 5% of cases and may require pharmacological reversal by means of intracavernosal drugs, such as metaraminol. For these various reasons this interesting therapeutic development requires very careful monitoring and should only be used in the context of thorough physical and psychological assessment. It is a cause of some concern that as a method of both diagnosis and treatment it is often being used in a somewhat haphazard fashion. Alternative methods of delivering appropriate drugs to the erectile tissues will obviously be sought. The transdermal route is one possibility, though it is not clear how possible it is to get drugs into the corpora cavernosa through this route. I have experimented with a synthetic prostaglandin which is a potent vasodilator and is well absorbed through the skin, but it was ineffective applied to the dorsum of the penis (unpublished observations). Amyl nitrite, applied to the penis transdermally has apparently been effective but at the cost of severe headaches (Morley, personal communication).

Oral drug treatment for erectile dysfunction

Most interest recently has been directed at yohimbine, an alpha$_2$ antagonist (see p. 125). A suggestion of therapeutic benefit for men with organic erectile dysfunction was reported by Morales et al (1982) in an uncontrolled study. It is slightly surprising that they should have directed their early efforts at organic dysfunction. If drugs such as yohimbine are effective, central mechanisms will probably be involved, hence the peripheral mechanisms should be intact if such effects are to be manifested. In a later placebo-controlled study of psychogenic dysfunction, the superiority of yohimbine over placebo was reported (Reid et al 1987), but unfortunately this study was confounded by an unsatisfactory design. Having randomly allocated patients to either yohimbine or placebo, they then crossed-over after the initial treatment period to the other treatment, but only for the placebo group and those of the yohimbine group who did not respond. Although the initial yohimbine group did better than the initial placebo group ($p<0.05$) there was much less response to yohimbine in the subjects who were crossed-over to active treatment. The results of this study are regrettably uninterpretable.

Drugs to enhance sexual interest

In Chapter 2 we considered the possible role of dopamine agonists in enhancing sexual motivation (see p. 125). We know that bromocriptine improves sexual interest in men with hyperprolactinaemia, but it is not yet clear whether this is due to lowering prolactin levels or to a direct dopaminergic action on the brain. Attempts to evaluate dopamine agonists such as bromocriptine for treatment of sexual dysfunction have not been successful so far, in part because of the level of side-effects with these drugs. No attempts to evaluate the effects of such drugs on the sexuality of women have been reported yet.

Drug treatment of premature ejaculation

Pharmacological inhibition of ejaculation has been exploited to treat premature ejaculation. Thioridazine and monoamine oxidase inhibitors have been used for this purpose, though the drug most widely used is clomipramine, a tricyclic antidepressant (Eaton 1973). In a controlled study this was shown to be significantly more effective than placebo in treating premature ejaculation (Porto 1980). However, there is no evidence as yet that such benefits continue after stopping the drug. These are powerful drugs with side-effects; alpha blockers, such as indoramin (Pentland et al 1981) might be preferable in this respect. But considering the range of side-effects of all these drugs, the apparent need for continued use and the relative efficacy of psychological methods of treatment, the indications for their use have not yet been properly established.

Anxiety-reducing drugs

The therapeutic value of anxiety drugs in the treatment of sexual dysfunction remains uncertain. The relationship between anxiety and sexual response was discussed at length in Chapter 2. In many cases the simple pharmacological reduction of anxiety may only succeed in reducing an accompanying symptom rather than the basic difficulty. Riley & Riley (1986) have shown that diazepam impairs the sexual response of normal women during masturbation. In addition anxiety reduction may in some cases interfere with counselling by making the source of sexual threat less apparent (see p. 498).

Hormonal treatment

The therapeutic role of hormones and antihormones has been considered more fully elsewhere in this book (see Chapters 2 and 5). In summary, the following points can be made.

In males low testosterone levels and/or raised prolactin may be associated with lowered sexual interest and ejaculatory failure. Correcting the hormonal abnormality with testosterone and bromocriptine respectively may help to solve the sexual problem. Erectile failure is unlikely to improve unless it is a psychological reaction to low sexual interest. Testosterone can be given orally as testosterone undecanoate, intramuscularly as esters (e.g. testosterone oenanthate, or Sustanon), or as implants.

Men with testosterone levels within the normal range who complain of low sexual interest sometimes benefit from additional testosterone (O'Carroll & Bancroft 1984). Such effects are usually modest, however, and will often need to be combined with counselling to make best use of them. Oral testosterone undecanoate will elevate circulating testosterone in eugonadal men, though the speed of absorption varies considerably (Davidson et al 1987). It is therefore a convenient method of administration in such cases.

Men aged 60 and over may have experienced a reduction in their levels of testosterone even when their levels remain within the laboratory normal range. Loss of sexual interest in this age group may respond to testosterone administration, but care should be taken because of possible adverse effects on blood lipids (hence increasing the risk of arterial disease) and on prostatic hypertrophy. Prostatic carcinoma should be excluded before embarking on such treatment.

In women, a small amount of oestrogen is necessary for normal vaginal function. If, following the menopause or oophorectomy, the circulating oestrogens fall sufficiently, problems of vaginal dryness and dyspareunia will result. This is highly likely to respond to oestrogen therapy, administered either systemically or by the vaginal route. In some women such oestrogen deficiency may also lead to loss of sexual interest and enjoyment which are not simply the consequences of vaginal dryness. The therapeutic administration of oestrogens to post-menopausal women, whether they have an intact uterus or not, poses various problems and uncertainties relating to risks of malignant disease and change in blood lipids. This is an issue surrounded with controversy, but at worst the risk must be assumed to be small unless a woman already falls into a high-risk group. Full discussion is beyond the scope of this book, but factors such as the type of oestrogen (i.e. natural or synthetic), the route of administration, whether given continuously or cyclically, or whether combined with a progestogen (which may counteract the sexually beneficial effects) all have to be taken into consideration. In general, one should aim for the smallest dose necessary to produce the desired effect.

The therapeutic role of androgens for either pre- or post-menopausal women remains obscure. Although there is evidence that androgens are related to certain aspects of sexuality, at least in some women (see Chapters 2 and 5) I have only rarely been successful in treating sexual problems in women with androgens. This is in contrast to a number of other clinical reports — though it may be relevant that all reports of clinical benefit from androgens in women have involved either intramuscular injections or implants. My experience has always been with sublingual testosterone or oral testosterone undecanoate. It may be therefore that the different routes of administration are of clinical significance, though, as reported in Chapter 2, both sublingual and oral routes produce massive increases in circulating testosterone above the normal male range for several hours. This issue remains an enigma and requires more research. Virilising effects are a hazard of androgen administration to women (and changes in blood lipids also occur) but troublesome side-effects are rarely reported.

Hyperprolactinaemia in women has a less certain relationship to sexual dysfunction than in men. Sexual improvement following dopaminergic drug therapy (e.g. bromocriptine) occurs in some cases but is relatively unpredictable (Lundberg et al 1986).

SEXUAL AIDS

A variety of mechanical devices intended to increase sexual response or enjoyment are commercially available (Roles 1972). They include devices which fit on the penis to give additional stimulation to the female partner, either clitorally or intravaginally; those which are inserted inside the vagina to increase muscle tone, artificial penises, vacuum pumps to increase the size of the penis and so on.

Only three such devices have received any serious attention or attempts at evaluation: the vibrator, the penile ring and the vacuum pump. The electrical vibrator has been mentioned several times earlier in the chapter. It is widely used as an adjunct to treatment for orgasmic difficulties in women (e.g. Riley & Riley 1978; Gillan et al 1980) as well as for inducing ejaculation in men. It is a powerful erotic stimulus, particularly for women when applied in the region of the clitoris. The frequency of vibrations varies according to the type of vibrator, and some frequencies are more effective than others (Gillan & Brindley 1979).

Vibrators may be particularly useful, when used in conjunction with counselling, in helping people to experience orgasm for the first time and reducing the subsequent inhibition. Some women learn to enjoy the vibrator stimulation to such an extent that they may be reluctant to abandon its use. In those circumstances the vibrator may come to represent a barrier between the woman and her partner, though it is perfectly possible to incorporate the vibrator stimulation into love-making.

The Blakoe suspensory energiser ring is a rectangular 'ring' made of ebonite which opens on a swivel to allow it to be fitted high up around the base of the penis and under the scrotum. It is made in various sizes to allow a close fit. It contains small metal plates on its surface which set up a mild but continuous electrical current when in contact with the moist surface of the genital skin. This current is said to have some stimulatory effect on the erectile mechanisms. Its use is advised whenever intercourse or masturbation is attempted. Cooper (1974) carried out a blind comparison of this ring with a placebo ring, constructed in the same way but without the metal plates. He found that both rings seemed to be beneficial but there was no difference between the two types. Whether the beneficial effect was due to mechanical or psychological factors is not clear. Apart from its harmlessness, this appliance has rather little to commend it.

Cooper (1987) has also evaluated the vacuum pump as a treatment for erectile failure finding that it is beneficial in some cases, though enthusiam for its use declines over time.

SURGICAL TREATMENT

At the present time two types of surgical treatment for sexual dysfunction in the male are attracting considerable interest: the surgical implantation of penile prostheses and revascularisation of the erectile tissues in the presence of peripheral arterial disease. For the female, apart from the surgical treatment of anatomical abnormalities such as congenital absence of the vagina or undue narrowing of the vaginal introitus, surgery is rarely being used for the treatment of female sexual dysfunction. The tendency to use Fenton's operation for the treatment of vaginismus is, or should be, now of historic interest only.

The use of antiandrogens, such as cyproterone acetate and medroxyprogesterone acetate, or psychotropic drugs such as benperidol to suppress sexual interest and unwanted sexual behaviour is discussed in Chapter 13.

Penile prostheses

The surgical implantation of plastic splints into the penis was first reported by Loeffler (1960) who used perforated acrylic for this purpose. Since then a variety of substances of different shapes and sizes have been used (Pryor

1979). Silastic is the most popular material. The original silastic rod (Small-Carrion type) was semi-rigid and hence produced a permanent erection. Modifications have involved a hinge at the base (Finney modification) or the use of central strands of silver wire which provide sufficient rigidity for intercourse but sufficient pliability to bend it out of the way when not in use (Jonas type).

A more sophisticated alternative was introduced by Scott et al (1973). This is a pair of inflatable penile implants connected to a small pump placed within the scrotum and also to a reservoir of hydraulic fluid placed in the prevesical space. To produce an erection the subject inflates the prosthesis by squeezing the pump mechanism in the scrotum. This process can be reversed by moving a valve on the pump which can be felt through the scrotal wall. Although this controllable erection has some advantages over the more or less permanent variety, the surgery involved is more complex, has a higher complication rate and is more expensive. The incidence of postoperative complications for these different devices appears to vary considerably from one report to another (Kolodny et al 1979).

Considering the extent to which men are prepared to part with their money in return for an effective erection, it is not surprising that considerable ingenuity has been applied to producing even more sophisticated varieties of inflatable devices. Three new devices are currently being used; the Hydroflex (American Medical Systems) and the Flexiflate (Surgitek) include their pump and fluid reservoir within the penile prosthesis, thereby simplifying the surgical insertion. The Omniphase (Dacomed) is a mechanical device which can be made rigid or flexible simply by manipulating it in a particular way. It is too early to know how effective these new devices will be (Krane 1986).

Penile implants are most commonly used for men whose erectile failure is thought to be of organic origin, though they are sometimes used for psychogenic cases who have been found to be resistant to psychological treatment. As a psychiatrist I have had to overcome prejudice before accepting that these devices have a proper place in the management of erectile dysfunction. To deal with erectile failure by implanting a plastic rod is, in my view, colluding with the assumption that good sex requires an erect penis, as well as the tendency to equate erectile function with masculinity and potency (Tiefer 1986). I am now beginning to accept that there is a place for such treatment, but we have a long way to go before we can say with confidence which type of man, with which type of partner (whose importance in the acceptance of these devices is often overlooked) is likely to benefit. Collins & Kinder (1984) reviewed the reports on outcome and satisfaction with penile prostheses. Whilst the majority of recipients reported being at least fairly satisfied with the outcome, the standard of enquiry in most of these follow-up studies is seriously deficient in many respects. These authors also found that less satisfaction was often expressed by the spouse when interviewed separately from the husband.

Steege et al (1986) contacted 85 men following the implantation of either Small-Carrion or Scott prostheses. They received questionnaires from 52 (61%). Whilst the majority were broadly satisfied with the operation, most of them regarded the post-implant erection as inferior to their normal erections; 75% believed that it was shorter than before and 65% reported decreased sensitivity of the erect penis. Whereas most were able to ejaculate, 52% reported a reduction in ejaculatory sensation. Evidence of additional tumescence in the glans or remaining part of the erectile spaces was reported by 58%, indicating that normal erectile capacity is not necessarily eliminated by this surgical procedure, though it is unlikely that normal erections could ever be obtained after insertion and removal of such a prosthesis.

What seems clear is that the use of these devices should be accompanied by appropriate counselling both before and after surgery, as described on p. 489. As yet few urological surgeons who insert these devices are working within an appropriately multidisciplinary team (Schover & van Eschenbach 1985) and I have come across men who have been offered surgical treatment without any attempt to assess the importance of psychological factors. This is a cause for concern. It is to be hoped that with the greater communication that is beginning between surgeons and sex therapists this will become less and less likely.

Vascular surgery for erectile failure

Increasing awareness of the association between arterial occlusion and erectile failure has led vascular surgeons to attempt revascularisation procedures. In some cases obstruction of the large pelvic arteries is recognised and may be treated by ilio-hypogastric anastomoses, endarterectomy or balloon transluminal angioplasty. Unfortunately, in most cases with large vessel obstruction there is also evidence of small vessel disease distal to the main obstruction. Various methods have been used to revascularise the corpus cavernosum in such cases (Michal 1978; Virag 1982): anastamosis of the inferior epigastric artery directly into the tunica albuginea, or end-to-end anastomosis to the dorsal penile artery, or end-to-side anastomosis to the dorsal penile vein associated with a venous anastomosis through the tunica. A section of the long saphenous vein may be used as a graft to connect the femoral artery to the penile vessels or directly into the corpus cavernosum. Given the subtle vascular mechanisms involved in normal erection (see p. 53), these methods must be seen as crude and as yet long-term results have not been encouraging.

Occasionally arteriovenous anastomoses are found to be the cause of erectile failure, preventing the intracavernosal pressure from building up sufficiently to produce rigidity (see p. 377). Surgical closure of such anastamoses can be attempted, though the results are less predictable than one might have expected (Ebbehøj & Wagner 1979).

MANAGEMENT OF THE TRANSSEXUAL PATIENT

The transsexual patient may present one of the most demanding challenges in clinical sexology, requiring the collaboration of behavioural, endocrinological and surgical specialists forming a clinical team. Although the surgical aspects are complex, it is the psychological management that is most time-consuming.

Transsexualism is an emotive subject. This is not only because of the difficulty people have in understanding the discrepancy between gender identity and anatomic sex. The use of surgical sex reassignment also generates much doubt. Is it morally acceptable (Bancroft 1981)? Is it colluding with psychosis? Is it a proper use of medical resources, particularly within the National Health Service?

The issue of surgery is indeed central to the whole topic. As discussed in Chapter 7, the existence of sex reassignment surgery, in spite of its considerable limitations, has provided a goal or a would-be solution for a wide variety of gender identity problems, sometimes referred to collectively as gender dysphoria. As we shall see, the well-being of the transsexual after sex reassignment depends only partly on the surgery. Yet this aspect looms large; many transsexual patients want nothing else and will go to great lengths to obtain surgery.

This is relevant to the clinician attempting to assess the transsexual patient. It is sometimes said that surgical reassignment should be confined to the 'true' or primary transsexual (Pauly & Edgerton 1986). In Chapter 7 we indicated that the true transsexual was difficult to define except in terms of his wish for sexual reassignment and his success in carrying through such a change. Roperto (1983) has reviewed the conceptual confusion that still prevails. Even if the true transsexual could be defined, the clinician would be hard-pressed to identify him with any confidence. The determination of transsexual patients, often combined with more than adequate intelligence, means that they probably know the literature on transsexualism as well as most clinicians and better than many. If it seems likely that their case will be more sympathetically received if their history conforms to a certain type, one should not be surprised to find that history forthcoming. Clinicians are used to this problem — psychiatrists at one time played a similarly absurd game with women wanting abortions.

The consequent difficulty in placing any reliance on past history has been one important reason why responsible clinicians have relied on the real-life test — the ability of the transsexual patient to cope with behavioural reassignment for a reasonable period of time before anything irreversible like surgery is undertaken. It is of particular importance to confront the patient with the fact that most of the problems of sex reassignment, being accepted as a member of that sex, working in that role, living from day to day as a woman rather than a man or vice versa, will not be solved by surgery — particularly genital surgery. Self-confidence may be increased, which undoubtedly helps. Intimate relationships may become possible and provide one of the most important consequences of the change. But the many day-to-day problems that must be overcome first require patience and relearning, not surgery. Thus it is important to demonstrate that these primary adjustments can be made before embarking on major irreversible steps. The transsexual who is likely to do badly after surgery is the one who sees most of the problems being solved by the surgery, with him playing a somewhat passive part. Such a person, faced with disillusionment after surgery, may seek more and more surgical change in search of well-being.

The main assessment of the transsexual patient is therefore a continuous one, in which the clinician gets to know the patient over a period of months, developing a sense of mutual trust. During that time the patient is trying out new behaviours, gradually working through a programme which will make it clearer to both the patient and the clinician whether a more permanent sex change is likely to be beneficial.

In the UK at the present time it is very difficult to obtain surgical re-assignment unless it is paid for privately. Surgery is available within the National Health Service in a few places, but remains a controversial matter within the profession. Unfortunately there are surgeons who, providing they are paid, operate without appropriate selection.

Most transsexuals contacting clinics are seeking help for reassignment. There are also some individuals who genuinely feel uncertain and who need time to explore the advantages and disadvantages. My policy is to make it clear from the outset that I am prepared to help with the non-surgical aspects of reassignment but that this takes time. Decisions about surgical help come much later and involve other people. This makes it easier for patients to express ambivalence, which would be less likely if they felt they had to present a consistent story before anyone was prepared to take them seriously. It is often said that there is no effective treatment for restoring a transsexual's comfort with his biological gender. This is to some extent true. A few case reports have indicated a response to behavioural or psychotherapeutic approaches leading to a reduction of transsexual feelings, mainly in adolescent transsexuals (Riseley 1986). In my view transsexualism is viewed too much as a static immutable condition. This is partly a function of the medical process; transsexuals need to present themselves that way or no one will contemplate surgery. Having known some patients over many years, it has become clear to me that the transsexual urge varies in intensity and may depend on situational factors, such as the views of the current sexual partner. This variable natural history warns us on the one hand to avoid rapid irreversible decisions and on the other to be cautious in interpreting reports of treatment which apparently removes transsexual feelings. But given a cautious and conservative approach I believe that there are some patients who will benefit from permanent sex reassignment, including surgery.

THE TREATMENT PROGRAMME

The initial contract

The extent to which the therapist is prepared to help should be made clear at the outset. Along the lines described above, it is emphasised that time will be needed, a trusting relationship between therapist and patient should be allowed to develop and nothing irreversible will be done for some time. The reasons for this cautious approach are given — principally that only some patients end up happier in the newly assigned role and that others change their mind before they get to that stage. Such a decision will eventually be irreversible and every care must be taken not only by the patient but also by the clinician to ensure that the correct choice is made.

At this stage the difficulties in obtaining surgery are stressed and the practical limitations of surgery discussed. Factual information about legal status (e.g. the inability to be legally married) and the biological possibilities (e.g. it will not be possible to have children in the new role) are pointed out. (See Graham (1986) for a useful summary of legal aspects.)

Usually the patient will accept such a contract, though the clinician may well find pressure for more rapid progress being brought to bear at an early stage. It is important to make the contract a two-way affair. It is unreasonable to expect the patient to wait months simply to provide the clinician with information to help him make up his mind. Something should be given in return.

Practical steps

From an early stage the patient who feels certain that he or she wants to change should be encouraged to spend more time 'passing' in the desired role, becoming increasingly ambitious and adventurous as time goes on. Initially this may mean going out at night cross-dressed and walking in the street. Later, people in shops should be approached and so on. The therapist can be giving useful advice about what to do and where to go, plus more tangible benefits, such as providing a letter for the patient to carry around, authorising the cross-dressing behaviour as part of a medically supervised treatment programme. This will often remove the fear of being harassed by the police.

When the patient feels ready, he or she can be invited to come to the clinic cross-dressed. The therapist can then provide more direct feedback about how effective the person is in that role.

Usually transsexuals are cut off from their own families, but occasionally it is helpful for the therapist to explain the nature of the problem to relatives, who sometimes provide extremely valuable support in the patient's future endeavours. It is particularly important to meet and get to know any sexual partners. These are much more likely to exist with female-to-male transsexual partners. They are important because often their attitude may play a major part in the patient's motivation for surgery. I have had experience with several female-to-male transsexuals whose strong desire to have surgery receded dramatically when they changed partners. Usually the issue is whether either the patient or the partner is prepared to accept the relationship as a homosexual rather than a heterosexual one.

Alongside more practical, positive advice, the therapist should be carrying out the continuous process of reality confrontation with both the patient and any partner who is involved. As trust in the therapeutic relationship develops, the therapist should be making sure the patient is aware of the enormous difficulties ahead. There is no place for false optimism, because it is vitally important, since the patient's (and the therapist's) ultimate decision depends on the patient's ability to overcome these problems. Physical appearance is a key factor. Some patients have no difficulty looking the part. For others it will remain a formidable problem, usually because of their facial structure. The older the person, the less of a problem this is likely to be.

In the male-to-female transsexual, beard growth is usually a problem, making effective facial make-up difficult. Facial electrolysis is the only real solution. This is a very time-consuming and expensive business. At a relatively early stage the patient can be advised to seek this treatment. At present it is difficult to obtain electrolysis within the National Health Service. In any case, it may be desirable to give the responsibility for this to the patient in the first instance. The treatment goes on for months, with one or two sessions per week. If the patient pays for these early sessions, later costs may possibly be met by the NHS when it becomes clearer that the treatment programme is going in the right direction. One advantage of electrolysis is that, though it is irreversible, it takes long enough for many uncertainties to be resolved and if sexual reassignment is eventually abandoned, loss of facial hair is not a major problem.

Alternatives to sex reassignment should periodically be reconsidered. The most important are the transvestite 'double role' (see Chapter 7) and the homosexual role. For many transsexuals, particularly female-to-male, life would be so much easier for them if they could accept and feel comfortable with a homosexual identity. Sometimes the extreme and rigid rejection of homosexuality reveals a personality which may not fare well after surgery (Morgan 1978).

In general one is looking for evidence that, apart from the gender dysphoria, the patient has a realistic view of the problems to be faced and of his or her abilities to overcome them.

More specific forms of training may be introduced stage by stage. Voice training is often helpful. Oates & Dacakis (1986) provide a useful review of the evidence of sex differences in speech and indicate that modification of speech needs to involve not only pitch and intonation pattern, but also vocal loudness, voice quality, vocabulary usage, articulatory precision and conversational style. Social skills training with video feedback may be useful in increasing the authenticity of gender role behaviour (Yardley 1976). Sometimes transsexuals caricature the role they seek and need to tone down mannerisms. Help with make-up and hairstyles is often needed.

At some stage the patient, if still intent on pursuing the programme, is encouraged to start living and working full-time in the new role. This usually means moving to a new place to live, and changing jobs. This is often the most difficult stage. Absence of any previous employment in the new role makes applying for jobs difficult as references cannot be supplied. The therapist can provide some help, e.g. by contacting the Disablement Resettlement Officer or arranging for a period of time on a government training scheme to learn some new skill. Medical reassurance can be given to the would-be employer. But the patient will have to take the main responsibility for finding employment.

For some female-to-male transsexuals, large breasts can make this stage particularly difficult, and mastectomy may have to be considered at this relatively early stage in the programme if further progress is to be made.

Hormone treatment

The use of hormones also requires careful thought. Although many of their effects may be reversible, this step should be seen as a definite move towards permanent reassignment which should not be started too early. In the male-to-female transsexual, oestrogens with or without progestagens are used. Their effects are difficult to predict with certainty but are likely to include some breast enlargement (usually not enough, so that mammoplasty will eventually be required), redistribution of fat of a more feminine type, softening of the skin and usually a reduction in sexual appetite. No effect on the voice is to be expected. Some authorities believe that the addition of progestagen to the oestrogen leads to more breast enlargement, but there is no evidence to support this view. Patients should be screened for contraindications to taking steroids (e.g. hypertension, liver disease, history of thrombotic disorders) and should be warned of the risks of taking hormones. It is sensible to carry out some endocrine investigations initially to establish a baseline. It is then advisable to start with a low dose and increase gradually in case of unpleasant side-effects, such as nausea. Ethinyloestradiol is the most widely used oestrogen and can be given in doses up to 0.05 mg daily. Meyer et al (1981) recommend starting with 0.05 mg daily and increasing to 0.1 mg daily if there has been no satisfactory response after 3 or 4 months. If progestagen is to be given, a combined oral contraceptive provides a convenient method, though before surgery it should be taken continuously. Antiandrogens may also be combined with oestrogens. They may further slow down hair growth and enhance breast growth, though a reduction in sexual interest is even more likely. Cyproterone acetate 50 or 100 mg daily is appropriate. It is sensible to stop steroids temporarily if surgery is to be carried out to reduce the risk of postoperative thrombosis.

For the female-to-male transsexual the appropriate hormone is testosterone. This can be expected to increase body and facial hair, though to what extent is difficult to predict, to cause some enlargement of the clitoris and probably increase clitoral sensitivity, increase muscle bulk and body weight and deepen the voice. Menstruation may be less heavy or stop and a slight reduction in breast size may occur but neither of these effects should be assumed.

Again it is advisable to build up the dose gradually. Sublingual testosterone 20–40 mg daily can be used initially. Once it is decided to continue with androgens, monthly injections (e.g. Sustanon 250), oral testosterone undecanoate (Restandol) 40–120 mg daily, or testosterone implants (at approximately 6-monthly intervals) can be used. Meyer et al (1981) recommend intramuscular testosterone cypionate every 2 weeks.

Surgery

After achieving a reasonably satisfactory and stable full-time adjustment in the new role for a minimum of 18 months, surgical reassignment can be seriously considered. For the male-to-female transsexual, this usually involves orchidectomy and penectomy, with preservation of scrotal and penile skin. The fashioning of a vaginal tube uses the penile skin and usually additional split-skin graft. The labia are fashioned out of the scrotal skin. The operation may be done in one or two stages. (For surgical details see Jones (1968), Wesser (1978) and McEwan et al (1986)). Postoperative complications are common and may be troublesome. Urethral stricture or urethrovaginal fistulae may occur. Most common is a fibrosis of the artificial vaginal barrel, leading to shortening or even closure. This can be corrected with further surgery (McEwan et al 1986). If successful, the vagina can eventually be used for sexual intercourse and pleasurable erotic sensations, including orgasm, may be experienced.

For the female-to-male transsexual the surgical options are less satisfactory. Mastectomy has already been mentioned. Hysterectomy and oophorectomy obviously present no surgical problems, but the creation of a penis or scrotum presents formidable difficulties. Although attempts have been made (e.g. Hoopes 1968; Noe et al 1978) results have been far from satisfactory with particular difficulty in avoiding urinary fistulae, and it is extremely doubtful whether they justify the time, expense and substantial risk of postoperative complications.

Postoperative care

The counselling relationship should obviously continue postoperatively and may well be needed for some considerable time. Hormones should also be continued, particularly if testes or ovaries are removed.

OUTCOME OF SEX REASSIGNMENT SURGERY

Adequate long-term follow-up studies of sex reassignment surgery are only recently appearing in the literature. There was a tendency in earlier reports to highlight the successes. In 1979 Meyer & Reter published a report from Baltimore, concluding that transsexuals who had received surgery were no better adapted than those who had not. This report had many deficiencies and has been justly criticised (e.g. Fleming et al 1980), as its main conclusions are not justified from the data. However, recent studies have pointed out that by no means all cases can be regarded as successes. Lundstrom et al (1984) reviewed the follow-up literature and reached the following conclusions:

1. An unsatisfactory result occurs in 10–15% of cases.
2. Approximately 5% of cases regret the surgery.
3. Female-to-male transsexuals fare somewhat better than male-to-female transsexuals.
4. Factors affecting outcome are complex, but include the functional effectiveness of surgery. Satterfield (1983) found a high correlation between postoperative satisfaction and the sexual functioning of the surgical vagina in male-to-female cases.
5. Personal and social instability preoperatively is associated with unsatisfactory postoperative outcome.
6. 'Secondary' transsexuals have poorer outcomes. According to Person & Ovesey's (1974) definitions, a 'primary' transsexual has had unambiguous cross-gender identity from a very early age; 'secondary' transsexuals develop their cross-gender identity much later (e.g. as part of the transvestite–transsexual shift or as a reaction to effeminate homosexuality). I have already commented on the difficulties in relying on the patient's retrospective history for making this distinction.
7. The younger the age at which reassignment is requested the better the outcome. This is probably related to the association between late presentation and 'secondary' transsexualism.

In more recent reports, Lindemalm et al (1986) followed-up 13 male-to-female transsexuals for an average of 12 years postoperatively. Only one-third had a functioning vagina and four individuals regretted the surgery. These poor results may reflect the less successful surgical techniques involved when these cases were treated. (There is little doubt that surgical skill is relevant; surgeons with little experience of these procedures should expect less good results.) Walters et al (1986), in contrast, reported on 68 male-to-female transsexuals operated on in Melbourne between 1976 and 1982, of which 56 were available at follow-up. Although 35% reported inadequate vaginas postoperatively, 80% were satisfied with the outcome.

Whilst good response to surgical reassignment is far from unusual, these varied results emphasise the point that surgery is only part of the reassignment process.

Those considered unsuitable for surgery

Transsexuals are often impatient in their pursuit of surgical treatment and if they believe that such help is not going to be forthcoming, they may well move on to seek help elsewhere. Those who have established a good relationship with a therapist, however, may well accept the decision not to pursue surgery and may strive for some other form of adaptation. Continuing support will still be required. Transsexuals need a great deal of help and the clinician is advised not to get involved with their management unless he is prepared to offer such long-term help and concern.

Standards of care

The Harry Benjamin International Gender Dysphoria Association recently published standards of care for hormonal and surgical reassignment (Walker et al 1985). Their main points include the following:

1. Clinical decisions about both hormonal and surgical reassignment should be made by clinical behavioural scientists with appropriate experience of the diagnosis and treatment of psychological and sexual problems, as well as experience of working with patients with gender dysphoria.
2. The wish for sex reassignment should have existed for at least 2 years.
3. The clinician should have known the patient for at least 3 months before recommending hormonal and 6 months before recommending surgical reassignment.
4. This recommendation should be supported by a second appropriately qualified clinical behavioural scientist.
5. The patient should have lived full-time in the preferred role for *at least* 1 year before surgery is recommended.

Appendix

Counselling notes for couples in sex therapy

Judy Greenwood and John Bancroft

HOW THE NOTES ARE USED

Once it has been decided to go ahead with couple therapy further time is spent by the therapist talking to each partner individually to get more background information. Whilst one partner is being interviewed, the other partner is given the notes and requested to read up to and including stage I. Then they change round and when the couple come back together to discuss with the therapist how to start the programme, they will both have read through these notes.

We first ask them for their reactions to the notes. This often provides important information, e.g. that the programme seems artificial or clinical, or that some point in the notes is particularly relevant to them. This can then be discussed. Finally the therapist goes over the details of stage I, making sure that the couple understand what is involved and agree to keep to the limits.

Subsequent stages are handed out, sheet by sheet, as the couple make progress through the programme.

When working as co-therapists we always interview the individual partners jointly, though the same sex therapist does most of the questioning. Some co-therapists prefer to split up at the individual stage. In that case the notes would obviously have to be used differently.

The couple are told: 'These notes are to help you understand more about why your sexual problems may have developed and why we advise you to tackle the problems in the way we do. By having these notes, you will be able to think over the main points at home and — most important — discuss them with your partner, as well as with your counsellor.'

WHY SEXUAL PROBLEMS ARISE

Sex is a natural function like digestion — and like digestion, can be upset by a whole variety of problems, usually not involving physical factors.

We all accept that faulty eating, feeling rushed, stressed, anxious or in a bad mood can lead to complaints like loss of appetite, indigestion, diarrhoea or constipation even though the body is basically healthy. We also know that if we eat normally and in a relaxed way, our digestive system works naturally and we enjoy our food.

In a similar way (though fewer people understand this), if sex is allowed to happen naturally and in a relaxed way our bodies will respond normally without any conscious effort on our part.

Common examples of problems or situations that can upset this normal sexual responsiveness are as follows:

1. *Misunderstanding or lack of information about sex*
   — not knowing what to expect or how to act
2. *Bad feelings about sex or its consequences*
   — fear of pregnancy or pain
   — fear of being caught, overheard or interrupted
   — fear of failing to perform normally or well
   — fear of losing control (becoming animal-like, undignified, incontinent or unattractive)
   — fear of your partner losing control
   — guilt (believing that sex is wrong)
   — disgust (feeling that sex is dirty or messy)
3. *Problems in the relationship*
   — feeling angry, bitter or resentful towards your partner
   — feeling insecure or frightened of being hurt
4. *Bad feelings about yourself*
   — feeling depressed, worthless, not deserving pleasure
   — feeling unattractive, unhappy with your body
5. *Unsuitable circumstances*
   — feeling too tired, or hurried, or preoccupied with other things
   — lack of comfort, warmth or privacy
6. *Alcohol, some drugs or medicaments*
   — these can interfere with normal responsiveness, though only temporarily
7. *Being in generally poor condition*
   — appetite for sex, like appetite for food, often (though not always) goes when you have been ill or had an accident. It returns gradually as you regain health.

HOW DO THESE PROBLEMS AFFECT SEXUAL RESPONSE?

It is well known that sexual problems are caused by inhibition of the natural response, but less well understood that it is usually performance anxiety that keeps the problem going. The original resentment or difficulty may be long past, but the vicious circle of worrying about your responses continues. You start to watch your performance as a spectator rather than being fully involved in it — and the more you watch, the less you respond.

In addition, if one partner fails to respond, then the other partner gets caught up in performance anxiety too, and doubts his or her abilities as a sexual partner. There is no such thing as an uninvolved partner, so don't make one of you the patient and the other the therapist — you are both involved in the problem.

BASIC PRINCIPLES

1. Improve communication within the relationship to help resolve the resentments and misunderstandings that keep a sexual problem going.
2. Correct ignorance and misunderstanding about sex.
3. Learn ways to avoid the 'spectator' role and allow yourself to relax and enjoy your natural sexual responses. Setting limits as to how far you go physically for an agreed time allows you to concentrate on and re-acquaint yourself with your body sensations with no goal in mind.

IMPORTANT POINTS

This approach is primarily educational — you are not curing an illness but learning new and more satisfactory ways of getting on with each other. Like any other learning process, the responsibility for change lies with you. If you are to make proper use of this advice, you will need to make a special joint effort to follow all the suggestions.

You will need to set aside time to be together — time to talk to each other without frequent interruptions from children or whatever. Try to find a regular half-hour (or longer) in the day that is exclusively for you.

You will also need to aim for at least three sessions a week for physical contact — although, of course, the more spontaneous and natural these occasions are, the better. You will need privacy (a lock on the bedroom door is not anti-social) and comfort. If sound-proofing is a problem, put the radio on. Going to bed earlier is the easiest way to find time for the sessions. A drink around bedtime may help. Several drinks won't.

Don't expect miracles at first. You may even have to force yourself to practise to begin with. This is not surprising if you have been put off sex for a long time — you will need to unlearn all your old habits and attitudes, wipe the slate clean and allow your natural feelings to re-emerge — that is, if you want them to.

Even if you are keen to have a baby, it is much wiser to delay getting pregnant until after you have had a chance of improving your sexual relationship. Therefore, we advise you to use an effective method of contraception whilst following these suggestions.

We suggest that you and your partner read these notes and decide *independently* whether you want to work on improving your relationship now, and whether you are prepared to make the full commitment in terms of setting aside time, making an effort and accepting agreed limits on your physical relationship for a short time.

COMMUNICATION

GUIDELINES

As mentioned in the introduction, sexual problems often stem from other problems in the relationship and even when they don't, they may lead to problems which in turn spoil the relationship and serve to keep the sexual difficulties going. It is therefore necessary to look carefully at your general relationship, particularly in the ways it may affect your sexual relationship.

There are two aspects of relating that are important to sex, but which, if improved, have more far-reaching benefits. These are good communication and the use of positive rather than negative reinforcement (i.e. praise, encouragement or rewarding acts rather than criticism, complaints or destructive gestures).

It is never too late to learn new ways of communication, however long you have been together, and in our experience improved communication is essential if a sexual problem is to be resolved.

Here are some basic principles of communication:

1. Aim to communicate with each other as two adults. In many marriages the husband communicates like a father and the wife like a child . . . and in others the wife behaves like a mother to her husband who reacts like a son Such 'parent and child' relationships do not promote or encourage healthy adult sexual responsiveness. The following points help to keep the status equal.

2. Teach yourself to self-assert and self-protect by using the expression 'I would like' or 'I feel hurt because' instead of the more traditional 'Should we' or 'Why don't you'. The usual method of communication (often thought to be unselfish) is to think or guess what your partner would like rather than putting your wishes first. This pattern can be fraught with all sorts of problems — you may always have been guessing wrong and your partner has never liked to tell you for fear of hurting you (being unselfish again), so that long-standing assumptions about what the other likes or dislikes may be quite incorrect. A much safer and less complicated way to communicate is to express your own thoughts and feelings and ideas and let your partner do the same thing. This keeps your own house in order by asserting and protecting yourself and lets your partner do the same, so that you are both equally represented and equally protected and the guesswork has gone out of the relationship.

3. Encourage your partner to use the term 'I' and allow him or her to express feelings of hurt without you reacting too violently and discouraging self-expression. You are both entitled to your own feelings and should be allowed to express them freely. Having respect for your own and each other's feelings is crucial. Feelings are real, whether you think they are justified or not. If they are not dealt with, by expressing them in a suitable way, they may become bottled up and can cause havoc in a relationship.

4. You will need to negotiate fairly on those occasions where each of you wants something different. For example, if one wants black and the other wants white, you have both declared yourselves. Rather than having grey each day it is far better to have black one day and white the next.

5. Praise and encouragement (positive reinforcement) work better than criticism. Work hard at noticing and commenting on the good things your partner does. This will have a much more positive effect than nagging about the bad things.

SEXUAL RESPONSES

These responses can result from all sorts of factors — from fantasies, from seeing an attractive person, hearing nice music, masturbating, touching, kissing and caressing each other and from full intercourse.

These bodily responses usually go through three phases:

1. Arousal or excitement.
2. Climax or orgasm.
3. Resolution or returning to where we started.

1. AROUSAL PHASE

In the man, erection of the penis may be the first thing to happen. As arousal is increased, he feels more excited, breathes more heavily and may feel tense and sweaty. In the woman, slight swelling of the outer lips of the vagina and increased lubrication inside the vagina occur at an early stage, as with the man's erection. Similarly, arousal as it increases involves other bodily responses and excitement.

The innermost part of the vagina 'balloons' slightly as arousal increases, so that only the lower part is in close contact with the man's penis during intercourse (an important point for men who worry about their penis being too small).

It does no harm to stop during the arousal phase before a climax occurs. Unpleasant frustration usually results from expecting more than you get (in other words, it's a psychological rather than a physical problem).

2. CLIMAX PHASE

As arousal increases, the man reachs a point of no return after which he will ejaculate, whatever happens. The fluid ejaculated can vary in quantity but is usually about a teaspoonful. It is perfectly clean and contains good things like sugar to feed the sperm. As he ejaculates so he experiences a climax, a sudden build-up and release of tension followed by a feeling of well-being and calm.

The woman may or may not come to orgasm or climax. She does not ejaculate like the man but she experiences a similar build-up and release of sexual tension — rather like a sneeze, though much more enjoyable. It lasts approximately 5–15 seconds. There are usually contractions of the vagina wall and surrounding muscle which the woman may be aware of. Most women need caressing of the clitoris before they reach a climax.

3. RESOLUTION PHASE

This is the lull after the storm when the body settles down and both partners feel fulfilled and calm, often pleasantly sleepy and relaxed. In the woman the feeling of fullness or congestion in her pelvis and her general sense of excitement may take longer to settle, particularly if she has not experienced a climax.

SOME MISUNDERSTANDINGS ABOUT SEXUAL RESPONSE

1. The penis can become erect at a very early stage, especially in a young man. This does not mean that he is necessarily ready for intercourse and he may start this far too soon — before his partner feels ready. She may become anxious because she feels she is keeping him waiting.
2. Vaginal lubrication may remain hidden inside the vagina, especially when the woman is lying down. Both partners may assume she is not responding when in fact she is. Remember that the penis gives a more obvious signal of response than the vagina.
3. Arousal comes in waves. Both the man and the woman may find that their arousal comes and goes, with increasing and decreasing erections and vaginal responses. This is quite normal. A decline does not mean something is wrong, so don't get filled with performance anxiety.
4. Premature ejaculation. 'Coming' too soon (i.e. before either partner wants to) is normal for young men, particularly when very sexually aroused and when there has been a long interval since the last ejaculation. You have to learn to control it. The notes given later will help you to learn that control. Too rapid ejaculation can also make the woman worry that she will take too long to reach her climax.
5. Many women never have an orgasm yet are otherwise fully responsive sexually. This does not mean they are frigid. In most early sexual relationships orgasms for the woman are unusual — yet both partners may become extremely anxious about this. Some women pretend to have orgasms to please their husbands. The more a man demands an orgasm from his wife, the less likely he is to get one. She needs to feel relaxed, trusting and free

from pressure. Whereas performance anxiety makes the man come more quickly, it has the opposite effect on the woman. There is no need for her to experience an orgasm every time.

6. The husband snoring one minute after ejaculating can produce resentment if his wife is still feeling the need for intimacy. Wake him up sometimes and let him sleep at other times. That way you both get what you want some of the time.

GUIDELINES TO HELP IMPROVE YOUR LOVE-MAKING

These should be used in conjunction with the guidelines about communication, which are equally important for improving sexual relationships.

Your counsellor will discuss the instructions for each stage with you before asking you to try them. We suggest you take them home, read through them carefully with your partner and talk about them. Discuss any difficulties in understanding them and any anxieties you may feel about following them so that you can discuss these with your counsellor at the next visit. Remember what we have said about communication. Only when you both feel comfortable with stage I will you be asked to go on to stage II and so on. Don't assume that you can miss out any stage. It is most important to work carefully through each. If, at any stage, you feel unrelaxed or tense then discuss your feelings, try again and if necessary go back to an earlier stage.

To start with we will be suggesting definite limits beyond which you should not go in a love-making session. At first this may seem a bit clinical, as though you were making love to doctor's orders, but this is a temporary phase. Before long you should be able to set yourselves limits when making love — to be able to say 'stop' without fearing that your partner will feel upset, angry or rejected. Only when you feel safe enough to stop will you really enjoy going on.

STAGE ONE

Sensate focus without genital contact — touching your partner for your own pleasure

This stage of the programme emphasises the importance of keeping safe within limits. *A formal agreement must be made between you to ban all attempts at intercourse or genital contact until you feel comfortable with these early stages of the programme.* This puts implicit trust in each partner to abide by the agreement and any attempt to sabotage the trust should be taken very seriously. This ban is essential if performance anxiety is to be reduced. It removes any particular goal, reduces the pressure in you to succeed, allows you to experience new feelings and lets physical contact become an end in itself.

You should aim for three sessions a week, each session being in two parts. Partner A (the male or the female) initiates the sessions when he or she wants to by saying to Partner B: 'I would like to touch or caress you' (or words to that effect). Partner B can accept the offer or decline as he or she wishes. If B accepts the invitation then the assumption is made that B will later in the same session want to caress A. On the next occasion it should be Partner B who initiates.

Important points to remember

1. If you are doing the caressing, assert yourself. Touch your partner where you want to touch (anywhere on the body except the genital area and breasts) in a way that is nice for you and for as long as you wish. Experiment and touch parts of the body that you have not touched before. Touching may include kissing.

2. If you are being caressed, relax. Protect yourself if you don't like what is being done to you (the easiest way to do this is to move your partner's hand elsewhere). You will need to recognise if and when you are 'spectatoring', which means watching your body being touched rather than participating fully by feeling the sensations that you are experiencing. Don't worry if this happens at first; you must learn to realise when you are doing it and learn ways to get out of it. There are two things to do: firstly, concentrate on relaxing your whole body and concentrate in addition on the sensations produced by your partner and secondly, stop caressing for a short time until you feel sufficiently relaxed and ready to start again.

3. It is nice to touch and feel close to your partner.

4. It is nice to be touched.

5. Aim for three sessions a week, taking it in turns to initiate the sessions with the initiator caressing first.

6. You may have to push yourself into starting a session, feeling little motivation or drive to begin. This is a common experience, partly because of the artificiality of the situation, partly because people feel a little embarrassed and awkward at first, perhaps because of long-standing resistance to body contact from previous experiences that have gone wrong. It is important to see this stage as a stepping stone towards a spontaneous sexual relationship.

7. Some people find this stage pleasantly relaxing, others find it arousing. It doesn't matter which, but it is important for you to recognise what you are feeling.

8. If after the session you find yourself very aroused and unable to settle, it is quite permissible to relieve your tension by masturbating — but you should do it to yourself at this stage, it should not be done to you by your partner. If you are quite clear about these limits you may well find that this relief of tension is not necessary.

STAGE TWO

Sensate focus without genital contact — touching for your own and your partner's pleasure

This stage is similar to stage one. Each session has two parts with one person starting to caress first in a way that is pleasing for him or her; in the second part his or her partner then caresses. But in addition you indicate to each other what you would like the other to do. If you are being caressed you must aim to (a) relax, (b) protect yourself — if you don't like what's being done, move your partner's hand elsewhere and (c) praise and encourage the things that you like — either in words or with grunts or by putting your partner's hand back for more (don't take over complete control though, that's your partner's responsibility). If something could be even nicer, put your hand on your partner's to demonstrate how you would like it (harder, softer, slower, more to the left etc.), then leave it to your partner. In this way the person caressing still maintains complete control but the person being caressed is beginning to give some feedback as to what is especially nice for him or her. But remember, it is up to the person caressing to choose what he or she does. Remember to discuss with each other how you felt after each session — self-assert and self-protect. Remember, it's nice to see your partner enjoy being touched by you.

STAGE THREE

Sensate focus with genital contact

Exactly the same basic principles apply for this stage of the programme.

1. A ban on intercourse persists but now genital contact with the hands and/or mouth is permitted.
2. Each session is in two parts as before: A caressing B — then B caressing A.
3. As before, alternate partners initiate the session, the initiator touching in the way he or she wants to touch, with the partner protecting himself or herself from anything that is disliked and guiding the hand to show what is particularly pleasurable. When genital contact occurs, subtle changes in pressure, speed or direction can have profound effects on the sensation received, so it is even more important to be able to communicate what is best for you and remember, it will not be the same for each session. Your body sensitivity can vary from day to day.
4. Do not concentrate solely on the genital regions; spend as much time as before on general body caressing and kissing as well.
5. The use of body lotions or KY jelly can enhance the pleasure both to the caressor and the caressed, especially when touching genital areas.
6. The only goal is to be able to relax and enjoy what is happening. Check for 'spectatoring' and learn ways of getting back to being fully relaxed and involved.
7. The partner being caressed may or may not become aroused and may or may not ejaculate or reach a climax. The response will vary from session to session and that is normal. Do not aim for a climax or orgasm but if it does occur it does not matter and need not mean the end of a session.
8. If premature ejaculation is a problem, you will be given additional suggestions on how to deal with this.

STAGE FOUR

Sensate focus with genital contact and simultaneous caressing

As caressing and genital contact become easier for both of you, you should now move on to simultaneous caressing so that both of you are giving and receiving physical pleasure at the same time — remembering all the principles you have learnt.

In particular remember:

1. Sex is a natural response if you let it happen.
2. Be on guard for 'spectatoring'.
3. Communicate to your partner when he or she is doing something particularly nice for you.
4. Protect yourself against things you don't like.

STAGE FIVE

Vaginal containment

Once sensate focus with genital contact is going well and the male partner is getting reasonably firm erections (and, if applicable, has begun to establish some control over ejaculations) you are ready to enter this stage of the programme.

As before, this stage is designed to allow the freedom to experience sensations of physical contact with each other without performance anxiety, i.e. failure to achieve a particular goal.

After a period of mutual caressing involving the genital area, when you (the woman) feel that you are ready, and when you feel your partner has a reasonably firm erection, you invite the penis into your vagina.

The easiest position is the female superior. In this position the man lies flat on his back. The woman kneels above him with her knees either side of his body more or less at the level of his nipples. In this position she is well placed, by lowering her bottom, to guide and insert his penis into her vagina. This means that the woman keeps full control over what is happening. The aim of this stage is to re-acquaint yourselves with the body sensation of a penis in a vagina. The woman should tighten and relax her vaginal muscles on the penis, which she may or may not be able to feel once it is inside the vagina. The penis itself is receiving little direct stimulation from this static position and the man may well find his erection gets less.

If you wish, you can then resume genital caressing and perhaps repeat the process over again. Remember that you are both to concentrate on the sensations you are feeling from your genital region and relax and not to start any thrusting movements.

Initially you should only allow vaginal containment for a brief period (say 15 seconds). The period of containment can be gradually lengthened on each occasion.

STAGE SIX

Vaginal containment with movement

It is important to re-emphasise at this stage that you use the same principles concerning your physical contact with each other as you used right at the start. You should be touching and being touched in a way that is pleasant for both of you and with no particular performance in mind other than that of giving and receiving pleasure.

As before, start with mutual caressing involving both non-genital and genital areas in a way that feels good for both of you and although the man may have an erection fairly quickly, it is important that both of you should feel aroused and receptive before vaginal entry takes place.

After a period of vaginal containment, you may try some limited thrusting movements to see how this affects your sensations. Only do this briefly to start with, but if you are both enjoying the feelings this produces, allow the movement to continue.

By this stage, it is essential that either of you can say 'stop' at any time. In this way you avoid the feeling that once vaginal intercourse has started you have to go on regardless. You are setting the limits for yourselves now. Practise this by saying 'stop'. Remember that even if you are enjoying love-making your partner may want to stop and needs to be able to without fearing that you will get angry. This is what a secure, safe sexual relationship is about — and when you feel really safe you'll usually want to carry on.

The movements of intercourse feel different in the different positions you can try and it is important to experiment to find ways that suit you both. You may find one position nicer for one of you and another position better for the other.

Your responsiveness will vary from session to session and month to month. This is normal for both sexes. Many women find that they respond better at a particular time of the month. Many women enjoy clitoral stimulation in addition to the thrusting of the penis and most find that they reach a climax most comfortably and pleasurably in this manner.

This is normal and not a sign that they are not fully aroused. Many women can also have a highly satisfactory and highly aroused sexual experience without a climax. It is an important rule to remember that provided physical contact is enjoyable, an orgasm is not necessary. It is also a myth that a joint climax is the ideal. Most people find it very pleasurable to enjoy the experience of their partner's climax, separate from their own, whilst on occasions they may enjoy coming together. These are all variations on the theme of making love and what you enjoy will depend on your feelings and state of mind at the time. The only goal is to enjoy yourselves — together.

PREMATURE EJACULATION

This problem can be first tackled during stage three (the sensate focus with genital contact stage of the programme). As mentioned earlier, every man has a point of no return after which he cannot avoid ejaculation. During your partner's caressing of your penis, you may feel yourself getting aroused to such a degree that you can predict that you will ejaculate shortly.

You must aim to stop your partner's caresses at a stage just short of the point of no return and allow your arousal level to subside slightly (say for half-a-minute) and then return to being caressed and repeat the process of stopping when you feel yourself near the point of inevitable ejaculation again. The difficulty at first is knowing when to ask your partner to stop.

This is a learning process which every male has to undertake at some stage in his life and it is never too late to learn control of ejaculation. It will, however, take time and practice and will require the full understanding and co-operation of your partner. Once your anxiety level begins to fall and your confidence builds up, you should find an increasing ability to control your ejaculation and once a slight improvement occurs your confidence will increase and anxiety will fall even more.

If you have difficulty in gaining control using this method (remember it will take time because you are changing what is probably a long-established pattern) then you can try the squeeze technique, which means that just before the point of no return you stop stimulation of the penis and either you or your partner grasps the tip of the penis between fingers and thumb at the point of attachment of the foreskin and squeezes firmly for 10 seconds or so. This reduces the reflex ejaculation response (and possibly the erection too) in the same way that biting your lip stops a sneeze. You can then resume stimulation and repeat the process if necessary.

Both the 'stop–start' and squeeze technique are effective in delaying ejaculation during manual stimulation of the penis or during sexual intercourse at a later stage in the programme.

REFERENCES

Annon J S 1974 The behavioral treatment of sexual problems, vol I. Brief therapy. Enabling Systems, Honolulu

Ansari J M A 1976 Impotence: prognosis (a controlled study) British Journal of Psychiatry 128: 194–198

Arentewicz G, Schmidt G 1983 The treatment of sexual disorders. Basic Books, New York

Balint M 1957 The doctor, his patient and the illness. Pitman Medical, London

Bancroft J 1971 The application of psychophysiological measures to the assessment and modification of sexual behaviour. Behaviour Research and Therapy 9: 119–30

Bancroft J 1974 Deviant sexual behaviour: modification and assessment. Clarendon Press, Oxford

Bancroft J 1981 Ethical aspects of sexuality and sex therapy. In: Bloch S, Chodoff P (eds) Psychiatric ethics. Oxford University Press, Oxford, pp 160–184

Bancroft J 1985 Letter to editor. British Journal of Sexual Medicine 12: 30–31

Bancroft J 1986 Sex therapy; education or healing. In: Dryden W (ed) Therapist's dilemmas. Harper & Row, London, pp 17–26

Bancroft J, Coles L 1976 Three years' experience in a sexual problem clinic. British Medical Journal 1: 1575–1577

Bancroft J, Dickerson M, Fairburn C G et al 1986 Sex therapy outcome research: a reappraisal of methodology. 1. A treatment study of male sexual dysfunction. Psychological Medicine 16: 851–863

Bandura A 1977 Social learning theory. Prentice-Hall, Englewood Cliffs, New Jersey

Barbach L G 1974 Group treatment of pre-orgasmic women. Journal of Sex and Marital Therapy 1: 139–145

Beck A 1976 Cognitive therapy and the emotional disorders. International Universities Press, New York

Birk L, Miller E 1970 Group psychotherapy for homosexual men by male–female co-therapists. Acta Psychiatrica Scandinavica 218 (suppl): 7

Blakeney P, Kinder B, Creson O, Powell L C, Sutton C 1976 A short-term intensive workshop approach for the treatment of human sexual inadequacy. Journal of Sex and Marital Therapy 2: 124–129

Brady J P 1966 Brevital–relaxation treatment of frigidity. Behaviour Research and Therapy 4: 71–77

Bramley H M, Brown J, Draper K C, Kilvington J 1983 Non-consummation of marriage treated by members of the Institute of Psychosexual Medicine: a prospective study. British Journal of Obstetrics and Gynaecology 90: 908–913

Brindley G S 1986 Maintenance treatment of erectile impotence by cavernosal unstriated muscle relaxant injection. British Journal of Psychiatry 149: 210–215

Carney A, Bancroft J, Mathews A 1978 Combination of hormones and psychological treatment for female sexual unresponsiveness: a comparative study. British Journal of Psychiatry 132: 339–346

Cole M 1985 Surrogate sex therapy. In: Dryden W (ed) Marital therapy in Britain, vol 2. Harper & Row, London pp 93–122

Collins G F, Kinder B N 1984 Adjustment following surgical implantation of a penile prosthesis: a critical overview. Journal of Sexual Marital Therapy 10: 255–271

Cooper A J 1969 Disorders of sexual potency in the male: a clinical and statistical study of some factors related to short term prognosis. British Journal of Psychiatry 115: 709–719

Cooper A J 1974 A blind evaluation for a penile ring — a sex aid for impotent males. British Journal of Psychiatry 124: 402–406

Cooper A J 1987 Preliminary experience with a vacuum constriction device (VCD) as a treatment for impotence. Journal of Psychosomatic Research 31: 413–418

Cotten-Huston A L, Wheeler K A 1983 Preorgasmic group therapy: assertiveness, marital adjustment and sexual function in women. Journal of Sexual and Marital Therapy 9: 296–302

Courtenay M 1968 Sexual discord in marriage. A field for brief psychotherapy. Tavistock, London

Crowe M J, Gillan P, Golombok S 1981 Form and content in the conjoint treatment of sexual dysfunction: a controlled study. Behaviour Research and Therapy 19: 47–54

Csillag E R 1976 Modification of penile erectile responses. Journal of Behavior Therapy and Experimental Psychiatry 7: 27–29

Csillag E R, Lord D J, Dunn J 1981 An in patient therapy programme for sexual dysfunction. Paper at 5th World Congress of Sexology, June 1981, Jerusalem

D'Ardenne P 1986 Sexual dysfunction in a transcultural setting: assessment, treatment and research. Sexual and Marital Therapy 1: 23–34

Davidson D W, O'Carroll R, Bancroft J 1987 Increasing circulating androgens with oral testosterone undecamoate in engonadal men. Journal of Steroid Biochemistry 26: 713–715

DeAmicis L A, Goldberg D C, LoPiccolo J, Friedman J, Davies L 1984 Three years follow up of couples evaluated for sexual dysfunction. Journal of Sexual and Marital Therapy 10: 215–228

DeAmicis L A, Goldberg D C, LoPiccolo J, Friedman J, Davies L 1985 Clinical follow up of couples after treatment for sexual dysfunction Archives of Sexual Behavior 14: 467–489

Dekker J, Everaerd W 1983 A long term follow up study of couples treated for sexual dysfunction. Journal of Sexual and Marital Therapy 9: 99–113

Dengrove E 1971 The mechano-therapy of sexual disorders. Journal of Sex Research 7: 1–12

Dicks H V 1967 Marital tensions. Routledge & Kegan Paul, London

Dow M G T 1983 A controlled comparative evaluation of conjoint counselling and self-help behavioural treatment for sexual dysfunction. Unpublished PhD thesis, University of Glasgow

Draper K 1983 Practice of psychosexual medicine. Libby, London

Dryden W 1985 Marital therapy — the rational–emotive approach. In: Dryden W (ed) Marital therapy in Britain, vol 1. Harper & Row, London, pp 195–221

Dryden W, Hunt P 1985 The therapeutic alliance. In: Dryden W (ed) Marital therapy in Britain, vol 1. Harper & Row, London, pp 121–166

Duddle C M 1975 The treatment of marital psychosexual problems. British Journal of Psychiatry 127: 169–170

Duddle C M, Ingram A 1980 Treating sexual dysfunction in couple groups. In: Forleo R, Pasini W (eds) Medical sexology. Elsevier/North Holland, Amsterdam, pp 598–605

Eaton H 1973 Clomipramine (Anafranil) in the treatment of premature ejaculation. Journal of International Medical Research 1: 432–434

Ebbehøj J, Wagner G 1979 Insufficient penile erection due to abnormal drainage of cavernous bodies. Urology 13: 507–510

Egan G 1975 The skilled helper : model skills and methods for effective helping. Brooks/Cole, Monterey, California

Ellis H 1915 Studies in the psychology of sex, vol 2. Sexual inversion. Davis, Philadephia

Ellis A 1962 Reason and emotion in psychotherapy. Lyle Stuart, Secaneus, New Jersey

Ellison C 1968 Psychosomatic factors in the unconsummated marriage. Journal of Psychosomatic Research 12: 61–66

Ersner-Hershfield R, Kopel S 1979 Group treatment of pre-orgasmic women: evaluation of partner involvement and spacing of sessions. Journal of Consulting and Clinical Psychology 47: 750–759

Everaerd W 1977 Comparative studies of short-term treatment methods for sexual inadequacies. In: Gemme R, Wheeler C C (eds) Progress in sexology. Plenum, New York, pp 153–165

Everaerd W, Dekker J 1982 Treatment of secondary orgasmic dysfunction. A comparison of systematic desensitisation and sex therapy. Behaviour Research and Therapy 20: 269–274

Eysenck H J 1964 The nature behaviour therapy. In: Eysenck H J (ed) Experiments in behaviour therapy. Pergamon, London, pp 1–15

Fleming M, Steinman C, Bocknek G 1980 Methodological problems in assessing sex-reassignment surgery: a reply to Meyer & Reters. Archives of Sexual Behavior 9: 451–456

Friedman D 1966 The treatment of impotence by brevital relaxation therapy. Behaviour Research and Therapy 6: 257–261

Geboes K, Steeno O, DeMoor P 1975 Primary anejaculation: diagnosis and therapy. Fertility and Sterility 26: 1018–20

Gillan P W 1977 Stimulation therapy for sexual dysfunction. In: Gemme R, Wheeler C C (eds) Progress in sexology. Plenum, New York, pp 167–172

Gillan P, Brindley G S 1979 Vaginal and pelvic floor responses to sexual stimulation. Psychophysiology 16: 471–482

Gillan P, Golombok S, Becker P 1980 NHS sex therapy groups for women. British Journal of Sexual Medicine 7(64): 44–47

Glover J 1983 Factors affecting the outcome of treatment of sexual problems. British Journal of Sexual Medicine 10: 28–31

Golden J S, Price S, Heinrich A G, Lobitz W C 1978 Group vs couple treatment of sexual dysfunction. Archives of Sexual Behavior 7: 593–602

Gordon P 1986 Sex therapy with gay men: a review. Sexual and Marital Therapy 1: 221–226

Graham D 1986 Legal aspects: should the law be changed? In: Walters W A W, Ross M W (eds) Transsexualism and sex reassignment. Oxford University Press, Oxford, pp 135–143

Greenwood J, Bancroft J 1988 Basic counselling and crisis intervention. In: Kendell R E, Zealley A (eds) Companion to psychiatric studies, 2nd edn. Churchill Livingston, Edinburgh

Hahlweg K, Jacobson N S 1984 Marital interaction: analysis and modification. Guilford, New York

Hamilton J B 1937 Induction of penile erection by male hormone substances. Endocrinology 21: 744

Hartman L M 1983 Effects of sex and marital therapy on sexual interaction amd marital happiness. Journal of Sexual and Marital Therapy 9: 137–152

Hastings D W 1967 Can specific training procedures overcome sexual inadequacy? In: Brecher R, Brecher E (eds) An analysis of human sexual response. Deutsch, London, pp 221–235

Hawton K 1982 The behavioural treatment of sexual dysfunction. British Journal of Psychiatry 140: 94–101

Hawton K 1985 Sex therapy: a practical guide. Oxford University Press, Oxford

Hawton K, Catalan J 1986 Prognostic factors in sex therapy. Behaviour Research and Therapy 24: 377–385

Hawton K, Catalan J, Martin P, Fagg J 1986 Long term outcome of sex therapy. Behaviour Research and Therapy 24: 665–675

Heiman J R, LoPiccolo J 1983 Clinical outcome of sex therapy. Archives of General Psychiatry 40: 443–449

Heiman J, LoPiccolo L, Lo Piccolo J 1976 Becoming orgasmic: a sexual growth program for women. Prentice-Hall, Englewood Cliffs, New Jersey

Heiman J R, LoPiccolo J, Hohan D, Roberts C 1985 Effectiveness of single therapist v co therapy teams in sex therapy. Journal of Consulting and Clinical Psychology 53: 287–294

Heisler J 1983 Sexual therapy in the National Marriage Guidance Council. NMGC, Rugby

Heller C G, Myers G B 1944 The male climacteric: its symptomatology, diagnosis and treatment. Journal of the American Medical Association 126: 472–7

Hoopes J E 1968 Operative treatment of the female transsexual. In: Green R, Money J (eds) Transsexualism and sex reassignment. Johns Hopkins, Baltimore, pp 335–352

Hunter R, MacAlpine I 1963 Three hundred years of psychiatry 1535–1860. Oxford University Press, London, pp 492–94

Jacobs M, Thompson L A, Truxan P 1975 The use of sexual surrogates in counselling. Counselling Psychologist 5: 73–77

Jacobson N S, Margolin G 1979 Marital therapy: strategies based on social learning and behavior exchange principles. Brunner/Mazel, New York

Johnson J 1968 Disorders of sexual potency in the male. Pergamon, Oxford

Jones H W 1968 Operative treatment of the male transsexual. In: Green R, Money J (eds) Transsexualism and sex reassignment. Johns Hopkins, Baltimore 313–322

Kaplan H S 1974 The new sex therapy. Brunner/Mazel, New York

Kaplan H S 1979 Disorders of sexual desire and other new concepts and techniques in sex therapy. Brunner/Mazel, New York

Kaplan H S, Kohl R N, Pomeroy W B, Offit A K, Hogan B 1974 Group treatment of premature ejaculation. Archives of Sexual Behavior 3: 443–452

Kelly H H, Thibaut J W 1978 Interpersonal relations. Wiley, New York

Keogh E J, Carati C J, Earle C M, Wiswiewski Z S, Lord D J, Tulloch A G S 1986 Comparison of intracavernosal papaverine v phenoxybenzamine in the treatment of impotence. Paper presented at 2nd World Meeting on Impotence, Prague June 1986

Kilmann P R, Mills K H, Cald C et al 1986 Treatment of secondary orgasmic dysfunction: an outcome study. Archives of Sexual Behavior 15: 211–230

Kockott G, Dittmar F, Nusselt L 1975 Systematic desensitisation of erectile impotence: a controlled study. Archives of Sexual Behavior 4: 493–499

Kolodny R C, Masters W H, Johnson V E 1979 Textbook of sexual medicine. Little, Brown, Boston

Krane R J 1986 Penile prosthesis in urology. Abstract for conference on the Scientific Basis of Sexual Dysfunction. NIDDICD & NIH, Baltimore

Lansky M R, Davenport A E 1975 Difficulties in brief conjoint treatment of sexual dysfunction. American Journal of Psychiatry 182: 171–175

Lazarus A A 1963 The treatment of chronic frigidity by systematic desensitisation. Journal of Nervous and Mental Disease 136: 272–278

Laughren T P, Kass D J 1975 Desensitisation of sexual dysfunction: the present status. In: Gurman A S, Rice D G (eds) Couples in conflict. Aronson, New York, pp 281–302

Leiblum S R, Ersner-Hershfield R 1977 Sexual enhancement groups of dysfunctional women: an evaluation. Journal of Sex and Marital Therapy 3: 139–152

Leiblum S R, Rosen R C 1979 The weekend workshop for dysfunctional couples: assets and limitations. Journal of Sex and Marital Therapy 5(1): 57–69

Leiblum S R, Rosen R C, Pierce D 1976 Group treatment format: mixed sexual dysfunctions. Archives of Sexual Behavior 5: 313–322

Liberman R P, Wheeler E G, deVisser L A J M, Kuehnel J, Kuehnel T 1980 Handbook of marital therapy; a positive approach to helping troubled relationships. Plenum, New York

Libman E, Fichten C S, Brender W, Burstein R, Cohen J, Binik Y M 1984 A comparison of three therapeutic formats in the treatment of secondary orgasmic dysfunction. Journal of Sexual and Marital Therapy 10: 147–159

Lindemalm G, Korlin D, Uddenberg N 1986 Long-term follow up of 'sex change' in 13 male to female transsexuals. Archives of Sexual Behavior 15: 187–210

Lobitz W C, Baker E L 1979 Group treatment of single males with erectile dysfunction. Archives of Sexual Behavior 8: 127–138

Loeffler R A 1960 Perforated acrylic implant in management of organic impotence. Journal of Urology 97: 716

Loewenstein J 1947 Treatment of impotence. Hamish Hamilton, London

LoPiccolo J 1977 Direct treatment of sexual dysfunction in the couple. In: Money J, Musaph H (eds) Handbook of sexology. Excerpta Medica, Amsterdam, pp 1227–1244

LoPiccolo J, Lobitz W C 1972 The role of masturbation in the treatment of orgasmic dysfunction. Archives of Sexual Behavior 2: 163–171

Lundberg P O, Muhr C, Hulter B, Brattberg A, Wide L 1986 Sexual libido in patients with hypothalamo-pituitary disorders. In: Kothari P (ed) Proceedings of the 7th World Congress of Sexology. Indian Association of Sex Educators, Counsellors and Therapists, Bombay, pp 126–128

Lundstrom B, Pauly I, Walinder J 1984 Outcome of sex reassignment surgery. Acta Psychiatrica Scandinavica 70: 289–294

McEwan L, Ceber S, Daws J 1986 Male to female surgical genital reassignment. In: W A W Walters, M W Ross (eds) Transsexualism and sex reassignment. Oxford University Press, Oxford, pp 103–112

Mackay D 1985 Marital therapy: the behavioural approach. In: Dryden W (ed) Marital therapy in Britain, vol 1 Harper & Row, London

McMullen S, Rosen R C 1979 Self-administered masturbation training in the treatment of primary orgasmic dysfunction. Journal of Consulting and Clinical Psychology 47: 912–918

McWhirter D P, Mattison A M 1980 Treatment of sexual dysfunction in homosexual male couples. In: Leiblum S R, Pervin L A (eds) Principles and practice of sex therapy. Guilford, New York

McWhirter D P, Mattison A M 1982 Psychotherapy of gay couples. In: Gonsiovex J C (ed) Homosexuality and psychotherapy. Haworth, New York

Marquis J N 1970 Orgasmic reconditioning: changing sexual object choice through controlling masturbation fantasies. Journal of Behavior Therapy and Experimental Psychiatry 1: 263

Masters W H, Johnson V E 1970 Human sexual inadequacy. Churchill, London

Masters W H, Johnson V E 1976 Principles of the new sex therapy. American Journal of Psychiatry 133: 548–554

Masters W H, Johnson V E 1979 Homosexuality in perspective. Little, Brown, Boston

Masters W H, Johnson V E, Kolodny R 1977 Ethical issues in sex therapy and research. Little, Brown, Boston

Masters W H, Johnson V E, Kolodny R C, Meyners J R 1983 Outcome studies at the Masters & Johnson Institute. Paper presented at 6th World Congress of Sexology, Washington, May 1983

Mathews A, Bancroft J, Whitehead A et al 1976 The behavioural treatment of sexual inadequacy: a comparative study. Behaviour Research and Therapy 14: 1861–1881

Mathews A, Whitehead A, Kellet J 1983 Psychological and hormonal factors in the treatment of female sexual dysfunction. Psychological Medicine 13: 83–92

Meichenbaum D 1977 Cognitive–behavior modification. Plenum, New York

Meyer J, Reter D 1979 Sex reassignment. Archives of General Psychiatry 36: 1010–1015

Meyer W J, Finkelstein J W, Stewart C A et al Physical and hormonal evaluation of transsexuals during hormonal therapy. Archives of Sexual Behavior 10: 347–356

Michal V 1978 Vascular surgery for treatment of impotence. British Journal of Sexual Medicine 5: 13–18

Mills K H, Kilman P R 1982 Group treatment of sexual dysfunction: a methodological review of the outcome literature. Journal of Sexual and Marital Therapy 8: 259–296

Milne H B 1976 The role of the psychiatrist. In: Milne H B, Hardy S J (eds) Psychosexual problems. Bradford University Press, Bradford

Morales A, Surridge D H C, Marshall P G, Fenemore I 1982 Non-hormonal pharmacological treatment of organic impotence. Journal of Urology 128: 45–47

Morgan A J 1978 Psychotherapy for transsexual candidates screened out of surgery. Archives of Sexual Behavior 7: 273–284

Munjack D, Cristol A, Goldstein A et al 1976 Behavior therapy of orgasmic function: a controlled study. British Journal of Psychiatry 129: 497–502

Munjack D J, Schlaks A, Sanchez V C, Usigli R, Zulueta A, Leonard M 1984 Rational–emotive therapy in the treatment of erectile failure. An initial study. Journal of Sexual and Marital Therapy 10: 170–175

Murphy C V, Mikulas W L 1974 Behavioural features and deficiencies of the Masters & Johnson programme. Psychological Record 24: 221–227

Nairne K D, Hemsley D R 1983 The use of directed masturbation training in the treatment of primary anorgasmia. British Journal of Clinical Psychology 22: 283–294

Noe J, Sato R, Coleman C, Laub D R 1978 Construction of male genitalia: the Stanford experience. Archives of Sexual Behavior 7: 297–304

Oates J M, Dacakis G 1986 Voice, speech and language considerations in the management of male to female transsexuals. In: Walters W A W, Ross M W (eds) Transsexualism and sex reassignment. Oxford University Press, Oxford

Obler M 1973 Systematic desensitisation in sexual disorders. Journal of Behavior Therapy and Experimental Psychiatry 4: 93–101

O'Carroll R, Bancroft J 1984 Testosterone therapy for low sexual interest and erectile dysfunction in men: a controlled study. British Journal of Psychiatry 145: 146–151

O'Gorman E 1978 The treatment of frigidity: a comparative study of group and individual desensitisation. British Journal of Psychiatry 132: 580–84

Patterson G R, Reid J B 1970 Reciprocity and coercion: two facets of social systems. In: Neuringer C, Michael J (eds) Behavior modification in clinical psychology. Appleton-Century-Crofts, New York

Pauly I B, Edgerton M T 1986 The gender identity movement: a growing surgical–psychiatric liaison. Archives of Sexual Behavior 15: 445–473

Pentland B, Anderson D A, Critchley J A J H 1981 Failure of ejaculation with indoramin. British Medical Journal 282: 1433–1434

Person E, Ovesey L 1974 The transsexual syndrome in males. 1. Primary transsexualism. American Journal of Psychotherapy 28: 174–193

Pincus L (ed) 1960 Marriage: studies in emotional conflict and growth. Institute of Marital Studies, London

Porto R 1980 Double-blind study of clomipramine in premature ejaculation. In: Forleo R, Pasini W (eds) Medical sexology. Elsevier/North Holland, Amsterdam, pp 624–628

Price S, Reynolds B S, Cohen B D, Anderson A J, Schochet B V 1981 Group treatment of erectile dysfunction for men without partners. Archives of Sexual Behavior 10: 253–268

Pryor J P 1979 The surgery of erectile impotence. British Journal of Sexual Medicine 6: 24–26

Reid K, Surridge D H C, Morales A et al 1987 Double-blind trial of yohimbine in the treatment of psychogenic impotence. Lancet ii: 421–423

Riley A J, Riley E J 1978 A controlled study to evaluate directed masturbation in the management of primary orgasmic failure in women. British Journal of Psychiatry 133: 404–409

Riley A J, Riley E J 1986 The effect of single dose diazepam on female sexual response induced by masturbation. Sexual and Marital Therapy 1: 49–54

Riseley D 1986 Gender identity disorders of childhood. Diagnostic and treatment issues. In: Walters W A W, Ross M W (eds) Transsexualism and sex reassignment. Oxford University Press, Oxford, pp 26–43

Roberto L G 1983 Issues in the diagnosis and treatment of transsexualism. Archives of Sexual Behavior 12: 445–473

Rogers C 1951 Client-centered therapy: its current practice, implications and theory. Houghton-Mifflin, Boston

Roles S 1972 A serious look at sexual aids. World Medicine October 4th: 17–22

Rosen I 1977 The psychoanalytic approach to individual therapy. In: Money J, Musaph H (eds) Handbook of sexology. Elsevier/North Holland, Amsterdam

Roughan P A, Kunst L 1981 Do pelvic floor exercises really improve orgasmic potential? Journal of Sexual and Marital Therapy 7: 223–229

Salmon U J, Geist S H 1943 The effects of androgens upon libido in women. Journal of Clinical Endocrinology 3: 235–238

Satterfield S 1983 Follow up of 25 transsexuals in the Minnesota program. In: Proceedings of the 8th International Gender Dysphoria Association, Bordeaux, France

Schellen M C M 1968 Further results with induction of ejaculation by electro vibration. Bulletin Society R. Belge. Gynecology & Obstetrics 38: 301–305

Schneidman B, McGuire 1976 Group therapy for non-orgasmic women: two age levels. Archives of Sexual Behavior 5: 239–248

Schover L R, van Eschenbach A C 1985 Sex therapy and the penile prosthesis; a synthesis. Journal of Sexual and Marital Therapy 11: 57–66

Schultz J H 1951 Autogenic training. Grune & Stratton, New York

Scott F B, Bradley W E, Timm G W 1973 Management of erectile impotence: use of implantable inflatable prosthesis. Urology 2: 80–82

Semans J 1956 Premature ejaculation: a new approach. Southern Medical Journal 49: 353–358

Skinner A C L 1976 One flesh, separate persons. Constable, London

Sloane R B, Staples F R, Cristol A H, Yorkston N, Whipple K 1975 Behaviour therapy v psychotherapy. Commonwealth Books, London

Snyder D K, Berg P 1983 Predicting couples' response to brief directive sex therapy. Journal of Sexual and Marital Therapy 9: 114–120

Sommers F G 1980 Treatment of the male sexual dysfunction in a psychiatric practice integrating the sexual therapy practitioner (surrogates). In: Forleo R, Pasini W (eds) Medical sexology. Elsevier/North Holland, Amsterdam, pp 593–598

Stackl W, Loupal G, Holzmann A 1986 Comparison of intracavernosal papaverine v phenoxybenzamine in the treatment of impotence. Paper presented at 2nd World Meeting on Impotence, Prague June 1986

Steege J F, Stout A L, Carson C C 1986 Patient satisfaction in Scott and Small-Carrion penile implant recipients. A study of 52 patients. Archives of Sexual Behavior 15: 393–400

Stone A, Levine L 1952 Group therapy in sexual maladjustment. American Journal of Psychiatry 197: 195–202

Stuart R B 1969 Operant interpersonal treatment for marital discord. Journal of Consulting and Clinical Psychology 33: 675–682

Stuart R B 1980 Helping couples change: a social learning approach to marital therapy. Guilford, New York

Taberner P V 1985 Aphrodisiacs. The science and the myth. Croom Helm, London

Tiefer L 1986 In pursuit of the perfect penis. The medicalisation of male sexuality. American Behavioral Scientist 29: 579–599

Treacher A 1985 Working with marital partners. Systems approach. In: Dryden W (ed) Marital therapy in Britain, vol 1 Harper & Row, London

Trudel G, Saint-Laurent S 1983 A comparison between the effects of Kegel's exercises and a combination of sexual awareness, relaxation and breathing on situational orgasmic dysfunction. Journal of Sexual and Marital Therapy 9: 204–209

Tullman G M, Gilner F H, Kolodny R C, Dornbush R L, Tullman G D 1981 The pre- and post-therapy management of communication skills of couples undergoing sex therapy at the Masters & Johnson Institute. Archives of Sexual Behavior 10: 95–110

Tunnadine P 1970 Contraception and sexual life. A therapeutic approach. Tavistock, London

Tunnadine P 1980 The role of genital examination in psychosexual medicine. Clinics in Obstetrics & Gynaecology 7: 283–291

Tunnadine P, Morrow C S, Hutchinson F D 1981 Sex problems in practice. Training and referral. Institute of Psychosexual Medicine, Margaret Pyke Centre, and Brook Advisory Centres. British Medical Journal 282: 1669–1672

Tuthill J F 1955 Impotence. Lancet i: 124

Tyndall N 1985 The work and impact of the National Marriage Guidance Council. In: Dryden W (ed) Marital therapy in Britain, vol 1. Harper & Row, London

Vansteenwegen A, Luyens M, Daelemans S 1983 Outcome of 10 years of residential and outpatient sex therapy. An exploratory and comparative study. Paper presented at 6th World Congress of Sexology, Washington, May 1983

Virag R 1982 Revascularisation of the penis. In: Bennett A (ed) Management of male impotence. Williams & Wilkins, Baltimore

Virag R, Frydman D, Legman M, Virag H 1984 Intracavernous injection of papaverine as a diagnostic and therapeutic method in erectile failure. Angiology 35: 79

von Schrenck-Notzing A 1895 The use of hypnosis in psychopathia sexualis with special reference to contrary sexual instinct. Translated by Chaddock C G, 1956. The Institute of Research in Hypnosis Publication Society and Julian Press, New York

Walker P A, Berger J C, Green R, Laub D R, Reynolds C L, Wollman L 1985 Standards of care: the hormonal and surgical sex reassignment of gender dysphoric persons. Archives of Sexual Behavior 14: 79–90

Walters W A W, Kennedy T, Ross M W 1986 Results of gender reassignment. Is it all worthwhile? In: Walters W A W, Ross M W (eds) Transsexualism and sex reassignment. Oxford University Press, Oxford, pp 144–151

Watson J P, Brockman B 1982 A follow up of couples attending a psychosexual problem clinic. British Journal of Clinical Psychology 21: 143–144

Warner P, Bancroft J 1986 Sex therapy outcome research: a reappraisal of methodology. 2. Methodological considerations — the importance of prognostic variability. Psychological Medicine 16: 855–863

Wesser D R 1978 A single-stage operative technique for perineoplasty in transsexuals. Archives of Sexual Behavior 7: 309–312

Whitaker C A 1975 A family therapist looks at marital therapy. In: Gurman A S, Rice D G (eds) Couples in conflict. Aronson, New York, pp 165–174

Whitehead A, Mathews A 1977 Attitude change during behavioural treatment for sexual inadequacy. British Journal of Social and Clinical Psychology 16: 275–81

Whitehead A, Mathews A 1986 Factors related to successful outcome in the treatment of sexually unresponsive women. Psychological Medicine 16: 373–378

Wolpe J 1969 The practice of behavior therapy. Pergamon, New York, pp 72–90

Wyatt G E, Strayer R G, Lobitz W C 1978 Issues in the treatment of sexually dysfunctional couples of Afro-American descent. In: LoPiccolo J, LoPiccolo L (eds) Handbook of sex therapy. Plenum, New York, pp 441–450

Yardley K M 1976 Training in feminine skills in a male transsexual: a pre-operative procedure. British Journal of Medical Psychology 49: 329–339

Yates A J 1970 Behavior therapy. Wiley, New York, p 18

Zilbergeld B 1975 Group treatment of sexual dysfunction in men without partners. Journal of Sex and Marital Therapy 1: 204–214

Zilbergeld B, Evans M 1980 The inadequacy of Masters & Johnson. Psychology Today, August, 29–43

Zorgniotti A W, LeFleur R S 1985 Autoinjection of the corpus cavernosum with a vasoactive drug combination for vasculogenic impotence. Journal of Urology 133: 39–41

11

Sexual aspects of medical practice

The wide variety of pathological and psychological mechanisms capable of interfering with sexual function were described in Chapter 8. Whilst it is probably true that for the majority of sexual problems the causes are not of medical relevance, there are few medical or surgical conditions which do not have sexual implications. In this chapter we aim to place these sexual aspects of clinical practice into perspective.

The physician or surgeon will be confronted with the sexual lives of his patients in a number of ways. A sexual problem may be the presenting symptom of an illness; impotence as the first evidence of diabetes mellitus is one example. The medical problem may be linked to sexual activity, a sexually transmitted infection being the most obvious example. In most acute illnesses sexual interest or enjoyment is likely to be impaired, if not abolished, but usually this is of little consequence in those circumstances. In the recovery phase, however, there may be concern or anxiety about when to resume sexual activity, whether it is safe to do so, and whether normal sexual function will be regained.

The possible effects of a clinical condition on a patient's sexuality can be summarised under the following headings:

1. The *direct physical* effects of the condition:
   a. specific interference with genital or other sexual responses, as with vascular impairment or neurological damage.
   b. non-specific effects, such as pain, general malaise, fatigue and lack of sexual desire, immobility with arthritis or spasticity making postural changes normally expected during sexual activity difficult or impossible.
2. The *psychological* effects of the condition:
   a. on the *individual*, such as embarrassment, feeling sexually unattractive, or generally experiencing a loss of self-esteem as a result of the condition.
   b. on the *relationship*. A man who is sexually disabled after an accident or stroke may become dependent on his wife in a number of ways, resulting in a relationship which is more like child–parent than the adult–adult relationship which existed before the accident. This may

make it difficult for either or both partners to continue with an active sexual relationship. The existence of a life-threatening illness, such as cancer, can also disrupt the sexual relationship because the healthy partner feels guilty about seeking sexual pleasure in such circumstances.

  c. concern about effects of sexual activity on the condition. The existence of ischaemic heart disease or severe hypertension may result in fear in either partner that sexual activity, particularly the excitement associated with orgasm, will be harmful.

3. The effects of *treatment* on sexuality:
  a. drug effects.
  b. effects of surgery, causing damage to genital structures or their neurological or vascular control.
  c. psychological effects of treatment, particularly surgery resulting in disfigurement.

Of particular importance are those conditions which result in chronic physical handicap. The extent to which sexual function is impaired by the handicap will vary, but sexual repercussions, depending often as much on psychological as physical factors, occur in a large proportion of the handicapped population. Stewart (1975) investigated a sample of 215 physically disabled individuals drawn from a survey of the general population, and representing a wide variety of physical problems and degrees of disability. Of this sample, 23% were unmarried compared with 16% of the same age group in the normal population; 54% of the disabled subjects were currently experiencing difficulties in their sexual lives. A further 18% had done so since the onset of their disability and had either overcome the problem or come to terms with it. In about 45% the sexual problem was attributed to physical factors; in 15% to predominantly psychological factors and in 30% to a combination of the two. Physical problems ranged from impairment of genital responses to mechanical difficulties in adopting suitable postures for love-making. Psychological reactions included unfounded fears about the consequences of sexual activity, loss of self-esteem and changes in the marriage, resulting from the handicap, that interfered with a good sexual relationship.

Obviously the needs of these patients include basic commonsense advice about overcoming practical problems, reassurance and encouragement to experiment. Such simple counselling should be based on a proper understanding of the sexual consequences of the condition in question as well as awareness of the psychological idiosyncrasies of the individual. One should not assume that a handicapped person wants or needs sex. On the other hand, the professional should create no barriers to discussing sexual matters. Fundamental to much of this simple counselling is 'giving permission' to approach love-making in ways which may be regarded as unconventional. Also important is the communication between the handicapped individual and the partner. Those without partners should not be ignored however. They also have their sexual needs and anxieties. They may need 'permission' to masturbate and in some instances practical help to do so, such as the woman who was unable to reach her genitalia because of severe arthritis but was able to use a vibrator with a special extension. One of the commonest barriers between the professional and the handicapped patient is the difficulty that non-handicapped people have in acknowledging that disabled people have sexual feelings. Obviously such attitudes have to be resolved before the professional can hope to help the patient in this area of his or her life.

In some cases, more substantial sexual counselling, as described in Chapter 10, will be required. Such counselling may be beyond the means available to the clinician. Nevertheless, any well organised clinical service for the handicapped should have access to such expertise for those who need it.

Those working in sexual dysfunction clinics must also be prepared to see many patients with physical disease which may or may not be relevant to their sexual problem. This is particularly likely to be the case with men presenting with erectile dysfunction. In the Edinburgh 3-year clinic survey (Warner et al 1988) 52% of those presenting with erectile problems had such a condition. The types of clinical problems encountered are shown in Table 11.1.

For the remainder of this chapter we will focus on a number of specific conditions. There are many more that could be considered but those selected cover most of the basic issues. (A more extensive review will be found in Kolodny et al 1979.)

Table 11.1 Evidence of organic disease in two series of men presenting with erectile dysfunction to (i) a regional service (Warner et al 1987) and (ii) a sexual problem clinic in a general hospital (Western General, Edinburgh).

	Regional Service 1981–84 n=262	General Hospital 1984–87 n=207
Type of organic problem	% with organic problem	
Arterial Disease	32	26
Neurological Disease	21	12
Urological Disease	29	43
Skeletal Problem	4	14
Diabetes Mellitus	19	13
Other endocrine disease	6	3
Infertility	4	7
Miscellaneous conditions	14	28
Any organic problem	52	73

GENERAL MEDICINE

DIABETES MELLITUS

Diabetes mellitus, whilst primarily an endocrine disorder resulting from an inadequate production of insulin, produces a wide variety of metabolic and degenerative effects, many of which are not understood. It has a particular tendency to damage peripheral and autonomic nerves and to cause degenerative changes in small blood vessels. As we shall see, there are various ways in which such changes may interfere with sexual function.

Sexual problems in male diabetics

The tendency for diabetic men to suffer from erectile dysfunction has been recognised for nearly 200 years. Surveys of diabetic men have consistently shown a high prevalence of erectile problems. Fairburn et al (1982) in their review listed seven studies. The prevalence of impotence ranged from 35% to 59%. In a Scottish study (McCulloch et al 1980), 563 males attending a diabetic outpatient clinic were interviewed. They were shown to be representative of the clinic population. In this group the prevalence of erectile problems of at least 6 months' duration was 35%. There was a clear relationship with age, showing a considerable amplification of the age-related pattern reported in non-diabetic men by Kinsey et al (1948) (see Fig. 11.1). There was an increasing prevalence of erectile failure with increasing duration of the diabetes. Whilst diabetics treated with diet alone were less susceptible, there was no obvious difference between those

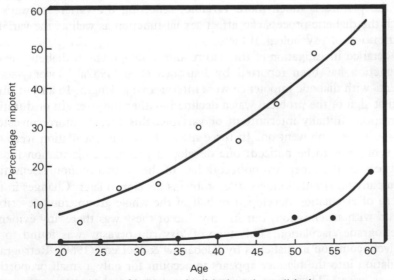

Fig. 11.1 The age incidence of impotence in diabetic and non-diabetic men.
○ = Diabetic men (McCulloch et al 1980); ● = non-diabetic men. (Kinsey et at 1948)

needing insulin and those using oral hypoglycaemic agents. There was an association between erectile failure and the presence of retinopathy, peripheral neuropathy and autonomic neuropathy. Erectile dysfunction was seen in all patients aged 50 years or more with proliferative retinopathy and in all those aged 35 or more with autonomic neuropathy. It was not, however, unusual to find erectile problems in men without any evidence of these diabetic complications. These authors concluded that diabetic erectile dysfunction has a multifactorial aetiology. They went on to follow up 466 of these patients over a 5-year period (McCulloch et al 1984). Of the 275 who were orginally free from erectile problems, 28% became dysfunctional during the follow-up period. Factors which predicted this deterioration included age, alcohol intake, initial glycaemic control, intermittent claudication and retinopathy, the appearance of neuropathic symptoms, and poor glycaemic control during the 5 years.

Of the 128 who were initially dysfunctional, only 9% remitted and they were young, with diabetes of short duration, and often with features suggesting psychogenesis. Also of interest was the finding that, of those without other diabetic complications to begin with, those with erectile problems were more likely to develop retinopathy or neuropathy than those with no erectile problems. This suggests that in some cases erectile failure is an early sign of other vascular or neurological damage. Jensen (1986) in a 6-year follow-up study of a smaller group of diabetic men, found some whose sexual dysfunction improved without treatment, in spite of evidence of peripheral or autonomic neuropathy.

There has been a tendency to attribute to diabetic impotence a rather predictable and consistent clinical picture. It is now increasingly recognised that the picture is much more variable, reflecting the variety of ways in which the diabetic process can affect sexual function as well as the variable contribution of psychological factors.

A detailed investigation of the nature and development of diabetic sexual dysfunction has been reported by Fairburn et al (1982a). Twenty-seven patients with diabetic impotence were interviewed at length. In all but three the first sign of the problem was a decline in either the strength or duration of erection. Initially intermittent or variable, this became more consistent and severe as time went on. In three men, changes in ejaculation were the first symptoms to be noticed; one developed premature ejaculation for no good reason, the other two noticed a loss of the normal pumping sensation accompanying ejaculation; erectile problems developed later. Changes in the pattern of ejaculation developed in half of the whole group; four described orgasm without emission, but in only one of these was there any evidence of retrograde ejaculation. This type of 'dry run orgasm' was found to be relatively common in diabetics by Klebanow & McLeod (1960). Retrograde ejaculation into the bladder appears to account for only a small proportion of these cases. There was no association between the pattern of sexual dysfunction and the presence of either retinopathy or autonomic neuropathy.

There was, however, a tendency for those men with obvious psychological problems to show a more classical psychogenic picture, i.e. loss of sexual interest but continuing morning erections. Certain distinct patterns of psychosomatic interaction emerged. In most, the initial erectile problem was followed by anxiety or distress. In some this anxiety gave way to a lessening of sexual interest and avoidance of sexual activity. In others, the couple worked through the anxious phase, came to accept that a physical factor was involved, and resumed sexual activity within the limits imposed by the erectile impairment. Some accepted the erectile failure with little apparent concern, as though it provided an escape from a sexual relationship that had not been particularly rewarding.

In most cases, declining sexual interest was understandable as a psychological reaction to the erectile problem. The form of such a reaction appears to reflect the importance of sexual function for that man's self-esteem or to his wife's sense of emotional security. In some men a limited amount of erectile impairment could produce sufficient performance anxiety to ensure total erectile failure. This could account for the continuation of morning erections in several men. It is therefore important when advising a diabetic with erectile problems to take these other confounding factors into account — a clear example of the need for a psychosomatic approach.

Some interesting evidence has come from psychophysiological studies of diabetic men with erectile failure. Kockott et al (1980) showed erotic films to diabetic and non-diabetic men with erectile failure, and normal controls. The occurrence of a normal blood pressure response in the diabetics was interpreted as evidence that a normal central process was operating and that the failure was peripheral. More recently, we measured erection, penile pulse amplitude and blood pressure response to erotic stimuli in three comparable groups (Bancroft et al 1985; see p. 436). The diabetic men were divided into those with and those without evidence of psychological causation. The psychogenic group showed significantly lower blood

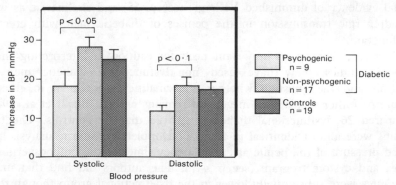

Fig. 11.2 Blood pressure response to visual erotic stimuli in two groups of diabetic dysfunctional men (with and without evidence of psychogenic causation) and a group of normal non-diabetic controls.(from Bancroft et al 1985)

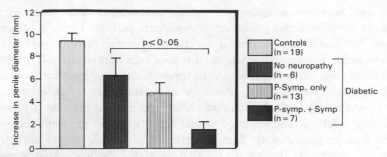

Fig. 11.3 Erectile response to visual erotic stimuli in diabetic dysfunctional men with and without autonomic neuropathy, and in normal non-diabetic controls. (from Bancroft et al 1985)

pressure but a significantly greater erectile response to the erotic stimuli than the non-psychogenic group, once again pointing to an impairment of central arousal in the psychogenic cases (see Fig. 11.2). It was also found that diabetics with evidence of both sympathetic and parasympathetic nerve damage (based on cardiovascular reflex tests; see p. 450) showed significantly greater impairment both of erection and penile pulse amplitude response when compared with the diabetics without any autonomic damage (see Fig. 11.3). The presence of severe (i.e. exudative or proliferative) retinopathy was associated with a significant reduction in penile pulse amplitude response but *not* erectile response. Thus in this study there was evidence of the importance of psychogenic factors, autonomic damage, and to a lesser extent vascular impairment in the development of diabetic erectile dysfunction.

There is more direct evidence of both autonomic and peripheral nerve damage in diabetic men with erectile failure (Ellenberg 1971; Faerman et al 1974). Melman and his colleagues (Melman & Henry 1979; Melman et al 1980) have reported diminished noradrenaline content of erectile tissue of at least some diabetic men with erectile dysfunction. Lincoln et al (1987) found evidence of diminished VIPergic (see p. 55) and cholinergic as well as adrenergic transmission in the penises of diabetic men with erectile dysfunction.

However, there is an important need for caution in interpreting these various studies. Few have used non-dysfunctional diabetic men as controls and the question whether abnormalities are related to erectile failure or rather to diabetes in general remains crucial. Buvat et al (1985) compared 26 dysfunctional diabetics with 26 diabetic controls. The two groups were almost identical in terms of Doppler wave form analysis and blood pressure of the penile arteries, latency time for the bulbocavernosus reflex and cystometrogram (see p. 447). The authors did find that urine flow rates were substantially lower in the dysfunctional group though they concluded that this may be a consequence of the sexual difficulty and the anxiety associated with it. They also found more consistent evidence of abnormalities on the MMPI which led them to conclude that neither neuropathic nor arteriopathic factors are a sufficient explanation, whereas psychogenic factors were at least contributory in about 50% of cases.

Schiavi et al (1985) measured sleep erections in diabetic men with and without erectile dysfunction and found that *both* groups were impaired in terms of maximum erection obtained, whereas the non-dysfunctional group were no different from the controls in the number and duration of episodes of nocturnal tumescence.

A comparable story can be told about possible endocrine factors. Some endocrine abnormalities have been identified, including abnormal response to LHRH stimulation and increased testosterone binding. But these abnormalities are found equally in diabetics with and without erectile problems (Fairburn et al 1982b).

In our present state of knowledge it is therefore sensible to conclude that erectile dysfunction in diabetic men is multifactorial in origin. Psychogenic factors are undoubtedly important, and in some cases may be the only cause. In others they may interact with physical factors along the lines described in Chapter 8. In some cases the physical damage is sufficient on its own. The relative importance of autonomic nerve, peripheral nerve and vascular damage remains a controversial issue, though neuropathic factors are likely to be most important in younger diabetics. There may be subtle changes in autonomic control of erection which precede overt erectile dysfunction (as shown in sleep tests). In turn, erectile failure may precede other clinical manifestations of autonomic neuropathy, such as postural hypotension, intermittent diarrhoea, diminished sweating in the legs, gustatory sweating, unawareness of hypoglycaemia and bladder dysfunction.

Peripheral neuropathy is manifested as numbness, paraesthesiae, burning pain or weakness and there is clinical evidence of diminished tendon reflexes, vibration and tactile sensation together with muscle-wasting in the lower limbs. Its functional significance in erectile failure is not clear except in causing diminished response to tactile stimulation. Ejaculatory disturbance is likely to result from neural dysfunction, which may be of a subtle kind. An association between ejaculatory and bladder dysfunction is to be expected because of their common neural control.

Peripheral arterial disease, as we shall see later, is commonly associated with erectile dysfunction in non-diabetic men. The vulnerability of the diabetic to both large and small vessel atherosclerosis makes it likely that vascular impairment at least contributes to erectile problems in some cases, and when severe enough may be a sufficient explanation, particularly in older diabetics.

Diabetes in women

Until recently, less attention has been paid to the sexual problems of diabetic women. Kolodny (1971) found a higher incidence of orgasmic dysfunction in diabetic women than in a control group (35 and 6% respectively). There is no obvious reason why orgasm per se should be affected by diabetes in either men or women. The dysfunction in women, equivalent to erectile failure in diabetic men, would be impaired vaginal lubrication and vulval tumescence. There was no evidence of such impairment in Kolodny's study. Other reports have indicated a high incidence of sexual problems in diabetic women but no comparison groups have been involved and the quality of diabetic control has been uncertain (Montenero et al 1973; Zrustová et al 1978).

Four further controlled studies have been reported in recent years (Jensen 1981; Tyrer et al 1982; Whitley & Berke 1984; Schreiner-Engel et al 1985). No association between diabetes and orgasmic dysfunction was found in any of the four studies, though in each there was some evidence of impaired vaginal lubrication, though usually insufficient to cause problems.

Ellenberg (1977) had earlier found no difference in sexual response between women with and without autonomic neuropathy, and this was the case also in the Danish (Jensen 1981) and Scottish (Tyrer et al 1983) studies. Whitley & Berke (1984), on the other hand, did find that women with autonomic neuropathy were more likely to report problems with vaginal dryness.

Schreiner-Engel and her colleagues (1985), whilst reporting little evidence of impaired sexual response, did find that their diabetic women showed lower levels of sexual desire and of a global measure of sexual functioning (as shown by the Derogatis sexual function inventory or DFSI) and less satisfaction with their relationships. These authors wondered whether the existence of a chronic disease like diabetes would have adverse effects on the dynamics of a long-term relationship. Somewhat in contrast, diabetic women in the Scottish study were more likely to report a beneficial effect of their diabetes on their marriage (21%) than a detrimental effect (9%). Jensen (1985), on the other hand, found that both men and women with diabetes were more likely to have sexual problems if they had made a poor psychological adjustment to their illness.

One difference between the study of Schreiner-Engel et al and the Danish and Scottish studies was that in the former both type I and type II diabetics were involved, whereas in the other two studies only type I cases were included. Schreiner-Engel et al (1986) went on to investigate the relevance of the type of diabetes in a further study of diabetic women. Type I (or insulin-dependent) and type II (or non-insulin-dependent) diabetes are also distinguished by their age of onset. In this study the type I group had an average age of onset of 17.6 years; for type II it was 35.9 years. Other potentially important differences were that the type II women were heavier and more likely to be post-menopausal than their age-matched controls. Using a similar method of assessment as in their previous study, they found that the type I women were virtually indistinguishable from their age-matched controls, whereas the type II women differed in a number of ways. These women rated themselves as less sexually attractive, less happy and satisfied with their sexual partners and sex life in general, less interested in and more likely to avoid sexual activity, less likely to lubricate and more likely to experience dyspareunia, and less likely to experience orgasm with their partners.

The orgasmic dysfunction was correlated with menopausal status, whereas none of the parameters correlated with weight. Although requiring replication, these interesting findings suggest that the stage of the life cycle and in particular of the relationship at the time the diabetes develops may be more important in relation to sexual function than the diabetic process itself — at least in women. The type I women would usually have been diagnosed before marriage and this would be reflected in their choice of partner, who would be likely to be caring and supportive. For the type II women there would be no such selection process to prepare the couple for a chronic illness.

Diabetic women are prone to vaginal infections when their diabetes is not well controlled. Reproduction is also surrounded with hazards. Not only is fertility impaired, there is also a tendency to spontaneous abortion, premature births and intrauterine death. Large babies are more common in diabetic (and pre-diabetic) women, increasing the likelihood of complications at delivery, as well as perinatal morbidity. Contraception also has its problems, as steroidal contraceptives may disturb the diabetic control.

It is therefore gratifying how well sexually adjusted most diabetic women are, and the weight of evidence points more to the psychological impact of the diabetes on the relationship than on the disease process itself as the cause of sexual problems when they occur. Although physical factors are more important in the male diabetic, it seems probable that these interpersonal factors are important for them also.

Management of sexual dysfunction in diabetic men

One should not, therefore, jump, to the conclusion that erectile failure in a diabetic is totally or even partially due to organic factors. The possible contribution of psychological and hence potentially reversible factors should be carefully considered in each case. The presence or absence of libido and/or morning erections is not sufficient evidence. Objective methods of investigation, such as recording nocturnal erections or other psychophysiological techniques, are discussed in Chapter 9. As yet they are of uncertain validity. In many cases, a course of counselling may be justified because even if no substantial improvement in the erectile function results, the couple may still be helped to adjust to the physical disability and to enjoy their sexual relationship within the physical limits. Such counselling is not basically different from that used for other types of sexual dysfunction, as described in Chapter 10.

In some couples, for whom the availability of an erect penis is of particular sexual importance, surgical techniques may be considered. They are also described in Chapter 10. In my view, they should not be used until a serious attempt at psychological treatment has been tried. This will in any case put the therapist in a much stronger position to judge the likely benefits of surgical treatment and to help the couple reach a well informed decision on the matter.

CARDIOVASCULAR DISEASE

Most disease of the cardiovascular system results from a variable combination of atheromatous degeneration and narrowing of the arteries, and raised blood pressure. Sometimes the arterial disease is confined to the heart, producing ischaemic heart disease with angina of effort and a predisposition to myocardial infarction. In other cases, the main effects are in more peripheral vessels causing ischaemic pain during exercise (intermittent claudication) and other peripheral manifestations. The importance of hypertension varies, but there is a marked tendency for raised blood pressure of any duration to be associated with arterial disease. The patient may present with symptoms of high blood pressure, of chronic arterial insufficiency or acutely, following a myocardial infarction. Association with sexual dysfunction is complex and once again, we need to consider both physical and psychological factors.

We will first consider the occurrence of sexual problems in men with known cardiovascular disease and then look at the evidence of cardiovascular pathology in men who present with sexual dysfunction.

Myocardial infarction

Most of the relevant evidence of the prevalence of sexual dysfunction is in relation to myocardial infarction. Several studies have shown that there is a persisting decline in sexual activity following a heart attack, with erectile impotence occurring in a substantial proportion (10–45%) of cases (Tuttle et al 1964; Bloch et al 1975). These problems are more likely, as one would expect, in the older patient. However, there is also evidence that sexual dysfunction is unusually prevalent in both men and women preceding a myocardial infarction. Wabrek & Burchell (1980) interviewed 131 men after acute infarction; two-thirds reported a significant sexual problem before the heart attack and of these, 64% had been impotent, 28% had experienced a substantial decrease of sexual interest and activity and 8% had experienced premature ejaculation. Abramov (1976) interviewed 100 women aged 40 to 60 shortly after admission to hospital with myocardial infarction, and compared them with 100 women of the same age who were hospitalised for other reasons. Of the women with infarcts, 65% reported sexual dissatisfaction prior to their heart attack, though in 60% of these, the problem was secondary to sexual dysfunction in the husband. In the control group, 24% reported sexual dissatisfaction, with again about two-thirds of these attributing the problem to their husbands. The importance of control groups is illustrated in a study by Dhabuwala et al (1986). They compared 50 men following myocardial infarction with 50 controls matched for age, hypertension, diabetes and smoking. They found little difference between the two groups in the incidence of sexual dysfunction. It is likely that the relevance of myocardial infarction is mainly based on fear of coital death, which can be largely dealt with by counselling.

Studies of men and women following coronary by-pass surgery have suggested that in women it is sexual desire that is most likely to be affected, whereas in men it is sexual arousal (in particular erection) (Althof et al 1984).

Hypertension

The effects of hypertension on sexual function are uncertain. In one study, treated hypertensives (i.e. receiving hypotensive drugs) were compared with untreated hypertensives and age-matched normotensive controls. The prevalence of erectile impotence in the three groups was 24.8%, 17.1% and 6.9% respectively; of ejaculatory failure, 25.6%, 7.8% and 0% (Bulpitt et al 1976).

We can consider the causes of these sexual problems under three headings:

1. direct effect of the disease process on sexual function;
2. the sexual consequences of treatment;
3. the psychological reactions to the disease.

In addition we must bear in mind the possibility that sexual problems may themselves contribute to the disease process.

The most obvious direct effect of cardiovascular disease is on the arterial supply to the erectile tissues and consequent erectile impairment (see Chapter 2). At the moment there is no reason to believe that hypertension per se will impair erectile function but the untreated hypertensive may well have some degree of peripheral arterial disease. Similarly, the person who suffers an acute myocardial infarct could have had peripheral arterial disease prior to the infarct.

As already mentioned, drugs used to lower blood pressure often appear to interfere with sexual function and these are considered more fully below. Digoxin, used to counteract heart failure and certain types of cardiac irregularity, may also interfere with sexual function (see below).

Psychological reactions to chronic or acute cardiovascular disease are obviously of crucial importance. The man who has had hypertension diagnosed may fear that sexual activity will raise his blood pressure to a dangerous level. The person with ischaemic heart disease who experiences angina during sexual activity may regard this as much more ominous than the angina he experiences with moderate exercise. The person who has experienced a life-threatening myocardial infarct may fear that his or her heart could not withstand the extra demands of sexual activity and excitement. In any of these cases, the anxiety of the spouse may be as important, if not more so. The prospect of one's partner dying during the process of making love is especially horrifying.

Sexual dysfunction is also stress-producing, especially in those for whom sexual potency has always been very important. Sexual problems may reflect more general marital discord, which in itself is a potent cause of stress. In either case, the resulting stress may contribute to the cardiovascular disease or to the acute episode.

In this, as in many other areas of medical care, the advice given to the patient with cardiovascular disease about his future sex life may be of crucial importance to his health, and even his survival. Before summarising the principles to follow in giving such advice, let us first consider the available evidence of the effects of sexual activity on cardiac function.

The most valuable data come from a study by Hellerstein & Friedman (1970). They monitored the cardiovascular function during a variety of activities in a number of men following myocardial infarction. In 14 of their subjects, sexual activity occurred during the monitoring period (carried out in their own homes). The increase in heart rate and blood pressure which was maximal around orgasm was somewhat less than that occurring during modest physical activity of a non-sexual kind. It is nevertheless important to remember that the degree of excitement and hence cardiovascular arousal may vary according to the circumstances of the sexual act. Ueno (1963) studied the circumstances of sudden death in Japan and found that death during sexual activity, whilst fairly rare (0.6% of sudden deaths) was much more likely to occur during extramarital sexual encounters. One should obviously be cautious in interpreting this data; the married woman whose husband dies during love-making may well conceal this fact. For the partner involved in an extramarital liaison, perhaps in a hotel room, concealment is much more difficult. But if there is any validity in this finding, it points to the extra exciting effects of novel or risky sexual situations. Some of the evidence of relatively high blood pressure and heart rate increases during sexual activity (e.g. Masters & Johnson 1966; see Chapter 2) could reflect the highly arousing (or anxiety-provoking) aspects of the laboratory testing situation. Hellerstein & Friedman's relatively modest changes occurred in a more familiar setting and are consistent with a further study cited by Wagner (1977). Ten young men were monitored during masturbation on three separate occasions. The cardiovascular changes were not only short-lived around the time of orgasm, but also were significantly reduced by the third session when they were becoming familiar with the circumstances. Comparable results were reported by Nemec et al (1976) from 10 normal men aged 26 to 40, monitored with portable electrocardiogram and blood pressure recorders in the home environment during sexual activity with their wives. The average resting heart rate rose from 60 to a maximum of 114 ($\pm$ 14) beats/min at orgasm. Within 120 s of orgasm the rate had fallen to 69 beats/min. Position during intercourse made no difference. Larson et al (1980) showed that sexual activity was comparable to exercise involving climbing 22 steps in normal men, and slightly less demanding than climbing steps in men following myocardial infarction.

Whilst familiarity in these circumstances is beneficial for the heart patient or hypertensive, it is also sensible to avoid more athletic sexual performances. Rhodes (1977) found that the female superior position during intercourse offered no apparent advantage over the male superior position in terms of cardiovascular changes. There is also likely to be reduced risk as the post-infarct patient becomes physically fitter. Stein (1977) found that men who underwent an exercise training programme after their myocardial infarct showed a decline in their peak heart rate during intercourse, compared with men who did not undergo such training.

Evidence of cardiovascular disease in men with sexual dysfunction

In recent years there has been increasing evidence of arterial disease in many men with erectile dysfunction, especially those in the older age groups. The association of erectile problems with aortoiliac stenosis has been recognised for many years, first described by Leriche (1940). The prevalence of erectile dysfunction in men with aortoiliac disease has varied from 40 to 80% (Michal 1982). However, it is usual in such cases to find that the erectile problem is just one among many and often not the most important. It is now increasingly recognised that erectile failure may be an early manifestation of arterial disease, and that the vessels supplying the penis may be especially vulnerable to atheromatous degeneration. It is worth bearing in mind that the penile arteries undergo frequent straightening and convoluting through the life cycle as erections come and go. Apart from the coronary arteries, there are probably no other medium size arteries which are submitted to so much mechanical distortion — a factor which could contribute to their vulnerability.

Michal (1982) has reviewed the various ways in which arterial disease can cause erectile dysfunction. He finds that in men assumed to have secondary psychogenic erectile failure, of those over 35 years of age, 88% had evidence of arterial stenosis or occlusion on angiography. One must be cautious in interpreting this figure. Since this series of cases had been referred to a vascular surgeon, they are not representative of erectile dysfunction in general. They presumably include many cases which failed to respond to pyschological methods of treatment. Nevertheless, Michal's findings are remarkable.

Virag et al (1985) investigated arterial risk factors in 222 men with erectile failure who were divided into two aetiological groups: organic and non-organic on the basis of such tests as the noctural penile tumescence (see p. 432). They then assessed the presence of four arterial risk factors; smoking, diabetes, hyperlipidaemia, and hypertension. Those without any of the four factors were equally likely to be in the organic or non-organic groups. Those with two or more risk factors were virtually all in the organic group. Again, one must be cautious with this evidence. In particular it should not be concluded that the presence of arterial disease is a sufficient explanation for the erectile failure, but it is likely to contribute in a substantial proportion of such cases. The onset of erectile dysfunction in those aged over 35 should generally be regarded as a possible warning sign of arterial disease.

Counselling the patient with cardiovascular disease

Some understanding of the significance of sexual activity to the particular patient and the partner is desirable. For this, there is a need to establish the level of sexual activity prior to the current medical problem and how the patient felt about it. Whereas one man may experience both frustration and loss of self-esteem at seeing his sexual activity curtailed, for another the 'excuse' of heart disease may provide a welcome relief from a sexual relationship that was unrewarding or even stressful.

Thereafter the resumption of sexual activity should be seen as comparable to other forms of physical activity. Gradual rehabilitation is advisable and if a patient is apprehensive about his or her performance on resuming sexual activity, it may help for him or her to masturbate alone in the first instance. In general, if moderate exercise such as climbing two flights of stairs or a short brisk walk can be managed without undue difficulty, sexual activity of a calm, non-athletic kind should be equally manageable.

The occurence of angina during sexual activity should be judged in the same way as angina occurring during exercise. Coronary dilators can be used before intercourse, although activity should not continue in the presence of persisting ischaemic symptoms. A short rest or even a slowing down may suffice in some instances. Sexual activity after substantial intake of food or alcohol should be avoided.

Although it is advisable to enquire about background factors with the patient alone, it is also important to discuss the same issues with the spouse and to go over the main points of sexual rehabilitation with the couple together.

In treating hypertension, the possibility of sexual side-effects of drugs should be discussed in a way not to alarm the patient or generate performance anxiety, but to point out that adjustment of the dosage or change of drug can be used if necessary to reduce such effects. If the patient is not told of these possible sexual side-effects, he may not only fail to mention them when they arise, but may cease to take the drug regularly because of them.

The investigation and possible treatment of arterial disease involving the erectile tissues is discussed in Chapter 9.

CHRONIC RENAL FAILURE

Men and women with chronic renal failure have a high prevalence of sexual problems. In some studies, 90% of men and 80% of women with uraemia have reported reduced sexual interest. A similar proportion complained of erectile difficulties or, in the case of women, difficulty in getting aroused or achieving orgasm (Kolodny et al 1979).

Whereas sexual interest may increase with the establishment of haemodialysis, sexual function usually does not and may even get worse. Levy (1973) found this deterioration with haemodialysis in 35% of men and 25% of women, whereas only 9% and 6% respectively improved. Procci (1984) on the other hand found his dialysis patients to be slightly more active sexually than pre-dialysis chronic renal failure patients. Successful renal transplantation more often leads to improvement, particularly in women, most of whom return to pre-illness levels of sexual functioning (Abram et al 1975). Improvement in men is less predictable (Levy 1973). Glass et al (1987) compared 13 men on dialysis with 13 after renal transplants. The dialysis subjects had a higher frequency of sexual problems. They also had less happy marriages and were less likely to show affection to their wives than the transplant patients. Once again it is difficult to know which is cause and which is effect. But we must take seriously the possibility that the interpersonal strain imposed by dialysis may be as important in disrupting the sexual relationship as any direct biochemical effect.

Fertility is usually impaired; uraemic women are often amenorrhoeic. On dialysis, they may show hypermenorrhoea but are seldom able to carry a pregnancy to term. Fertility in women improves substantially after renal transplantation. In men, spermatogenesis is impaired and testicular atrophy is common. Haemodialysis does not improve their fertility.

The prevalence of sexual problems is sufficiently high in this group of patients to indicate some specific effects of the renal disease on sexual function. The nature of such effects is not yet clear and is likely to be multifactorial. Renal failure is an end state of a variety of diseases, many of which may take their toll of sexual function. Furthermore, the degree of incapacity and uncertain life expectancy must have their effects on the marital relationship. Home dialysis, with the unique demands that it places on the spouse, must create special problems in the relationship. Psychological factors are therefore likely to be substantial. Nevertheless, the tendency during dialysis for sexual interest to improve whilst sexual function worsens suggests that there is some physiological effect involved. Evidence for its nature is so far lacking.

Lowered sexual interest is not only likely as a reaction to the psychological factors, but also to the general metabolic disturbance and malaise that accompany uraemia. This non-specific metabolic factor should be largely eliminated by dialysis, but the endocrine status of the dialysed patient is still likely to be abnormal. Results of endocrine studies have been variable and inconsistent, indicating no inevitable hormonal consequences, but impairment of steroidogenesis as well as spermatogenesis appears to be common (Holdsworth et al 1977). Thus gonadotrophins are often raised, follicle-stimulating hormone more so than luteinising hormone, and testosterone levels may be low (Lim & Fang 1976). Prolactin may also be raised (Hagen et al 1976). This rather variable endocrine picture is reflected in the sexual response to different forms of treatment. Thus improvement has been reported with clomiphene (Lim & Fang 1976) and bromocriptine (Bommer et al 1979; Vircburger et al 1985). According to Kolodny et al (1979) testosterone treatment itself does not improve erectile or ejaculatory problems though it may increase libido. This is consistent with the role of androgens discussed in Chapter 2. Most of the reports do not make a sufficiently clear distinction between libido and genital response to be certain on this point. If erectile failure is secondary to loss of libido, then it may be expected to improve as the libido increases. However, as already mentioned, erectile failure may persist or even worsen as libido improves, suggesting some specific effect on genital responses. Antoniou (1977) reported a controlled study of dialysed men in which erectile problems were improved by the administration of zinc through the dialysis machine. In this study the men were found to be deficient in zinc. This metal is known to feature in many enzyme systems. In certain parts of the world dietary zinc deficiency has been found to cause impairment of sexual development but its precise relevance to sexual function remains obscure and it is not known how common zinc deficiency is amongst dialysis patients.

It is to be hoped that with further research these various uncertainties will be resolved. This will not only be important for the clinical management of these unfortunate patients, but may throw some useful light on metabolic or endocrine determinants of sexual function.

OBESITY AND ANOREXIA

The relationship between abnormal body weight and sexuality presents us with one of the most puzzling riddles of psychosomatic medicine. We have to consider overeating and obesity on the one hand and anorexia and weight loss on the other. In between these two contrasting states is the use of vomiting or purging as a method of losing weight, or if associated with episodes of overeating, avoiding weight gain. In most respects, we do not understand the origins of the more extreme forms of eating disorders. Obesity and anorexia are occasionally caused by endocrine or neurological disease. Genetic factors are sometimes important, particularly for obesity, and early childhood patterns of eating may influence later body weight by determining the number of fat cells that develop in the body. In the majority of cases, however, there is no obvious physical explanation and psychological factors are often assumed to be paramount.

Body shape has obvious sexual connotations. Being overweight or abnormally thin is likely to be seen as sexually unattractive by most people. Grossly fat people in particular may become stigmatised because of their size and have difficulty in finding sexual partners. Those who do may have sexual difficulties of a mechanical kind because of their size.

For young women in particular, body shape becomes central to their self-image as sexually attractive females. According to Crisp (1979), 70–80% of young women are preoccupied with attempts to reduce their weight by dieting, mainly by restricting carbohydrates. At the same time, the traditional role of women in our society is to prepare and provide food for others. Thus, in recent years fat has become a feminist issue (Orbach 1981). Conflict between being fat, motherly and caring and slim and sexually attractive is seen as an important aspect of the problems that stem from society's stereotyped sex roles. Whilst this almost universal concern with keeping or becoming slim can be seen as part of a search for sexual success by young women, a continuation of slimming to the point of being grossly underweight may also be understood as an avoidance of the sexually attractive or sexually mature role. At what point losing weight changes from the pursuit of sexual attractiveness to its avoidance is another matter. Fashions of ideal body shape, which have changed fairly dramatically over the past 50 years, are obviously important though not well understood.

These ideas have nevertheless led some authorities to conclude that severe anorexia and obesity are methods of avoiding normal sexuality. How often this is the case is uncertain, but it remains an intriguing possibility.

Also to be considered are the sexual connotations of eating. Some patterns of eating, e.g. the binge episodes where short bouts of impulsive overeating occur, can be seen as acts of oral self-gratification. They are usually carried out in private with a feeling of guilt or shame. There is an increasing tendency for them to be countered by subsequent vomiting. The similarity between this type of oral gratification and masturbation is striking but once again we do not know whether this is simply analogy of description or whether the sexual symbolism in any way determines the eating behaviour. Beumont et al (1981) found that amongst patients with anorexia nervosa, those whose weight loss relied on vomiting and purging rather than dieting were more sexually active prior to the onset of the weight loss. Further evidence of this kind relating the pattern of eating disturbance to the type of sexual development may throw more light on this issue.

The psychosomatic complexity is increased by the endocrine correlates of abnormal weight. In the male, obesity is associated with somewhat low testosterone levels and raised oestrogens. The level of sex hormone-binding globulin, however, is usually low rather than raised, so that in only exceptionally fat men is the free testosterone likely to be significantly lowered. The mechanisms underlying this endocrine pattern are not understood, but there is no clear evidence that obese men are prone to low sexual interest (Amatruda et al 1978; Schneider et al 1979). In women obesity is associated with menstrual dysfunction and some impairment of fertility. In the so-called polycystic ovary syndrome (Yen 1980) excess weight is associated with oligomenorrhoea or amenorrhoea, raised plasma androgens and often hirsutism. In one small study (Gorzynski & Katz 1977) women with this condition were found to be more sexually assertive. Whilst this would be an understandable effect of raised androgens, the obesity and the hirsutism are likely to have somewhat contrary effects on female sexuality. More evidence of the psychological characteristics of these women is therefore required. In contrast to this complex and ill-understood condition, there is a more general tendency for obese women to show increased peripheral conversion of androgens (in particular androstenedione) to oestradiol in their adipose tissue. The behavioural consequences of this, if any, are not known. In general we know very little about the sexuality of obese women.

In anorexia and associated weight loss, the endocrine and reproductive consequences are much more striking. There is obviously a basic relationship between body weight and reproductive function. It makes biological sense for fertility to require adequate nutritional status of the would-be mother. In fact if body weight falls too much, women tend to become infertile with anovular cycles and often amenorrhoea. Conversely, restoring body weight is likely to restore fertility and menstrual function. One of the puzzling aspects of so-called anorexia nervosa is that the amenorrhoea often precedes the more dramatic weight loss and may only be reversed long after normal body weight is regained. It is thus often assumed that a different or at least additional mechanism interfering with hypothalamic function is involved in anorexia nervosa compared with the amenorrhoea of simple weight loss. However, in most respects the hormonal profiles are indistinguishable with low non-cyclical gonadotrophins and gonadal steroids.

Evidence from rodents shows that lesions in certain parts of the hypothalamus may lead either to regulated eating which maintains a substantially low but stable body weight, or self-starvation (Anand & Brobeck 1951; Powley & Keesey 1970). The neural substrates controlling eating and reproductive function are obviously close both anatomically and functionally in the rat and may well be so in the human. It is therefore tempting to see disorders such as anorexia nervosa as resulting primarily from hypothalamic malfunction (Russell 1970). On the other hand, the behavioural and emotional aspects of the condition are often gross. Elaborate deception may be used to avoid food intake or conceal vomiting and there is often a fixed determination to avoid regaining normal weight. Also the condition not infrequently follows some psychologically or sexually traumatic experience (Beumont et al 1981). This leads other authorities to see the psychological process as being of primary importance, with the hypo-thalamic malfunction as a secondary effect (Crisp 1980). There are few conditions where there is such polarisation of views between psychogenic and somatic aetiologies, reflecting the basic mystery of the condition. Part of the problem is our lack of understanding of the likely psychological or behavioural manifestations of hypothalamic malfunction.

In the meantime, anorexia nervosa poses formidable treatment problems as in its more severe forms it seriously threatens life. But the motivation for weight gain is usually lacking, representing the essence of the condition. More physically oriented regimes which concentrate on increasing food intake and body weight are often sabotaged by the psychological com-plexities of the patients, whilst psychodynamic approaches may uncover rich and seemingly highly relevant material without necessarily leading to physical improvement. There are occasional successes with both approaches but the mystery and uncertainty largely remain.

ARTHRITIS

Ferguson and Figley (1979) found that 54% of women and 56% of men with arthritis that they studied experienced sexual problems, involving pain, weakness, fatigue and limited movement. In a study of 60 patients with either rheumatoid arthritis or ankylosing spondylitis, Navon et al (1982) found that fatigue was a more important limiting factor on sexual activity than pain or restricted joint movement.

CEREBROVASCULAR ACCIDENTS

Return of sexual function after stroke has received little attention. Hawton (1984) in a follow-up study of 50 male stroke victims with an average age of 49 years found that sexual interest and erectile function usually returned 6 to 7 weeks after the stroke. The best predictor of sexual activity after the stroke was the level of sexual activity preceding it. Mechanical problems due to weakness or spasticity were not uncommon but were usually over-come by modifying sexual technique. Counselling for couples after strokes is indicated for those who were previously sexually active.

EPILEPSY

A link between epilepsy and sexuality featured in the medical writings of antiquity. Sexual behaviour, particularly masturbation, has in the past been seen as a cause of epilepsy (Money & Pruce 1977). The similarity between orgasm and an epileptic seizure has often received comment. Kinsey et al (1953) made a serious comparison between these two equally mysterious neurophysiological phenomena.

In modern medicine, the sexual implications of epilepsy are threefold:

1. *The sexual manifestations of epileptic attacks.* Sexual feelings or gestures as part of an epileptic attack are probably rare, though genital sensations or orgasm-like experiences have been reported (Currier et al 1971; Scott 1978).
2. *The provocation of an attack by sexual activity.* This is also rare though there are some well-known cases in the literature (Mitchell et al 1954; Hoenig & Hamilton 1960).
3. *The sexuality of epileptic individuals in between their attacks.* Much more common is the occurrence of chronic sexual problems in epileptics, usually low sexual interest but sometimes abnormal sexual preferences. In most studies the association has been with temporal lobe epilepsy. Gastaut & Collomb (1954) found that 26 of 36 patients with temporal lobe epilepsy had 'hyposexuality', not only a lack of interest in sexual intercourse but also lack of sexual curiosity, erotic fantasies or sensual dreams. Usually this became evident after the onset of the epilepsy. Blumer (1970) reported that 29 out of 50 patients with temporal lobe epilepsy showed 'global hyposexuality' and often an inability to achieve orgasm. Taylor (1969) studied 100 temporal lobe epileptics who underwent temporal lobectomy. Before the operation, 56% had sexual problems, usually reduced sexual activity and indifference with 'a bland denial of interest in sex'. Money & Pruce (1977) have suggested that the association between sexual disorders and temporal lobe epilepsy rather than other types of epilepsy is an artefact of the selection of cases; severe temporal lobe epilepsy is more likely to be seen by the neurosurgeons and psychiatrists who have carried out these surveys. However, Kolarsky et al (1967) used a register of a central epileptic clinic of Prague and intensively investigated a group of 86 males. Sixteen (19%) were hyposexual and this was usually associated with temporal lobe epilepsy.

Occasionally hypersexuality is reported. It is usually episodic and most often is manifested as excessive masturbation (Taylor 1969; Blumer 1970). The association between epileptic disorder and fetishism and transvestism has already been mentioned (see Chapter 7) and other types of abnormal sexual preference may be more common in epileptics, especially those with temporal lobe focus (Kolarsky et al 1967).

The reasons for these connections between epilepsy and sexual disturbance are likely to be complex. Epilepsy carries considerable stigma, even nowadays, and children with epilepsy are more likely to be overprotected and to have personality problems for this reason alone. They may lack self-confidence, fear rejection or failure, and, particularly when with another person, fear the effects of sexual excitement because of its similarity to epileptic phenomena. Sexual disturbance is more likely to arise on this basis if the onset of the epilepsy is in childhood rather than if it occurs after normal adult sexual development is established (Taylor 1972). The available evidence supports this; Kolarsky et al (1967) found in particular an association between sexual deviation and early onset of temporal lobe epilepsy. But the very early onset in many of these cases may also indicate a direct neurological interference with normal sexual development. The importance of the limbic system as the neural substrate of sexuality is not disputed, though its precise role is far from clear (see Chapter 2). It has been suggested that excessive neuronal activity of the limbic portions of the temporal lobe produce a suppression of sexual behaviour whereas lack of such activity leads to increased sexuality. This is supported by the characteristics of the Kluver-Bucy syndrome, a state produced by surgical removal of both temporal lobes. This condition has been studied in primates, and something comparable has been observed in humans (Terzian & Orr 1955). Amongst a number of other bizarre features, there is a tendency to hypersexuality, usually in the form of masturbatory or aimless sexual mounting behaviour.

Although lack of sexual appetite is the most commonly reported problem in epileptics, there is also evidence that women have difficulty in responding to sexual stimulation with increased arousal and men have problems establishing normal erections (Lundberg 1977). This could also reflect impairment of limbic function. In humans there is some evidence of improvement in hyposexuality as fits are brought under control. The effects of unilateral temporal lobectomy on the characteristic hyposexuality are rather less predictable. Some patients improve, whereas others get worse (Taylor & Falconer 1968; Blumer 1970). Recent evidence of the effects of anti-convulsants on endocrine status, described in Chapter 2, now increases the likelihood that a substantial amount of the hyposexuality in epileptics (at least in men) is iatrogenic. Further evidence from Denmark supports this view. Jensen et al (1987), in a study of outpatient epileptics, found that the prevalence of low sexual interest and erectile problems was no greater than in their control group. This is in apparent contrast with previous studies. However almost all of their epileptic subjects were using carbamazepine as an anti-convulsant. This does not increase sex hormone binding globulin in the way that most earlier anti-convulsants, such as phenytoin do. The subjects in this study were endocrinologically normal. Thus the higher incidence of sexual problems in other series could be due to the endocrine effects of other anti-convulsants.

Thus it seems appropriate at our present stage of knowledge to consider neurophysiological, endocrine and psychosocial factors to be important. Further studies of the types of sexual abnormality and the locus of the epileptic discharge in both males and females may throw more light on the role of the neurophysiological mechanisms.

MULTIPLE SCLEROSIS

In multiple sclerosis (MS), the basic lesion is demyelination of nerve fibres. It can affect subjects at any age from 12 to 60, but most commonly has its onset in the 20s or 30s. It is about twice as common in women as in men. Its basic cause is not known, but may involve an abnormality of the immune response of the nervous system, with abnormal reactions to certain virus infections. Demyelination can occur anywhere in the nervous system, hence the manifestations of the disease are protean. MS may be quite localised; it has a tendency to come and go, leading to remissions and relapses. The prognosis is extremely uncertain, as there must be many people who have had mild or transient forms of this disease and have never seen a neurologist. In a proportion of cases, however, impairment becomes permanent and may be severe.

Sexual problems are common in MS patients. They may stem from the non-specific consequences of physical handicap and the strains that these impose on sexual relationships. Also, sufferers from MS may be particularly prone to anxiety and depression which will take their own toll of sexual happiness (Burnfield 1979). But specific effects of the disease on sexual function are also to be expected. Impairment of peripheral autonomic nerves or their spinal pathways may lead to failure of genital responses such as erection, similar to the neural effects of diabetes. Lundberg (1977) made the interesting observation that in some MS sufferers erection to fantasies or other centrally mediated stimuli was lost whilst erection and response to genital touch continued. This suggests selective impairment of the pathways involved in psychic erection — perhaps the thoracic sympathetic outflow (see Chapter 2).

Ejaculation may be impaired in the presence of normal erections. Sensation may also be affected, resulting in diminished response to tactile stimulation or sometimes hypersensitivity which can make either genital touch or orgasm unpleasant (Lundberg 1980). Spasticity, particularly of the leg adductors in women, may interfere with normal love-making in a distressing fashion.

Sexual problems are associated with disturbances of bladder function or other peripheral autonomic symptoms more commonly than with more central lesions causing ocular or cerebellar disturbance or upper motor neurone disease (Lundberg 1978). Sexual difficulties may arise in some whose other manifestations of the disease are mild or negligible. In others, the sexual problem may be the first manifestation of the disease. The onset of sexual dysfunction may be quite rapid and, consistent with the general pattern of the disease, may fluctuate in severity or remit.

Lilius et al (1976) gave a questionnaire to 302 men and women with moderately severe MS: 64% of the men and 39% of the women reported sexual problems or cessation of sexual activity. Of the men with problems, 80% had erectile difficulties and 56% diminished libido. General weakness, spasticity of limb muscles and loss of genital sensation were given as reasons by some of the men. Of the women with problems, 48% reported low interest in intercourse, 49% diminished clitoral sensitivity and 57% difficulty in attaining orgasm. Spasticity and dryness of the vagina were also mentioned.

Vas (1969), investigating men with mild MS, found 47% with erectile problems. This was commonly associated with disturbance of body sweating. Lundberg (1980) compared 25 women with established MS but minimal disability with 25 migraine sufferers of similar age. Thirteen (52%) of the MS women had sexual problems compared with 3 (12%) of the control group. Reduced libido, orgasmic difficulty and altered genital sensitivity were the most common complaints. Other reports showing a substantial prevalence of sexual problems include those by Ivers & Goldstein (1963) and Miller et al (1965).

The reasons for reduced libido in MS are not clear. Impaired sensation may be relevant as sexual appetite is often activated by awareness of one's genitals. Central neural pathological mechanisms may also be involved. But it is probably most often a psychological reaction to the sexual problem or to other aspects of the condition.

SPINAL INJURIES

Spinal injuries, mainly from war and traffic accidents, are tragic and all too common. In the USA there are approximately 100 000 individuals with such injuries (Higgins 1979). About 85% are men. They tend to be young, and with modern methods of treatment have good life expectancy with no particular risk of progression of the disability. Their sexual capacity is therefore of considerable importance. Sexual enjoyment, if still possible, may be an important option for someone with an otherwise severely restricted life. The married paraplegic or quadriplegic, largely dependent on the spouse for so many things, may both want and need to give sexual pleasure to his or her partner. Self-esteem may be severely affected by the physical incapacity, particularly in a man who relied on his physical prowess before the injury. The retention of potency may have extra importance for such a person. Potent male paraplegics were found by Berger (1952) to have higher self-esteem than those who were impotent. Lindner (1953) found that those who were impotent had more physical complaints and bodily preoccupations. In some cases the need for sexual activity produces difficulties in the marital relationship; the partner may sometimes resent having to be available sexually as well as taking so many other responsibilities.

In recent years there has been an increasing number of reports on the sexuality of people with spinal injuries. Earlier studies mainly involved men, but a few reports on females have appeared. As yet most evidence is on the sexual consequences of the injuries; there is relatively little information on the effects of counselling or treatment. Useful reviews are provided by Cole (1975), Higgins (1979) and Brindley (1982). There is some uncertainty about the effects of spinal injuries on sexual interest or appetite, though the most widely held view is that for the majority, sexual appetite is unimpaired (Higgins 1979) and this may be particularly so in women (Fitting et al 1978). If so, this is of some interest when compared with other forms of disability, where secondary loss of sexual interest is common and usually assumed to be psychologically determined (e.g. male diabetes, multiple sclerosis). It appears that for many if not most people with spinal injuries, sex remains an important aspect of their limited lives. It is therefore important to develop as much understanding as possible of the nature of the sexual deficits so that appropriate counselling can be given.

Evidence of the relationship between the type of sexual impairment and type of injury is not only of clinical importance but also of theoretical interest as a source of understanding of the neuroanatomy and neurophysiology of sexual response. Unfortunately, much of the evidence is too vague or too inadequately defined to be conclusive in this respect. But some useful and interesting generalisations are possible.

Sexual effects in the male with spinal injuries

Erection

It is helpful to distinguish between psychic and reflexive erections (see p. 53). In men with complete cord lesions who have recovered from the initial phase of spinal shock, some reflex erection is to be expected, providing that the sacral segments of the cord are not destroyed. In general, the higher the level of the lesion, the more likely there are to be reflexive erections (Higgins 1979). The completeness and duration of such erections do vary, however, and may be partly due to variable degrees of damage. Psychic erections, by contrast, are more likely to continue with lower lesions, and with incomplete rather than complete lesions, though usually they are also associated with reflexive responses. There are, however, a number of men described in the literature with lesions below the level of T8 who have psychic erections in the absence of reflexive responses (Higgins 1979). This is understandable if we accept the hypothesis, discussed in Chapter 2, that psychic erections are mediated by the thoracic sympathetic outflow, whilst reflexive erections require the sacral outflow.

Many men with spinal injuries are therefore able to have vaginal intercourse using either psychic or reflexive erections. The definition of successful intercourse is usually lacking in the literature but its incidence in different series is said to range from 5 to 56% (Higgins 1979).

Ejaculatory capacity tends to be more impaired than erection. It is unlikely in men with complete lesions (ranging from 0–7% in different series) but with incomplete lesions ejaculatory failure is present in about a third of cases. It is more likely to occur with lower than with upper motor neurone lesions, and with lower than with higher level lesions, though the evidence is far from conclusive (Higgins 1979). It is even more difficult to be certain about the incidence of orgasm as this has seldom been defined adequately in the various studies reported. Lack of awareness of any pelvic sensations must make recognition of orgasm difficult. Many paraplegic men do describe orgasmic experiences. These are often followed by a period of comfortable resolution, comparable to that of a normal orgasm (Cole 1975). Those few men with upper motor neurone lesions and spasticity of the lower limbs who do ejaculate may experience considerable reduction in the spasticity following ejaculation, which can be gratifying (Bors & Comarr 1960). Our lack of understanding of the relative importance of central and spinal mechanisms for the experience of normal orgasm and its associated refractory period was discussed in Chapter 2. It is possible that a central component of the orgasm could be experienced by some of these men, particularly if they can receive enough erotic stimulation from the intact parts of their body. A heightening of erotic sensitivity in areas above the lesion is not unusual, though the neurophysiological mechanism involved is not understood (Bors & Comarr 1960; Cole 1975; Kolodny et al 1979). In some men with cord injuries above the fourth thoracic vertebra sexual stimulation may lead to excessive excitation of the autonomic nervous system — so-called autonomic dysreflexia. This may lead to a marked rise in blood pressure and headache or flushing, sweating and cardiac arrhythmia (Kolodny et al 1979).

Spinal injuries in women

The limited evidence so far suggests that the sexuality of women with spinal injuries is somewhat less affected than it is in men. Weiss & Diamond (1966) found no evidence of a reduction in sexual desire or sexual fantasies. Bregman (1975) interviewed 31 women with spinal injuries. All reported some sexual experience after the injury. Twenty-seven reported vaginal lubrication and most of the subjects felt that their injuries had not affected sexual arousal and lubrication. It was not clear how many of these women experienced orgasm. Fitting et al (1978) investigated 24 women; 20 (85%) had had sexual relationships since the injury and 13 (54%) were involved in a relationship at the time of the interview. Thirteen women had complete spinal lesions and of these, seven found sexual relations to be 'very enjoyable'. Eight of the 11 women with incomplete lesions reported the same. The subjective feelings expressed by the women did not appear to correlate with the level of injury. Although it was not stated, one assumes that these women had little or no awareness of genital sensations. Six of them spontaneously mentioned experiencing orgasm, though differing from their preinjury experiences. One woman described her orgasm as 'a fusebox gone haywire'. Two-thirds stated that concern about their bowel and bladder dysfunction had interfered with sexual expression. Spasticity may occasionally cause problems, particularly if the adductors are involved (Cole 1975). The impression from these reports is that, in spite of radical changes in the capacity for normal sexual experience, many women with spinal injuries have been able, usually after a period of difficult adjustment, to reestablish rewarding sexual relationships and maintain positive feminine identities.

Fertility and spinal injuries

Fertility in women with spinal injuries is relatively unaffected. Menstruation usually resumes within 6 months of the injury. Pregnancy may occur and continue to normal delivery, although there is an increased risk of urinary infection, anaemia and premature labour (Griffith & Trieschmann 1975). Contraception is therefore an important issue in these women if they are sexually active. Steroidal contraceptives are probably contraindicated because of the increased risk of thrombosis. Diaphragms are impractical and intrauterine devices have to be used with extra caution because of the absence of pelvic sensation and the small risk of uterine perforation or pelvic infection. The appropriateness of sterilisation should not be assumed, however, as many women have coped with motherhood from a wheelchair when provided with additional support (Cole 1975).

For the male with spinal injuries, fertility is much less likely. As mentioned above, few ejaculate and among those who do, spermatogenesis is not always normal. This could be related to scrotal temperature which is notably higher than in normal men (Brindley 1982). The endocrine status of cord-injured men is usually normal (Kolodny et al 1979). Artificially induced ejaculation may be possible and, if the ejaculate is fertile, may be used for artificial insemination. Ejaculation can be induced by intrathecal neostigmine but this carries a significant risk of unpleasant and even dangerous side-effects. Electroejaculation, though less predictably successful, is safer; details of the method, which involves inserting electrodes into the rectum and positioning them appropriately, are given by Brindley (1982). Ejaculation has occasionally been obtained by applying a vibrator to the penis.

Counselling men and women with spinal injuries

Most of the issues involved in counselling people with spinal injuries are common to the general field of physical handicap, discussed earlier in this chapter. The younger age of this population compared with some other disabled groups is associated with a relatively high level of sexual awareness and interest, the importance of sexuality for self-esteem and concern with fertility. More specific issues are often of a practical, commonsense nature, involving catheters, sphincter control, spasticity and physical positioning during love-making (Cole 1975). It is important in the early stages not to reach conclusions about sexual impairment before sufficient time has elapsed to judge the degree of recovery. Whilst it is important to accept the realities of an irreversible and static disability, there does seem to be scope for developing and enhancing new forms of sexual pleasure. An approach to love-making involving exploration and discovery is therefore required. Encouragement or even 'permission' to do this may be needed.

MALIGNANT DISEASE

When considering the sexual implications of malignant disease, the multi-factorial issues, discussed on p. 552, are of special importance. First there are the various ways the illness can directly affect well-being. Secondly, there are the psychological reactions to the illness by both the patient and spouse. Malignancy, whatever its realistic prognosis, is regarded as life-threatening. This often leads to an increased need for physical intimacy or closeness with the partner, whilst the desire for sexual activity is reduced (Leiber et al 1976). There are the effects of treatment: surgery, radio-therapy and cytotoxic drugs can all take their toll sexually and in a variety of ways. Last and not least, there is the reaction of the medical profession who also tend to focus on the life-threatening aspects and pay insufficient attention to less immediate issues. As the effectiveness of treatment for malignant disease increases, so it will be necessary to pay more attention to the quality of life during and following treatment. In this respect, the role of the health professional in helping the patient and partner to maintain a worthwhile sexual relationship should be fairly high on the agenda.

The literature has been well reviewed by Kolodny et al (1979) and only a few of the types of malignant disease will be considered here; some others will be referred to elsewhere in the chapter (e.g. gynaecological disease).

BLOOD DYSCRASIAS

The prognosis for several forms of leukaemia and for Hodgkin's disease is improving with modern forms of treatment. This mainly involves the use of cytotoxic drugs and their effects on sexuality are therefore becoming increasingly important. In men loss of sexual desire following chemotherapy is common and may persist in 40 to 50% of cases (Chapman et al 1979a). The reasons for this are not always clear. Although spermatogenesis (and fertility) are usually impaired, testosterone levels typically remain normal. In women, on the other hand, suppression of ovarian function induced by cytotoxic drugs appears to be important in causing loss of sexual desire as well as menopausal-type symptoms, such as vaginal dryness (Chapman et al 1979b). This is of importance clinically as there is no reason why such women should not receive hormone replacement.

TESTICULAR NEOPLASMS

The treatment of malignant testicular tumours in men may involve surgery, irradiation and cytotoxic drugs. Of particular interest is the surgical dissection of retroperitoneal lymph nodes when secondary deposits are suspected. Bilateral dissection usually results in failure of seminal emission (i.e. 'dry-run' orgasm; see p. 384), though not usually erectile failure. This typically occurs in men following cystectomy or total prostatectomy which is sometimes necessary because of local spread of the tumour (Fraley et al 1979).

MASTECTOMY

Breast cancer is the commonest form of malignancy in women and, compared with many other forms of cancer, carries a relatively poor prognosis. It has been estimated that a 20-year-old white American woman has an 8% probability of developing breast cancer in her lifetime (Kolodny et al 1979).

Mastectomy with or without radiotherapy or chemotherapy is still the commonest method of treatment, though there is controversy as to whether the more radical surgical methods improve the prognosis. Nevertheless, many women who are found to have evidence of malignancy at biopsy will emerge from the operating theatre with a breast removed.

Maguire et al (1978) assessed women prior to biopsy for suspected breast cancer, and then followed them up after biopsy. The authors compared those women who were found to have malignancy and received mastectomy with those whose breast lumps were found to be benign. After 1 year, significantly more of the mastectomy women (33%) had substantial sexual problems (i.e. had stopped intercourse, or had ceased to enjoy it) than did the benign group (8%). Before the biopsy, the incidence was 8% in both groups. Comparable findings were reported by Kolodny et al (1979) who also found that there was commonly avoidance of breast stimulation or coital positions that emphasised breast shape (e.g. the female superior position). Undoubtedly, mastectomy produces an adverse effect on a woman's sexual self-image and secondarily, on her sexual relationship. In the past this has received inadequate attention and more discussion of these issues pre-operatively as well as postoperatively is desirable. Increasing attention is being paid to the possibility of reconstructive mammoplasty (Kolodny et al 1979) but as yet we do not know whether this will be effective in preventing these sexual repercussions.

Few studies have looked at the sexual implications of cytotoxic or endocrine-based treatments (Bransfield 1982). The sexual consequences of ovarian suppression, referred to earlier in relation to Hodgkin's disease, makes it particularly important to identify effectively those malignant cell types which are hormone-dependent and which therefore require suppression of ovarian function for control of the malignancy. In those cases which are not hormone-sensitive, ovarian suppression and its sexual consequences are unwanted by-products of chemotherapy which are potentially reversible with hormone replacement.

GENERAL SURGERY

OSTOMIES

The surgical formation of permanent openings of the bowel on to the abdominal wall is a common component of treatment for a variety of bowel disorders. Inflammatory diseases of the bowel such as ulcerative colitis or Crohn's disease usually require removal of the entire colon and much if not all of the rectum when surgery is indicated. This requires an ileostomy, an opening of the ileum on to the abdominal wall through which liquid faeces escape into a collecting bag. Other conditions, in particular carcinoma of the lower colon or rectum, may require less of the bowel to be removed, leaving the patient with a colostomy (i.e. an opening of the colon). The inflammatory diseases are more likely to arise in younger age groups, whereas malignant disease of the lower bowel and rectum is more common in the elderly.

The direct effects of the surgery on sexual function depend to a large extent on whether the rectum and surrounding tissues have to be removed. As described in Chapter 2, the sympathetic fibres of the hypogastric nerves supplying the genitalia are usually scattered and unpredictably placed in the pelvis so that it is easy to damage them during surgical resection in this area. Devlin et al (1971) reported on 68 heterosexual men who had received surgical treatment of anorectal cancer. Sixty-three of them had been sexually active before surgery, but less than half were postoperatively. Those who had a colostomy were more likely to be impotent than those receiving restorative surgery. Of 12 women in this series who were sexually active pre-operatively, only half remained so afterwards.

Burnham et al (1977) surveyed by questionnaire a one-in-ten sample of married members of the Ileostomy Association of Great Britain. They had 128 male and 175 female respondents: 19% of the men and 12% of the women had married *after* receiving the ileostomy; 33% of men and 10% of women had had children since their ileostomies. In those cases where the rectum had not been excised, there were no instances of postoperative sexual dysfunction. Only 8% of this group found the stoma a problem during love-making, although embarrassment or a reduced sense of sexual attractiveness was reported by 30% of them. In those whose rectum was removed, 29% of the men reported sexual dysfunction. This was age-related; in men aged 35 or less, 8% had partial erectile failure and 15% had ejaculatory failure. In the 36–45-year age group, a third had erectile problems and amongst those over 45 years, more than half had erectile problems, 17% with total impotence. Several patients reported that sexual function improved for up to 2 years after operation. In the women, rectal excision was followed by dyspareunia in 30%; this is usually due to a fibrous plaque behind the vagina with consequent loss of mobility, making deep thrusting painful. Interestingly, as with diabetes and multiple sclerosis damage to the pelvic autonomic nerve supply does not produce obvious sexual dysfunction in women as it does in men. Fortunately, greater recognition of the sexual consequences of rectal excision is now being made by surgeons and techniques of resection are being devised which reduce the likelihood of nerve damage or vaginal deformities (Lee & Dowling 1972), though the results are likely to be better in experienced hands.

Apart from such physiological and anatomical damage, there are obvious psychological problems to be considered in relation to ostomies. The new form of spout ileostomies, which are much more satisfactory from the point of view of stoma control, have a somewhat off-putting, almost phallic appearance, which creates problems for some patients or their spouses. In general, there is the understandable feeling of mutilation plus the chronic fear that one's ostomy may leak or emit smells during love-making. Sometimes orgasm causes ileostomies to empty reflexly. Positions during intercourse may have to be adjusted to avoid pressure on the ileostomy bag and each couple needs to work out methods of dealing with the ileostomy which are acceptable to them and which interfere as little as possible with their sexual enjoyment (Devlin & Plant 1979). The reaction of the partner to the ostomy is often crucial. Although the majority react positively, Gloeckner (1983) found 30% of her ostomy subjects had partners who had reacted negatively, most often expressing 'fear of hurting me'. Obviously there is much psychological work to be done by a couple in coming to terms with this state of affairs, but with appropriate counselling before and after operation and the support of such organisations as the Ileostomy Association, most patients effectively resolve these problems.

PROSTATECTOMY

In the majority of men beyond their mid-40s, there is an enlargement of the suburethral glands surrounding the prostatic part of the urethra. In approximately 10% of these men, this will cause some narrowing and obstruction of the urethra as well as compression of the normal prostatic tissue. In time, this may lead to incomplete emptying of the bladder with loss of bladder tone, back pressure effects on the kidney and the risk of infection. This is the commonest indication for prostatectomy. Less common and more serious is malignant change in the prostate. Chronic prostatitis is also sometimes treated by surgical removal of the gland. None of these conditions in themselves should interfere with sexual function, but it is often assumed that surgical treatment will.

There are four types of operation:

1. *Transurethral prostatectomy* is the most widely used method and carries the lowest morbidity when used by experienced surgeons. The adenom-

atous tissue is removed through a special endoscope inserted along the urethra (Notley 1979).
2. *Suprapubic prostatectomy*, the earliest form of operation to be used, involves an abdominal incision and access to the prostate through the bladder.
3. *Retropubic prostatectomy*, now more favoured than the suprapubic approach, also involves an abdominal incision but gains access to the prostate and bladder neck by passing between the pubic bone and the bladder.
4. *Perineal prostatectomy* involves access through a perineal incision. This is usually confined to radical removal for prostatic carcinoma as more extensive clearance is possible.

The incidence of erectile problems is lowest after transurethral resection (approximately 5%) and slightly higher (10–20%) for the suprapubic and retropubic methods. In all three, however, disturbance of ejaculation is usual, resulting in retrograde ejaculation in 30–90% of cases (Kolodny et al 1979; Pearlman 1980). The perineal operation, particularly when of a radical kind, is much more likely to interfere with the neural control of erection and loss of erectile capacity occurs in almost all cases. Also, if the operation is for prostatic carcinoma, additional treatment with oestrogens, anti-androgens or bilateral orchidectomy may be used as prostatic carcinoma is androgen-dependent. Consequently, loss of sexual interest from this androgen-reducing treatment is to be expected (see Chapter 2).

There is no particular reason why the first three methods of prostatectomy should affect erectile function. In one study, however (Madorsky et al 1976), men undergoing transurethral resection had their nocturnal erections measured in the sleep laboratory before and after the operation. About half of them showed some impairment of sleep erections postoperatively. It is difficult to interpret this finding as we do not understand sufficiently the psychophysiological basis of nocturnal erections (see Chapter 10) but this finding deserves further study. Most people assume that when erectile failure does arise, it is psychologically determined. As most men undergoing this operation are elderly it would not be surprising to find some of them had abandoned sexual activity before the operation. Failure to establish this fact would create an impression of postoperative sexual dysfunction, particularly in those men who might find the operation a convenient excuse for their sexual incapacity. In others, sexual problems may be anticipated and lead to expectation of failure which can so easily become a self-fulfilling prophecy. Retrograde ejaculation may also incur adverse psychological reactions in some men, particularly if they are not expecting it and do not understand its significance. There is undoubtedly an important need for adequate counselling pre-operatively as well as the opportunity for discussing sexual function in the postoperative recovery period.

GYNAECOLOGY

Gynaecology has in the past been a predominantly surgical specialty. That situation is changing: with increasing emphasis on the diagnosis and treatment of pelvic infections, endocrine abnormalities of the reproductive system and infertility, the medical aspects of gynaecology are growing in importance.

The most important gynaecological symptom, from the sexual point of view, is pain. A number of gynaecological conditions causing pain during sexual activity have been mentioned earlier (see p. 420). Similarly, the reproductive endocrine disorders are dealt with in Chapter 2, and infertility in Chapter 12. Here we will consider gynaecological malignancies and the common surgical procedures of hysterectomy and vaginal repair.

GYNAECOLOGICAL MALIGNANCY

The four most common malignancies of the genital tract are carcinoma of the endometrium, ovary, cervix, and vulva. Endometrial carcinoma is important sexually mainly because of its oestrogen dependency, with the need for oophorectomy and the consequent hormonal deficiency. The cause of ovarian carcinoma is ill understood. It is difficult to diagnose and is often identified in an advanced stage of the disease. Hence the prognosis tends to be much worse than for the other three types. Its relevance to sexuality is mainly because of the hormonal implications of ovarian removal and the major threat to life that is involved.

The sexual implications of carcinoma of the cervix and vulva are more complex. Cervical carcinoma is the end state of a sequence which starts with dysplasia, passes through carcinoma in situ to reach its invasive form. The dysplasia is believed to be caused, in the majority of cases, by a sexually transmitted factor, probably a virus. Genital herpes and the virus of genital warts have been implicated. The risk of cervical dysplasia is increased when sexual activity starts before the age of 17 (Rotkin 1973) and is proportional to the number of sexual partners a woman has had (Martin 1967). This issue is gaining in prominence in the debate for and against teenage sexuality. One consequence is that cervical carcinoma is developing an emotive dimension beyond its threat to life. Women who are diagnosed as having cervical dysplasia often suffer a deterioration in their sexual lives.

The method of treating cervical carcinoma is also a controversial issue. The cure rate for surgery and radiotherapy is similar, so that the implications of the two methods for quality of life have gained in importance. Several studies have suggested that radiotherapy causes ovarian decline, soreness of the vagina with a risk of stenosis and more sexual problems than occur with surgical treatment. But overall the evidence is conflicting and this remains an important unresolved issue (Andersen 1984).

Vulval carcinoma, which tends to occur in older women than do the other forms of malignancy, commonly effects the labia (70%) and less commonly the clitoris (13%). Its treatment is noteworthy because of its mutilating nature. Radiotherapy is seldom used because of the intense irritation it causes. Surgery usually includes removal of all labial tissue and the clitoris. The impact of such a procedure on the woman's sexuality is likely to be considerable. Andersen (1984) studied 15 such women post-operatively and found evidence of a reduced capacity for sexual arousal, though, interestingly, orgasmic capacity was retained in some women, even those who had their clitoris removed. Similarly, Weijmar Schultz et al (1986) studied 10 women postoperatively and found that half made a satisfactory sexual recovery, including orgasm.

With all types of gynaecological malignancy, therefore, many women will need postoperative counselling to enable them to return to a rewarding sexual life (Andersen 1984).

Hysterectomy

For many years it has been widely believed that hysterectomy carries a high psychiatric morbidity and consequent sexual repercussions (Barker 1968; Richards 1973). However, the evidence on which this assumption was based has been unsatisfactory for a variety of reasons. In view of the commonness of this operation, it is of some importance to clarify these issues. In the last few years, adequately designed prospective studies have largely rejected the idea that hysterectomy per se is psychologically or sexually harmful. Gath et al (1982a, b) found that the incidence of psychiatric morbidity was high *before* hysterectomy for benign conditions and the predominant postoperative change was one of improvement. The explanation for this pre-operative morbidity was not clear, but it was not apparently related to the presence or absence of pathology in the uterus. Hence there was no support for the idea that dysfunctional uterine bleeding without objective pathology is a somatic manifestation of a psychological state. Sexually, this group of women showed significant improvement, both in terms of enjoyment and frequency of intercourse, following the operation.

McFarlane & Kincey (1981) followed up 98 women in a prospective study of hysterectomy: 44% reported an improvement in their sex lives, 31% no change, and 19% had deteriorated. For most of these the deterioration had been 'loss of libido'. In neither this study nor that of Gath and his colleagues has a clear distinction been made between hysterectomy with or without oophorectomy. It is possible that the hormonal effects of bilateral oophorectomy, discussed in Chapter 5, account for most of the sexual deterioration that follows hysterectomy. These two studies are concerned with hysterectomy via the abdominal route. There is no reason, however, to believe that hysterectomy via the vagina will cause any more sexual problems. Jackson (1979) received questionnaires from 33 women who had undergone vaginal hysterectomy about 1 year previously and who had been given an explanatory booklet before the operation: 42% reported an improvement and 52% no change in their sexual enjoyment. The few women who reported deterioration had also received vaginal repairs (see below).

There are no mechanical or physiological reasons why hysterectomy per se should impair sexual response. As mentioned in Chapter 2, the cervix, which is removed during hysterectomy, is not necessary for adequate vaginal lubrication. Obviously time must be allowed for adequate healing of the vaginal vault, and a recovery period of 6 weeks is recommended before intercourse is resumed. Initially the vagina may seem somewhat shrunken or shortened and this may be more marked if postoperative sepsis has been troublesome. But a cautious return to intercourse will gradually stretch the vaginal tissues (Amias 1975).

Adverse sexual reactions may occur for psychological reasons. Hysterectomy results in irreversible sterilisation; as discusserd in Chapter 12, this occasionally causes problems in women for whom fertility is an important component of their sexual identity. This type of reaction may be more common in women from other cultures, though no such evidence is available. The spouse may also react adversely to the operation; lack of understanding may lead to fear that his partner has been physically weakened or altered in a way that he finds difficult to assess. In couples where sex has been unrewarding or continued with a sense of obligation to normality, the operation may be used as an excuse to bring the sex life to an end. But apart from these various and occasional possibilities we can reasonably conclude that hysterectomy has no adverse effects on the sexuality of women and may, because of its beneficial effects on health and pelvic symptoms, lead to an enhancement of the woman's sexual life.

Vaginal operations

Surgical repair of the vagina is indicated when there is a degree of prolapse. In the less severe forms, the bladder is prolapsed, producing a cystocele interfering with bladder emptying. The rectum is less often prolapsed — a rectocele. These conditions result from weakening of the pelvic supporting tissues, and occur in older women who have borne children. Further weakening of the supporting tissue which accompanies ageing often leads to a progression of the prolapse which in its more extreme form results in complete eversion of the vagina and descent of the uterus, so-called procidentia.

Surgical repair involves either the anterior wall of the vagina (anterior colporrhaphy), the posterior wall and perineum (posterior colpoperineorrhaphy) or a combination of the two procedures. Sometimes a vaginal hysterectomy is carried out in addition.

Interference with sexual functioning after these operations may result from undue narrowing of the vaginal introitus, shortening of the vagina or the presence of tender scar tissue. Francis & Jeffcoate (1961) followed up 243 women after vaginal repairs: 177 had had anterior and posterior repairs; 140 of these women had continuing opportunities for sexual activity, but only half of them reported trouble-free sexual intercourse. Of the others, most had stopped having intercourse altogether whilst the remainder had little interest or found attempts at intercourse painful. Of these women, 40% gave evidence that their sexual activity was considerably reduced before the operation. On examination, however, the majority of them were found to have anatomical deficiencies which would have made satisfactory intercourse unlikely. One can conclude on the basis of this evidence that about one-fifth of women receiving this operation regret the loss of sexual function that follows, and for those who have no regret, the lack of use of the vagina during coitus ensures its narrowing and fibrosis, making later attempts at intercourse impossible or difficult in any case. Forty-four women in this study received only an anterior repair. The prevalence of sexual difficulty was substantially less in this group, and when present was unlikely to be due to an anatomical defect. In fact none of these women was found to have undue narrowing of the vagina. Francis & Jeffcoate therefore concluded that posterior repair should be avoided if possible, particularly in women who hope for continuing sexual activity. Narrowing of the vaginal introitus is the most likely consequence; shortening of the vagina may occur, whereas tender scar tissue is in their view unusual. Formation of a posterior 'skin bridge' commonly causes dyspareunia, however. The anterior repair, whilst producing some degree of vaginal shortening, is much less likely to cause narrowing of the vagina and does not produce the posterior skin bridge (Amias 1975). With either operation, if intercourse is to be resumed, it should begin reasonably soon (say after 6 weeks) and should be seen as an important part of the vaginal rehabilitation process.

SEXUALLY TRANSMITTED DISEASES AND GENITAL INFECTIONS

A wide variety of pathogens are involved in sexually transmitted disease, including bacteria (e.g. gonococcus), spirochaetes (e.g. *Treponema pallidum*), parasites (e.g. *Trichomonas*), fungi (*Monilia*) and viruses (e.g. herpes simplex, HIV).

In most cases the effects of infection are local, causing genital or perineal lesions or pelvic infection. Such infections may cause discomfort and interfere with normal sexual function, but they have a particularly emotive significance because they can be transmitted between sexual partners. As a consequence, such venereal diseases have strong connotations of illicit or immoral sex and carry considerable social stigma as well as potentially horrifying medical consequences. As we shall see, the justification for such stigma varies considerably, but it is nonetheless important. In some countries, certain diseases are legally designated as venereal. In the UK this only applies to syphilis, gonorrhoea and chancroid.

Organisms causing infection may be normal inhabitants of the bowel or skin which gain access to inappropriate places as a result of sexual activity, or become established because of some alteration in the local conditions such as following the use of broad-spectrum antibiotics. They may be inevitably pathogenic organisms transmitted from the infected person to the recipient during sexual contact, the classical venereal infection. But often infections that arise non-venereally may be kept going venereally by being passed back and forth within a stable sexual partnership. Promiscuity or infidelity is not therefore necessarily involved, but is often implied.

Sexually transmitted infections are not confined to the genitalia. Oral–genital contact may result in pharyngeal infection by organisms from the genital region and vice versa. The apparent increase in oral sex (see Chapter 4) is reflected in an increase in such infections. Similarly, anal intercourse allows infection of the anal region by genital organisms and vice versa. Both types of cross-infection are particularly important for gay men.

In some instances the local consequences of infection are much less important than the systemic disease that may follow. Thus gonococcal infection can cause arthritis. But the most important infections in this respect are syphilis and AIDS.

In the early 20th century, when syphilis was rife, the protean manifestations of the disease, especially as it affected the cardiovascular and central nervous systems, provided much of the florid pathology of clinical practice. Today AIDS has taken its place and is beginning to dominate clinical medicine not only with its appalling threat to world health but also with its rich if morbid insights into abnormalities of the immune system and

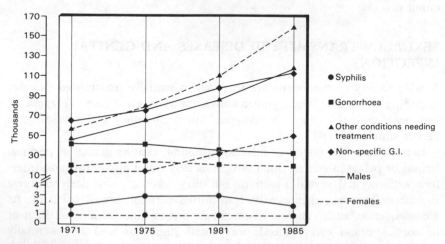

Fig. 11.4 Sexually transmitted diseases in new patients attending hospital clinics in the UK. (from Ramprakash & Daly 1981; Griffin & Morris 1987)

tumour formation. We will consider AIDS in greater detail; it is probably the single most important infectious disease of our time.

In the past, sexually transmitted diseases increased in incidence during war time, with its widespread movement of people and lowering of social constraints on sexual behaviour. Syphilis showed worldwide peaks of incidence associated with the First and Second World Wars. There was a decline during the 1950s and a further rise in the 1960s in many countries, including the UK. Gonorrhoea also showed a post-war decline but by the early 1950s its incidence was rising again. In the 1960s there was a dramatic rise in gonorrhoea in the USA and Scandinavia whilst that in the UK was more modest (Idsoe et al 1973). Trends for the UK since the early 1970s are shown in Figure 11.4. Syphilis and gonorrhoea remained relatively stable for several years. Both have been common in gay men. Now with the exponential increases in AIDS we are beginning to see major changes in sexual practices amongst gay men (see p. 596), which is reflected in a recent decline in syphilis and gonorrhoea. Other infections, such as non-gonococcal urethritis, genital herpes and genital warts are still increasing.

COMMON INFECTIONS IN WOMEN

Infections of the vulva, vagina and urinary tract are common in women. The shortness of the female urethra and its anatomical position make it vulnerable to ascending infection in women who are sexually active. The normal vagina has a varied bacterial flora, mainly of non-pathogens, and an acidic pH which inhibits the growth of most pathogenic varieties. In a study of a large number of women attending a family planning clinic, 21% were found to have yeasts or fungi in the vagina, presumably most of them asymptomatically; 1% had *Trichomonas* present, usually associated with a vaginal discharge. Oral contraceptive users, contrary to earlier reports, did not have a higher incidence of pathogenic organisms (Goldacre et al 1979). It remains possible, however, that they may be more vulnerable to such organisms when present.

The importance of local infection in causing pain and disrupting the psychosomatic circle of sex was emphasised in Chapter 8. In addition, offensive discharges or unpleasant-looking lesions may distract sexually for aesthetic reasons. Of particular importance are the more long-term and generalised consequences of some of these infections. Thus infection ascending into the pelvic cavity may cause deep dyspareunia as well as infertility, and in pregnant women may lead to neonatal infection which can be serious or even fatal for the infant.

Recurrent urethritis and cystitis

Faecal organisms (e.g. *Escherichia coli*) which gain access to the urethra may cause urethritis or ascend to cause cystitis. Such access may result from sexual activity. An increase in the bacterial counts in the urine after sexual intercourse has been reported (Buckley et al 1978). This underlies the condition known as 'honeymoon cystitis', painful and frequent urination that comes on after intercourse, classically in the sexually inexperienced woman. The post-menopausal woman is particularly prone to this problem, perhaps because her oestrogen-deficient vagina has poor lubrication and does not engorge sufficiently to cushion the urethra against the buffeting of the anterior vaginal wall (see p. 291).

Until recently the increasingly common non-specific urethritis (or non-gonococcal urethritis, NGU) in women and men (see Fig. 11.4) was of uncertain aetiology. It is now clear that at least half of cases are due to *Chlamydia trachomatis*. This is an important pathogen in women, as in addition to cervicitis and urethritis, it is a common cause of pelvic imflammatory disease and subsequent infertility. *Ureaplasma urealyticum* is also commonly implicated. These infections are responsive to tetracyline treatment.

Trichomonas vaginitis

This is one of the commonest of sexually transmitted diseases. *Trichomonas* is a parasitic organism that typically causes a painful vaginitis and profuse, frothy and offensive discharge. The onset is often acute and commonly affects young women a week or so after their first sexual experience (Catterall 1972). The infection is often asymptomatic in the male, who therefore should be treated routinely in order to eliminate the infection from the couple. Metronidazole (Flagyl) is an effective treatment.

Monilial vulvovaginitis (thrush)

Monilia are commonly present in the vagina and may proliferate if the normal flora is eliminated by broad-spectrum antibiotics. Monilial infections are also more common in diabetics, the obese and during pregnancy. The main symptom is an intense burning or itching of the vagina and vulval region. A thick curd-like discharge may occur. Once again, the partner may harbour the infection. It has been suggested that at least 10% of cases are sexually transmitted and in about one-fifth of infected women, cure is only obtained if the male partner is also treated (Harris 1977). Fungicides, such as nystatin, can be used, though recurrences are common.

Genital herpes

Human herpes simplex is of two types — i and ii. Type i is common around the oral cavity, causing cold sores. Type ii causes genital herpes, typically a cluster of ulcerating vesicles on the labia and/or the cervix. Not only may these be very painful, particularly during the first acute outbreak, but they are notoriously difficult to treat. In a characteristic herpetic fashion, the virus lies dormant in the dermal cells or possibly within the nervous system, breaking out in recurrent vesicles from time to time and often causing serious sexual disability. The primary infection is commonly subclinical. The virus is highly transmissible through sexual contact during the primary acute attack, somewhat less transmissible during recurrences, and relatively little during the quiescent phases. About 15% of cases involve type i virus and may well be transmitted by oral–genital contact. The herpes simplex virus has been implicated as a possible causative factor in cervical cancer. Infection of the neonate by active lesions in the mother can also be extremely serious. The presence of genital herpetic vesicles in the latter stages of pregnancy is probably grounds for a Caesarean delivery.

The number of new cases of genital herpes presenting at sexually transmitted disease clinics is rising steadily. In the UK there were 9576 new cases in 1979 and nearly 20 000 in 1984. According to Katchadourian (1985) the number of cases in the USA has increased amost 100-fold between 1966 and 1979 and an estimated 1 in 5 American adults has genital herpes.

Treatment with oral acyclovir is relatively effective in shortening an attack (Riley 1984).

Genital warts

Genital warts or condylomata acuminata, are caused by the papilloma virus and most commonly appear on the vulva, less often inside the vagina. They are unsightly and itch. Treatment is chemical (podophyllin) or by laser surgery.

Genital warts are also on the increase (in the UK there were 27 654 new cases in 1979; 49 884 in 1984; Communicable Diseases Scotland Weekly Report, 1986). As with genital herpes, the increase has been greater amongst women. The most important aspect of this virus is its assumed causative link with cervical dysplasia. Women who have been infected should have regular cervical screening. Although the overall death rate for cervical carcinoma has fallen, in women under 30 the death rate has increased fourfold, possibly reflecting the increase in genital warts.

Gonorrhoea

Gonococcus is typically transmitted sexually. It is a sensitive organism which does not flourish in the acidic vaginal environment, hence in women infection is initially in the cervical canal or urethra. Early gonococcal infection in women is usually symptomless, so that a woman may be an active carrier without realising it. Furthermore the infection can ascend the reproductive tract; salpingitis and pelvic inflammatory disease occurs in about 10% of cases, frequently leading to permanent infertility. In certain parts of the world gonococcal salpingitis is a major cause of infertility and declining birth rate. Acute pelvic infection can lead to various manifestations of the 'acute abdomen'. Pharyngeal and rectal gonococcal infections can also occur. The organism is usually sensitive to penicillin and hence gonorrhoea, if diagnosed, is highly treatable. In some countries however, due to casual use of antibiotics, penicillin-resistant strains of gonococcus are common.

Syphilis

The primary lesion of syphilis, the chancre, occurs on the genitals or perianal region. Though often noticeable, it is relatively symptomless and does not interfere with sexual activity. The significance of syphilitic infection is that it spreads rapidly through the body, causing a generalised infection and fever, usually associated with a rash. This occurs within 6 to 8 weeks of the appearance of the primary lesion. If untreated, this infectious second stage may continue in a remitting and relapsing fashion for 2 years or more. Thereafter the disease becomes latent and no longer contagious. Subsequently, and usually after many years, the tertiary stage presents itself as damage to the cardiovascular system or central nervous system or by the presence of gummatous tumours.

COMMON INFECTIONS IN MEN

Non-specific (i.e. non-gonococcal) urethritis

This presents with dysuria and purulent urethral discharge in which no gonococci can be found. The two organisms, *Chlamydia trachomatis* and *Ureaplasma urealyticum* are most commonly responsible. This condition is more difficult to eradicate than the gonococcal variety, and recurrences after intercourse are common.

Gonorrhoea

In the majority of cases of gonorrhoea in men, the infection is confined to the urethra, causing urethritis with dysuria and purulent discharge. Occasionally cystitis or prostatitis and generalised infection or arthritis may occur. In male homosexuals, anorectal infections are common. In general the consequences are more serious for the female than the male, though the initial infection is more obvious in the male.

Genital herpes

As in the female, ulcerating and sometimes extremely painful vesicles arise on the genitals, mainly the glans penis, and are likely to recur.

Trichomonas and Monilia

Trichomonas infections in men are usually asymptomatic, though urethritis may occur. Nevertheless, the success of treating the female patient is much enhanced if the male is also treated to prevent re-infection. Monilial infections in the male may cause itching and soreness of the penis.

Syphilis

The features of syphilitic infection are basically the same as for the female. The primary lesion, or chancre, is typically found on the penis or, in the case of homosexuals, at the anal margin.

Acquired immune deficiency syndrome (AIDS)

The story of AIDS started in 1981. Two reports appeared from California and New York of gay men with a rare and lethal form of pneumonia (*Pneumocystis carinii* or PCP) and/or Kaposi's sarcoma, a malignant condition of the skin. This was the start of an epidemic which is rapidly spreading worldwide.

It is now known that this condition is the result of a retrovirus which has attracted a variety of names since it was first identified. It is now most widely called HIV (human immune deficiency virus) but is sometimes referred to as HTLV–III (human T-lymphotrophic virus type III), LAV (lymphadenopathy-associated virus) or ARV (AIDS-related virus).

Retroviruses have the ability to incorporate a DNA copy of their RNA genome into the DNA of the host cell. Some retroviruses contain a DNA sequence which results in the rapid development of malignancy in the host. Some forms of leukaemia and lymphoma are caused in this way. The HIV virus infects a subset of peripheral lymphocytes, called the T helper cells, which play a crucial role in orchestrating the immune defences of the body. Infection with this virus therefore damages the immune system, leading to susceptibility to other pathogens, causing so-called 'opportunistic' infections. This immune defect also leads to certain kinds of tumour, notably Kaposi's sarcoma (Miller et al 1985).

The initial infection with HIV may cause an acute illness of glandular fever-type, though this may pass unnoticed (reminiscent of primary syphilis). Once established, infection with HIV is likely to go through various stages, often with a long latency before clinical manifestations are recognised.

The commonest early clinical manifestation is a persistent generalised lymphadenopathy (PGL) which is thought to be the direct result of HIV itself rather than opportunistic infection. The prognosis at that stage is very unclear; perhaps 5 to 25% will ultimately develop AIDS.

The AIDS-related complex (ARC) is infection with HIV leading to symptoms such as malaise, loss of weight, unexplained diarrhoea and fever, together with PGL, but without evidence of opportunistic infection or tumour formation.

This may give way in due course to full-blown AIDS which has three principal types of manifestation:

1. Opportunistic infection, mainly pulmonary (e.g. PCP) or gastrointestinal.
2. Kaposi's sarcoma (usually affecting the skin but sometimes arising in other organs).
3. AIDS encephalopathy, presenting a picture similar to pre-senile dementia and evident in up to 40% of AIDS sufferers.

Once full-blown AIDS with opportunistic infections has developed survival beyond 2 years is unlikely.

Mode of transmission

Up to now in the western world, and in particular in the USA the most important mode of transmission has been anal intercourse between gay men. Semen and blood can transmit the virus, but it is not yet clear whether oral ingestion of either fluid when infected causes transmission. Saliva and tears may contain the virus but as yet there is no evidence that transmission occurs via those body fluids.

On the African continent AIDS is spreading rapidly, predominantly by heterosexual intercourse. A high proportion of female prostitutes in some African countries have evidence of infection with HIV. As yet the real prevalence in Africa is unknown because of the lack of screening and diagnostic facilities. But the number of infected cases could be astronomical and growing.

Transmission by blood or blood products is another important cause of infection. Before this was realised a substantial number of haemophilia sufferers, both adults and children, became infected by their supplies of factor VIII, and some other cases resulted from infected blood transfusions. That source of infection should now have been eliminated. A further mode of transmission is by the sharing of needles and syringes by intravenous drug misusers. In Edinburgh 50% of intravenous drug misusers were found to have serological evidence of HIV infection. There is now evidence of a growing epidemic of AIDS amongst drug misusers in Europe (SHHD 1986). Many drug misusers not only have heterosexual partners but also resort to prostitution to finance their habit. They therefore present a serious source of infection for the heterosexual community.

There are several persisting mysteries about the transmission of HIV. Compared with other viruses, such as hepatitis B, infectivity is low. In spite of the fact that in the early days of the AIDS epidemic a viral cause was not suspected, infection as a result of laboratory, medical or nursing procedures has been virtually unknown. A recent case was reported of a nurse with a skin disease seroconverting after being splashed with the blood of an AIDS sufferer.

There is increasing evidence that amongst gay men it is receptive anal intercourse (Kingsley et al 1987), and in particular the more extreme forms of anal stimulation such as 'fisting' (see p. 322) which leads to transmission of the virus (see below). This has raised the possibility that tissue damage increases the risk of transmission either by facilitating entry of virus into the blood stream or by provoking the immune system in some way.

The female partners of infected men have shown a relatively low incidence of infection — though it has been estimated that such women become infected at a rate of 3–5% per year (SHHD 1986). However, as many as 50% of infants born to infected women are likely to be infected, with a high mortality.

A striking contrast to this picture is the predominantly heterosexual transmission in the African continent. Whereas in the UK the male proportion of cases is 96%, and in the USA 93%, in Africa the sex ratio is almost equal. The discrepancy has not yet been explained. A different virus is one not very likely possibility. Alternatively other genital infections (e.g. gonorrhoea) which might predispose to HIV infection, could be more prevalent in African women.

The classical epidemic growth rate of AIDS cases and deaths in the UK is shown in Figure 11.5. By May 1987, the World Health Organisation reported more than 43 000 cases throughout the world, with 31 382 of those in the USA. The stated figure of 2804 for Africa is almost certainly a gross underestimate, for reasons given earlier. The number of reported cases per

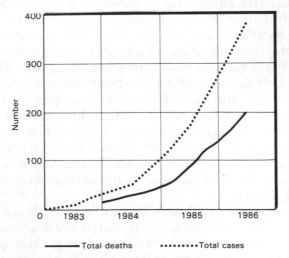

Fig. 11.5 Acquired immune deficiency syndrome (AIDS) total cases and deaths reported to the UK Communicable Disease Surveillance Centre. (from Griffin & Morris 1987)

million of population in 1985 was 48.4 in the USA, 9.7 in Switzerland, 7.0 in France and 3.1 in the UK (Griffin & Morris 1987).

Screening

Some time after the acute infection (which could be several months) antibodies appear in the blood. This is the basis of the serological screening for AIDS. The very low rate of positive tests in the large numbers screened as blood donors indicates that false positives are rare. But false negatives can occur, particularly if the screening is carried out too early after infection.

At the present time, the presence of positive serology has to be interpreted as evidence of infection and hence potential infectivity. A number of cohort studies of gay men show that when sero-positive individuals are followed, the annual incidence of clinical disease after a latent period of 2 to 3 years is up to 10% (SHHD 1986; Polk et al 1987).

Psychological consequences of AIDS and its impact on sexual behaviour

It is difficult to exaggerate the impact that AIDS has had on gay male communities. In areas such as California or New York, where the epidemic was first established, bereavement of lovers and friends is a recurring experience comparable to war time. Added to such losses is the fear of developing the disease and the often protracted and unique problem of living with and trying to support an AIDS sufferer who will surely die.

A further unique aspect of this epidemic is the problem of the individual who has positive HIV serology but no manifestations of the disease. He is in an extremely difficult situation. He may or may not develop the disease, and could do so several years hence. He may well be a source of infection to other people. Such difficulties, already affecting large numbers of gay men and many drug misusers, often require counselling help. The approach to such counselling has been well described by Miller et al (1985), including education about the virus and safe sex. The principles of safe sex were summarised by the authors as follows: reduce the number of partners — to one if possible; avoid anal sex altogether — if not, at least use a condom and extra lubrication, though that does not guarantee safety; do not transfer body fluids (e.g. 'deep kissing'); discuss safe sex guidelines with prospective partners; keep to body rubbing and mutual masturbation; have regular venereological screening.

Other important advice to seropositive men includes; do not give blood; do not carry an organ donor card; inform doctors and dentists, particularly when invasive procedures are being undertaken; do not have acupuncture, or share razors, toothbrushes or anything likely to be contaminated with blood; do not be shaved at the barbers; know what to do if blood is spilt (wash surface with 1 in 10 household bleach); do not share syringes or needles if injecting drugs.

Seropositive individuals can be reassured that there is no risk to others from casual contact, shaking hands, kissing on the cheek. The toilet, wash-basin and bath present no risk to others. The virus is not airborne and cannot be caught from cups, cutlery or crockery (Miller et al 1985).

In addition to the needs and anxieties of the seropositive individuals, there are also the 'worried well' — people who fear they may have contracted AIDS. This is not a new phenomenon; phobias about catching venereal disease have always occurred and are often particularly intractable and unhelped by reassurance and negative tests. We may nevertheless expect an increase in this particular form of neurotic reaction as a result of the AIDS scare.

There is already evidence that in the gay community sexual behaviour is changing as a result of the epidemic. McKusick et al (1985) surveyed 655 gay men in San Francisco regarding their sexual practices during the previous month and the same month one year previously. They were recruited from gay bathhouses, gay bars, and through gay organisations. The bathhouse group, probably those at highest risk, reported little change in their number of sexual partners. The other groups showed substantial reductions in casual sexual contacts, whereas men in monogamous relation-ships showed little change in sexual behaviour within their relationships. Martin (1985) assessed a cohort of 745 initially AIDS-free gay men, assessing their behaviour both before and after they became aware of the AIDS epidemic. Knowledge of AIDS was associated with a substantial reduction in the number of sexual partners and certain forms of sexual activity, in particular ingestion of semen (anally or orally), anal genital sex, oral–anal sex, and number of sexual partners. There was even a 50% reduction in sexual kissing. In a further longitudinal study in the Nether-lands (Tielman & van Grieusven 1985) a cohort of 750 gay men were assessed every 6 months. Indulgence in passive anal intercourse was found to be highly predictive of HIV positive serology, whereas mutual mastur-bation showed a negative association with positive serology. The number of partners was only a risk factor when it related to sexual techniques used (i.e. many partners only involving mutual masturbation would not increase the risk). More evidence of this kind will be emerging from the various cohort studies in the near future. The reduction in other kinds of sexually transmitted disease in gay men, referred to earlier, is additional though indirect evidence of a change in the pattern of gay male sexuality.

The impact of the AIDS epidemic on the heterosexual community is as yet much more difficult to assess. The British government's campaign to promote safe sex was clearly aimed at the heterosexual as well as the homosexual populations. But it may be that little change will occur amongst heterosexuals until there is more obvious evidence of spread of AIDS by heterosexual activity.

The social and sexual ramifications of AIDS will nevertheless be far-reaching. Already there is a greater preparedness to educate young people about sex. At the same time there is a hardening of prejudice and stigmatising attitudes towards homosexuality. It is nevertheless to be hoped that various benefits will emerge from this awful epidemic. Already gay communities are demonstrating exemplary and responsible community action. Attitudes to death and the dying, still a taboo subject for many, will be exposed and reappraised. We must hope that before long there will be effective methods of both prevention and cure, and we can at least expect that in searching for such methods we will learn a great deal of useful information about the defence systems of the human body.

Psychological and sexual implications of sexually transmitted diseases other than AIDS

Schofield (1977) has emphasised three distinguishing characteristics amongst those attending clinics for venereal infection: general social maladjustment, promiscuity without other obvious maladjustment and resort to occasional sexual contacts outside their stable relationships in those who are not promiscuous. In a random sample of men attending a special clinic in Australia, 16% had had more than three partners in the past 6 months, 31% had had casual partners but less than three in that period of time, 23% had regular partners with a recent episode of 'extramarital' intercourse and 28% only had sex with their regular partners (Pamnany 1980). Whereas syphilis and gonorrhoea are unlikely to be contracted without some new sexual contact, non-specific urethritis, trichomoniasis or moniliasis may develop within a stable sexual relationship. Nevertheless, the stigma associated with venereal disease may make attendance at a special clinics threatening for such non-promiscuous individuals, in spite of the use of clinic names such as 'genitourinary medicine'. It is difficult to escape from the implication of sexual misdemeanour. For those with regular partners who have had other contacts, there is likely to be considerable anxiety and guilt about the possibility of infecting one's partner or of the interpersonal crisis that may follow. The policy of contact tracing, whilst highly desirable for health care and usually carried out with considerable tact and sensitivity, nevertheless confronts the clinic attender with the interpersonal implications and may accentuate anxiety and guilt. The more promiscuous or socially irresponsible clinic attenders are said to be relatively unaffected by guilt or anxiety when attending these clinics (Schofield 1977).

In general, for those who attend a clinic at a reasonably early stage, concerns about the infections themselves are short-lived because of their treatability. Some infections, such as non-specific urethritis and genital herpes, may cause more psychological repercussions because of their frequently intractable and relapsing course.

Homosexuals present a special case. As discussed in Chapter 6, the homosexual world has provided opportunities for casual sex to an extent that is unusual for most heterosexuals. Although the incidence of homosexuality in the community is uncertain, homosexuals have featured disproportionately as clinic attenders and this proportion was rising (McMillan & Robertson 1977) until the recent AIDS-related decline. The pattern of infection reflects the nature of homosexual contact, with rectal and oral infections being relatively more common than amongst heterosexuals. What is difficult to explain is the link between homosexual contact and both syphilis (Morton 1977) and viral hepatitis B infections (Harris 1977).

In view of the rather chaotic sexual lives of many clinic attenders, it would not be surprising to find that sexual problems are common amongst those seeking treatment. Catalan et al (1981) found that one-fifth of males and about one-quarter of females attending a clinic for sexually transmitted diseases were experiencing sexual dysfunction of one kind or another. Although there was no comparison group in this study, such evidence that we have from other clinic and non-clinic populations (see Chapter 8) suggests that this group of patients is not particularly prone to sexual difficulties. Nor, on the basis of Pamnany's (1980) survey, do they appear to be unusually sexually active or likely to participate in unusual types of sexual practice.

Certain types of psychological problems may be peculiar to people attending these clinics. Phobias about catching venereal disease have already been mentioned. Rodin & Goldmeier (1976) described the 'Bangladeshi syndrome' affecting Bangladeshi men in the East End of London. These are usually young, married Muslims who have left their families in Bangladesh to come to this country and earn money. They commonly present with urethral discharge, noticeable mainly at the end of micturition or whilst straining at stool. Usually they do not show evidence of infection and Rodin & Goldmeier attribute this symptom to a 'physiological prostatovesicular overflow' stemming from their sexual continence. It is not clear whether this is a distinct entity, or whether this explanation has any validity, but these symptoms may be part of a more general tendency to preoccupation with sexual health that is common amongst Asian men.

Contraception and sexually transmitted diseases

It has been suggested that the increasing use of oral contraceptives has contributed to the rise in sexually transmitted diseases (Morton 1971). Three explanations for this link have been proposed. Oral contraception may increase the amount of sexual activity and numbers of partners involved. This issue was discussed more fully in Chapter 4 and the evidence was found to be unclear. But in any case, Juhlin & Lidén (1969) found that the incidence of gonorrhoea amongst their female patients was the same whether or not they were taking the pill. Oral contraceptives may, by altering the vaginal environment, increase the likelihood of pathogenic organisms being present. The best evidence on this issue, already mentioned (Goldacre et al 1979), does not support this suggestion though it is still possible that when present, pathogens are more likely to cause an acute infection. The use of oral contraceptives leads to a reduction in the use of barrier methods such as the condom which may also provide a barrier to infection. There is more evidence in support of this suggestion. Condoms used effectively do provide protection against transmission of infection (Ekstrøm 1970) and the use of condoms amongst those attending special clinics appears to be low ranging in different clinic studies from 3 to 20% (Pamnany 1980; see Chapter 12). This advantage of the condom is now being widely stressed in relation to AIDS. Whether oral contraceptives or other methods such as intrauterine devices influence the susceptibility to AIDS infection is an important question that has not yet been answered.

SEXUAL SIDE-EFFECTS OF THERAPEUTIC DRUGS

Much more attention has been paid to the sexual side-effects of drugs in the last few years. This is to be welcomed, as it is obviously a priority to minimise iatrogenic disability. Not only may distressing problems be avoided, but patients are more likely to use drug treatment properly if these aspects are satisfactorily managed. However, evaluation of this kind of drug effect is not easy. As yet, we have many case reports but very little substantial or relevant evidence. Such evidence that is available is largely confined to men. It is not clear whether women suffer less obvious sexual side-effects or that, more simply, they are not asked about them. Proper evaluation should be possible with appropriate methodology and provided that a number of complexities are taken into consideration. Most fundamental is the difficulty in attributing a sexual problem to a drug rather than to other causative factors. The basic disease for which the drug is prescribed may itself cause sexual problems not elicited in the pre-drug history. Psychological reactions to either the basic illness or its need for treatment may lead to sexual anxiety and failure in vulnerable individuals. The patient or doctor may prefer to blame a drug rather than be confronted with other possibly more threatening alternative explanations. Whilst it often helps to stop the drug and re-start it, the psychological reactions to the initial drug effect may continue after the drug is stopped and serve to keep the problem going (see Chapter 8).

In appraising the likelihood of a drug-induced sexual effect, the following questions should be asked:

1. What proportion of people taking the drug are affected in this way? The number of drugs for which there is good evidence of a high proportion affected is small. Much more commonly, we have evidence of assumed side-effects in a small proportion, say 5–10%. Obviously the higher the

proportion, the more likely it is that the drug is responsible. But we have to allow for the possibility of relatively idiosyncratic reactions to a drug, as well as for variability in the functional importance of a particular pharmacologically sensitive mechanism.

2. How specific is the observed effect? If interference with a discrete mechanism is repeatedly observed, a drug effect is more likely. The best example of this is the selective blocking of seminal emission by certain alpha adrenergic blockers, leaving orgasm, erection and sexual interest unaffected (see below). Unfortunately, it is unusual for investigators to ask sufficiently careful questions to distinguish between failure of emission and failure of orgasm. Inhibition of both could result from some central impairment of sexual arousability or even as a non-specific effect of general sedation. Erectile failure could be due to a peripheral or a central pharmacological effect or alternatively result from a psychological reaction to some other effect, such as ejaculatory failure. It is particularly difficult to distinguish between pharmacological and psychological mechanisms when loss of sexual interest is the problem.

3. Is there a pharmacological basis for the suspected drug effect? Here we are hampered by both our lack of understanding of the neurotransmitters involved in sexual response and the relatively mixed pharmacological action of so many modern drugs. Once again, we are on strongest ground with ejaculation in the male. The weight of evidence favours adrenergic mediation of seminal emission and the frequency of ejaculatory failure with adrenergic blocking drugs reinforces this view. But the neurotransmitters involved in orgasm in either the male or female are not known. Erection is also more complex in this respect than is often recognised. It has been widely assumed that erection depends on cholinergically mediated arteriolar dilatation. As a result, it is frequently asserted that anti-cholinergic drugs may impair erection. Yet is is difficult to find any evidence of such an effect. Wagner & Brindley (1980) demonstrated that erections to psychogenic and reflexive stimuli continued in normal men under the influence of atropine, probably the most potent anti-cholinergic drug in use. Ironically, there is much more evidence of erectile problems in men taking adrenergic blocking drugs, as we shall see.

As discussed in Chapter 2, understanding of the biochemical determinants of sexual appetite and central arousal is negligible. Whereas sex steroids are probably important, their effects are likely to be mediated by cerebral amines or other neurotransmitters. Drugs may therefore produce central effects by altering sex steroids or other hormones such as prolactin, or more directly by altering cerebral amines or neurotransmitter metabolism.

Such effects are made much more difficult to investigate by the pharmacological complexity of many modern drugs. Whilst there are some which have relatively specific anti-cholinergic or alpha or beta adrenergic blocking effects, many, particularly psychotropic and anti-depressant drugs, have much more complex pharmacological effects. Drugs also vary in the extent to which they cross the blood–brain barrier.

With these unavoidable complexities, we should not expect straightforward evidence, and as yet there is very little to find. But with greater attention to these details we can justifiably expect more satisfactory evidence in the future. Let us in the meantime review some of the available evidence, concentrating on those drugs which have been commonly implicated.

DRUGS USED FOR THE TREATMENT OF HYPERTENSION

Bulpitt et al (1976) compared three groups of men: hypertensives receiving hypotensive drug treatment, hypertensives before receiving any treatment and normotensive controls. The proportions reporting erectile impotence in each group were 24.6, 17.1 and 6.9% respectively. There were significantly more impotent men in the treated hypertensive group than amongst the controls; the untreated group came midway but was not significantly different from either. Ejaculatory failure was reported by 25.6, 7.3 and 0% respectively. The treated group showed significantly more ejaculatory problems than either of the other two. From this evidence it seems likely that ejaculatory problems result from drug treatment, whereas erectile problems could result either from the hypertension itself or from the treatment. Erectile problems may result not only from the pharmacological effect of the drug but also from the lowering of blood pressure if it falls below that necessary to maintain supply through narrowed vessels in the erectile tissues. Erectile failure is also more likely than ejaculatory failure to result from psychological factors.

Comparing the incidence of sexual problems with the pharmacological characteristics of the drug proves to be informative. Ganglion blockers such as hexamethonium or pentolinium, which block both sympathetic and parasympathetic post-ganglionic fibres, predictably produce complete erectile and ejaculatory failure. They are seldom used now except for the management of acute hypertensive crises. Adrenergic neurone blocking drugs, such as guanethidine or bethanidine, depress the function of post-ganglionic adrenergic nerves, affecting both alpha and beta mechanisms. Their use is associated with erectile problems in 40–67% and ejaculatory problems in 40–79% of patients (Pritchard et al 1968; Bulpitt & Dollery 1973). Unfortunately in these studies it was not established whether failure of ejaculation was also associated with failure of orgasm. Money & Yankowitz (1967) however described clearly the occurrence of orgasm without ejaculation in men taking guanethidine.

Methyldopa is a different form of hypertensive agent which has marked central as well as peripheral anti-adrenergic effects. Erectile and ejaculatory problems occur significantly less often than with the adrenergic neurone blockers (Pritchard et al 1968; Bulpitt & Dollery 1973) but loss of libido has been reported in up to 25% of men and women using this drug, depending on the dosage involved (Kolodny et al 1979). This would be consistent with the central effect but also may be secondary to a general sedating effect; tiredness is the commonest side-effect with this drug. The adrenergic neurone blocking drugs are seldom used nowadays, and methyldopa is also being used less often.

Beta adrenergic blockers (e.g. propanolol) are probably the most widely used hypotensives at the present time. The occurrence of side-effects is much less with these drugs. Warren & Warren (1977) reported 5 out of 95 men taking 120 mg or more propanolol daily who had erectile failure, though they were not able to show convincingly that the drug was to blame. Idiosyncratic reactions may have been involved however. Riley (1980a) describes a man who experienced erectile failure within two days of starting propanolol which was reversed as quickly on stopping the drug. He reacted similarly to further propanolol, but not to acebutolol. Both drugs are beta blockers but only propanolol crosses the blood–brain barrier, suggesting that in this case erectile problems resulted from some central pharmacological effect. Labetolol is a hypotensive drug that acts by both alpha and beta blockade. Riley & Riley (1983) in controlled studies with volunteers have demonstrated that it increases the time taken to reach orgasm in women and ejaculation in men, without affecting erection in the male subjects.

In a multicentred study of hypertensive treatment, sexual side-effects were somewhat more common with the diuretic used bendrofluaside than with the beta blocker (propanolol) (Medical Research Council Working Party 1981).

Alpha blockers have not been blamed for erectile problems, but may interfere with ejaculation. Dibenzyline, an early alpha blocker used for hypertension, was liable to block ejaculation (Green & Berman 1954). More recently, indoramin, an alpha blocker used not only for hypertension but also for asthma and migraine, has been reported to interfere with ejaculation in two-thirds of men using it, whereas in the same study, no such effect was produced by clonidine or placebo. In this study, all men affected described normal erections and orgasms in spite of the ejaculatory failure (Pentland et al 1981).

Sexual problems have been attributed to other hypotensive agents such as clonidine, reserpine, and even diuretics. But as yet the evidence is far from conclusive. Spironolactone has also been implicated as causing loss of libido in men and menstrual irregularities in women. This could be related to interference with androgen function or to some progestational effects (Kolodny et al 1979).

Further systematic studies of these various effects will not only be valuable for the clinical management of the hypotensive patient, but may also throw further light on sexual physiology.

PSYCHOTROPIC DRUGS

Drugs used to influence psychological states are particularly difficult to evaluate from the sexual point of view. The psychological states for which they are prescribed are likely to have sexual repercussions and most of the drugs used today have a rich mixture of pharmacological actions. Psychotropic drugs can be considered under three broad headings – minor tranquillisers, sedatives and hypnotics; major tranquillisers; anti-depressants.

Minor tranquillisers, sedatives and hypnotics

The benzodiazepines are the most commonly used drugs in this category, both as tranquillisers (e.g. chlordiazepoxide, diazepam) and hypnotics (e.g. nitrazepam). Riley & Riley (1986), in a placebo-controlled study of normal volunteers, found that a single dose of diazepam delayed orgasm in women. It is not known whether this effect would occur in anxious women. Barbiturates are seldom prescribed as sedatives nowadays except for short-term use. They will be considered further under the sections on anticonvulsants and drug of addiction.

Major tranquillisers

The principal groups of drugs in this category are the phenothiazines and butyrophenones, used for more severe states of agitation or psychotic disturbance. Impairment of sexual interest has often been noted in patients using these drugs, but usually it is difficult to distinguish between a specific or non-specific drug effect and the condition being treated. Fluphenazine enanthate, a long-acting phenothiazine, has been advocated as a drug suitable for controlling unwanted sexual behaviour (Bartholomew 1968) though without adequate controlled evidence of its efficacy. Thioridazine, a piperidine phenothiazine, has frequently been reported as blocking ejaculation (Kotin et al 1976). With usual therapeutic doses, the commonest effect is increased time before orgasm occurs, followed by a normal orgasm but without ejaculation. With lower doses, only the delay is experienced (Segraves 1977). (Comparable effects in women have also been reported (Segraves 1985).) This is likely to be a specific drug effect. It has been suggested that it is due to retrograde ejaculation into the bladder, resulting from drug interference with sphincter control. However, no evidence of sperm in the post-orgasm urine has been found in such cases (Kedia & Markland 1975) and a direct inhibition of emission is more likely.

Benperidol is a butyrophenone which is marketed specifically for controlling unwanted sexual behaviour. In one controlled study, it was found to reduce self-rated sexual interest more than either chlorpromazine or placebo, though it did not alter the psychophysiological responses to erotic stimuli (Tennent et al 1974). As yet, there is no convincing evidence that other butyrophenones, such as haloperidol or triperidol, which are commonly used as major tranquillisers, produce the same effects.

Phenothiazines are dopamine antagonists and alpha adrenergic blockers as well as having anti-histaminic and anti-cholinergic effects. It is thus difficult, if not impossible to account for any observed sexual effects on the basis of their pharmacological characteristics. The inhibition of ejaculation could, for example, be a peripheral alpha adrenergic blockade or a central dopamine blockade (Segraves 1979). Butyrophenones have similar pharmacological effects to phenothiazines, though probably with less anti-adrenergic, anti-histaminic and anti-cholinergic effects. Both groups of drugs may cause a rise in prolactin, presumably as a consequence of their dopamine antagonism. As discussed in Chapter 2, the effects of prolactin on sexual function are not understood but an association between hyperprolactinaemia and impaired sexual appetite is well described in men and may also occur in women (Jacobs 1979). Galactorrhoea and menstrual irregularities, probably due to a prolactin rise, do occur in some patients using either phenothiazines or butyrophenones (Beumont et al 1974). The reduction of sexual interest produced by benperidol (Tennent et al 1974) was not associated with any alteration in plasma testosterone or luteinising hormone (prolactin assays were not available at that time). The pattern of behavioural effects produced by benperidol was similar to those produced by cyproterone acetate and ethinyloestradiol in a parallel study, though the endocrine effects were different (Murray et al 1975). It is possible that the basic mechanism of all these drugs depends on an alteration of cerebral amine action, with benperidol altering this directly, and the anti-androgen and oestrogen indirectly via the steroid modulation of cerebral amines (see Chapter 2).

Anti-depressants

There are two principal types of anti-depressant — the monoamine oxidase inhibitors (e.g. phenelzine, tranylcypromine) and the tricyclics (e.g. imipramine, amitryptyline).

Monoamine oxidase inhibitors (MAOIs), as the name suggests, lead to increased concentrations of cerebral amines in the brain (i.e. noradrenaline, dopamine and 5-hydroxytryptamine (5HT); see p. 122) though it is not clear to what extent these changes account for their anti-depressant effects. Some, like tranylcypromine, have additional amphetamine-like effects. The most convincing sexual effect of these drugs is ejaculatory failure, probably similar to that produced by adrenergic blocking drugs, or thioridazine. Also a number of case reports have been published of women using MAOIs having difficulty achieving orgasm (Segraves 1985). It has been suggested that this effect is more likely with the irreversible hydrazine inhibitors, such as phenelzine, than with the reversible inhibitors such as tranylcypromine (Rees 1983).

The tricyclic anti-depressants have pharmacological properties similar to the phenothiazines, with additional effects in inhibiting presynaptic uptake of cerebral amines which may account for their anti-depressant action. The pharmacological nature of this uptake inhibition varies from one anti-depressant to another. The most carefully controlled evaluation of the effects of anti-depressants on sexual function was reported by Harrison et al (1985). They studied 36 men and 47 women who were clinically depressed. Each person received phenelzine, imipramine or placebo, in increasing dosage. Decrease in sexual function occurred in 8% of men and 16% of women on placebo, 80% of men and 57% of women on phenelzine and 50% of men and 27% of women on imipramine. For men the differences between active drug and placebo were significant for both anti-depressants; for women, only for phenelzine.

Clomipramine has received special attention in this respect. Everitt (1979) found that the sexuality of female rhesus macaques was 'switched off and on' within 3 days of starting and stopping clomipramine. This anti-depressant is regarded as an inhibitor of re-uptake of 5HT as well as noradrenaline. This results in the accumulation of 5HT and noradrenaline at the synapse and a prolongation of the post-synaptic effect. As discussed in Chapter 2, there is some evidence from subprimates that 5HT inhibits sexuality in males and females. A comparable effect could be operating in these rhesus monkeys and may also be relevant to human subjects. But, once again, the best documented effect of clomipramine is inhibition of ejaculation or inhibition of female orgasm (Segraves 1985), and it is not clear how the above pharmacological processes could account for that.

OTHER DRUGS

Anti-convulsants

As described earlier in this chapter, sexual problems, particularly those stemming from lack of interest, are common amongst epileptics. Endocrine effects of anti-convulsants, including phenobarbitone, have been recognised. These probably stem mainly from enzyme induction effects in the liver which alter the metabolism of steroids and may lead to increased production of sex hormone-binding globulin. Several studies have shown that raised sex hormone-binding globulin levels are common in epileptics taking most types of anti-convulsants and are usually associated with increased total testosterone as well as luteinising hormone, sometimes to very high levels (Victor et al 1977; Barragry et al 1978; Toone et al 1980). There is now evidence that free testosterone is lowered in some cases, in spite of normal or raised total testoterone, and lack of desire or impairment of sleep erections is related to these low free T levels (Toone et al 1983; Fenwick et al 1986). Carbamazepine, an anti-convulsant which does not have this effect on testosterone levels, appears to be relatively free from such adverse sexual effects (see p. 573).

Hormones

The effects of hormones used therapeutically are discussed elsewhere in this volume (see Chapter 2).

Digoxin. This cardiac glycoside may produce endocrine changes. Raised levels of oestradiol and lowered levels of testosterone and luteinising hormone have been reported in men taking digoxin (Stoffer et al 1973; Neri et al 1987). In one study, 14 men on long-term digoxin therapy were compared with 12 men of similar age and cardiac functional capacity. The digoxin users had significantly raised oestradiol and lowered testosterone and luteinising hormone and also reported significantly greater reduction in sexual interest and sexual activity (Neri et al 1980). This was replicated in a further study (Neri et al 1987).

Metoclopramide. This is a dopamine receptor antagonist used as an antiemetic and for other upper gastrointestinal tract disorders. As a result of its anti-dopaminergic effect prolactin levels are raised. In one study of five normal volunteers, metoclopramide was administered for 6 weeks. Four of the five men reported decrease in libido and three, loss of spontaneous erections. This was an uncontrolled study and no details were given of how the sexual effects were measured. If, however, there was a genuine drug effect, it remains uncertain whether it was a direct result of dopamine antagonism or of the raised prolactin (Falaschi et al 1978).

Cimetidine. This drug is a histamine H2 receptor antagonist which is widely used for the treatment of peptic ulceration. A few reports of sexual side-effects have appeared (e.g. Peden et al 1979; Wolfe 1979) but as yet the evidence is inconclusive. However, the endocrine effects of cimetidine are complex and as yet ill-understood and may prove to be relevant to sexual side-effects. Anti-androgenic activity has been demonstrated in rodents, though such effects have not been convincingly shown in humans so far. Gynaecomastia does occur, however, in a proportion of subjects (Riley 1980b). In view of the wide use of this drug, often for inadequately defined clinical indications, it is important that these possible side-effects should be properly studied.

Fenfluramine, an anorectic drug which releases 5HT, is associated with reduced sexual desire in as many as 85% of women taking it. (Pinder et al 1982).

DRUGS THAT MAY ENHANCE SEXUAL EXPERIENCE

The search for an effective aphrodisiac has a very long history. Our erotic susceptibility to suggestion has created the impression of effectiveness of a variety of substances, but as yet no such effect has been convincingly demonstrated.

Observations that parkinsonian patients reported increased sexual appete when treated with L-dopa created a certain interest. As yet no specific sexual effects of L-dopa have been demonstrated in humans (Everitt 1979) but such an effect is compatible with animal evidence that in males dopamine facilitates sexual behaviour; L-dopa is a precursor of dopamine (see Chapter 2). Conversely, 5HT is believed to have sexual inhibiting effects and there is some evidence that drugs which block synthesis of 5HT from tryptophan, such as PCMA (p-chloromethamphetamine) or PCPA (p-chlorophenylalanine) increase sexual activity at least in the presence of androgens (Everitt 1979). Benkert (1973) failed to demonstrate any such effects in men in a controlled comparison with placebo, however. Such drugs, particularly PCMA, are potentially neurotoxic, so it is unlikely that we will get more human evidence of this kind until a safer specific 5HT inhibitor is available.

Amylnitrite, a vasodilator used principally for angina, is said to enhance the orgasmic experience of some men and women but there is no convincing evidence to support this claim and the drug is not without its risks.

Cocaine and marijuana have been claimed to enhance sexual desire in some users; these will be considered in the section on drugs of addiction.

SEXUAL ASPECTS OF ALCOHOL AND DRUG ADDICTION

ALCOHOL AND ALCOHOLISM

Beliefs about the relationship between alcohol and sex are widespread. Many regard alcohol in moderate doses as an aphrodisiac, or at least a disinhibitor that allows one's natural sexual feelings freer expression. In the Psychology Today survey (Athanasiou et al 1970), 45% of male and 68% of female respondents said that alcohol enhanced their sexual enjoyment; 42% and 21% respectively said that it decreased enjoyment. The apparent difference between men and women was taken to support the notions that alcohol reduces sexual inhibition and women are more often inhibited than men. Klassen & Wilsnack (1986) reported a 1981 national survey of drinking and sexuality amongst 917 American women: 60% said that alcohol made them feel less inhibited sexually; 45% found alcohol made sex more pleasurable and in 62% it made them feel closer to their drinking partner. Only 22% said they became 'sexually forward' when drinking, whereas 60% said that someone else had been sexually aggressive towards them whilst drinking. The lighter drinkers and abstainers were more likely to report apparent 'traditional sexuality'.

It is also widely believed that however much alcohol may enhance sexual desire, too much will impair performance. Men may therefore be more susceptible because of their vulnerability to erectile failure. Masters & Johnson (1970) emphasised the importance of alcohol in causing secondary erectile impotence. Typically, an episode of acute alcohol intoxication results in erectile failure, which then generates performance anxiety which may be compounded by the use of further alcohol to lessen the anxiety. What should have been a transient pharmacological interference with erectile function becomes established as psychogenic impotence in a susceptible individual. Masters & Johnson (1970) identified this process in 16% of their cases of secondary impotence. In Klassen & Wilsnack's (1986) survey of women, the moderate drinkers had lower levels of sexual dysfunction than either the light or heavy drinking groups. The heavy drinkers had the highest rates of lifetime lack of sexual interest and orgasm.

Although it is commonly assumed that chronic alcoholics have a high incidence of sexual problems, good evidence to support this is hard to find. Lemere & Smith (1973) state that of 17 000 alcoholics treated in their centre, 'at least 8% of males were impotent and in approximately 50% of these the impotence persisted after years of sobriety'. This does not sound like a high incidence, but no details were given of how they arrived at these figures and at best they should be regarded as a rough estimate. Whalley (1978) compared 50 hospitalised male alcoholics with 50 controls, matched for age and social class and recruited through a trade union. Significantly more of the alcoholics (54%) reported erectile problems than did the controls (28%) but this was based on the question 'Have you ever suffered from erectile impotence?'. The numbers who had more or less permanent impotence were not given. There was no difference in the two groups in reported loss of libido. The alcoholics did indicate significantly less satisfaction with their sexual relationships. Jensen (1979) gave questionnaires to 100 male alcoholics attending a treatment centre; 63% reported sexual problems. Types of sexual problems were not clearly defined but difficulties with erection and reduced libido seemed to be the commonest. There is even less systematically collected evidence about sexual problems amongst female alcoholics.

The relationship between chronic alcoholism and sexuality is complex. The reasons for abusing alcohol in the first place may be important. In some cases, alcohol is used to cope with sociosexual anxieties in people who are prone to develop sexual problems for personality reasons. What proportion of alcoholics comes into this category is not known and not easy to establish. The consequences of alcoholism on sexual relationships and marriage are likely to be considerable. Not only may marital and sexual conflict result from heavy drinking, but the development of such conflict will have an adverse effect on the subsequent drinking pattern (Orford et al 1976); alcoholics often drink to cope with the problems produced by their alcoholism. The sexual relationship is bound to suffer in many such cases and marital breakdown is high amongst alcoholics.

Against this background of psychological and interpersonal complexity, we need to consider not only the pharmacological effects of alcohol intoxication on sexual function, but also the more long-term toxic effects of alcohol on the nervous system, liver and endocrine system and their sexual consequences.

The pharmacological effects of alcohol

Alcohol is a central nervous system depressant that impairs sensorimotor performance in a dose-related manner (Wallgren & Barry 1970). It is widely assumed that the so-called disinhibiting sexual effect of alcohol derives from a modest depressant effect of low doses, and a failure of genital response from the depressant effects of higher doses. Fortunately we have a valuable series of experiments, well reviewed by Wilson (1977, 1984), that address this issue. Farkas & Rosen (1976) measured erectile response to erotic films in male social drinkers, varying the dose level of alcohol so that mean blood alcohol concentrations (BACs) of 0, 25, 50 and 75 mg% were obtained. They found a slight though non-significant facilitation of erection with the low (25 mg) BAC but thereafter a progressive decline in erectile response with increasing alcohol concentration. These results are at least consistent with the disinhibition effect of moderate alcohol doses described above. Briddell & Wilson (1976) in a comparable experiment achieved slightly different BACs (0, 35, 67.5 and 95 mg%) and also attempted to manipulate expectancies. Half of the subjects were told that alcohol would enhance their response, half that it would impair it. They found no significant expectancy effect, and no apparent facilitation of erection at low doses, which they attributed to the dose being slightly higher than that in the first study. Wilson & Lawson (1976a) then carried out a similar experiment with female social drinkers with similar results. Using vaginal photometry as an indicator of vaginal response to erotic films, they found the response to be diminished with increasing levels of blood alcohol (0, 26, 49 and 79 mg%). Of additional interest was the finding that in spite of this decrement of physiological response, the women tended both to predict and subsequently to report higher levels of sexual arousal with increasing levels of alcohol intoxication. It is possible that whereas a man's expectation of a sexual enhancing effect of alcohol is going to be rudely challenged at high dose levels by a very tangible failure of erection, such expectation in a woman will be less challenged because her genital responses are less tangible, particularly with the blurred perception of alcohol intoxication.

Wilson & Lawson (1976b) then proceeded with a crucial experiment. They divided their male subjects into two expectancy groups, one expecting that they would receive alcohol (vodka and tonic), the other that they would receive tonic only. Half of each group were then given a standard dose of vodka and tonic and half were given tonic only — in other words in half of each group their expectations were met and in half they were not. The average BAC obtained was about 40 mg%. In this study there was no apparent effect of alcohol on erection, whereas those who thought they were taking alcohol showed stronger erections than those who thought they were only drinking tonic. If we accept this evidence, it suggests that the disinhibition effect of alcohol is not pharmacologically induced but results from the individual's learned expectations of alcohol effects. Wilson (1977) went further and suggested that this assumed pharmacological effect of alcohol may be used to justify bebaviour which would be unacceptable in a sober state. This was further supported by a study of Briddell et al (1978) in which male social drinkers listened to different types of erotic tapes, including descriptions of mutually enjoyable heterosexual intercourse and forcible rape. Subjects who *believed* they had consumed alcohol showed higher levels of erectile response to the rape stimulus than those who believed they had not. The authors concluded: 'These findings suggest that normal males who have been drinking (or believe they have been drinking) may exhibit sexual arousal patterns indistinguishable from those reported for identified rapists' (see p. 686). Other studies have suggested that this effect of belief about drinking is most marked in individuals with high sex guilt (Wilson 1984). These findings are relevant to sexual offences committed under the influence of alcohol (see Chapter 13) and may also be relevant to understanding the effects of other pharmacological agents on sexuality.

Alcohol also increases, in a dose–response fashion, the latency to ejaculation in men and orgasm in women (Malatesta et al 1979, 1982). Interestingly, the men also reported decreased subjective arousal, reduced pleasure and less intense orgasm as the dose levels increased. By contrast, the women, whilst experiencing longer latencies to orgasm, reported greater sexual arousal and more enjoyable orgasm with higher dose levels.

The direct pharmacological inhibiting effect of alcohol on genital and orgasmic responses would appear, on the basis of these various studies, to arise at blood alcohol levels higher than 40 mg%.

Apart from possibly direct effects on sexual responses, alcohol may also inhibit sexual arousal by impairing the cognitive processes that mediate arousal (Wilson 1984).

Male chronic alcoholics were tested by Wilson et al (1978) and were found to show the same susceptibility to erectile failure at higher blood levels of alcohol. Tolerance, therefore, does not apparently protect against these negative effects. The chronic alcoholic, however, may have to contend with less reversible consequences of alcohol either on the nervous or endocrine systems.

Long-term toxic effects of alcohol

A variety of effects of long-term alcohol abuse on the central nervous system have been described (Lees 1967). The commonest neurological manifestation, however, is peripheral neuropathy. The aetiological mechanisms are not properly understood but, at least in some cases, thiamine deficiency is a contributory factor. Peripheral neuropathy may affect sexual function directly by impairing sensory input and hence tactile erotic sensitivity. Autonomic nerves may also be damaged (Novak & Victor 1974) and this could result in the same type of impairment of erection and ejaculation that occurs with diabetic autonomic neuropathy.

The endocrine effects of alcohol are complex and have been reviewed by Van Thiel & Lester (1979). Either alcohol or its principal metabolite acet-aldehyde are toxic to the testis. After intoxication sufficient to produce a hangover, plasma testosterone was decreased to 20% of control values within 12 to 20 hours after ingestion (Ylikahri et al 1974). Mendelson et al (1977) showed that in non-problem drinkers, as blood alcohol levels rose, plasma testosterone fell whilst luteinising hormone remained unchanged. With the highest levels of alcohol the luteinising hormone rose, indicating that the alcohol was having its effect on the testis, not the hypothalamo-pituitary axis. If such lowering of testosterone levels is prolonged, then it is conceivable that an impairment of sexual interest could result. As yet there is no evidence directly linking the two phenomena.

Similar toxic effects may also occur in women. Ovarian atrophy is commonly found at autopsy in the female alcoholic (Van Thiel & Lester 1979) and may be related to the menstrual irregularity and infertility that are common amongst such women. Altered steroid production may affect women's vaginal responsiveness or appetite but as yet relevant information is lacking.

More permanent testicular damage does occur in men, leading to testicu-lar atrophy and the usual signs of hypogonadism. More common is a finding of raised oestrogen and lowered testosterone with raised sex hormone-binding globulin. This may be associated with gynaecomastia and certainly could lead to loss of sexual interest if sufficiently marked. The precise mechanisms are not understood. Alcohol-induced liver disease is also common and in the past it has been assumed that the liver damage is responsible for the endocrine changes in alcoholism. Whilst this is likely to be relevant in some cases, it is now doubted that this is the usual expla-nation (Van Thiel & Lester 1979).

MARIJUANA

Marijuana is commonly regarded as a sexually enhancing drug. There is a definite association between marijuana use and early onset of sexual activity amongst young people (Goode 1972; Plant 1975). But this is likely to reflect some common determinant, such as a more liberal attitude, than any causal link between the two. As with alcohol, many marijuana users see the drug as enhancing their sexual experiences. In the Psychology Today survey (Athanasiou et al 1970), about 25% of the total sample had experienced intercourse under the influence of marijuana and four-fifths of these reported increased enjoyment. Plant (1975) concluded from his interviews of English drug-takers that the main effect reported was a reduction of inhibition. Kolodny et al (1979) reported that of the marijuana users seen at their institute, 83% of men and 81% of women experienced enhanced sexual enjoyment. However, the positive effects described were not increased desire or improved erections or orgasm, but rather 'an increased sense of touch, a greater degree of relaxation (both physically and mentally) and being more in tune with one's partner'. Also, if their partner wasn't 'high' at the same time, the effect was if anything unpleasant or disruptive. They also found a relatively high incidence of impotence (20%) in men using marijuana on a daily basis.

As with alcohol, it is difficult to distinguish between genuine pharmacological effects and expectation. On balance, evidence of a pharmacological enhancing effect on sexuality is lacking (Taberner 1985). Long-term adverse effects on sexual function may be related to endocrine changes. Although there is some contradictory evidence, Kolodny et al (1979) reviewed several studies showing lowered testosterone and inhibited spermatogenesis in men and lowered gonadotrophins and altered menstrual cycles in women.

OPIATES

People addicted to heroin and opiates present a similarly complex picture of background factors and secondary social and intrapersonal problems as is found with chronic alcoholics. Many have had major intrapersonal problems and sexual difficulties prior to their addiction. Those with established addiction may use sexual encounters as a means of making money to obtain drugs. Nevertheless, there is much more consistent evidence that opiates, particularly heroin and morphine, have a marked inhibiting effect on both male and female sexuality, often demonstrated by a noticeable improvement sexually once the drugs have been withdrawn, or the addict moves on to a less inhibiting drug, such as methadone. There is also an interesting parallel, if only symbolic, between the 'high' and following calm of the intravenous opiate experience and the sexual orgasmic experience that it appears to replace.

Cushman (1972) studied four groups of men: heroin addicts, addicts maintained on methadone, abstainers and controls. The heroin addicts claimed normal sexual function before becoming addicted, but two-thirds of them reported reduced sexual drive, two-thirds a delay in ejaculation time beyond 25 minutes and nearly half some erectile difficulty whilst on heroin. These problems usually disappeared as the drug was withdrawn, leading to striking increases in sexual activity. Similar improvement occurred in those moving from heroin to methadone maintenance, through delayed ejaculation often persisted. Gossop et al (1974) found slightly more sexual disturbance in female narcotic addicts than males, though the difference was not significant. Mintz et al (1974) found that opiate addicts were likely to report premature ejaculation during drug-free periods. It was not clear if this was a withdrawal effect or represented their usual response. This study also found that erectile problems and delayed ejaculation were common during both heroin and methadone use, though less severe with the latter.

Because of the consistency of this inhibitory effect, and the apparent rebound of sexuality after opiate withdrawal, the underlying mechanism is of considerable theoretical interest. Evidence of endocrine effects of opiate addiction is somewhat conflicting. Some studies have found lowered plasma testosterone and gonadotrophin levels, whilst others have found no such effect (Kolodny et al 1979). More recently Carani et al (1986) found lowered *free* testosterone in young male heroin addicts and this could contribute to the loss of sexual desire. In women, amenorrhoea and infertility are common (Bai et al 1974; Santen et al 1975). A direct inhibiting effect of opiates on sexual response has been suggested by the finding of spontaneous erections in normal men taking opiate antagonists (see p. 126 and Mendelson et al 1979).

Cocaine

Cocaine is rapidly increasing in importance as a drug of abuse. It has a complicated and unusual pharmacological action, combining local anaesthetic and central stimulant properties. Its principal action within the central nervous system is to prevent the re-uptake of noradrenaline. This is assumed to be the basis for the increased mental activity, restlessness and euphoria that cocaine produces. In spite of the widely held belief that cocaine enhances sexual performance or pleasure, there is no evidence to support the idea. In fact chronic cocaine use seems to be commonly associated with loss of sexual desire as well as other adverse effects on health and well-being (Taberner 1985).

Other drugs

The effects of amphetamine addiction on sexuality are not clear. Bell & Trethowan (1961) found that most of a small series of amphetamine users had some form of sexual problem, though it was not clear to what extent this resulted from amphetamine use. Gossop et al (1974) found that female amphetamine users showed significantly more sexual difficulties than male users. Amphetamine is a dopamine releaser and there is some evidence from lower animals that dopamine facilitates male sexual behaviour and female proceptive sexuality (see Chapter 2).

LSD has attracted unsubstantiated claims that it has sexually enhancing effects. Kolodny et al (1979) found that of 85 men and 55 women passing through their institute who had used LSD on three or more occasions, less than 15% of each sex reported any such effects.

SEXUAL PROBLEMS IN PSYCHIATRIC ILLNESS

It is often assumed that sexual problems lie in the province of the psychiatrist. In many medical schools, the psychiatric department takes responsibility for teaching human sexuality. Often sexual problem clinics are based in psychiatric departments. In spite of this the association between sexual problems and psychiatric illness has not been well studied. To what extent do people suffering from psychiatric illness experience sexual difficulties? Conversely, do people with sexual problems have a greater likelihood of psychiatric illness?

Crisp (1979) has presented a rough assessment of the presence of sexual deterioration in a group of 375 consecutive new psychiatric outpatients. He found that people with endogenous depression, alcoholism, or the presence of anxious or sad moods or tension were significantly more likely to report a reduction of sexual activity since the onset of their problem, whereas those with conversion hysteria, obsessional neurosis or paranoid psychosis were significantly less likely to do so.

As yet there is very little systematic evidence of the incidence of psychiatric problems in patients attending sexual problem clinics. The relevance of neuroticism to sexual difficulties was discussed in Chapter 8 and the relationship between anxiety, anger and sexual response looked at in some detail. Depression remains an important issue. Watson (1979) estimated that 30% of women and 14% of men attending his sexual problem clinic had a present or past psychiatric illness, usually affective in type.

DEPRESSION AND SEXUALITY

Beck (1967) found that loss of sexual interest was reported by 61% of severe depressives compared with 27% non-depressed controls. In factor analytic studies of depressive phenomenology, he found that loss of libido tended to be associated with fatiguability, loss of appetite, weight loss and insomnia and he inferred that the sexual change was part of a more general biological component. Cassidy et al (1957) found that in a group of patients suffering from manic depressive psychosis, sexual activity had decreased in 63% compared with 39% of medically sick, non-depressed controlled subjects. Reduced libido affected 83% of the depressed males and 53% of the females. Sexual dysfunction, such as erectile impotence, occurs less commonly. Woodruff et al (1967) found impotence in 23% of men with a primary affective disorder. Mathew & Weinman (1982) found significantly more loss of sexual interest in a group of drug-free depressed men and women than in their control group. They did not find differences in genital dysfunctions. More recently, Schreiner-Engel & Schiavi (1986) studied men and women with low sexual desire as their primary problem. They found that although not depressed at the time of assessment, the low sexual desire group had a significantly higher incidence of depressive illness in the past. Also the initial episode of depressive disorder almost always coincided with or preceded the onset of loss of sexual desire. Sleep erections have also been shown to be impaired in depressed men (Roose et al 1982; Thase et al 1987).

An association between depressed mood and reduced sexual appetite is not surprising. In Chapter 2, we considered mood change during the menstrual cycle. Women's self-ratings of sexuality are influenced by their general feelings of well-being (Sanders et al, 1983). Sexuality is most readily expressed at times when the individual is feeling generally well. The presence of negative thoughts about self and low self-esteem is likely to lower the individual's sense of sexual worth. This is presumably a non-specific effect and we should expect it to operate during more prolonged states of depressed mood. There may however be a more specific link. As yet, the biochemical basis of mood change, whether of the normal variety during the menstrual cycle, or the more severe kinds in depressive illness, is not understood, though there is no shortage of biochemical theories. A common biochemical change in cerebral amine function may link mood with sexuality, but as yet we can only speculate on its nature.

Depression is also commonly related to marital problems and in many of these the sexual relationship may be disturbed or may be the main cause of the marital difficulty. In such cases, we should expect a depressed mood to arise as a reaction to the sexual or marital problem. As discussed on page 605, the picture is further complicated by the sexual side-effects of drugs used to treat depression.

Occasionally depressed people show a paradoxical increase in sexual activity. This reaction has not been well documented and may reflect more of an anxious search for reassurance or intimacy than a genuine increase in sexual desire or response (Mathew & Weinman 1982).

Sexual interest and activity are often increased in states of mania or hypomania. Disinhibited sexual behaviour leading to promiscuity or socially inappropriate actions is quite common in this condition (Clayton et al 1965) though diminished sexual interest can also occur. Once again, we have to consider at least two possibilities — that the increased sexuality reflects the general increase in well-being and energy, a non-specific effect, or that the biochemical basis may have a parallel effect on sexuality. Again, we can only speculate, though more detailed studies of these associations and their response to treatment in both depressive and manic states may throw further light on this very fundamental issue.

SCHIZOPHRENIA

Changes in behaviour, emotional reactions and thought processes that manifest the schizophrenic state are often so gross and so pervading that it would be surprising if sexual repercussions did not occur. If schizophrenia occurs early, then the alteration of personality is likely seriously to impair the development of normal sexual relationships. According to Gittleson and his colleagues, both male and female schizophrenics show less reduction of sexual interest than do patients with other types of psychiatric illness, though the female schizophrenics show more loss of interest than the males (Gittleson & Levine 1966; Gittleson & Dawson-Butterworth 1967). Friedman & Harrison (1984) in a small, controlled study of schizophrenic women found that sexual dysfunction was more common amongst the schizophrenic women, both before and after the onset of the psychosis. Of the schizophrenics, 60% had never experienced orgasm and the psychotic group reported a higher incidence of sexual abuse during childhood.

The psychotic phenomena of schizophrenia in many cases have a sexual content. In one study of males, hallucinations involving the genitalia occurred in 30%, delusions of genital change in 20% and of sex change, or being no longer a man, in 27% (Gittleson & Levine 1966). The figures for female schizophrenics were very similar (36, 24 and 25% respectively; Gittleson & Dawson-Butterworth 1967). According to Connolly & Gittleson (1971), these sexual hallucinations are significantly associated with gustatory and olfactory hallucinations. They made the interesting suggestion that some disorder of the temporal lobe could be the common factor.

The continuation of sexual interest in the presence of bizarre sexual ideas or highly abnormal patterns of personal interaction may account for the psychotic sexual behaviour or sexual attacks that accasionally occur in schizophrenics.

Few schizophrenics nowadays escape the effects of long-term phenothiazine treatment. As discussed on page 604, it has additional, probably inhibitory effects on sexual expression. Sexual dysfunction or loss of appetite in the well controlled schizophrenic may well be due to such medication.

HYSTERIA

In spite of the contrary finding of Crisp (1979), mentioned above, hysteria is widely believed to be associated with sexual problems, sexual indifference and dyspareunia being the commonest cited (Purtell et al 1951).

Few concepts in psychiatry have generated more controversy than hysteria. There is still considerable disagreement about its definition or even its existence as a distinct entity. Perhaps the most authoritative view is that there are certain hysterical mechanisms, in particular dissociation and conversion, which may arise in anyone if sufficiently stressed, but which are particularly likely to arise in susceptible individuals whether in states of illness or other crises (Reed 1971). The relationship between this susceptibility to such mechanisms and the so-called hysterical personality is very unclear, and confusion between the two concepts is widespread.

It is conceivable that in those who are predisposed to react with hysterical mechanisms, dissociation leading to sexual anaesthesia or conversion leading to dyspareunia may arise as a reaction to a sexual conflict or difficulty, but this must be regarded as speculative.

SEXUALITY AND MENTAL HANDICAP

Approximately 3% of the population are mentally handicapped. We know remarkably little about the sexuality of these individuals, though there has been no shortage of beliefs and assumptions. They are believed to show uncontrolled sexuality which in the case of males leads to sexual offences, and in females, promiscuity. Until recently, many parents of the handicapped and most professionals looking after them were unable to acknowledge the acceptability of any form of sexual depression. To some extent these assumptions become self-fulfilling prophecies because with segregating the mentally handicapped, separating the sexes and giving them no opportunity to learn appropriate sexual expression, they are more likely to manifest their sexuality inappropriately, with public displays of masturbation or unsolicited sexual approaches.

There has been in the past a particular fear that 'national degeneracy' would increase by overbreeding of the 'mentally defective', a term often used to cover a wide variety of unfortunates (Craft & Craft 1978). This has reinforced the repressive attitudes to sexual expression and has frequently led to policies of involuntary sterilisation for the institutionalised. By the mid 1940s, this attitude was changing as people began to realise that only a small proportion of mental handicap is genetically determined and this group has in any case a low fertility (Hall 1975).

The limited available evidence suggests that the mentally handicapped are somewhat less sexually active than those with more normal intelligence and that the greater the degree of handicap, the less sexual they are likely to be (Hall 1975). Gebhard (1973) reported 84 mentally handicapped men and compared them with a control group of men who had never been convicted of crime or sent to a mental institution. Evidence of prepubertal sex play indicated somewhat less heterosexual experience but somewhat greater homosexual experience for the handicapped than for the controls. The proportion (4%) who as children had contacts with adults was very similar in the two groups. Almost half of the retarded men had engaged in prepubertal masturbation, compared with a third of the control men. But after puberty, the incidence in the two groups was very similar. However, for each post-pubertal age group, the frequency of masturbation was less for the retarded men than for the controls. Not surprisingly, the retarded men had less post-pubertal heterosexual experience. Their greater incidence of homosexual experience was only noticeable up to the age of 15. This tendency may well reflect the lack of any opportunity or encouragement to explore heterosexual relationships.

The mentally handicapped may be more prone to get involved in sexual offences for a number of reasons. Their natural tendency to relate to people of similar mental age may result in their making sexual approaches to children. Gebhard et al (1965) found that the 'feeble-minded' (i.e. IQ less than 70) were somewhat over-represented in those committing non-violent offences against female children, incest with adults, peepers, and exhibitionists. They were not over-represented amongst the sexual aggressors.

The mentally handicapped are usually naive and vulnerable hence easily exploited; they may also act impulsively. However, their difficulties with sex derive less from poor self-control than from lack of appropriate learning. For reasons already described, most institutions for the mentally handicapped have in the past been sexually repressive and over-protective. As a consequence, such individuals have had very few opportunities to explore and learn about close personal relationships, particularly with members of the opposite sex. Typically they have been given no sex education, on the basis that a little information would cause more problems than it would solve. Whereas the normal child can often compensate for lack of sex education by finding out for himself, from peers or by reading, the mentally handicapped person remains virtually cut off from useful information.

Yet mentally handicapped people have special educational needs. Because of their very limited intelligence, information must be given in extremely simple terms, and because of their very short attention span, in small amounts and repeatedly. They need to learn clear and simple rules which allow for sexuality in its proper place. The fact that sex should be in private is especially important, as is the need for proper consent for involving any would-be sexual partner. Handicapped girls have a special need to learn about menstrual hygiene. Given such clear rules and limits, sexuality may provide one of the few pleasures in the extremely limited lives of these unfortunate people. It is a particularly cruel world that denies them even that.

The limitations of the handicapped do not affect their capacity for love, though they may need opportunities to learn how to express that love. Marriage may be successful not only in enhancing the well-being of the couple but also in reducing the need for institutional care. Mattinson (1975) investigated 32 married couples living in the community, all of whom had been regarded as subnormal before marriage. Nineteen couples felt their partnership to be supportive and affectionate. In six, there was no obvious resentment but there were signs of marital stress; in four, one partner was over-dependent and there was expressed resentment and the other three had obviously unsatisfactory marriages. Craft & Craft (1978) studied a further group of such married couples. Some were living in institutions, some in hostels, some in the community with fairly regular support and some were leading independent lives. They found no correlation between the degree of handicap and the success of the partnership.

The question of children in such marriages is a controversial one. It is widely assumed that children in these circumstances will be handicapped and their parents unable to care for them. Neither assumption is necessarily true. Reed & Reed (1965), in an extensive follow-up study, found that where both parents had IQs of less than 70, 40% of the children born to them were retarded but the mean IQ of those children was 74. Where only one parent had an IQ of less than 70, then 15% were retarded and 54% had IQs greater than 90. There was thus the expected tendency to 'regress towards the mean'. In Mattinson's 32 couples, the average number of children was 1.5, lower than the national average for the same age group. Only 7.5% of the children were retarded.

Many handicapped couples use contraception or choose to be sterilised. For the unmarried, contraception is more problematic. For those who are unreliable in their use of oral contraceptives, long-acting injectible progestagens or intrauterine devices are sometimes used. This raises ethical issues which have to be taken seriously.

REFERENCES

Abram H S, Hester L R, Sheridan W F, Epstein G M 1975 Sexual function in patients with chronic renal failure. Journal of Nervous and Mental Disease 160: 220–226
Abramov L S 1976 Sexual life and sexual frigidity among women developing acute myocardial infarction. Psychosomatic Medicine 38: 418–425
Amatruda J M, Harman S M, Pourmotabbed G, Lockwood D H 1978 Depressed plasma testosterone and fractional binding of testosterone in obese males. Journal of Clinical Endocrinology and Metabolism 47: 268–271
Amias A G 1975 Sexual life after gynaecological operations. British Medical Journal 2: 608–609; 680–681
Anand B K, Brobeck J R 1951 Localisation of a feeding centre in the hypothalamus of the rat. Proceedings of Society of Experimental Biology (NY) 27: 323
Andersen B C 1984 Psychological aspects of gynaecological cancer. In: Broome A, Wallace L (eds) Psychology and gynaecological problems. Tavistock, London, pp. 117–141
Antoniou L D, Shalhoub R J, Sudbaker T, Smith J C 1977 Reversal of uraemic impotence by zinc. Lancet 2: 895–898
Athanosiou R, Shaver P, Tavris C 1970 Sex. Psychology Today 4 July: 39–52
Bai J, Greenwald E, Caterini H, Kaminetzky H A 1974 Drug-related menstrual aberrations. Obstetrics and Gynecology 44: 713–719
Bancroft J, Bell C, Ewing D J, McCulloch D K, Warner P, Clarke B F 1985 Assessment of erectile function in diabetic and non-diabetic impotence by simultaneous recording of penile diameter and penile arterial pulse. Journal of Psychosomatic Research 29: 315–324
Barker M G 1968 Psychiatric illness after hysterectomy. British Medical Journal 2: 91–95
Barragry J M, Makin H L J, Trafford D J H, Scott D F 1978 Effects of anticonvulsants on plasma testosterone and sex hormone binding globulin levels. Journal of Neurology, Neurosurgery and Psychiatry 41: 913–914
Bartholomew A A 1968 A long acting phenothiazine as a possible agent to control deviant sexual behaviour. Americal Journal of Psychiatry 124: 917–923
Beck A T 1967 Depression. Clinical, experimental and theoretical aspects. Staples Press, London
Bell D S, Trethowan W H 1961 Amphetamine addiction and disturbed sexuality. Archives of General Psychiatry 4: 74–78
Benkert O 1973 Pharmacological experiments to stimulate human sexual behaviour. In: Ban T A et al (eds) Psychopharmacology, sexual disorders and drug abuse. North Holland, Amsterdam
Berger S 1952 The role of sexual impotence in the concept of self of male paraplegics. Dissertation Abstracts International, p 12
Beumont P J V, Gelder M G, Friesen H G et al 1974 The effects of phenothiazines on endocrine function. I. Patients with inappropriate lactation and amenorrhoea. British Journal of Psychiatry 124: 413–419
Beumont P J V, Abraham S F, Simson K G 1981 The psychosexual histories of adolescent

girls and young women with anorexia nervosa. Psychological Medicine 11: 131–140

Bloch A, Maeder J P, Haissly J C 1975 Sexual problems after myocardial infarction American Heart Journal 90: 536–537

Blumer D 1970 Hypersexual episodes in temporal lobe epilepsy. American Journal of Psychiatry 126: 1099–1106

Bommer J, Ritz E, Del Pezo E, Bommer G 1979 Improved sexual function in male haemodialysis patients on bromocriptine. Lancet ii: 496–497

Bors E, Comarr A E 1960 Neurological disturbances of sexual function with special reference to 529 patients with spinal cord injury. Urological Survey 10: 191–222

Bransfield D D 1982 Breast cancer and sexual functioning: a review of the literature and implications for future research. International Journal of Psychiatry in Medicine 12: 197–211

Bregman S 1975 Behaviors relating to unfeminine attractiveness and sexual adjustment among women with spinal cord injuries. Unpublished Masters' thesis, cited in Fitting et al 1978

Briddell D W, Wilson G T 1976 The effects of alcohol and expectancy set on male sexual arousal. Journal of Abnormal Psychology 35: 225–234

Briddell D W, Rimm D C, Caddy G R, Krawitz G, Sholis D, Wunderlin R J 1978 Effects of alcohol and cognitive set on sexual arousal to deviant stimuli. Journal of Abnormal Psychology 87: 418–430

Brindley G S 1982 Sexual function and fertility in paraplegic men. In: Hargreave T (ed) Male infertility. Springer Verlag, Berlin

Buckley R M Jr, McGuckin M, MacGregor R R 1978 Urine bacterial counts after sexual intercourse. New England Journal of Medicine 298: 321–324

Bulpitt C J, Dollery C T 1973 Side effects of hypotensive agents evaluated by a self-administered questionnaire. British Medical Journal 3: 485–490

Bulpitt C J, Dollery C T, Carne S 1976 Change in symptoms of hypertensive patients after referral to hospital clinics. British Heart Journal 38: 121–128

Burnfield P 1979 Sexual problems and multiple sclerosis. British Journal of Sexual Medicine 6 (50): 33–38

Burnham W R, Lennard-Jones J E, Brooke B N 1977 Sexual problems among married ileostomists. Gut 18: 673–677

Buvat J, Lemaire A, Buvat-Herbaut M, Guien J D, Bailleul J P, Fossati P 1985 Comparative investigation of 26 impotent and 26 non-impotent diabetic patients. Journal of Urology 133: 34–38

Carani C, Zinin D, Caricchioli F et al 1986 Effects of heroin addiction on the endocrine control of sexual function in young men. In: Kothari P (ed) Proceedings of the seventh world congress of sexology. IASECT, Bombay, pp 160–163

Cassidy W L, Flangan N B, Spellman M, Cohen M E 1957 Clinical observations in manic depressive disease. Journal of American Medical Association 164: 1535–1546

Catalan J, Bradley M, Gallwey J, Hawton K 1981 Sexual dysfunction and psychiatric morbidity in patients attending a clinic for sexually transmitted diseases. British Journal of Psychiatry 138: 292–296

Caterall R D 1972 Trichomoniasis, venereal disease. Medical Clinics of North America 26: 496–497

Chapman R M, Sutcliffe S B, Malpas J S 1979a Cytotoxic induced ovarian failure in women with Hodgkin's disease. II Effects on sexual function. Journal of American Medical Association 242: 1882–1884

Chapman R M, Sutcliffe S B, Rees L H, Edwards C R, Malpas J S 1979b Cyclical combination chemotherapy and gonadal function. Retrospective study in males. Lancet i: 285–289

Clayton P J, Pitts F N Jr, Winokur G 1965 Affective disorders. IV. Mania. Comprehensive Psychiatry 6: 313–322

Cole T M 1975 Sexuality and physical disabilities. Archives of Sexual Behavior 4: 389–401

Communicable Diseases Scotland Weekly Report 1986 Sexually transmitted disease surveillance, United Kingdom 1984. Comunicable Diseases Scotland Weekly Report CDS 86/31

Connolly F H, Gittleson N L 1971 The relationship between delusions of sexual change and olfactory and gustatory hallucinations in schizophrenia. British Journal of Psychiatry 119: 443–444

Craft M, Craft A 1978 Sex and the mentally handicapped. Routledge & Kegan Paul, London

Crisp A H 1979 Sexual psychopathology in the psychiatric clinic. British Journal of Clinical Practice (suppl) 4: 3–11

Crisp A H 1980 Anorexia nervosa; let me be. Academic Press, London

Currier R D, Little S C, Suess J F, Andy O J 1971 Sexual seizures. Archives of Neurology 25: 260–264

Cushman P 1972 Sexual behavior in heroin addiction and methadone maintenance. New York State Journal of Medicine 72: 1261–1265

Devlin H B, Plant J 1979 Sexual function — an aspect of stoma care. Part II. British Journal of Sexual Medicine 6(46): 22–26

Devlin H B, Plant J A, Griffin M 1971 Aftermath of surgery for anorectal cancer. British Medical Journal 3: 413–418

Dhabuwala C B, Kumar A, Pierce J M 1986 Myocardial infarction and its influence on male sexual function. Archives of Sexual Behavior 15: 499–504

Ekstrom K 1970 Patterns of sexual behaviour — relation to venereal disease. British Journal of Venereal Disease 46: 93–95

Ellenberg M 1971 Impotence in diabetes: the neurological factor. Annals of Internal Medicine 75: 213–219

Ellenberg M 1977 Sexual aspects of the female diabetic. Mount Sinai Journal of Medicine 44: 495–500

Everitt B J 1979 Monoamines and sexual behaviour in non-human primates. In: Sex, hormones and behaviour. Ciba Foundation Symposium 62 (New Series). Excerpta Medica, Amsterdam, pp 329–348

Faerman I, Glocer L, Fox D, Jadzinsky M N, Rapaport M 1974 Impotence and diabetes. Histological studies of the autonomic nervous fibres of the corpora cavernosa in impotent diabetic males. Diabetes 23: 971–976

Fairburn C G, Wu F C W, McCulloch D K et al 1982a The clinical features of diabetic impotence: a preliminary study. British Journal of Psychiatry 140: 447–452

Fairburn C G, McCulloch D K, Wu F C 1982b The effects of diabetes on male sexual function. Clinics in Endocrinology and Metabolism 11: 749–768

Falaschi P, Frajese G, Sciarra F, Rocco A, Conti C 1978 Influence of hyperprolactinaemia due to metoclopramide on gonadal function in men. Clinical Endocrinology 8: 427–433

Farkas G M, Rosen R C 1976 The effect of alcohol on elicited male sexual response. Journal of Studies of Alcohol 37: 265–272

Fenwick P B C, Mercer S, Grant R et al 1986 Nocturnal penile tumescence and serum testosterone levels. Archives of Sexual Behavior 15: 13–22

Ferguson K, Figley B 1979 Sexuality and rheumatic disease: a prospective study. Sexuality and Disability 2: 130–138

Fitting M D, Salisbury S, Davies N H, Mayclin D K 1978 Self concept and sexuality of spinal cord injured women. Archives of Sexual Behavior 7: 143–156

Fraley E E, Lange P H, Kennedy B J 1979 Germ-cell cancer in adults. Part 2. New England Journal of Medicine 301: 1420–1426

Francis W H, Jeffcoate T N A 1961 Dyspareunia following vaginal operations. Journal of Obstetrics and Gynaecology of the British Commonwealth 68: 1–10

Friedman S, Harrison G 1984 Sexual histories, attitudes and behavior of schizophrenic and 'normal' women. Archives of Sexual Behavior 13: 555–568

Gastaut H, Collomb H 1954 Etude du comportement sexuel chez les épileptiques psychomoteurs. Annals Medico-Psychologigues 112: 657–696

Gath D 1980 Psychiatric aspects of hysterectomy. In: Robins L, Clayton P, Wing J (eds) The social consequences of psychiatric illness. Brunner/Mazel, New York

Gath D, Cooper P, Day A 1982a Hysterectomy and psychiatric disorder. I Levels of psychiatric morbidity before and after hysterectomy. British Journal of Psychiatry 140: 335–342

Gath D, Cooper P, Bond A, Edmonds G 1982b Hysterectomy and psychiatric disorder. II Demographic, psychiatric and physical factors in relation to psychiatric outcome. British Journal of Psychiatry 140: 343–350

Gebhard P H 1973 Sexual behavior of the mentally retarded. In: de la Cruz F F, La Veck G D (eds) Human sexuality and the mentally retarded. Brunner-Mazel, New York, pp 29–49

Gebhard P, Gagnon J, Pomeroy N, Christenson C 1965 Sex offenders. Harper Row, New York
Gittleson N L, Dawson-Butterworth K 1967 Subjective ideas of sexual change — female schizophrenics. British Journal of Psychiatry 113: 491–494
Gittleson N L, Levine S 1966 Subjective ideas of sexual change in male schizophrenics. British Journal of Psychiatry 112: 779–782
Glass C A, Fielding D M, Evans C, Ashcroft J B 1987 Factors related to sexual functioning in male patients undergoing hemodialysis and with kidney transplants. Archives of Sexual Behavior 16: 189–208
Gloeckner M R 1983 Partner reaction following ostomy surgery. Journal of Sexual and Marital Therapy 9: 182–190
Goldacre M J, Watt B, Loudon N, Milne L J R, Loudon J D O, Vessey M P 1979 Vaginal microbial flora in normal young women. British Medical Journal 1: 1450–1453
Goode E 1972 Drug use and sexual activity on a college campus. American Journal of Psychiatry 128: 1272–1276
Gorzynski G, Katz J L 1977 The polycystic ovary syndrome: psychosexual correlates. Archives of Sexual Behavior 6: 215–222
Gossop M R, Stern R, Connell P H 1974 Drug dependence and sexual function: a comparison of intravenous users of narcotics and oral users of amphetamines. British Journal of Psychiatry 124: 431–434
Green M, Berman S 1954 Failure of ejaculation produced by dibenzyline. Connecticut State Medical Journal 18: 30–33
Griffin T, Morris J 1987 Social trends no 17. HMSO, London
Griffith E, Trieschmann R B 1975 Sexual functioning in women with spinal cord injury. Archives of Physical Medicine and Rehabilitation 56: 18–21
Hagen C, Ølgaard K McNeilly A S, Fisher R 1976 Prolactin and the pituitary–gonadal axis in male uraemic patients on regular dialysis. Acta Endocrinologica 82: 29–38
Hall J E 1975 Sexuality and the mentally retarded. In: Green R (ed) Human sexuality. A health practitioner's texts. Williams & Wilkins, Baltimore, pp. 181–195
Harris J R W 1977 Other sexually transmitted disease. In: Money J, Musaph H (eds) Handbook of sexology. Excerpta Medica, Amsterdam, pp 1023–1036
Harrison W M, Stewart J, Ehrhardt A A et al 1985 A controlled study of the effects of antidepressants on sexual function. Psychopharmacological Bulletin 21: 85–88
Hawton K 1984 Sexual adjustment of men who have had strokes. Journal of Psychosomatic Research 28: 243–249
Hellerstein H K, Friedman E H 1970 Sexual activity and the post-coronary patient. Archives of Internal Medicine 125: 987–999
Higgins G E 1979 Sexual response in spinal cord injured adults: a review. Archives of Sexual Behavior 8: 173–196
Hoenig J, Hamilton C M 1960 Epilepsy and sexual orgasm. Acta Psychiatrica Neurologica Scandinavica 35: 449–456
Holdsworth S, Atkins R C, De Kretser D M 1977 The pituitary–testicular axis in men with chronic renal failure. New England Journal of Medicine 296: 1245–1249
Idsoe O, Kiraly K, Causse G 1973 World Health Organization Chronicle 27: 413
Ivers R R, Goldstein N P 1963 Multiple sclerosis: a current appraisal of symptoms and signs. Mayo Clinic Proceedings 38: 457–466
Jackson P 1979 Sexual adjustment to hysterectomy and the benefits of a pamphlet for patients. New Zealand Medical Journal 90: 471–2
Jacobs H S 1979 Prolactin and sexual function. British Journal of Sexual Medicine 6 (47): 3–6
Jensen S B 1979 Sexual customs and dysfunction in alcoholics. I & II. British Journal of Sexual Medicine 6 (53): 20–32; (54): 30–34
Jensen S B 1981 Diabetic sexual function: a comparative study of 160 insulin treated diabetic men and women and an age-matched control group. Archives of Sexual Behaviour 10: 493–504
Jensen S B 1985 Sexual relationships in couples with a diabetic partner. Journal of Sexual and Marital Therapy 11: 259–270
Jensen S B 1986 Sexual dysfunction in insulin treated diabetics: a 6 year follow up study of 101 patients. Archives of Sexual Behaviour 15: 271–284

Jensen P, Jensen S B 1987 Sexual dysfunction in epileptic patients. Paper presented at 13th Annual Conference, International Academy of Sex Research, Tutzing, West Germany

Juhlin L, Lidén S 1969 Influence of contraceptive gestogen pills on sexual behaviour and the spread of gonorrhoea. British Journal of Venereal Disease 45: 321–324

Katchadourian H A 1985 Fundamentals of human sexuality, 4th edn. Holt, Rinehart & Winston, New York

Kedia K, Markland C 1975 Effects of sympathectomy and drugs on ejaculation. In: Sciarra J J, Markland C, Speidel J J (eds) Control of male fertility. Harper Row, New York

Kincey J, McFarlane T 1984 Psychological aspects of hysterectomy. In: Broome A, Wallace L (eds) Psychology and gynaecological problems. Tavistock, London, pp. 142–160

Kinsey L A, Detels R, Kaslow R et al 1987 Risk factors for Sero conversion to human immunodeficiency virus among male homosexuals Lancet 1: 345–348

Kinsey A C, Pomeroy W B, Martin C F 1948 Sexual behavior in the human male. Saunders, Philadelphia

Kinsey A C, Pomeroy W B, Martin C E, Gebhard P H 1953 Sexual behavior in the human female. Saunders, Philadelphia

Klassen A D, Wilsnack S C 1986 Sexual experience and drinking among women in a US national survey. Archives of Sexual Behavior 15: 363–392

Klebanow D, MacLeod J 1960 Semen quality and certain disturbances of reproduction in diabetic men. Fertility and Sterility 11: 255–261

Kockott G, Feil W, Ferstl R, Aldenhoff J, Besinger U 1980 Psychophysiological aspect of male sexual inadequacy: results of an experimental study. Archives of Sexual Behavior 9: 477–494

Kolarsky A, Freund K, Machek J et al 1967 Male sexual deviation: association with early temporal lobe damage. Archives of General Psychiatry 17: 735–743

Kolodny R C 1971 Sexual dysfunction in diabetic females. Diabetes 20: 557–559

Kolodny R C, Masters W H, Johnson V E 1979 Textbook of sexual medicine. Little, Brown, Boston

Kotin J, Wilbert D E, Verburg D, Soldinger S M 1976 Thioridazine and sexual dysfunction. American Journal of Psychiatry 133: 82–85

Larson J L, McNaughton M W, Ward Kennedy J, Mansfield L W 1980 Heart rate and blood pressure response to sexual activity and a stair climbing test. Heart and Lung 9: 1025–1030

Lee E C G, Dowling B L 1972 Perimuscular excision of the rectum for Crohn's disease and ulcerative colitis. British Journal of Surgery 59: 29

Lees F 1967 Alcohol and the nervous system. British Journal of Hospital Medicine December: 264–272

Lemere F, Smith J W 1973 Alcohol-induced sexual impotence. American Journal of Psychiatry 130: 212–213

Leriche R 1940 De la résection du carrefour aorticoiliaque avec double sympathectomie lombaire pour thrombose artéritique de l'aorte; le syndrome de l'oblitération terminoaortique par artérite. Presse Médicale 48: 601–604

Levy N B 1973 Sexual adjustment to maintenance haemodialysis and renal transplantation: a national survey by questionnaire. Preliminary report. Transactions of American Society for Artificial Internal Organs 19: 138–143

Leiber L, Plumb M M, Herstenzang M L, Holland J 1976 The communication of affection between cancer patients and their spouses. Psychosomatic Medicine 38: 379–389

Lilius H G, Valtonen F J, Davis F A 1976 Sexual problems in patients suffering from multiple sclerosis. Journal of Chronic Diseases 29: 65–73

Lim V S, Fang V S 1976 Restoration of plasma testosterone levels in uremic men with clomiphene citrate. Journal of Clinical Endocrinology and Metabolism 43: 1370–1377

Lincoln J, Crowe R, Blackley P F, Pryor J P, Lumley J S P, Burnstock G 1987 Changes in VIPergic, cholinergic and adrenergic innervation of human penile tissue in diabetic and non-diabetic impotent males. Journal of Urology 137: 1053–1059

Lindner H 1953 Perceptual sensitisation to sexual phenomena in the chronically physically disabled. Journal of Clinical Psychology 9: 67–68

Lundberg P O 1977 Sexual dysfunction in patients with neurological disorders. In: Gemme R, Wheeler C C (eds) Progress in sexology. Plenum, New York

Lundberg P O 1978 Sexual dsyfunction in patients with multiple sclerosis. Sexuality and Disability 1: 218–222

Lundberg P O 1980 Sexual dysfunction in women with multiple sclerosis. In: Forleo R, Pasini W (eds) Medical sexology. Elsevier/North Holland, Amsterdam

McCulloch D K, Campbell I W, Wu F C, Prescott R J, Clarke B F 1980 The prevalence of diabetic impotence. Diabetologia 18: 279–283

McCulloch D K, Young R J, Prescott R J, Campbell I W, Clarke B F 1984 The natural history of impotence in diabetic men. Diabetologia 26: 437–440

McKinsick L, Horstman W, Coates T J 1985 AIDS and sexual behavior reported by gay men in San Francisco. American Journal of Public Health 75: 493–496

McMillan A, Robertson D H H 1977 Sexually transmitted diseases in homosexual males in Edinburgh. Health Bulletin 35: 266–271

Madorsky I L, Ashamalla M G, Schussler I, Lyons H R, Miller G H Jr 1976 Postprostatectomy impotence. Journal of Urology 115: 401–403

Maguire G P, Lee E G, Bevington D J, Kücheman C S, Crabtree R J, Cornell C E 1978 Psychiatric problems in the first year after mastectomy. British Medical Journal 1: 963–965

Malatesta V J, Pollack R H, Wilbanks W A, Adams H E 1979 Alcohol effects on the orgasmic–ejaculatory response in human males. Journal of Sex Research 15: 101–107

Malatesta V J, Pollack R H, Crotty T D, Peacock L J 1982 Acute alcoholic intoxication and female orgasmic response. Journal of Sex Research 18: 1–17

Martin E M 1967 Marital and coital factors in cervical cancer American Journal of Public Health 57: 803–814

Martin J L 1986 Psychological, social and serological correlates of sexual behavior change among gay men: a life stress and illness perspective. Paper at 11th Annual Conference International Academy Sex Research, Amsterdam, Netherlands

Masters W H, Johnson V E 1966 Human sexual response. Churchill, London

Masters W H, Johnson V E 1970 Human sexual inadequacy. Churchill, London

Mathew R J, Weinman M L 1982 Sexual dysfunction in depression. Archives of Sexual Behavior 11: 323–328

Mattinson J 1975 Marriage and mental handicap, 2nd edn. Tavistock, London

Melman A, Henry D 1979 The possible role of the catecholamines of the corpora in penile erection. Journal of Urology 21: 419

The Medical Research Council Working Report on Mild to Moderate Hypertension 1981. Adverse reactions to bendrofinazide and propanolol for the treatment of mild hypertension, Lancet ii: 539–543

Michal V 1982 Arterial disease as a cause of impotence. Clinics in Endocrinology and Metabolism 11: 725–748

Miller H, Simpson C A, Yeates W K 1965 Bladder dysfunction in multiple sclerosis. British Medical Journal 1: 1265–1269

Miller D, Weber J, Green J (eds) 1985 The management of AIDS patients. Macmillan, London

Mintz J, O'Hare K, O'Brien C P 1974 Sexual problems of heroin addicts. Archives of General Psychiatry 31: 700–703

Mitchell W, Falconer M A, Hill D 1954 Epilepsy fetishism relieved by temporal lobectomy. Lancet 2: 626–630

Money J, Pruce G 1977 Psychomotor epilepsy and sexual function. In: Money J, Musaph H (eds) Handbook of sexology. Excerpta Medica, Amsterdam

Money J, Yankowitz R 1967 The sympathetic inhibiting effects of the drug Ismelin on human male eroticism, with a note on Melleril. Journal of Sex Research 3: 69–82

Montenero P, Donatone E, Magi D 1973 Diabète et activité séxuelle chez la femme. Journal Annelles Diabetologia de l'Hôtel-Dieu 11–13: 91–103

Morton R S 1971 Sexual freedom and venereal disease. Peter Owen, London

Morton R S 1977 Venereal disease. In: Money J, Musaph H (eds) Handbook of sexology. Excerpta Medica, Amsterdam, pp 1009–1022

Murray M A F, Bancroft J H J, Anderson D C, Tennent T G, Carr P J 1975 Endocrine changes in male sexual deviants after treatment with anti-androgens, oestrogens or tranquillisers. Journal of Endocrinology 67: 179–188

Navon S, Caspi D, Fishel B, Fishel R, Yaron M 1982 Sexual problems in patients with rheumatic disease. British Journal of Sexual Medicine 9 (86): 12–15

Nemec E D, Mansfield L, Ward Kennedy J 1976 Heart rate and blood pressure responses during sexual activity in normal males. American Heart Journal 92: 274–277

Neri A, Aygen M, Zukerman Z, Bahary C 1980 Subjective assessment of sexual dysfunction of patients on long-term administration of digoxin. Archives of Sexual Behavior 9: 343–347

Neri A, Zukerman Z, Aygen M, Lidor Y, Kaufman H 1987 The effect of long term administration of digoxin on plasma androgen and sexual dysfunction. Journal of Sexual and Marital Therapy 13: 58–63

Notley R G 1979 Transurethral resection of the prostate. British Journal of Sexual Medicine 6: (55); 10–15; 26

Novak D J, Victor M 1974 Vagus and sympathetic nerves in alcoholic neuropathy. Archives of Neurology 30: 273–284

Orbach S 1981 Compulsive eating in women. British Journal of Sexual Medicine 8:(70); 42–43

Orford J, Oppenheimer E, Egert S, Hensmen C, Guthrie S 1976 The cohesiveness of alcoholism-complicated marriages and its influence on treatment outcome. British Journal of Psychiatry 128: 318–339

Pamnany L J 1980 Sexual behaviour of young males attending an STD clinic. British Journal of Sexual Medicine 7: 12–19

Pearlman C K 1980 Sex and prostatectomy patient. British Journal of Sexual Medicine 7: (59); 31–35

Peden N R, Cargill J M, Browning M C K, Saunders J H B, Wormsley R G 1979 Male sexual dysfunction during treatment with cimetidine. British Medical Journal 1: 659

Pentland B, Anderson D A, Critchley J A J H 1981 Failure of ejaculation with indoramin. British Medical Journal 282: 1433–1434

Pinder R M, Brogden R N, Sawyer P R et al 1982 Fenfluramine: a review of its pharmacological properties and therapeutic efficacy in obesity. Drugs 10: 241–323

Plant M A 1975 Drug takers in an English town. Tavistock, London, pp 188–204

Polk B F, Fox R, Brookmeyer R, et al 1987 Predictors of the acquired immunodeficiency syndrome developing in a cohort of seropositive homosexual men. The New England Journal of Medicine 316: 61–66

Powley T L, Keesey R E 1970 Relationship of body weight to the lateral hypothalamic feeding syndrome. Journal of Comparative and Physiological Psychology 70: 25

Pritchard B N C, Johnston A N, Hill I D, Rosenheim M L 1968 Bethanidine, guanethidine and methyldopa in treatment of hypertension: a within-patient comparison. British Medical Journal 1: 135–144

Procci W R 1984 Male sexual functioning and maintenance hemodialysis: a prospective study. Dialysis and Transplantation 13: 100–104

Purtell J J, Robins E, Cohen M E 1951 Observations on clinical aspects of hysteria. Journal of the American Medical Association 146: 902–909

Ramprakash D, Daly M 1981 Social trends no 11. HMSO, London

Reed J L 1971 Hysteria. British Journal of Hospital Medicine February: 237–246

Reed E W, Reed S C 1965 Mental Retardation. Saunders, Philadelphia

Rees J M H 1983 Sexual dysfunction and prescribed psychotropic drugs. In: Wheatley D (ed) Psychopharmacology and sexual disorders. Oxford University Press, Oxford, pp 138–147

Rhodes E D 1977 Blood pressure and heart rate responses during sexual activity. Cited in Wagner 1977

Richards D H 1973 Depression after hysterectomy. Lancet ii: 430–432

Riley A 1980a Antihypertensive therapy and sexual function. British Journal of Sexual Medicine 7: 23–27

Riley A 1980b The sexual side effects of drugs used in the treatment of peptic ulceration and dyspepsia. British Journal of Sexual Medicine 7: (64); 12–16

Riley A J 1984 Treating genital herpes. British Journal of Sexual Medicine 11 (109): 169–170

Riley A J, Riley E J 1983 Cholinergic and adrenergic control of human sexual response. In: Wheatley D (ed) Psychopharmacology and sexual disorders. Oxford University Press, Oxford, pp 125–137

Riley A J, Riley E J 1986 The effects of single dose diazepam on female sexual response induced by masturbation. Sexual and Marital Therapy 1: 49–54

Rodin P, Goldmeier D 1976 Sexual problems seen by venereologists. In: Crown S (ed)

Psychosexual problems: psychotherapy, counselling and behavioural modification. Academic, London

Roose S P, Glassman A H, Walsh B T, Cullen K 1982 Reversible loss of nocturnal penile tumescence during depression: a preliminary report. Neuropsychobiology 8: 284–288

Rotkin I D 1973 A comparison review of key epidemiological studies in cervical cancer related to current searches for transmissible agents. Cancer Research 33: 1353–1367

Russell G F M 1970 Anorexia nervosa: its identity as an illness and its treatment. In: Price J H (ed) Modern trends in psychological medicine. Butterworth, London

Sanders D, Warner P, Backström T, Bancroft J 1983 Mood, sexuality, hormones and the menstrual cycle I. Changes in mood and physical state: description of subjects and method. Psychosomatic Medicine 45: 487–507

Santen R J, Sofsky J, Bilic N, Lippert R 1975 Mechanism of action of narcotics in the production of menstrual dysfunction in women. Fertility and Sterility 26: 538–548

Schiavi R C, Fisher C, Quadland M, Glover A 1985 Nocturnal penile tumescence: evaluation of erectile function in insulin dependent diabetic men. Diabetologia 28: 90–94

Schneider G, Kirschner M A, Berkowitz R, Ertel N H 1979 Increased estrogen production in obese men. Journal of Clinical Endocrinology and Metabolism 48: 633–638

Schofield C B S 1977 Psychological and sociological consideration of diseases of the genital tract. In: Money J, Musaph H (eds) Handbook of sexology. Excerpta Medica, Amsterdam, pp 985–1007

Schreiner-Engel P, Schiavi R C 1986 Lifetime psychopathology in individuals with low sexual desire. Journal of Nervous and Mental Diseases 174: 646–651

Schreiner-Engel P, Schiavi R C, Vietorisz D, Eichel J deS, Smith H 1985 Diabetes and female sexuality: a comparative study of women in relationships. Journal of Sexual and Marital Therapy 11: 165–175

Schreiner-Engel P, Schiavi R C, Vietorisz D, Smith H 1986 The differential impact of diabetes type on female sexuality. Journal of Psychosomatic Research 31: 23–33

Scott D 1978 Psychiatric aspects of sexual medicine. Epilepsy. British Journal of Sexual Medicine 5: (33); 17–18; (34); 12–14

Segraves R T 1977 Pharmacological agents causing sexual dysfunction. Journal of Sexual and Marital Therapy 3: 157–176

Segraves R T 1979 Sexual dysfunction and psychotropic drugs. British Journal of Sexual Medicine 6: (52); 51–52

Segraves R T 1985 Psychiatric drugs and orgasm in the human female. Journal of Psychosomatic Obstetrics and Gynaecology 4: 125–128

SHHD 1986 HIV infection in Scotland. Report of the Scottish Committee on HIV infection and intravenous drug misuse. Scottish Home and Health Department, Edinburgh

Stein R A 1977 The effect of exercise training on heart rate during coitus in the post-myocardial infarction patient. Circulation 55: 738–740

Stewart W F R 1975 Sex and the physically handicapped. National Fund for Research in Crippling Diseases, Horsham

Stoffer S S, Hynes K M, Jiany N S, Ryan R J 1973 Digoxin and abnormal serum hormone levels. Journal of American Medical Association 225: 1643–1644

Taberner P V 1985 Aphrodisiacs. The science and the myth. Croom Helm, London

Taylor D C 1969 Sexual behaviour and temporal lobe epilepsy. Archives of Neurology 21: 510–516

Taylor D C 1972 Psychiatry and sociology in the understanding of epilepsy. In: Mandelbrote B M, Gelder M G (eds) Psychiatric aspects of medical practice. Staples, London

Taylor D C, Falconer M A 1968 Clinical, socio-economic, and psychological changes after temporal lobectomy for epilepsy. British Journal of Psychiatry 114: 1247–1261

Tennent G, Bancroft J, Cass 1974 The control of deviant sexual behavior by drugs: a double-blind controlled study of benperiodol, chlorpromazine and placebo. Archives of Sexual Behavior 3: 261–271

Terzian H, Orr G D 1955 Syndrome of Klüver and Bucy reproduced in man by bitemporal removal of the temporal lobes. Neurology 5: 363–380

Thase M E, Reynolds C F, Glanz L M et al 1987 Nocturnal penile tumescence in depressed men. American Journal of Psychiatry 144: 89–82

Tielman R A P, van Grieusven G J P 1986 The impact of AIDS on homosexual lifestyle:

methods and results of a panel study. Paper presented at 11th Annual Conference, International Academy Sex Research, Amsterdam, Netherlands

Toone B K, Wheeler M, Fenwick P B C 1980 Sex hormone changes in male epileptics. Clinical Endocrinology 12: 391–395

Toone B K, Wheeler M, Nanjee M, Fenwick P, Grant R 1983 Sex hormones, sexual drive and plasma anticonvulsant levels in male epileptics. Journal of Neurology, Neurosurgery and Psychiatry 46: 824–826

Tuttle W, Cook W, Fitch E 1964 Sexual behavior in post-myocardial infarction patients. American Journal of Cardiology 13: 140–153

Tyrer G, Steel J M, Ewing D J, Bancroft J, Warner P, Clarke B F 1983 Sexual responsiveness in diabetic women. Diabetologia 24: 166–171

Ueno M 1963 The so-called coition death. Japanese Journal of Legal Medicine 17: 333–340

Van Thiel D, Lester R 1979 The effect of chronic alcohol abuse on sexual function. Clinics in Endocrinology and Metabolism 8: 499–510

Vas C J 1969 Sexual impotence and some autonomic disturbances in men with multiple sclerosis. Acta Neurologica Scandinavica 45: 166–182

Victor A, Lunberg P O, Johansson E D B 1977 Induction of sex-hormone-binding globulin by phenytoin. British Medical Journal ii: 934

Virag R, Bouilly P, Frydman D 1985 Is impotence an arterial disorder? Lancet i: 181–184

Vircburger M I, Prelevic G M, Peric L A, Knesevic J, Djukanovic L 1985 Testosterone levels after bromocriptine treatment in patients undergoing long-term haemodialysis. Journal of Andrology 6: 113–116

Wabrek A J, Burchell R C 1980 Male sexual dysfunction associated with coronary heart disease. Archives of Sexual Behavior 9: 69–75

Wagner N N 1977 Sexual behavior and the cardiac patient. In: Money J, Musaph H (eds) Handbook of sexology. Excerpta Medica, Amsterdam, pp 959–967

Wagner G, Brindley G 1980 The effect of atropine, α and β blockers upon human penile erection — a controlled pilot study. In: Zorgniotti A (ed) First international conference on vascular impotence. Charles C Thomas, New York

Wallgren H, Barry H 1970 Actions of alcohol. Elsevier, Amsterdam

Warren S C, Warren S G 1977 Propranolol and sexual impotence. Annals of Internal Medicine 85: 682–683

Warner P, Bancroft J and members of Edinburgh Human Sexuality Group 1987 A regional clinical service for sexual problems: a 3-year study. Sexual and Marital Therapy 2: 115–126

Watson J P 1979 Sexual behaviour, relationship and mood. In: British Journal of Clinical Practice (suppl) 4: 23–26

Weijmar Schultz W C M, Wijma K, Van de Wiel H B M, Bouma J, Janssens J 1986 Sexual rehabilitation of radical vulvectomy patients. A pilot study. Journal of Psychosomatic Obstetrics and Gynaecology 5: 119–126

Weiss A, Diamond D 1966 Sexual adjustment identification and attitudes of patients with myelopathy. Archives of Physical Medicine and Rehabilitation 47: 245–250

Whalley L J 1978 Sexual adjustment of male alcoholics. Acta Psychiatrica Scandinavica 58: 281–298

Whitley M P, Berke P 1984 Sexual response in diabetic women. In: Woods N F (ed) Human sexuality in health and illness. C V Mosby, Missouri, pp 328–340

Wilson G T 1977 Alcohol and human sexual behavior. Behaviour Research and Therapy 15: 239–252

Wilson G T 1984 Alcohol and sexual function. British Journal of Sexual Medicine 11(105): 56–60

Wilson G T, Lawson D M 1976a The effects of alcohol on sexual arousal in women. Journal of Abnormal Psychology 85: 489–497

Wilson G T, Lawson D M 1976b Expectancies, alcohol and sexual arousal in male social drinkers. Journal of Abnormal Psychology 85: 587–594

Wilson G T, Lawson D M, Abrams D B 1978 Effects of alcohol on sexual arousal in male alcoholics. Journal of Abnormal Psychology 87: 609–616

Wolfe M M 1979 Impotence on cimetidine treatment. New England Journal of Medicine 300: 94

Woodruff R A, Murphy G E, Herjanic M 1967 The natural history of affective disorders: I. Symptoms of 72 patients at the time of index hospital admission. Journal of Psychiatric Research 5: 255–263

Yen S S C 1980 The polycystic ovary syndrome. Clinical Endocrinology 12: 177–208

Ylikahri R, Huttunen M, Harkonen M et al 1974 Low plasma testosterone values in men during hangover. Journal of Steroid Biochemistry 5: 655–658

Zrustová M, Rostlapil J, Kabrhelová A 1978 Sexualni Poruchy u žen s úplaricic cukrovon. Cs Gynekologie 43: 277–280

12

Sexual aspects of fertility, fertility control and infertility

The most important consequence of heterosexual activity is pregnancy. What effect does pregnancy have on the sexual relationship? The avoidance of unwanted pregnancy is crucial if the non-reproductive benefits of human sexuality are to be exploited. For health professionals, their involvement in the provision of fertility control provides one of the main opportunities for discussing the sexual problems of their clients and patients. In addition, sexual problems may arise as a consequence of fertility control. There is therefore a fundamental need to understand the sexual implications and consequences of fertility regulation. It is an unfortunate fact that of the huge sums of money that have been spent on developing and evaluating methods of fertility control, a negligible proportion has gone on appraising their effects on sexual behaviour. This is surprising considering that if it were not for sexual activity, fertility control would be unnecessary; also surprising when the major obstacle to world population control lies not in a lack of suitable technology but in the low level of acceptance of the various effective methods that are already available. And yet we know virtually nothing about the importance of sexual factors in producing this low acceptance and usage. In this chapter we will consider fertility control under three headings: contraception, sterilisation and induced abortion. Avoidance of unwanted pregnancy is not the only issue, however. Inability to conceive is a source of much distress in many would-be parents and high rates of infertility are a cause of social concern in certain parts of the world. We will therefore consider the sexual aspects of infertility. But first let us consider pregnancy.

PREGNANCY AND THE PUERPERIUM

In Chapter 2 we considered the decline in sexual interest and activity that typically accompanies pregnancy (see p. 111). White & Reamy (1982) in their review of the literature concluded: 'the first trimester is usually accompanied either by a decrease in sexual activity or by little or no change . . . in the second trimester there is either an increase in sexual feelings or behaviours or the more frequent finding of a continued decline in libido and sexual activity. Lack of sexual interest and reduced sexual activity as pregnancy nears completion appear to be the predictable pattern for most pregnant women'.

Ford & Beach (1952) showed how taboos against sex during pregnancy are widespread across cultures, though varying in severity and extent. Various reasons for such taboos are put forward, principally fear of harming the fetus. Such fears are common though not institutionalised in our own culture.

Is there any medical evidence that sexual activity during pregnancy can harm the fetus? There have been some reports suggesting this might be the case, in particular leading to fetal distress (Grudzinskas et al 1979), infection or antepartum haemorrhage (Naeye 1979, 1980) and premature labour (Goodlin 1969). The evidence for such claims has been disputed and the weight of current opinion is that in the absence of obvious contraindications, sex and orgasm during pregnancy are not only safe but often advantageous for the well-being of the family unit (White & Reamy 1982; Reader & Savage 1983). Typical advice is to avoid intercourse or orgasm during the first trimester when previous miscarriages have been attributed to congenital uterine defects or uterine fibroids, and in the second trimester in cases of cervical incompetence, at least until the defect has been surgically corrected. For the third trimester it is recommended that coitus and orgasm should be avoided in women with obvious obstetric complications such as bleeding, ruptured membranes, premature dilatation of the cervix or threatened premature labour (White & Reamy 1982).

In the post-partum period, Robson et al (1981) found that nearly all women had resumed sexual intercourse by the 12th week, and a third had done so by the sixth week. Grudzinskas & Atkinson (1984) found 51% of 328 women had resumed intercourse when interviewed between 5 and 7 weeks post-partum.

An important factor influencing the quality of the early post-partum sexual experience is pain, particularly in those women who have had an episiotomy — a procedure for cutting the perineum so as to avoid uncontrolled tearing during delivery. This is commonly done, especially for women undergoing their first delivery. It is carried out in about two-thirds of all deliveries in the USA (Reamy & White 1987).

Beischer (1967) studied the effects of this procedure and its subsequent repair on sexual function. In one Australian hospital episiotomies were performed in 30% of deliveries. Ninety per cent of these were repaired by medical students. Post-partum, 39% of the women with episiotomies had experienced dyspareunia, persisting 3 months after delivery in 23%. This was unrelated to the time of resuming intercourse. In 6% the dyspareunia was severe and in those cases there was usually some narrowing of the vaginal introitus or the creation of a skin bridge due to inappropriate repair. Garner (1982) studied 204 women following their second delivery in an English maternity hospital. Thirty per cent of the women with episiotomies and 30% of those with perineal tears reported interference with their sex lives. Of interest was the finding that these sequelae were less common in women who had forceps deliveries. This was attributed to the involvement of more skilled personnel at the repair stage in such cases.

Some attention has also been paid to the positioning of episiotomies, with suggestions that midline episiotomies cause less problems subsequently than the more usual mediolateral incisions (Reamy & White 1987). The midline incision is usually avoided in case it extends into a third degree tear involving the anal sphincter. But clearly these almost routine procedures and the rather casual manner in which they are often repaired require careful reappraisal.

BREASTFEEDING

As discussed in Chapter 2, the main determinant of the hormonal status of the woman in the puerperium is her method of infant-feeding. The fully breastfeeding woman is likely to have ovarian suppression, raised prolactin levels and relative oestrogen deficiency. We considered some evidence that sexual difficulties, especially dyspareunia, are more common in the fully breastfeeding woman. Hormonal factors, such as oestrogen lack or low testosterone, might play a part (Alder et al 1986; see p. 114), but there are obviously other factors to be taken into account. Breastfeeding is associated with more disrupted sleep for the mother and hence greater fatigue. The psychological implications of breastfeeding for both the mother and her partner are complex and may be important. For some mothers there is an erotic aspect to breastfeeding. For some, such a reaction makes them feel uncomfortable and may lead to their giving up breastfeeding. Some men are disturbed by the sight of their partner breastfeeding (Reamy & White 1987). Full breastfeeding may make it difficult for the mother to carry out all her other usual commitments, leading in some cases to tension or resentment in the spouse or other family members. We found no evidence that women who persist with breastfeeding have more negative or inhibited attitudes towards sex prior to the breastfeeding experience (Alder & Bancroft 1988). When making the decision whether to breastfeed and for how long, a variety of costs and benefits have to be taken into account. There is a tendency at the present time for health professionals to convey the impression to mothers that failing to breastfeed is in some sense giving the baby a less than ideal start in life, and many women who are unable to breastfeed feel guilt or failure for that reason. In developing countries the advantages of breastfeeding to the health of the infant are undisputed. In our society, the advantages are not so clearcut and have to be weighed against the disadvantages. Whilst stressing that breastfeeding is perfectly compatible with a good sexual relationship, there is some suggestion that the fully breastfeeding woman may take longer to return to her pre-pregnancy levels of sexual enjoyment and interest (Alder & Bancroft 1988).

CONTRACEPTION

The use of different methods of fertility control varies enormously from one culture to another, and to a lesser extent within cultures according to age and social class.

Figures for married women in the UK for the years 1970, 1975 and 1983 are given in Table 12.1 showing that in 1975 and 1983 oral contraception was the most widely used method in the UK, whereas barrier methods, such as the diaphragm and condom were being used less. The main difference in the 1983 General Household Survey compared to 1975 was the continuing increase in sterilisation of women in the 30–44 age group.

It is important to point out that the 1983 survey was carried out shortly before the 1983 'pill scare' and hence may have been followed by more dramatic changes. It is also a consistent finding that single women are nearly twice as likely to use oral contraception than married or cohabiting women.

Table 12.1 Contraceptive use in the UK amongst fertile married women, not pregnant and not trying to conceive. Figures for 1970 and 1975 are for women aged under 41 (Bone 1978); Figures for 1983 are for women aged under 44 (General Household Survey 1983)

Current method	1970 (n = 1895) %	1975 (n = 1655) %	1983 (n = 1917) %
Withdrawal	19	7	10
Pill	25	42	40
Intrauterine device	5	9	12
Diaphragm	6	3	3
Condom	36	25	28
Safe period	6	1	3
None	7	11	8

There have been changes in the usage of the pill in relation to social class. These are shown in Figure 12.1, with Social class V married mothers being the least likely pill users in 1967–1968, but the most likely in 1984. There has also been a relative increase in intrauterine device (IUD) usage by Social classes I and II women between 1975 and 1984 (Cartwright 1987).

There remains a marked difference amongst age groups, particularly in pill usage, reflecting the concern about health risks for older women on the pill (Fig. 12.2). There is reason to think that middle-class women, the first to adopt oral contraception, are showing the earliest abandonment of this method for fear of the associated health hazards. This trend is being accompanied by an increased use of the medically safe barrier methods (Kleinman 1980). The number of women attending family planning clinics in the Lothian area of Scotland and using diaphragms or cap has shown a steady increase since 1977, when the percentage of registered patients using this method was 5.1%. By 1986 it had risen to 10.6%.

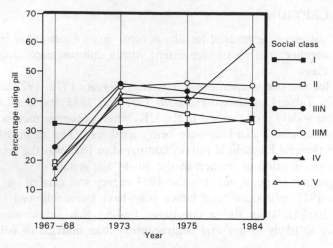

Fig. 12.1 Pill use by social class. (from Cartwright 1987)

There are likely to be substantial increases in the use of the condom or sheath as a result of the AIDS scare, though this will probably be more evident among the unmarried. As yet, evidence for such change is not available.

An estimate of worldwide use of different methods is shown in Table 12.2. Most of the variation in usage of these different methods depends on varying criteria of acceptability, which in turn reflect sociocultural and religious influences. Before considering each method, there are certain general comments that can be made about the acceptability of fertility control methods. Some concern physical effects; most are related to their psychological or social implications. Of enormous importance is the morality of contraception. The Roman Catholic Church, in particular, deems any artificial method of avoiding conception to be immoral

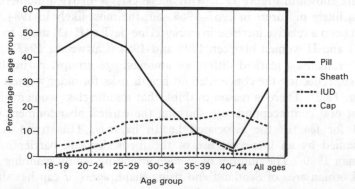

Fig. 12.2 Current use of contraception by women in 1976 in England, Scotland and Wales, by age. (Dunnell 1979)

Table 12.2 Estimated worldwide use of fertility control methods (Djerassi 1979a)

Methods	Millions of users
Prolonged lactation	50–100
Oral contraceptives	50–80
Abortion	30–55
Sterilisation	15–30
Condoms	15–20
Intrauterine devices	15
Diaphragm	2–3
Coitus interruptus	?
Rhythm method	?

(Humanae Vitac 1968), a dictate which is being strongly reinforced by the current Pope, John Paul II. In the face of changing modern attitudes, and the inescapable fact of world over-population, an increasing number of Catholics are rejecting this particular part of the Church's teaching (Westoff & Jones 1977). (Orthodox Jewry also oppose contraception, though with the constant threats to the survival of the Jewish race this is perhaps more understandable (Parrinder 1987).) One hopes that the price they pay in terms of religious conflict and guilt is small in comparison with the appalling consequences that so many, particularly women and their children, suffer as a result of unwanted pregnancies or the fear of them. Nevertheless the subservience of sex to reproduction, which biologically disappeared at a much earlier stage of human evolution, is still fostered by such religious beliefs and goes deep in many individuals. Thus for some, most commonly women, sex requires at least the possibility of conception for it to be fully enjoyed. Methods of contraception which are foolproof such as steroidal contraceptives, or irreversible, such as sterilisation, may thus be unacceptable. For others, the associated conflict may make it difficult for the individual to take active responsibility for contraception, particularly that which has to be repeatedly exercised, such as taking a pill each day or inserting a diaphragm. In such cases 'medical' methods, such as IUDs, the fitting of which is the responsibility of the doctor, may hold special appeal.

Problems may reflect difficulties in male/female relationships. Thus conflict may lead to reluctance in one or other partner to take responsibility. A women may decline oral contraception because she resents her partner's failure or refusal to take a share of responsibility. But there are also factors which reflect individual personality differences more than sociocultural influences. Barrier methods, such as the condom or diaphragm, are disliked by some because of their interference with the spontaneity of love-making or the physical barrier they present between partners. For others, this same barrier may be an added attraction; the man or woman who dislikes mess may prefer ejaculate to be captured in a sheath rather than allowed to 'run free'. The protection afforded by the sheath against sexually transmitted disease is one increasingly important consideration for some. Any method of contraception which substantially alters the enjoyment or interest of the user may cause repercussions in the sexual relationship. A woman whose sexuality has been inhibited for years by fear of pregnancy, once started on effective contraception may find that her sexual awakening leads to anxieties or sexual failure in her partner, who cannot cope with the apparent increase in sexual demands upon him.

It is difficult to dispute the idea that modern methods of fertility control have contributed to the changing status of women who can now decide whether to have children and to some extent, when. They are much less likely to be trapped in traditional female roles by unplanned pregnancies. The social impact of this is and will continue to be considerable. And yet, on an individual level, such freedom can be threatening. In its most extreme form, this threat may be linked with a fear of losing one's female identity or of becoming promiscuous. In the case of oral contraception, this can be compounded by a fear of anything that changes one's internal chemistry and hence one's behaviour. Some people dislike taking any kind of drug which alters their internal state in an unpredictable way. Women with such personalities may find oral contraceptives difficult to tolerate.

In Chapter 4 we considered the incidence of sexual activity amongst teenagers. The risk of pregnancy in this group is of obvious importance and yet the factors influencing the use of contraception are complex. Unprotected sexual intercourse in this age group is common. Kantner & Zelnik (1973) found that nearly half of the sexually active girls in their sample were not using any method of contraception. Of those that were, the commonest method was coitus interruptus. Findings from a number of studies are consistent with this, and show that whilst many sexually experienced adolescents have used contraception at some stage, regular use is considerably less frequent (McCormick et al 1977; Ryde-Blomqvist 1978).

Lindemann (1977), in an interesting discussion, suggested three stages of birth control behaviour: the natural stage when no contraceptives are used; the peer stage, when methods learned from peers are used; and the expert stage, when experts or professionals are consulted. In the natural stage, she suggests, 'the very nature of sexual activity is not conducive to the use of contraceptives'. Intercourse is unplanned, and hence unpredictable and, at this stage, usually infrequent. Spontaneous sex is seen as natural; contraception is artificial. There is in any case a generally low level of awareness of the possibility of pregnancy which may be perpetuated by the experience of sexual activity which does not lead to pregnancy. To some extent this may be less unrealistic than it seems for the young adolescent girl who may still be in a phase of relative adolescent infertility (see p. 234). At some point, determined by such factors as a delayed period, or pregnancy of a friend, or even in herself, awareness of the need for contraception develops. It is difficult to know what effects sex education has on this process. Knowledge may be acquired, but not seen to be of personal relevance. A number of studies have shown that teenagers who get pregnant are often aware of various methods of contraception but have not made use of that knowledge (Ryde-Blomqvist 1978). Sack et al (1985) found that the best predictor of whether a female student used effective contraception was whether her friend also did so.

At the peer group stage of introducing contraception, understanding normal fertility and its relevance to the risk of conception is important, particularly if artificial methods of contraception are seen to be inaccessible. In Kantner & Zelnick's (1973) study, the understanding of the times of maximum fertility during the menstrual cycle was generally poor. The commonest fallacy was that conception was most likely just before, during or after menstruation. Recent attempts to evaluate the efficacy of educational programmes aimed at teenagers have shown some success particularly when attention is focused on 'Communication and problem-solving skills' (Beck & Davies 1987).

It is at this stage in the girl's life that the commitment to sexual activity becomes of crucial significance. For a girl to take the decision to use contraception, particularly methods such as the pill which imply long-term needs, may be much more difficult than her becoming involved periodically and 'in the heat of the moment' in unprotected sexual activity. As Lindemann says, commitment to sex gets focused on birth control rather than on sex itself. It is in this respect that social attitudes to the adolescent male are so negative and unhelpful. For an adolescent boy, to obtain a condom represents much less of a threat of sexual commitment than for a girl to start on the pill. The condom may even be carried around as a kind of status symbol without being used (Coles 1978). Only recently has attention started to be paid to fostering responsibility for contraception in the adolescent male, which if successful, would not only reduce the likelihood of unprotected intercourse but also reinforce more responsible, caring and less exploitative attitudes in male sexuality. Very little research has been done on the factors influencing the contraceptive behaviour of teenage boys, especially those in the high-risk 12–16 age group. Parental attitudes are also highly relevant. Many girls will participate in sexual intercourse but avoid the use of contraceptives in case their parents find out. The double standard which is so prevalent in parental attitudes will encourage boys to see the responsibility for contraception as being with the girl. Educational programmes which aim to involve either the boyfriend or the family may be more effective in changing behaviour (Beck & Davies 1987).

Part of the girl's conflict about commitment to sex reflects a concern to retain her virgin status (see p. 232) or at least avoid being labelled as sexually promiscuous. Thus at the early stage of a sexual relationship, the girl may fear that evidence of preparedness on her part will be construed by the boy as evidence of lax sexual morals and hence reduce her attractiveness as a potential wife.

Another aspect which was discussed in Chapter 2 is the need for the adolescent girl to demonstrate her fertility, particularly in those social settings which provide the developing female with few sources of self-esteem other than motherhood and marriage. The 'bundling' system of premarital sex until pregnancy, proving the girl's suitability for marriage (see p. 221), incorporated this theme, which probably still lingers in many teenage girls, albeit unwittingly. It is far from unusual to find teenage girls living in deprived families or communities and falling pregnant with apparent satisfaction, and yet accepting termination of pregnancy when it is offered to them. It is as though they need the reassurance of proving their fertility and the status that goes with it, rather than the mothering of the child. Concern about fertility is not of course confined to the adolescent. Married women may be reluctant to delay starting their family for this reason and particular concern about the effect of oral contraceptives on fertility has been common, though as yet unfounded. One of the most popular attempts to account for contraceptive risk-taking was presented by Luker (1975) based on her study of young women following termination of pregnancy. Her model was an example of 'SEU theory' (i.e. subjective expected utility). The likelihood of risking pregnancy is seen as a product of the balance of costs and benefits of both avoiding pregnancy and getting pregnant for a particular woman. Crosbie & Bitte (1982) sought evidence to support this theoretical model but failed. They concluded that humans are 'unable to choose consistently in the face of even moderate complexity or uncertainty'.

Certainly we can conclude that contraceptive use amongst adolescents is far from being a straightforward matter of availability and common sense.

With these general considerations in mind, let us look at the various methods of fertility control in more detail.

STEROIDAL CONTRACEPTION

The mechanism and physical effects of steroidal contraception are well covered in many other texts but it is necessary for our present purposes to consider briefly the different types of steroidal contraceptives and their presumed mechanism of action and hormonal effects.

Most steroidal contraceptives are taken orally, made possible by the development of synthetic oestrogens and progestagens with much greater potency than the natural steroids (Djerassi 1979a; see Fig. 12.3). Oral contraceptives are of three main types: combined, sequential and progestagen only. Combined pills contain both oestrogen (most commonly ethinyloestradiol) and progestagen (usually either norethisterone or levonorgestrel). They are taken for 21 days, followed by 7 pill-free days during which the exogenous steroid levels fall in the blood and there is a monthly withdrawal bleed. The early forms of sequential pill aimed to mimic the normal cycle by giving only oestrogen during the first part of the cycle and then an oestrogen–progestagen combination in the second half. These early versions were withdrawn from the market, partly because of slightly lower efficacy than the combined form, but also because of concern about possible long-

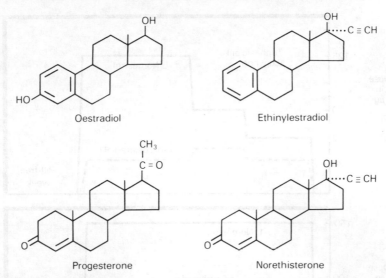

Oestradiol

Ethinylestradiol

Progesterone

Norethisterone

Fig. 12.3 Oral contraception became a possibility because of the synthesis of oestrogens and progestagens, which were much more potent and resistant to metabolic degradation than natural steroids. This allowed sufficient absorbtion from the gut to be effective. The structures of a commonly used oestrogen and progestagen are shown here together with natural oestradiol 17β and progesterone.

term effects of the constituents used. There are now several new versions, e.g. the tri-phasic pill, in which for the first 6 days of the pill cycle, a very low dose of progestagen is combined with a low dose of oestrogen. For the next 5 days, there is a slight increase in the dosage of both constituents and then for 10 days there is a further increase in the progestagen and a return of the ocstrogen to its initial low level. There are then the usual 7 pill-free days. Comparison of the hormonal profile of a combined and a tri-phasic pill is shown in Figure 12.4.

Both combined and sequential types are believed to work by suppressing ovulation, though other effects on the cervical mucus, reducing sperm penetration, and elsewhere on the reproductive tract, may also inhibit fertility. The progestagen only pills are less predictable in inhibiting ovulation and rely primarily on their endometrial effects (Hawkins & Elder 1979). Whereas the combined and sequential pills are taken cyclically, leading to predictable withdrawal bleeds, the progestagen only preparations are taken continuously and menstrual bleeding may be irregular or 'break-through' bleeding may occur. This affects the acceptability of the method for many women.

In recent years, there has been a sustained attempt to reduce the steroidal constituents of oral contraceptives to the minimum necessary for contra-ceptive effectiveness, in the belief that harmful effects will thereby be reduced. There has been particular concern with the oestrogenic compo-nent. Whereas early contraceptives contained the equivalent of 100 μg of

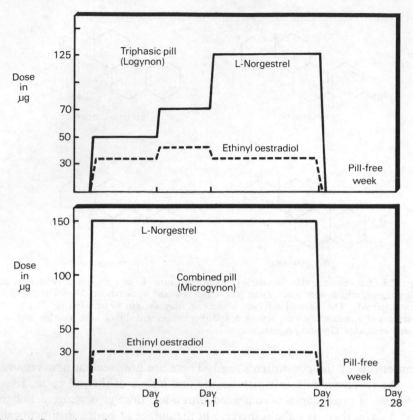

Fig. 12.4 Comparison of combined and tri-phasic oral contraceptives.

ethinyloestradiol or more, 50 μg pills were used for many years and have now largely given way to 30–35 μg preparations. The progestagenic component has been receiving similar attention more recently in the combined and progestagen only methods. With the new tri-phasic pills an attempt has been made to reduce both constituents to a minimum.

The injectable forms of steroidal contraceptives have mainly contained progestagen only, e.g. medroxyprogesterone acetate (Depo-Provera). They have the advantage of long-term efficacy and may be particularly useful in women who are incapable of taking responsibility for daily oral medication. Such use raises ethical problems, however, and there is continuing uncertainty about possible long-term effects, which makes the use of these injectables controversial. Recently, vaginal rings containing slowly released progestagens have been introduced, but it is too early to comment on their value or efficacy. Progestagen contraception may have a special place for the breastfeeding woman as oestrogens are likely to inhibit lactation. However injectable progestagens are more likely to appear in the milk and oral preparations are therefore to be preferred.

The effects of steroidal contraceptives on sexual behaviour

The early literature on this subject can best be described as confused. As most of it concerns oral contraceptives which are no longer in use we will not consider it in detail here (for fuller reviews see Glick 1967; Bardwick 1973; Bancroft 1974; Bragonier 1976; Kane 1976.)

Several large-scale studies (e.g. Westoff et al 1976) have shown that the frequency of coitus was higher in women on the pill than in those using other methods or no methods at all. Whilst one can take some overall reassurance from such evidence, there are a number of difficulties in interpreting it. First, women who choose oral contraceptives may be different in their pattern of sexuality to those who prefer other methods. Secondly, a proportion of women may cease to use oral contraceptives because of sexual difficulties. One can say nothing from such evidence of the likely numbers so affected. Thirdly, coital rates tell us very little about the quality of the sexual experience. Adoption of an effective method may remove obstacles to the male's sexual demands; coital frequency might therefore increase even with a reduction in the woman's spontaneous interest. It is relevant that in one study (Gambrell et al 1976) increase in sexual interest and activity whilst on the pill was more likely to be reported by single than married women. Single women also reported having more sexual partners; possibly the greater sexual freedom that these women experienced as a result of the oral contraceptive had a libido-enhancing effect; they were in a position to choose. Consequences for the married women may have been less exciting. In most previous studies, the concept of libido has been ill-defined, making recognition of subtle but important effects difficult.

According to a large survey in general practice, women using oral contraceptives were four times more likely to complain of sexual difficulties than women using other methods (Royal College of General Practitioners 1974). Once again we must be cautious in interpreting this evidence. The provision of oral contraception provides a better opportunity for talking about sexual problems than most other reasons for attending the general practitioner.

In Chapter 2 I stressed the important relationship between mood and sexuality as they change through the menstrual cycle. This association is highly relevant when considering the effects of oral contraceptives on behaviour. Early pill studies reflected this association, though the evidence for a relationship between pill constituent and mood change was inconsistent. Herzberg et al (1971) found that women stopping the pill because of loss of libido were also significantly more depressed than those who continued. Grant & Pryse-Davies (1968) in their study of the effects of oral contraceptives made a combined rating of depression and loss of libido, and found that this combined variable was more adversely affected the higher the progestagen content of the pill. Kutner & Brown (1972) in relation to depression (sexuality was not assessed) found the reverse: pills containing high doses of progestagen were associated with less severe depression. In one of the better studies, Cullberg (1973) varied the progestagen dosage in a controlled way. He found that all the active pills used produced significantly more psychological side-effects than the placebo preparation, but these effects did not vary with the progestagen dosage (but see below). He found sexual impairment to be slight and concluded that when it occurred it was secondary to mood change.

Morris & Udry (1972) found in a placebo-controlled study that women did not show a different pattern of well-being through the cycle whilst taking oral contraceptives, compared with placebo cycles. Interestingly, in both conditions the women tended to feel worst premenstrually or during menstruation (see below). Udry et al (1973), reporting on the same women, did find a difference in the pattern of sexuality between the pill and placebo cycles. Although the overall frequency of sexual activity was similar, there was a decline in the latter part of the placebo cycle which was not evident in the pill cycle.

In a large-scale retrospective study, readers of a monthly women's magazine completed a questionnaire about menstrual health (Warner & Bancroft 1988). They were asked, amongst other things, to indicate where in their last cycle their well-being and their sexual interest were at their highest and lowest. They could choose between 'week before period', 'during period', 'week after period', 'other times' or 'never'. The distribution for the highs and lows for pill-using and non-pill-using women are shown in Figure 12.5. Ther was a strong association between well-being and sexual interest in both groups, with the week after the period being the best time for both groups and both variables. But the two groups did differ significantly from each other; the pill-using women were less likely to report either highs or lows, and more likely to report high sexual interest either *during* menstruation or *the week before*. This difference between the groups in the timing of sexual interest could not be attributed to differences

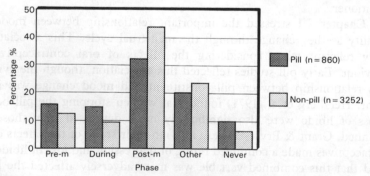

Fig. 12.5 Timing of high sex interest during the menstrual cycle by pill and non-pill users. Women were asked to indicate the week before the period (pre-m), during the period, the week after the period (post-m) or at other times. (Warner & Bancroft 1988)

in the timing of highs and lows of well-being. The pill appeared to be having a direct effect on sexuality independently of its effects on mood.

If the constituents of the pill are having a direct effect on how the woman feels, then a comparison of the different pill regimes could be fruitful (see Fig. 12.4). One such study using the original sequential pills was reported by Bardwick (1973). In this study, women not using oral contraceptives were compared with those using either combined or sequential preparations. Only mood was measured, not sexuality, but the results showed that the women using the sequential pill had a cyclical pattern of mood change similar to the non-pill-taking women and different to those using the combined preparation.

We now have comparable evidence from the newer generation of triphasic and combined pills. In the previously mentioned retrospective study (Warner & Bancroft 1988) we were able to compare low dose combined with tri-phasic pill users. The tri-phasic group came midway between the combined pill and the non-pill groups in their distribution of highs and lows of both sexuality and mood, differences that were significantly different. We

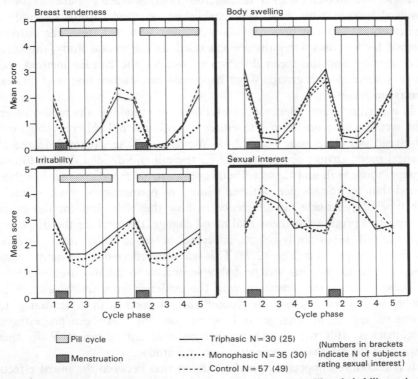

Fig. 12.6 The timing of four changes, breast tenderness, body swelling, irritability and sexual interest through two menstrual cycles in three groups of women, triphasic pill users, monoplasic (Combined) pill users and non-pill controls. Each cycle is divided into five phases according to the varying dose levels of the triphasic pill regime. Only breast tenderness showed any difference between the groups. (Walker & Bancroft 1988)

then examined this further in a prospective study in which three groups of women (tri-phasic, combined and non-pill-using groups, matched for age and parity) completed daily ratings of mood, sexuality and other changes for three consecutive cycles (Walker & Bancroft 1988). The most striking thing about this study was the degree of similarity of the three groups, raising the question of how important a normal ovulatory cycle is for the perimenstrual changes that women commonly experience.

Sexuality and mood were closely related to each other in all three groups, and the groups did not differ significantly from each other in either variable. They were also strikingly similar in their pattern of cyclical bloating. The one variable to show clear differences was cyclical breast changes; the non-pill and tri-phasic users were indistinguishable in this respect, whereas the combined pill users reported significantly fewer breast changes (Fig. 12.6). The differences between groups which were observed and found to be significant in the larger retrospective study were noticeable in this prospective study but were of modest degree and did not reach statistical significance.

These two studies (Walker & Bancroft 1988; Warner & Bancroft 1988) involved women who were well established on their current method of contraception. In the first study any woman who had used her current method for less than 6 months was excluded. In the second study, the same limit applied and the mean duration of use for the current method was about 4 years in each group. What happens when women first start on oral contraceptives?

In a further study (Bancroft et al 1987) we randomly allocated women who were to start on the pill to either a combined pill (Microgynon) or a tri-phasic pill (Logynon; Fig. 12.4). We assessed the women's degree of cyclical mood change before starting on the pill and divided them into two groups, those with and those without premenstrual mood change. We then found that for the women with *no* history of premenstrual mood change, the type of pill made no difference to how they felt. But for the other group, with previous premenstrual mood change, those taking the tri-phasic pill showed significantly more lowering of mood than those on the combined preparation (Fig. 12.7). This was also reflected in the daily sexual interest ratings, but this was probably secondary to the mood effect.

These findings are consistent with the evidence from Cullberg's (1973) study, mentioned earlier. He found that women with a tendency to premenstrual mood change did worse on the oestrogen/progestagen combination with the lowest progestagen content (comparable in that respect to the tri-phasic preparation on our study).

It is therefore important to make a distinction between the initial effects of starting on the pill (e.g. Morris & Udry 1972; Cullberg 1973, Bancroft et al 1987) and the much later effects of the pill on women who are long established on that contraceptive regime (e.g. Walker & Bancroft 1988; Warner & Bancroft 1988). In between these early and late time periods two

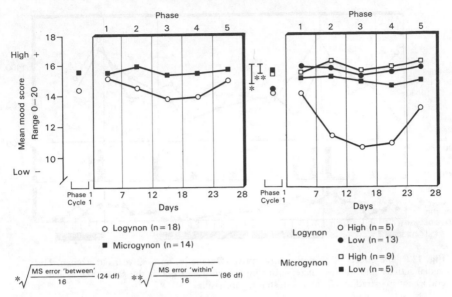

Fig. 12.7 Mood ratings during five phases of the second cycle of women after starting on either a triphasic (Logynon) or monophasic (Microgynon) oral contraceptive. On the left there is no significant difference between the two groups. On the right women are divided into those with and without a history of premenstrual mood change before starting the pill. ('High' & 'low' respectively). The high premenstrual mood change group women, using the triphasic pill, showed significantly lower mood during the cycle (Bancroft et al 1987)

things may have happened. Some women will have discontinued the pill, often because of side-effects. (Discontinuation rates within the first year of pill use have varied between 27% (Royal College of General Practitoners 1974) and 45% (Melton & Shelton 1971).) They will have selected themselves out of the 'stable state' studies. Secondly, women staying on the pill will have adjusted to the new hormonal regime. The initial phase can be likened to a mini-adolescence, when the body, and in particular the brain, is required to adjust to a new cyclical hormonal regime. As yet we do not know how long this period of adjustment takes but it is certainly likely to be at least 2–3 months.

Thus it would seem that oral contraceptives may have an adverse effect during the initial phases dependent on characteristics, firstly of the women (e.g. whether she is prone to perimenstrual mood change) and secondly, of the particular pill. Some women will accommodate these initial effects and settle satisfactorily on the pill; others may find them sufficiently persistent and troublesome to persuade them to abandon that method of contraception. Although the evidence is far from conclusive as yet, it seems that oral contraceptives can influence a woman's sexuality directly, in addition to indirect effects via her mood.

In what way might the pill directly affect sexuality? As we have seen, the commonest pattern is for sexual interest to be maximal in the post-

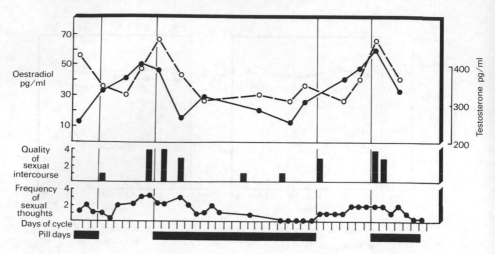

Fig. 12.8 The effects of an oral contraceptive (Ovranette) on a 32-year-old women. Her sexual activity and interest increase during the pill-free week at the same time as her endogenous oestradiol 17β and testosterone are rising.

menstrual week in both pill- and non-pill-taking women. Sometimes sexual interest and activity become restricted to that relatively brief part of the pill cycle, presenting as a problem of insufficient sexual desire. An example of this is shown in Figure 12.8, which also illustrates how in some pill-taking women both oestradiol and testosterone increase during the pill-free week. Could the relative suppression of these steroids at other times in the pill cycle be contributing to the altered pattern of sexual activity? In an earlier study, we explored the possibility that loss of sexual desire in pill-takers could be due to lowered androgen levels (Bancroft et al 1980). We compared women with sexual problems attributed to the pill with women without such problems but taking the same contraceptive preparations. The androgen levels were similarly low in *both* groups, making an androgen explanation unlikely. Furthermore, a placebo-controlled evaluation of androgen administration to the women with problems produced no benefit.

The mechanisms by which oral contraceptives affect sexuality therefore remain obscure. It would seem that in the majority of women such effects are absent or negligible. What proportion of women are adversely affected is not yet known, but in some this may depend on their susceptibility to pill-induced mood change and in others on a more direct sexual effect. The role of the premenstrual syndrome in this picture also remains unclear. For many women cyclical symptoms are *reduced* by oral contraceptives (e.g. Andersch 1980). But for some, their pattern of cyclical symptoms are aggravated by the pill, often making this method of contraception unacceptable for them. This is an important area which requires further research.

INTRAUTERINE DEVICES (IUDs)

There is little evidence of the effects of IUDs on sexuality. Herzberg et al (1971), comparing women using IUDs with those on the pill, found that in the first group there was a steady increase in sexual interest, frequency of intercourse and sexual satisfaction. This may well have reflected a growing confidence in the safety of the method with continuing use plus a reduction in the menstrual disturbance (i.e. intermenstrual bleeding, increased menstrual blood loss and pain) that often occurs for the first few cycles after IUD insertion. There are indirect effects to be considered resulting from pelvic inflammatory disease, of which there is an increased risk, particularly in young nulligravid women who have had numerous sexual partners (Booth et al 1980; Vessey et al 1981; Tatum & Connell 1986). But apart from this, there is no reason to think that IUDs will adversely affect sexuality in women who can physically tolerate them. IUDs have the advantage, important for some women, that the responsibility for their fitting is taken by a doctor, after which no positive action on the part of the woman is required.

THE DIAPHRAGM

This form of barrier method, which is reasonably effective if used conscientiously and in combination with a spermicidal cream, is probably the safest method of contraception for the health of the woman. For many, however, it is unacceptable. It requires frequent handling of the genitalia, which may cause concern. More important is its potential interference with spontaneity. The diaphragm is fitted every day, which is tiresome, or it is fitted in anticipation of intercourse, which some women are reluctant to reveal, or it is fitted after love-making has started. Occasionally the male partner finds the presence of the diaphragm uncomfortable during intercourse, or, if the diaphragm is too large, the woman may find that her sexual enjoyment is impaired.

NATURAL METHODS

The various rhythm methods which avoid conception by avoiding intercourse during the fertile period of the woman's cycle, are the only methods of fertility control acceptable to the Roman Catholic Church. The two commonest methods involve taking a daily temperature and identifying the day of ovulation by the rise in temperature, or the ovulation method in which the woman learns to observe the nature of her cervical mucus, and by this means, to recognise when she is getting close to ovulation (Billings & Billings 1973). Intercourse is then avoided until the safe period is reached. Unfortunately, this method has an unacceptably high failure rate and in a five-centre World Health Organization (WHO) study there was an annual rate of 19.4 pregnancies per 100 women years, though according to the WHO report, this was mainly due to a failure to abstain, rather than failure to recognise the fertile period (WHO 1978). The extent of abstinence required is considerable; in the first half of the cycle, intercourse has to be avoided on alternate days so that the partner's semen does not obscure the mucus changes. Then, with the change in consistency of the mucus, abstinence may be required for 7 to 14 days before the next safe period prior to menstruation is reached. It is notable that the instructions on this method distributed by Catholic agencies seem to be as much concerned with the spiritually uplifting effects of self-imposed abstinence as on the avoidance of conception. There is no suggestion that other forms of sexual stimulation, such as oral or manual, leading to orgasm with ejaculation well away from the vagina, might be used instead of vaginal intercourse. It may well be that for such reasons this method has not been adequately explored. According to the evidence presented in Chapter 2, there is no obvious peak of female desire around ovulation, so that limitation of sexual activity around this time may not be as physiologically contradictory as it first seems. As it is, such methods may hold appeal for couples whose level of sexual appetite is modest and who may welcome a good reason for restricting their sexual activity.

The infertility associated with breastfeeding is probably the most natural method of birth spacing. Whilst breastfeeding is by no means a foolproof contraceptive, there is little doubt that reduction of breastfeeding and increased use of artificial methods of feeding has led to reduced birth intervals in many parts of the world (Short 1976). The contraceptive effect may depend on the nutritional status of the mother. There is some evidence that if the mother is undernourished, her prolactin levels will be higher as part of a process of ensuring adequate nutrition in the breast milk for the infant. These higher prolactin levels have the added biological advantage of preventing ovulation. If the mother is well nourished, the prolactin levels are not so high and inhibition of ovulation is less certain. Not everyone accepts this interpretation of the evidence (Bongaarts 1980). As discussed in Chapter 2, the suckling frequency is also relevant; ovulation becomes more likely if the frequency of suckling declines and supplementary feeds are introduced.

THE MALE METHODS

Both the two methods for which the male is responsible, coitus interruptus and the condom, have long histories. Coitus interruptus, or withdrawal, has often been blamed as a cause of sexual problems, though there is no convincing evidence that this is so. There is little doubt, however, that for most people the degree of vigilance that is required and the inevitable interruption of intercourse that ensues detracts from the enjoyment of lovemaking. But there may be some for whom controlled withdrawal presents no problems and others for whom the avoidance of intravaginal ejaculation may be welcomed for aesthetic rather than contraceptive reasons. It should not therefore be assumed that coitus interruptus will always spoil sexual enjoyment. With the condom, the most obvious disadvantage is its interference with normal tactile sensations of the penis, though with modern technology thinner sheaths are being produced to minimise this effect. Another problem frequently cited is the interference with the spontaneity of love-making. The condom, however, has become something of a sexual symbol; the used sheath floating in the river conjures up images of illicit sex which may be quite erotic. In recent years, condoms have been marketed in a much more imaginative fashion, not only with alluring packaging, but also with exotic colours for the condoms themselves and added structures like delicate rubber ribs which are intended to enhance stimulation of the woman during intercourse. Condoms have some obvious advantages. They are easily distributable and hence are particularly suitable for young sexually uncommitted couples. They act as a barrier against venereal infection and are now being widely recommended as the method for reducing the risk of infection with HIV virus (see p. 596). Also, as mentioned earlier, they provide the male with an opportunity to be sexually responsible. Cultural differences in the acceptability and use of condoms are an interesting comment on the varying attitudes to male sexual responsibility. According to Djerassi (1979a), men in Arab countries and the macho cultures of Latin America are unlikely to use them. In other countries, like Bangladesh, they are quite popular.

Attempts to develop other effective and acceptable male contraceptives continue. One that has been used in China since the 1950s is a phenolic compound called gossypol. This directly interferes with spermatogenesis. It is not, however, free from side-effects — fatigue, gastrointestinal symptoms and decreased sexual desire (5% of cases) are the most frequent (Liu 1981). So far, attempts to produce less toxic variants have not succeeded and gossypol has not found favour in the western world.

Most current efforts are being directed at the hormonal control of spermatogenesis (WHO 1982). The main problem is to suppress spermatogenesis without also suppressing testosterone and hence sexual desire. LHRH agonists, for example, produce both effects (Linde et al 1981). It is possible that the combination of such regimes with a supply of testosterone may achieve one effect without incurring the other, but it remains to be seen how feasible this is, and how acceptable a regime that would provide. There is also the possibility that in the future developments with inhibin may prove to be fruitful in this respect (see p. 25).

STERILISATION

Surgical methods of contraceptive sterilisation are now becoming of worldwide importance. In the female, various techniques can be employed but the most widely used nowadays is tubal diathermy or the application of clips or rings through a laparoscope. In the male, vasectomy is normally carried out under local anaesthetic and is a relatively simple and quick surgical procedure.

There has been a dramatic increase in the incidence of these procedures. In the UK, female sterilisation has risen most markedly since 1967, vasectomy since 1970. In 1970 in 4% of couples where the wife was aged under 41 years, one of the couple had been electively sterilised. By 1973, the figure had risen to 13% (Bone 1978). In the General Household Survey of 1983, 22% of couples (with the female partner aged 18–44) had been sterilised: 11% of the women and 10% of the men. There is also an increasing tendency for younger couples with fewer children to elect for sterilisation. At the present time this is the one method of fertility control showing a continuous upward trend.

This increase has been noted in many countries. According to Population Reports (1978) there was an estimated 3.4 million surgical sterilisations worldwide in 1950, 20 million in 1970 and 65 million in 1975. By 1983 the estimated figure was 135 million (95 million females and 40 million males; Population Reports 1985).

In 1982 female sterilisation was the most widely used method of fertility control in the USA, employed by more than 17%, compared with a pill use of 14% and vasectomy, 10%.

The decision whether it should be the man or woman who is sterilised is associated with some interesting cultural and social class differences. In the UK the ratio is now close to parity (see above). In the USA this is also the case amongst whites, though the better educated couples show a preference for male sterilisation. Black Americans are strikingly different, though the difference is getting less. In 1970 the female to male ratio was 22.5:1; in 1976, 6.4:1 (Hollerbach & Nortman 1984). In Australia male exceeded female sterilisation by 1.2:1 in 1974. In India the ratio is 4 men to 1 woman (Newman & Leavesley 1980). By contrast, in Mexico the number of female sterilisations rose from 4000 in 1978 to 250 000 in 1981, with vasectomy representing only 1% of all sterilisation operations (Johnson 1983).

Surgical sterilisation is to a large extent irreversible. Though reversal techniques are being developed and improved, the success rate is still low and the operative procedure highly skilled and time-consuming, particularly where the female is concerned. The long-term consequences of this more or less irreversible procedure are therefore of increasing social importance.

FEMALE STERILISATION

There has been a trend in recent studies towards a more favourable outcome and follow-up, and this may reflect a change in the type of person being sterilised and in particular, a decreasing proportion of women being sterilised on medical grounds or as a condition of termination of pregnancy. There is general agreement that such indications are more likely to be followed by psychological repercussions, whereas women who clearly elect for contraceptive sterilisation are unlikely to regret the operation. In recent studies the percentage regretting sterilisation has usually been in single figures and it is uncertain how many of these would actually choose to have the operation reversed if they had the opportunity. One of the most obvious reasons for regret is marital breakdown and the wish for further children with a new partner (Alder 1984a). Given the steady increase of marital breakdown (see Chapter 4), this issue is likely to be of growing importance.

Also relevant is the psychological need for fertility, the unfulfilled parental role. Although some studies have indicated that regret is most likely in women sterilised young and with relatively few children (e.g. Wilson et al 1977), the pattern is probably changing. There is an increasing number of women who are clear that they want few (say two) children and are happy to limit their maternal role to that extent. They are likely to accept sterilisation with few regrets. Nulliparous women who seek sterilisation are perhaps those with the least need for the maternal role. In one follow-up study of such women, the incidence of regret was no different from that expected with parous women (Benjamin et al 1980). There is no reason to believe that female sterilisation procedures have any direct effect on sexual function. There is some evidence, though as yet inconclusive, and disputed by some workers, that menstruation may become heavier after sterilisation (Kasonde & Bonnar 1976; Noble 1978; Alder et al 1981), and may interfere secondarily with the woman's sex life. Adverse effects, when they occur, are more likely to stem from psychological reactions to the sterilisation, either in the woman or her spouse. These may reflect the need to link sex with potential reproduction or conversely, the freedom from the fear of pregnancy may increase the woman's enjoyment and interest in sex and put pressure on the husband who reacts adversely. In most studies, the majority of women report no change in their sexual relationships; improvement is relatively common and deterioration usually occurs in no more than 3 to 5%. In contrast to most reports is a study from India (Khorana & Vyas 1975) which, whilst methodologically sound, reported an extremely high incidence of mild psychological reactions. Most women (88%) were re-interviewed 3 to 6 months after the operation. In 65% sexual desire had declined and 29% were still abstaining from sexual intercourse. In spite of these complaints, only 8% of the women were dissatisfied with the operation. It is difficult to interpret these results as, clearly, cultural factors are operating which make them of limited relevance to western women. In a British study, at 1 year follow-up, 58% of women reported no change in their sexual satisfaction, 34% said it was better and 8% worse (Smith 1979).

In Germany, 95% of 2000 sterilised women were followed up by questionnaire and interview: 64% reported no change in the quality of their sex lives and 34% felt more adequate sexually. Of the husbands, 99% considered their partners at least as attractive after the sterilisation as before. Thus only 2% reported any adverse sexual effects (Rönnau 1980).

Cooper et al (1982), in a prospective study of 201 women, found that the frequency of sexual intercourse remained unchanged in 46% with equal numbers reporting an increase or a decrease. Sexual enjoyment was unchanged in 76%, increased in 22% and decreased in 6%. Although 11% reported dissatisfaction with their sexual relationship post-operatively, most had also been dissatisfied before the operation.

Cliquet et al (1981) found 1 year post-operatively that 8% of sterilised women reported reduced sexual interest, 10% reduced frequency of sexual intercourse and 7% reduced orgasm. But the majority of couples reported an improvement, usually attributing it to the removal of the fear of pregnancy. Bean et al (1980) found an increase in sexual desire following sterilisation that was significantly more frequent in the wives of vasectomised men than in the women who had themselves been sterilised (see below).

MALE STERILISATION

It is generally believed that vasectomy will not produce any adverse physiological effects on sexual function. Whilst local post-operative complications are common, they are usually mild and transient. On the basis of some animal evidence, anxiety has been expressed that vasectomy may lead to long-term impairment of cardiovascular function. But the weight of evidence from human studies, which now include some with a relatively long follow-up, is reassuring. Massey et al (1983) administered a comprehensive health questionnaire to more than 10 000 vasectomised men and an equal number of matched controls and found no difference in the incidence of cardiovascular disease (see also Linnet et al 1982; Petitti et al 1982a,b).

At an earlier stage, before vasectomy was so widespread, opinions about the psychologically castrating effects of vasectomy were often expressed (Wolfers 1970) and there was a tendency to be suspicious about the type of man who asked for the operation (Rodgers et al 1967). But even the early follow-up studies failed to support these gloomy views (Ferber et al 1967).

There have now been several large scale follow-up studies using relatively superficial assessments of sexual effects. They have all been reassuring in their findings. The Simon Population Trust (1969) followed up 1092 vasectomised men with questionnaires and obtained a 93% response: 73% reported an improvement in their sexual lives, 79% an improvement for their wives. In 25% of the men and 20% of the women there was no change; 1.5% and 0.5% respectively reported a deterioration. The Margaret Pyke Centre (1973) also reported on 1000 vasectomies studied prospectively: 460 men were sent follow-up questionnaires 1 year after the operation and 271

replied (60% response rate). Of those replying, 62% reported an improvement in their sexual life, 34% no change and 4% some deterioration. Very
similar figures were reported at 6 months' follow-up by Hart & Deane
(1980). Newman & Leavesley (1980) compared 50 married couples where
the husband had been vasectomised with 50 couples using other methods
of contraception. They found that significantly more of the vasectomy
couples reported increased sexual satisfaction and libido since the vasectomy, when compared to changes in the sexual relationships of the control
group.

Howard (1978) reported on the reasons given by men for seeking vasectomy. Prevention of further pregnancies because of completed family size
and protection of the wife from the health hazards of other contraceptive
methods, from the dangers of child-bearing or from the fears of pregnancy
were the principal reasons. However, many couples added that they hoped
for an improvement in their sex life, and in some cases this was the principal reason. This was particularly so in couples aged 35 and over. Vasectomy requests after the age of 40 seemed to have little to do with the
avoidance of pregnancy. Also of interest was the finding that most of the
men had small families and had tended to use male methods of contraception in the past.

The relative merits of male and female sterilisation are issues of considerable importance in advising couples seeking sterilisation, though they have
received little attention so far. Alder et al (1981) compared a small but
representative sample of sterilised women with the wives of vasectomised
men, matched for age and social class. It was noticeable that whereas most
of the vasectomy couples had been counselled before the decision to carry
out vasectomy was finalised, for most of the sterilised women discussion had
been minimal and the husband was hardly involved in the decision-making.
It was thus of interest to find that the sterilised women reported a significantly lower frequency of sexual intercourse and more sexual problems
than the wives of the vasectomised men. It was not clear whether this
reflected a difference in the quality of the sexual and marital relationships
before the operation, or rather a consequence of the different methods of
sterilisation. The results did suggest, however, that in the marriages of the
sterilised women, the wife's responsibility for fertility control was more
likely to be taken for granted, whereas with the vasectomy couples the
husband was more involved in sharing responsibility. The differing qualities
of relationship implicated may have accounted for the sexual differences in
the two groups. This interpretation is similar to that reached by Bean et
al (1980). In general it would seem desirable to encourage couples to
consider carefully the advantages and disadvantages of male and female
methods of sterilisation before making their decision. It would also be
encouraging if the usual degree of concern about the possible adverse effects
of vasectomy on men could also be directed at women before they are
sterilised.

INDUCED ABORTION

Termination of pregnancy by therapeutic abortion remains an important and widely used method of controlling fertility. In Britain the abortion rates per conception rose from 5.8 per 1000 women aged 15–44 in 1969 to 11.8 in 1978 and has remained relatively stable since then (12.8 in 1984; Cartwright 1987). It has been estimated that 8 of every 100 fertile women in the world have an abortion in any 1 year (Djerassi 1979a). There is evidence that in most parts of the world the use of legal abortion is increasing. There are, however, some important and interesting social and cultural differences in this usage. It has been suggested that abortion, as a 'curative' approach to unwanted pregnancy, is more likely to be relied on in conditions of socioeconomic deprivation. As conditions improve, 'preventive' methods become more and more widely used (Requena 1969). Whereas there may be some truth in this, it is clearly an over-simplification. Other factors influence the use of legal abortion. In general, the Communist countries have relied more on abortion, perhaps because as part of state policy of a pronatalist kind, methods of contraception were relatively unavailable. State control of such methods has been used deliberately to influence the birth rate, though the factors controlling the population growth are too complex to be manipulated in such a relatively simple fashion. Djerassi (1979a) describes such a situation in Romania. Until 1966, this country had the highest number of legal abortions anywhere in the world, nearly four for each live birth. The Romanian Government, concerned about the rapidly falling birth rate, introduced a very restrictive abortion law following which the birth rate rose dramatically by 150% in 1 year. Thereafter the Romanian population apparently adjusted to the changed circumstances with an increased use of other methods of fertility control and since then there has been a further continuing decline in the birth rate. A salutary lesson from the Romanian experience is that the restriction of legal abortion was followed by an increased use of illegal abortion and a substantial rise in maternal deaths from abortion. Communist China, where an ideologically based pronatalist policy was pursued for some time in the face of enormous over-population problems, has in more recent years adopted an active and so far moderately successful anti-natalist strategy. Legal abortion, it would appear, is one part of this broadly based programme.

It is also striking that in the USA and western Europe, abortion is primarily used by the unmarried, whereas in Eastern Europe and the Third World, it is primarily married women with several children who are involved. This confronts us again with one of the more fundamental cultural differences in human sexuality, the apparently much greater level of premarital and adolescent sexuality in western countries. One of the reasons why Requena's socioeconomic model of abortion breaks down is that it is in relatively affluent western countries that legal abortion is being increasingly used to cope with unwanted teenage pregnancies, which as we have already discussed, stem from an underuse of contraceptive methods rather than simply their unavailability.

As with sterilisation, earlier reports were full of gloom about the psychiatric and sexual consequences of abortion (Simon & Senturia 1966). It is of course difficult to distinguish between the effects of the abortion per se and the impact of an unwanted pregnancy. Follow-up studies, however, have consistently failed to find evidence of adverse psychiatric consequences (Pare & Raven 1970; Hamill & Ingram 1974; Greer et al 1976; Brewer 1977), though short-lived emotional reactions may be common (Ashton, 1980; Broome 1984). Unfortunately, very little information is available about the sexual consequences. Greer et al (1976) interviewed 360 women shortly before legal abortion. Whereas 91% were contacted 3 months later, this dropped to 60% at the final follow-up, 15 months to 2 years after the abortion. The proportion of women whose sexual adjustment was rated as satisfactory rose from 59% before the abortion to 74% 3 months later. They comment that improvement was maintained up to 2 years after termination. Ashton (1980) interviewed 64 women 8 weeks after abortion. Of those with a continuing sexual relationship, 61% reported no change in the quality of their sexual fulfilment, 36% that it had improved and 19% that it had deteriorated. Some 12% attributed sexual deterioration to the abortion. The available evidence, whilst mostly reassuring, is nevertheless extremely limited. It is not unusual to find a woman presenting at a sexual problem clinic for whom an earlier abortion had been followed by some sexual difficulties. It remains a possibility that for some women, the experience of abortion leads to some problematic changes in their sexual self-image. One should not necessarily attribute this to the abortion itself; it is difficult to know what the sexual consequences would have been if the pregnancy had continued and these consequences may have been much worse. But the whole experience, occurring at a time when the young woman's sexual self-esteem is still precarious, would have been best avoided. It is to be hoped that more attention will be paid to the sexual consequences of legal abortion in future studies. In the meantime, we can continue to use this procedure with no particular fear that psychological harm will follow. But we should not lessen our attempts to avoid unwanted pregnancies in the first place by doing our best to ensure that if sexual activity occurs, it is protected by appropriate contraception.

INFERTILITY

The average time required for pregnancy to occur in normal couples not using contraception is 5.3 months. After 1 month of unprotected intercourse, 25% will have conceived; after 6 months, 63% and after 1 year, 80%. After 1 year of unsuccessful attempts to conceive, therefore, a couple may be regarded as potentially infertile. Between 10 and 15% of couples of fertile age remain unable to have children (Kolodny et al 1979). For many such couples the infertility is cause of considerable distress.

In order to appreciate the psychological and sexual significance of infertility, we first need to understand why it is important or desirable to have children. Motivation for parenthood has received little attention from behavioural or social scientists (Bell et al 1985). This in part reflects the general tendency to assume that having children is the norm — there is little need to question it (McCormick et al 1977). But in the face of changing circumstances this exceedingly important question is now beginning to receive some attention. It is often assumed that the desire for children is innate, biologically determined. The dramatic changes in birth rate and family size that have occurred over the past two centuries indicate how susceptible to social factors this process is. More recently the general shift towards a preference for two-children families has been accompanied by an increase in voluntary childlessness. People are now beginning to question whether it is pathological not to want any children. Economic factors are probably important. Whereas in the past, children were often seen as a material resource, they are now widely regarded as a major expense. Whereas the rewards of parenthood may have increased to some extent, particularly for fathers, the costs of having children are rising steadily and inexorably. The benefits of children are therefore receiving closer scrutiny by would-be parents. But also involved, and germane to our subject, is the increased availability of alternative roles for the woman. Whereas being a mother has figured largely in the expectations and ambitions of most women in the past, it is now competing with other potentially rewarding roles. Such changes are not universal, however, and in many situations, as discussed earlier, motherhood still presents one of the most powerful sources of self-esteem for women. Nevertheless it is reasonable to assume that in societies where the opportunities for women are improving, there will be an increasing proportion of infertile women who accept their infertility with little distress. For those who do not, we must expect either that acceptable alternative roles are not available or that there are other more powerful reasons for wanting children. For men, the reliance on the role of father for self-esteem has never been so obvious. And yet it may be that fatherhood is important for a man's sense of masculinity (Humphrey 1977). The sense of immortality that children provide their parents with is important for some and may be manifested in the pressure that older parents put on their adult children to give them grandchildren. Pressures may come from within the marriage with one partner feeling he or she is letting the other down by being infertile.

Sexual difficulties are common amongst infertile couples. Steele (1976) reported sexual or marital problems in 37% of 500 couples attending an infertility clinic. Mai et al (1972) found infertile women to have more disturbances of sexual identity and problems of sexual adjustment. Rubinstein (1980) found that 50% of couples with primary infertility had 'a fearful approach to sex which caused a problem in marital relations'.

In a proportion of cases the infertility is likely to be a direct consequence of the sexual problem. Dubin & Amelar (1972) concluded that in 5.5% of their series of infertile couples, a sexual difficulty was a primary cause of the infertility. Any problem which interferes with the deposition of semen in the vagina will obviously impair, if not entirely prevent, fertility. Non-consummation, vaginismus or erectile impotence, inability to ejaculate inside the vagina or severe premature ejaculation occurring usually before vaginal entry are obvious examples. The role of more subtle changes in sexual response is not so clear. The frequency of sexual intercourse is relevant. Too frequent intercourse or ejaculation may lead to a reduction in sperm count. Intervals between ejaculation of less than 12 hours or greater than 7 days result in reduced fertility of the ejaculate (Eliasson 1965; Mortimer et al 1982), even to the extent of reducing sperm penetration (Rogers et al 1983). Macleod & Gold (1953) estimated that within a 6-month period, the relationship between coital frequency and conception would be 84% conception for a frequency of four or more per week, 32% for once but less than twice per week, and 17% for less than weekly. Obviously reduced frequency, if otherwise unrelated to the timing of ovulation, will reduce the likelihood of intercourse occurring during the fertile period.

Does the coital frequency influence the woman's fertility? In a series of studies Cutler and her colleagues have proposed that it does; that if intercourse is less than once weekly the likelihood of ovulatory cycles is reduced (Cutler et al 1979, 1980, 1985). Their evidence is suggestive but not conclusive. What is lacking is evidence that by changing coital frequency, the ovarian cycle is affected. Without such evidence one is left with the possibility that the coital frequency is in some way a *consequence* of the woman's reproductive physiology rather than a cause of it (Bancroft 1987).

The importance of the female orgasm to fertility has also been much discussed. It is obvious that orgasm is not necessary for conception; the question is whether it may increase its likelihood. Three aspects of female genital physiology have been considered: the suction of semen into the uterus, the pooling of semen close to the cervix and the alteration of pH of the vagina to make it less hostile to sperm. Masters & Johnson (1966) studied six women by placing radiopaque liquid, similar in consistency to semen, close to the cervix and then asking the women to masturbate to orgasm. In no case did they find any evidence of the radiopaque material in the uterine cavity after orgasm. They therefore concluded that uterine 'insuck' did not occur and considered that the pattern of orgasmic contraction of the uterus, starting as it does in the fundus, is more likely to produce positive pressure within the uterus. Fox et al (1970) used a radio-telemetric capsule placed inside the uterus of one woman. This measured intrauterine pressure during coitus and orgasm. A positive pressure was recorded during orgasm and was followed by a sharp fall to a negative pressure after the orgasm. They concluded on this basis that a uterine 'insuck' does occur. Masters & Johnson (1966) reported that the ballooning of the inner third of the vagina during sexual arousal leads to a pooling of semen after intercourse, reducing its drainage from the vagina. This, they suggested, might facilitate conception. They also described the vaginal environment as hostile to sperm because of its normally acidic pH. Vaginal fluid arising during sexual arousal raises the pH and hence makes the vagina more suitable for sperm (Levin 1980). The male ejaculate also has a buffering effect on the vaginal pH which is probably sufficient to safeguard the spermatozoa. It is possible that in some infertile men, this buffering effect is inadequate, in which case the effects of the vaginal response will become more important (Fox et al 1973). It nevertheless seems unlikely that any of these three mechanisms are of much importance to fertility, but they may make a difference in those couples whose fertility is marginal for other reasons.

It is a common clinical impression that when stress, which might be associated with a sexual problem, declines, conception occurs. There is some evidence that ovulation can be delayed by stress of various kinds (Peyser et al 1973). But the importance of such a mechanism to infertility remains very uncertain. If it is relevant, then one might expect to find conception occurring in some couples when their general sexual relationship improves. It is therefore of interest that in Rubinstein's study (1980), 32 of the 40 couples with sexual anxieties felt more relaxed and enjoyed sex more after sexual counselling and 18 of the women conceived.

The adverse effects of infertility on the sexual relationship also have to be taken into consideration. The potential importance of fertility to one's gender identity has already been mentioned. Berger (1980) interviewed 16 married couples after the diagnosis of azoospermia had been made. Ten of the men suffered a period of erectile failure, usually starting within 1 week of being informed of the diagnosis. Hostility and guilt were also quite common in the wives. Humphrey (1984) has been unable to replicate these rather negative findings. But it would not be surprising if the discovery that one's partner is sterile leads to tensions which in turn have adverse effects on the sexual relationship. It is commonplace to find that infertile couples, once they have started to strive to conceive, find that their sexual enjoyment is impaired. This can be particularly marked if the couple are concentrating on the fertile period, producing the 'this is the night' syndrome (Kaufman 1969). This problem may come to light when arranging post-coital tests, which find the man unable to respond or to ejaculate at the appropriate time. Certainly any tendency to sexual dysfunction in either partner is likely to be aggravated by following such a timetable of optimal coitus. This should be taken into consideration when recommending such an approach to the infertile couple. It is particularly important to avoid long periods of such striving as the damage to the sexual and marital relationship may not be so easily reversed.

AID, or artificial insemination using the semen of a donor, requires special consideration as a method of dealing with male infertility. The procedure remains controversial, though compared with the initial, very negative attitudes of the Church and medical profession, there is growing acceptance of its use (Snowden & Mitchell 1980). The ethical issues have been highlighted in the controversy over the use of AID for lesbian women who wish to be mothers. The legal complexities remain unresolved; the child of an AID conception is illegitimate. With all this ethical uncertainty, it would not be surprising to find that some couples making use of AID experience psychological or sexual repercussions. So far the limited evidence is reassuring. Short-term adverse effects on the marital and sexual relationship may occur but it is not always clear whether this stems from the AID or the infertility itself (Alder 1984b).

Whilst infertility and the attempts to treat it may cause substantial upset to many couples, we should not assume that such effects will necessarily be permanent. Some marriages may break up as a consequence. Others will eventually work through this crisis and may end up with their relationship strengthened. The weight of evidence suggests that in the long term, childless couples are physically and psychologically as well off, if not better off, than couples with children (Humphrey 1975).

REFERENCES

Alder E 1984a Sterilisation. In: Broome A, Wallace L (eds) Psychology and gynaecological problems. Tavistock, London, pp 1–17
Alder E 1984b Psychological aspects of AID. In: Emery A E H, Pullen I M (eds) Psychological aspects of genetic counselling. Academic, London, pp 187–199
Alder E, Bancroft J 1988 The relationship between breast feeding persistence, sexuality and mood in the post-partum woman. Psychological Medicine 18: 389–396
Alder E, Cook A, Gray J et al 1981 The effects of sterilisation: a comparison of sterilised women with the wives of vasectomised men. Contraception 23: 45–54
Alder E, Cook A, Davidson D, West C, Bancroft J 1986 Hormones, mood and sexuality in lactating women. British Journal of Psychiatry 148: 74–79
Andersch B 1980 Epidemiological, hormonal and water balance studies in premenstrual tension. MD Thesis, University of Göteborg
Ashton J R 1980 The psychosocial outcome of induced abortion. British Journal of Obstetrics and Gynaecology 87: 1115–1122
Bancroft J 1974 The effects of fertility control on human sexual behaviour. In: Parry H B (ed) Population and its problems. Clarendon Press, Oxford, pp 322–353
Bancroft J 1987 Hormones, sexuality and fertility in women. Journal of Zoology (London) 213: 445–454
Bancroft J, Davidson D W, Warner P, Tyrer G 1980 Androgen and sexual behaviour in women using oral contraceptives. Clinical Endocrinology 12: 327–340
Bancroft J, Sanders D, Warner P, Loudon N 1987 The effects of oral contraceptives on mood and sexuality: a comparison of triphasic and combined preparations. Journal of Psychosomatic Obstetrics and Gynaecology 7: 1–8
Bardwick J 1973 Psychological factors in the acceptance and use of oral contraceptives. In: Fawcett J T (ed) Psychological perspectives on population. Basic Books, New York, pp 274–305
Bean F D, Clark M P, South S et al 1980 Change in sexual desire after voluntary sterilisation. Social Biology 27: 186–193

Beck J G, Davies D K 1987 Teen contraception: a review of perspectives on compliance. Archives of Sexual Behavior 16: 337–368

Beischer N A 1967 The anatomical and functional results of mediolateral episiotomy. Medical Journal of Australia 2: 189–195

Bell J S, Bancroft J, Philip A 1985 Motivation for parenthood: a factor analytic study of attitudes towards having children. Journal of Comparative Family Studies 16: 111–119

Benjamin L, Rubinstein L M, Kleinitopf V 1980 Elective sterilisation in childless women. Fertility and Sterility 34: 116–120

Berger D M 1980 Impotence following the discovery of azoospermia. Fertility and Sterility 34: 154–156

Billings J, Billings E L 1973 Determination of fertile and infertile days by the mucus pattern: development of the ovulation method. In: Urrichio W A, Williams M K (eds) Natural family planning. The Human Life Foundation, Washington, DC

Bone M 1978 The family planning services: changes and effects. OPCS Social Survey Division. HMSO, London

Bongaarts J 1980 Does malnutrition affect fecundity? A summary of evidence. Science 208: 564–569

Booth M, Beral V, Guillebaud J 1980 Effect of age on pelvic inflammatory disease in nulliparous women using a Copper 7 intrauterine contraceptive device. British Medical Journal 281: 114

Bragonier J R 1976 Influence of oral contraception on sexual response. Medical Aspects of Human Sexuality October: 130–143

Brewer C 1977 Incidence of post-abortion psychosis: a prospective study. British Medical Journal i: 476–77

Broome A 1984 Termination of pregnancy. In: Broome A, Wallace L (eds) Psychology and gynaecological problems. Tavistock, London, pp 60–76

Cartwright A 1987 Family intentions and the use of contraception among recent mothers 1967–84. Population Trends 49: 31–35

Cliquet R L, Thiery M, Stailens R, Lambert G 1981. Voluntary sterilisation in Flanders, Journal of Biosocial Science 13: 47–67

Coles R 1978 Acceptability and use-effectiveness of contraception for teenagers. Journal of Biosocial Science (suppl) 5: 159–170

Cooper P, Gath D, Rose N, Fieldsend R 1982 Psychological sequelae to elective sterilisation in women: a prospective study. British Medical Journal 284: 461–464

Crosbie P V, Bitte D 1982 A test of Luker's theory of contraceptive risk taking. Studies in Family Planning 13: 67–78

Cullberg J 1973 Mood changes and menstrual symptoms with different gestagen/estrogen combinations. Acta Psychiatrica Scandinavica (suppl) 236

Cutler W B, Garcia C R, Krieger A M 1979 Luteal phases defects: a possible relationship between short hyperthermic phase and sporadic sexual behaviour in women. Hormones and Behaviour 13: 214–218

Cutler W B, Garcia C R, Krieger A M 1980 Sporadic sexual behaviour and menstrual cycle length in women. Hormones and Behaviour 14: 163–172

Cutler W B, Preti G, Huggibs G R, Erickson B, Garcia C R 1985 Sexual behavior frequency and biphasic ovulatory type menstrual cycles. Physiology and Behaviour 34: 805–810

Djerassi I C 1979a The politics of contraception. Vol I, the present. The Portable Stanford, Stanford Alumni Association, Stanford, California

Djerassi I C 1979b The politics of contraception. Vol II, the future. The Portable Stanford, Stanford Alumni Association, Stanford, California

Dubin L, Amelar R D 1972 Sexual causes of male infertility. Fertility and Sterility 23: 579–582

Dunnell K 1979 Family formation 1976. HMSO, London

Eliasson R 1965 Effect of frequent ejaculation on the composition of the human seminal plasma. Journal of Reproduction and Fertility 9: 331–336

Ferber A S, Tietze C, Lewit S 1967 Men with vasectomies: a study of medical, sexual and psychosocial change. Psychosomatic Medicine 29: 354–366

Ford C S, Beach F A 1952 Patterns of sexual behaviour. Eyre & Spottiswoode, London

Fox C A, Wolff H S, Baker J A 1970 Measurement of intravaginal and intrauterine pressures during human coitus by radio-telemetry. Journal of Reproduction and Fertility 22: 243–251

Fox C A, Meldrum S J, Watson B W 1973 Continuous measurement by radio-telemetry of vaginal pH during human coitus. Journal of Reproduction and Fertility 33: 69–75

Gambrell D, Bernard D M, Sanders B I, Vanderburg N, Buxton S J 1976 Changes in sexual drives of patients on oral contraceptives. Journal of Reproductive Medicine 17: 165–171

Garner P 1982 Dyspareunia after episiotomy. British Journal of Sexual Medicine 9(86): 11–12

General Household Survey 1983, 1985. OPCS. HMSO, London

Glick I D 1967 Mood and behavioural changes associated with the use of oral contraceptive agents. Psychopharmacologia 10: 363–374

Goodlin R C 1969 Orgasm and premature labour. Lancet ii: 646

Grant E C G, Pryse-Davies J 1968 Effect of oral contraception on depressive mood change and on endometrial monoamine oxidase and phosphatase. British Medical Journal 3: 777–780

Greer H S, Lal S, Lewis S C, Belsey E M, Beard R W 1976 Psychosocial consequences of therapeutic abortion. Kings' termination study III. British Journal of Psychiatry 128: 74–79

Grudzinskas J C, Atkinson L 1984 Sexual function during the puerperium. Archives of Sexual Behavior 13: 85–92

Grudzinskas J C, Watson C, Chard T 1979 Does sexual intercourse cause foetal distress? Lancet ii: 692–693

Hamill E, Ingram I M 1974 Psychiatric and social factors in the abortion decision. British Medical Journal i: 229–232

Hart A J L, Deane R F 1980 A retrospective study of 100 vasectomies carried out at the FPA. British Journal of Sexual Medicine 7 (67): 10–14

Hawkins D F, Elder M G 1979 Human fertility control, theory and practice. Butterworth, London, pp 98

Herzberg B N, Draper K C, Johnson A L, Nicol G C 1971 Oral contraceptives, depression and libido. British Medical Journal 3: 495–500

Hollerbach P E, Northman D L 1984 Sterilisation. In: Emery A E H, Pullen I M (eds) Psychological aspects of genetic counselling. Academic, London, pp 169–186

Howard G 1978 Motivation for vasectomy. Lancet i: 546–548

Humphrey M 1975 The effect of children upon the marriage relationship. British Journal of Medical Psychology

Humphrey M 1977 Sex differences in attitude to parenthood. Human Relations 30: 737–749

Humphrey M 1984 Infertility and alternative parenting. In: Broome A, Wallace L (eds) Psychology and gynaecological problems. Tavistock, London, pp 77–94

Johnson J H 1983 Vasectomy: an international appraisal. International Family Planning Perspectives 9: 96–99

Kane F J 1976 Evaluation of emotional reactions to oral contraceptive use. American Journal of Obstetrics and Gynecology 126: 968–972

Kantner J F, Zelnik M 1973 Contraception and pregnancy: experience of young unmarried women in the United States. Family Planning Perspectives 5: 21

Kasonde J M, Bonnar J 1976 Effect of sterilisation on menstrual blood loss. British Journal of Obstetrics and Gynaecology 83: 572–575

Kaufman S A 1969 Impact of infertility on the marital and sexual relationship. Fertility and Sterility 20: 380–383

Khorana A B, Vyas A A 1975 Psychological complications in women undergoing voluntary sterilisation by salpingectomy. British Journal of Psychiatry 127: 67–70

Kleinman R 1980 Family planning handbook for doctors. IPPF Publication, London

Kolodny R C, Masters W H, Johnson V E 1979 Textbook of sexual medicine. Little, Brown, Boston

Kutner S J, Brown S L 1972 Types of oral contraceptives, depression and pre-menstrual symptoms. Journal of Nervous and Mental Disorders 115: 153

Levin R J 1980 Physiology of sexual function in women. Clinics in Obstetrics and Gynaecology 7: pp 213–252

Linde R, Doelle G C, Alexander N et al 1981 Reversible inhibition of testicular steroidogenesis and spermatogenesis by a potent GnRH agonist in normal men. New England Journal of Medicine 305: 663

Lindemann C 1977 Factors affecting the use of contraceptives in the non-marital context. In: Gemme R, Wheeler C C (eds) Progress in sexology. Plenum, New York, pp 397–408

Linnet L, Møller N P, Bernth-Petersen P, Ehlers N, Brandslund I, Svehag S E 1982 No increase in arteriosclerotic retinopathy or activity in tests for circulating immune complex 5 years after vasectomy. Fertility and Sterility 37: 798–806

Liu G Z 1981 Clinical study of gossypol as male contraceptive. Reproduction 5: 189–193

Luker K 1975 Taking chances: abortion and the decision not to contracept. University of California Press, Berkeley, California

McCormick E P, Johnson R L, Friedman H L, David H P 1977 Psychosocial aspects of fertility regulation. In: Money J, Musaph H (eds) Handbook of sexology. Elsevier/North Holland, Amsterdam

Macleod J, Gold R Z 1953 The male factor in fertility and sterility. Fertility and Sterility 4: 10–14

Mai F M M, Munday R N, Rump E E 1972 Psychiatric interview comparisons between infertile and fertile couples. Psychosomatic Medicine 34: 431–440

Margaret Pike Centre 1973 One thousand vasectomies. British Medical Journal 4: 216–221

Massey F J Jr, Bernstein G S, Schuman L M, O'Fallon W M 1983 The effects of vasectomy on the health status of American men. Fertility and Sterility 40: 414–415

Masters W H, Johnson V E 1966 Human sexual response. Little, Brown, Boston

Melton R J, Shelton J D 1971 Pill versus IUD: continuation rates of oral contraceptive and Dalkon shield use in Maryland clinics. Contraception 4: 319–326

Morris N M, Udry J R 1972 Contraceptive pills and day-by-day feelings of well being. American Journal of Obstetrics and Gynecology 113: 763–765

Mortimer D, Templeton A A, Lenton E A, Coleman R A 1982 Influence of abstinence and ejaculation-to-analysis delay on semen analysis parameters of suspected infertile men. Archives of Andrology 8: 251–256

Naeye R L 1979 Coitus and associated amniotic fluid infections. New England Journal of Medicine 301: 1198–1200

Naeye R L 1980 Coitus and antepartum haemorrhage. British Journal of Obstetrics and Gynaecology 88: 765–770

Newman P, Leavesley J H 1980 Medicine in Australia — a review of vasectomy in general practice. British Journal of Sexual Medicine 7 (64): 48–56

Noble A D 1978 Female sterilisation: long term effects. In: Sciarra J J, Zatuchni G I, Speidel J J (eds) Risks, benefits and controversies in fertility control. Harper & Row, Maryland

Pare C M B, Raven H 1970 Follow up of patients referred for termination of pregnancy. Lancet i: 635–638

Parrinder G 1987 A theological approach. In: Geer J H, O'Donohue W T (eds) Theories of human sexuality. Plenum, New York, pp 21–48

Petitti D, Klein R, Kipp H, Kahn W, Siegelaub A B, Friedman G D 1982a A survey of personal habits, symptoms of illness and histories of disease in men with and without vasectomies. American Journal of Public Health 72: 476–480

Petitti D, Klein R, Kipp H, Kahn W, Siegelaub A B, Friedman G D 1982b Physiologic measures in men with and without vasectomies. Fertility and Sterility 37: 438–440

Peyser M R, Ayalon D, Harell A, Toaff M, Cordova T 1973 Stress-induced delay of ovulation. Obstetrics and Gynecology 42: 667–671

Population Reports 1978 M/F sterilisation. Special topic monograph no 2. Department of Medical and Public Affairs, Washington, DC

Population Reports 1985 Female sterilisation. Series c, no 9. Johns Hopkins University, Baltimore

Reader F, Savage W 1983 Sexual activity during pregnancy: giving advice. British Journal of Sexual Medicine 10(103): 23–27

Reamy K J, White S E 1987 Sexuality in the puerperium: a review. Archives of Sexual Behavior 16: 165–186

Requena M 1969 Chilean program of abortion control and fertility planning: present situation and forecast for the next decade. In: Behrman S J, Corse L, Freedman R (eds) Fertility and family planning. University of Michigan Press, Ann Arbor p 485

Robson K M, Brant H A, Kumar R 1981 Maternal sexuality during first pregnancy and after childbirth. British Journal of Obstetrics and Gynaecology 88: 882–889

Rodgers D A, Ziegler F J, Levy N 1967 Prevailing cultural attitudes about vasectomy: a possible explanation of post-operative psychological response. Psychosomatic Medicine 29: 367–375

Rogers B J, Perreault S D, Bentwood B J, McCarville C, Hale R W, Soderdahl D W 1983 Variability in the human-hamster in-vitro assay for fertility evaluation. Fertility and Sterility 39: 204–211

Rönnau H J 1980 The psychologic influence of female sterilisation on sexology and family structure. In: Forleo R, Pasini W (eds) Medical sexology. Elsevier/North Holland, Amsterdam, pp 378–380

Rubinstein I 1980 Sterility caused by sexual disturbance. In: Forleo R, Pasini W (eds) Medical sexology. Elsevier/North Holland, Amsterdam, pp 364–66

Royal College of General Practitioners 1974 Oral contraceptives and health. Pitman, London

Ryde-Blomqvist E 1978 Contraception in adolescence — a review of the literature. Journal of Biosocial Science (suppl) 5: 129–158

Sack A R, Billingham R E, Howard R D 1985 Premarital contraceptive use: a discriminant analytic approach. Archives of Sexual Behavior 14: 165–182

Short R V 1976 The evolution of human reproduction. In: Short R V, Baird D T (eds) Contraceptives of the future. Royal Society, London

Simon N M, Senturia A G 1966 Psychiatric sequelae of abortion: review of the literature 1935–1964. Archives of General Psychiatry 15: 278–289

Simon Population Trust 1969 Vasectomy: follow up of 1000 cases. Simon Population Trust, Cambridge

Smith A H W 1979 Psychiatric aspects of sterilisation: a prospective study. British Journal of Psychiatry 135: 304–309

Snowden R, Mitchell G D 1980 A sociological view of artificial insemination by donor. British Journal of Family Planning 6: 45–49

Steele S J 1976 Sexual problems related to contraception and family planning. In: Crown S (ed) Psychosexual problems. Academic Press, London, pp 383–401

Tatum H J, Connell E S 1986 A decade of intrauterine contraception 1976–1986. Fertility and Sterility 46: 173–192

Udry J R, Morris N M, Waller L 1973 Effects of contraceptive pills on sexual activity in the luteal phase of the human menstrual cycle. Archives of Sexual Behavior 2: 205–214

Vessey M, Yeates D, Flavel R, McPherson K 1981 Pelvic inflammatory disease and the intrauterine device. Findings in a large cohort study. British Medical Journal 282: 855–857

Walker A, Bancroft J 1988 Cyclical changes in mood, sexuality and physical symptoms in women on triphasic, monophasic and non-steroidal contraceptives. (in press)

Warner P, Bancroft J 1988 Mood, sexuality, oral contraceptives and the menstrual cycle. Journal of Psychosomatic Research. (in press)

Westoff C F, Jones E F 1977 The secularisation of US Catholic birth control practices. Family Planning Perspectives 9: 204

Westoff C F, Bumpass L, Ryder N B 1976 Oral contraception, coital frequency and the time required to conceive. Social Biology 16: 1–10

White S E, Reamy K J 1982 Sexuality and pregnancy: a review. Archives of Sexual Behavior 11: 429–444

Wilson K, Abramovich D, Thompson B 1977 Follow-up of women sterilised under age 25. Fertility and Contraception 1: 62–66

Wolfers H 1970 Psychological aspects of vasectomy. British Medical Journal 4: 297–300

World Health Organization 1978 Special programme of research, development and research training in human reproduction, 7th annual report. November 1978. WHO, Geneva

World Health Organization 1982 Hormonal contraception for men; acceptability and effects on sexuality. Studies in Family Planning 13: 328–342

13

Sexual offences

The one common factor in the variety of sexual offences is that each breaks the law. The law can be seen to have three functions in this respect. First, to protect the individual, secondly to avoid social disruption caused by explicit sex in public places and thirdly the 'declarative' function, or the discouragement of certain forms of behaviour considered for one reason or another to be undesirable.

Protection of the individual is concerned not only with assault, the use of physical force or the threat of it to achieve sexual ends, but also with exploitation. Protection against assault is in itself not controversial. The main problems are associated with evidence, particularly in cases of rape and with the controversy over the legal status of assault or rape of a woman by her husband. More recently a fierce debate has started about evidence of the sexual abuse of children. These issues will be discussed further below. Protection against exploitation raises more dispute. It is accepted in principle, but the definition of exploitation poses many problems, most notably in relation to age of consent.

The second function, avoidance of social disruption, is likely to continue in some form. The imposition of social constraints on public sexuality appears to be a universal of human societies, though there have been certain exceptions when public orgies were allowed on specific days.

It is the third, 'declarative' function, that is the most controversial and which has shown and will continue to show the most change. There has been long-standing controversy over the use of the law in this way. John Stewart Mill (1859) considered that 'the only purpose for which power can be rightfully exercised over any member of a civilised community against his will, is to prevent harm to others'. Many years later, in a similar vein, the Wolfenden Committee (1957) asserted: 'it is not the duty of the law to concern itself with immorality as such . . . it should confine itself to those activities which offend against public order and decency, or expose the ordinary citizen to what is offensive or injurious'. These views, needless to say, have not been the prevailing ones. The more recent but inconclusive debate on this issue has been well summarised by Freeman (1979). In fact, both the Church, through the ecclesiastical courts of earlier times, and the

664

more recent legal system, have consistently punished immorality, though what constitutes punishable immorality has changed dramatically, often reflecting the prevailing norms of the establishment. Adultery or fornication has in the past been punishable in western societies and still remains proscribed in some states of the USA. Though such law is seldom if ever used in Christian countries, there are still some cultures, e.g. Islamic, where it is applied with considerable severity. The most recent example of such a change in the western world concerns homosexuality and on this there are comments in Chapter 6. The law involving sexual obscenity and the pureying of pornography provides some of the more striking inconsistencies of the system at the present time.

Legal proscription of certain forms of sexual behaviour also has indirect consequences that are undesirable. When the proscribed behaviour is a source of pleasure, a black market develops based on organised crime. Not infrequently, the sexually deviant individual becomes involved in an escalation of deviant activities which has been described as secondary or amplified deviance (Lemert 1967). Thus in weighing up the pros and cons of legislation against immorality, we have to consider the extension of other criminal behaviour that may result. Also, as much of the behaviour that is proscribed on grounds of immorality rather than the protection of others does not involve a victim or a complainant, the police are more likely to resort to entrapment techniques. These are themselves of very dubious morality and bring discredit to the legal and police systems.

When considering those acts which, in my view, are unequivocally the proper concern of the law — the protection of the victim against sexual assault or exploitation — we have to consider the importance of non-sexual motives. There is a general tendency for sexual offenders to be convicted of other non-sexual crimes. Part of this is due to the secondary deviance already mentioned, but probably of greater importance is the incorporation of sexual behaviour into a more general antisocial lifestyle, or alternatively the use of sexually offensive behaviour as a way of dealing with non-sexual conflicts or crises. The importance of sexual reward in determining sexually offensive behaviour is thus variable and often obscure and we will consider this more closely when dealing with some of the specific types of sexual offence.

TYPES OF SEXUAL OFFENCE

If a man or woman commits a sexual offence, at least one of the following conditions apply (Walmsley & White 1979):

1. The sexual behaviour takes place without the consent of the other party (and the aggressor is not married to the other party);
2. The sexual behaviour takes place with a person under the age of consent (16 for heterosexual, 21 for homosexual behaviour);

Table 13.1 Indictable sexual offences (from Honoré 1978; Walmsley & White 1979)

Category of offence	Proportion indicted	Maximum sentence	Median length of custodial sentence*	Proportion receiving custodial sentence†
Rape	96%	Life	3–4 years	92%
Indecent assault on a female	18%	Female under 13 — 5 years Female over 13 — 2 years	1–1½ years	14%
Unlawful sexual intercourse with girl aged under 13	87%	Life	2–3 years	57%
Unlawful sexual intercourse with girl aged 13–15	94%	2 years	½–1 year	23%
Gross indecency with children	15%	2 years	1 year	9%
Incest	96%	Under 13 — life Over 13 — 7 years	2–3 years	72%
Buggery	96%	Under 16 — life Under 21 — 5 years Both under 21 — 2 years	1½–2 years	59%
Attempted buggery and indecent assault on a male	29%	Under 16 — 10 years Under 21 — 5 years Both under 21 — 2 years	1½–2 years	19%
Indecency between men	8%	Partner under 21 — 5 years Both over 21 — 2 years	1–1½ years	1%
Procuration	77%	2 years	1–1½ years	58%

* Based on 1975 figures (Honoré 1978).
† Based on 1973–1978 figures (Walmsley 1980).

3. The sexual behaviour itself is prohibited by law, i.e. incest, bestiality, buggery with a female or intercourse with a mentally defective person;
4. Homosexual behaviour between males not committed in private;
5. Homosexual behaviour by a male who is himself under the age of consent.

It is noteworthy that the last four categories apply even when both parties consent to the behaviour.

Although the above criteria apply in most countries, the precise categories of sexual offence vary, making comparative statistics difficult. In England and Wales, most categories of sexual offence are indictable, i.e. tried in a Crown Court in front of a jury. Other offences are not indictable and are tried summarily in a Magistrate's Court. A proportion of indictable offences may be tried summarily in certain circumstances, depending on a number of factors such as the age of the offender. The various categories of indictable sexual offences in England and Wales are shown in Table 13.1.

Non-indictable sexual offences include brothel-keeping, living on prostitute's earnings, soliciting and male importuning, and indecent exposure.

Rape is sexual intercourse by a male with a female, not his wife*, who at the time does not consent. Some degree of vaginal penetration by the penis has to occur before the act is defined as rape. For some anachronistic reason, a boy under 14 is deemed in English law to be incapable of rape, though capable of indecent assault†. Consent of a female who is under the age of consent is a defence against a charge of rape, but not of unlawful sexual intercourse. Indecent assault on a female does not necessarily involve force, but rather any form of physical contact which is indecent or sexual in purpose and which is without her consent. A girl under the age of 16 cannot in law consent to such contact.

The term 'buggery' covers both anal intercourse and sexual contact with animals. The former, whilst predominantly homosexual, is also a hetero-sexual offence even between husband and wife. In 1973 10% of convictions for buggery were heterosexual (Walmsley & White 1979). Homosexual buggery above the age of consent and in private is no longer illegal, whereas it remains so for heterosexual couples — one of the many inconsistencies of this area of the law.

Below the homosexual age of consent (i.e. 21), consent has no bearing on the category of offence, whereas with heterosexual intercourse, it makes a crucial difference between rape and unlawful sexual intercourse. Never-theless, consent and the age of the victim do have a bearing on the sentences usually imposed. Indecent assault on a male is comparable to that on a female. For this purpose, 16 is also the age below which boys cannot legally consent, emphasising the illogicality of calling 21 years the age of consent for homosexual acts.

Indecent assault on a male can of course be carried out by a woman but this is relatively unusual. Some cases of 'rape' of men by women have attracted interest, in particular as to whether such an act involving vaginal penetration is possible. In English law it would be regarded as indecent assault and not rape.

The use of the term 'indecency' to describe homosexual offences causes some confusion. In males aged over 16, any form of sexual interaction short of buggery, if carried out in a public place, can be regarded as 'gross indecency'; actual physical contact is not necessary; masturbation by one man in front of another would come into this category. However when a person is too young to give legal consent (under 16), any such physical contact by the offender would be regarded as assault. If only the child does the touching (e.g. masturbates the man) or if no actual physical contact ensues (e.g. the man masturbates in front of the child) then the act is called gross indecency.

Procuration is another somewhat confused category. Obviously intended originally to inhibit prostitution, it is deemed an offence to procure (i.e.

* This does not apply is Scotland where several husbands have been prosecuted for the rape of their wives (Chambers & Millar 1983).
† In Scotland boys under 14 can be prosecuted for rape (Chambers Millar 1983).

to persuade, cause or encourage) a woman to act as a prostitute. But it is also a crime to procure any woman under the age of 21 to engage in unlawful sexual intercourse with a third person, whether for money or not. For that purpose, the only lawful form of heterosexual intercourse is within marriage. What applies to heterosexual acts involving women under 21, applies to *any* homosexual act. It is therefore criminal to procure or attempt to procure someone to engage with a third person in a homosexual act which is not in itself an offence.

INCIDENCE OF SEXUAL OFFENCES

In considering trends in the statistics for sexual offences it is important to bear in mind that changing statistics may reflect changes in reporting or recording of crimes rather than their actual occurrence. As we shall see, this is particularly relevant to rape.

In England and Wales, from 1946, when there were 9329 indictable sexual offences, the annual number has increased by about 2.5 times, reaching a peak in 1971 of 23 621. Since then the numbers have fallen slightly (see Fig. 13.1). This can be compared with the figures for crimes of violence against the person which increased steadily from 4062 in 1942 to 127 000 in 1985, a 30-fold increase. The total for all indictable offences increased nearly eightfold during the same period, from 472 489 to 3 611 900. Thus sexual offences in general, whilst on the increase, have not shown as much increase as crime in general. The secular trends in some of the more important categories of sexual offence are shown in Figures

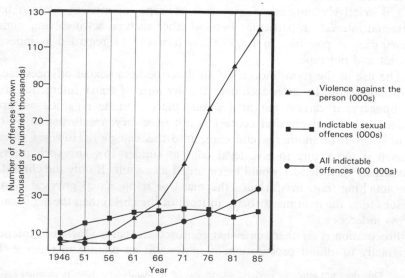

Fig. 13.1 Offences known to the police. 1946–1985. (Criminal Statistics for England and Wales 1985)

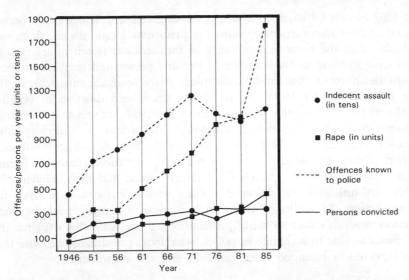

Fig. 13.2 Incidence of rape (and attempted rape) and indecent assault on females from 1946–1985. Offences known to the police and persons convicted. (Criminal Statistics for England and Wales 1985)

13.1–13.3. As we shall see, trends in rape, sexual assault and sexual abuse of children show differences which will need to be considered in more detail.

An example of the distorting effect on criminal statistics of the prosecuting procedure is shown in the figures for persons convicted of indecency between men (see Fig. 13.3). Walmsley (1980) has pointed out that since

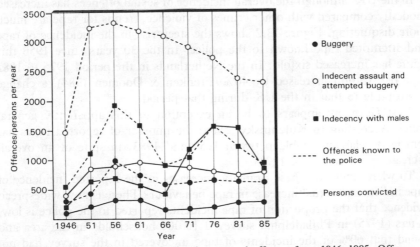

Fig. 13.3 Incidence of buggery and other homosexual offences from 1946–1985. Offences known to the police and persons convicted. (Criminal Statistics for England and Wales 1985)

the 1967 Sexual Offences Act, which for England and Wales made homosexual acts between consenting adults in private no longer illegal, there was a doubling of the recorded incidence of indecency between males (i.e. in public), a trebling of the number of persons prosecuted for that offence, whilst the number convicted quadrupled. After reaching this peak in the late 1970s and early 1980s the trend has since been downwards (Griffin & Morris 1987). One other consequence of the 1967 Act was that indecency between males became triable summarily. According to Walmsley, this paradoxical trend is a direct consequence of the new Act. The Wolfenden Report (1957), he suggests, threw some doubt on the illegality of homosexual behaviour, whilst the 1967 Act clearly stated that such behaviour *in public* was unlawful, providing the police with a less equivocal basis for taking action. In addition, the introduction of summary trial for such offences made it easier to bring prosecution. Thus Walmsley explains the difference as due to a change in police behaviour, presumably not one that was expected or intended when the 1967 Act was drawn up.

INCIDENCE OF RAPE AND SEXUAL ASSAULT AND COMPARISON WITH THE USA AND OTHER COUNTRIES

It has been estimated that American women are 12 times more likely to be raped than women in England and Wales, and even more so than those in other European countries (Katz & Mazur 1979). Rape is the most rapidly increasing crime of violence in the USA. Reported cases were 17 190 in 1960 and 82 088 in 1980, nearly a fivefold increase in 20 years; this is an increase three times greater than that of other major crimes of violence (Katchadourian 1985).

In the UK, although the overall incidence of sexual offences has increased modestly compared with other crimes of violence, trends for rape are much more disquieting. Figure 13.2 shows the steep rise in the incidence of rape and attempted rape known to the police. In the 30 years since 1956 this figure has increased sixfold. In the Netherlands in the period 1975 to 1982 rape registration increased by 40% (Frenken & Doomen 1984), a change comparable to that in the UK during that period.

West Germany appears to be an exception to this apparently general trend. According to Kutchinsky (1985) the number of reported rapes has remained relatively stable between 1959 and 1983, in spite of an overall increase in all crimes of 127%.

To what extent do these dramatic increases in the reported incidence of rape indicate an actual increase in rape behaviour? There is now widespread evidence that the proportion of rape incidents reported to the police is low. Peters (1975) in Philadelphia surveyed 10 000 households in the area and found that 60% of the incidents of rape uncovered in the survey had not been reported. In Scotland, the British Crime Survey discovered that only 7% of sexual assaults uncovered by the survey had been reported to the police (Chambers & Millar 1983). Approximately 45% of women contacting Rape Crisis Centres in Britain have not reported their experiences to the police. It is therefore possible that the increase in reported cases is an increase in reporting rather than an increase in rape. Against this explanation is the finding in the Netherlands that the willingness to report sexual offences in general decreased from 21% in 1980 to 8% in 1982, though it is not clear what the figure is for rape specifically. Frenken & Doomen nevertheless concluded from the Dutch figures that there has been a *real* increase in sexual offences in the Netherlands.

Population surveys report a disturbingly high proportion of women who have been victims of sexual assault at some time. In census surveys of American cities, Hindlelang & Davis (1977) found that for every 100 000 females aged 12 and over, 315 reported being the victim of rape or attempted rape during the previous 12 months. Koss & Oros (1982) surveyed American university students and found that 6% of a sample of 2000 females had been raped at some time and 18% had been subjected to attempts at intercourse under the threat of physical force. Russell (1982) interviewed 930 married Californian women in a carefully executed, randomly sampled study. She found that 14% had been raped by their husbands or ex-husbands and a remarkable 44% had been subjected to at least one rape or attempted rape in the course of their lives.

The reasons why so many rape victims do not report their experiences are well recognised. The victims often receive very unsympathetic if not humiliating treatment at the hands of the police and the courts, and not infrequently feel stigmatised by the experience in the eyes of their spouses or families. Chambers & Millar (1983) carried out an in-depth study of the police methods of investigating sexual assaults in Scotland. They found grounds for criticism of police methods on a number of counts. The collection of evidence was often carried out insensitively at a time of considerable emotional distress. This tended to be justified or at least defended on the grounds that the first priority was to catch the offender. Some CID officers clearly saw it as their job to challenge the truth of the victim's story as a way of testing its validity, little realising that they were probably reducing its validity in the process, an approach which, in any case, would seldom be used with the victims of other types of crime. Police officers were often unaware of the up-to-date interpretations of the law on rape, and there was a tendency to apply stricter standards of evidence than were actually required to prove a case. Almost one-quarter of the cases studied were 'no-crimed' by the police. This involves amending the initial crime report after a judgement has been made that no crime has been committed. Such cases do not appear in the official statistics of crimes reported to the police. Decisions to 'no-crime' a case were often taken by relatively junior or inexperienced officers. The 'no-crime' rate found by Chambers & Millar (1983) is considerably higher than that reported for crime in general. Other studies have found comparable 'no-crime' rates for sexual assault, e.g. in

England 24%, USA 18% and 20%. Chambers & Millar discussed in some detail the criteria used to reach a 'no-crime' decision. They concluded with a number of recommendations for improving investigative procedure in ways which would increase the likelihood of victims reporting the experience.

Investigation by the police is only one of the deterrents to reporting. The legal process is another off-putting experience. As Chambers & Millar (1986) found in Scotland, one-third of cases reported to the Procurator Fiscal were not prosecuted, the principal reason being the lack of independent third-party evidence. To have one's case turned down for lack of such evidence must be extremely distressing for genuine victims. Rules about corroboration of evidence are more stringent in Scotland than in England.

Most women were not only anxious about going to court, they also found the experience worse than they had expected. This was due in particular to the cross-examination which often made the complainant feel that her own character was on trial. The defence often used tactics to discredit the complainer and rarely did the judge intervene to protect the complainer from such lines of questioning. In general, women were inadequately prepared for the experience in court. The 1976 Sexual Offence Act made evidence of the previous sexual history of the complainant with other men inadmissible in the course of a rape trial except with the leave of the trial judge. This was intended to reduce the extent that the woman rather than the defendant was being put on trial. But Chambers & Millar (1986) and others have concluded that this Act has done little to reduce the humiliation of rape victims by the judicial procedure.

To some extent this highly unsatisfactory situation for the victims of rape stems from the potential severity of the sentence if the defendant is convicted. The maximum sentence for rape is life imprisonment, though as we shall see the average sentence is 3 to 4 years. Occasionally false accusations of rape are made. There is therefore an understandable desire on the part of the police and judiciary to ensure that no one is unjustly convicted, and an undue tendency not to prosecute if the evidence is not 'cast-iron'. To some extent this problem would be lessened by a reform of the criminal law which abolished the category of rape per se, and instead involved a general category of sexual assault. As it is, a case of indecent assault can be much more horrific than a case of rape, but for technical reasons it falls into a category with a much lighter maximum sentence. In the USA the Michigan Penal Code has adopted a sexual assault law which recognises assault on either sex, placing each offence on a continuum depending on lethality and degree of coercion used. In the state of Nebraska, sex law is based on the concept of sexual penetration, which includes fellatio, anal intercourse, and the intrusion of anything into the victim's anus or vagina. In Canada rape is now treated as a subcategory of assault and not as an illegal sexual act (Chambers & Millar 1983). In such ways the sentences, if conviction occurs, can be as severe as the circumstances justify but there would be less reluctance to prosecute (West 1984).

Thus it would seem that there is a need for major changes not only in the legal definition of sexual assault, but also in the ways that cases are investigated by the police, how decisions to prosecute are made, and the judicial procedure itself. Until such changes are made the consequences of reporting rape will effectively deter many genuine victims from reporting their ordeal, and this is a most unsatisfactory state of affairs.

Incidence of non-indictable sexual offences

The number of people convicted for the main non-indictable offences over a 10-years period are shown in Table 13.2.

The only non-indictable offence to show any increase during this time period is soliciting by prostitutes. The commonest sentence for non-indictable offences is a fine. In 1975, 50% of solicitings and 54% of indecent exposures were fined; the proportion receiving custodial sentences were 5 and 2.5% respectively (Honoré 1978).

Table 13.2 Numbers of persons convicted of non-indictable sexual offences during 1965, 1970 and 1975 (Honoré 1978)

	1965	1970	1975
Brothel-keeping	154	140	99
Living on prostitutes' earnings	227	219	130
Soliciting etc. by prostitute	1532	2347	3292
Importuning by men	820	451	591
Indecent exposure	2496	2862	2490

THE PENALTIES FOR SEXUAL OFFENCES WITH REFERENCE TO AGE OF VICTIM AND CONSENT

Whilst the maximum penalty for a particular offence indicates the legal seriousness of the offence, the maximum penalties are rarely used, as shown in Table 13.1.

The severity of sentences clearly relates to the issue of consent, and for those below the age of consent, the difference between the age of the victim and of the offender also has an effect (Walmsley & White 1979). Thus whilst consent if given by someone under the age of consent is not a defence, the penalties for rape of a 15-year-old girl are much heavier than those for unlawful sexual intercourse (i.e. with her consent). Similar differences, although less marked, apply to homosexual offences. There is however a striking difference between homosexual and heterosexual offences in the proportion which are consensual (see Table 13.3). These figures emphasise the extent to which the law concerns itself with consensual homosexual behaviour.

Table 13.3 Persons convicted of indictable sexual offences with victims/partners aged 10 or over: homosexual and heterosexual behaviour and consent (Walmsley & White 1979)

	Homosexual (%)	Heterosexual (%)
Consensual	80	34
Non-consensual	20	66

Table 13.4 Age of victims/partners of persons convicted of indictable heterosexual offences in 1973 (Walmsley & White 1979)

Age of victim/ partner (years)	Rape (%) (n = 321)	USI (%) (n = 709)	Indecent assault (%) (n = 2551)	Incest (%) (n = 129)
0–4	—	—	3.2	—
5–9	4.7	2.7	24.8	7.8
10–12	2.8	13.8	15.4	19.4
13–15	24.3	83.5	26.2	45.7
16–17	23.1	—	7.1	12.4
18–20	15.0	—	7.8	7.0
21–29	20.6	—	9.9	4.7
30+	9.7	—	5.6	3.1

USI = unlawful sexual intercourse.

Whilst the law distinguishes between girls aged under 13 and those under 16, Walmsley & White (1979) have shown that in sentencing practice, the crucial age for girls is 12. Most girls below 12 are prepubertal and there is an important association with the age of the offender in this group. In two-thirds of cases involving girls aged under 12, the offender was *over* 25; for girls over 12 but under 13, two-thirds of the offenders were *under* 25. The age of 12 is probably important in distinguishing paedophiliac offenders from others. The comparable age for boys, below which sentences

Table 13.5 Age of victims/partners of persons convicted of indictable homosexual offences in 1973 (Walmsley & White 1979)

Age of victim/ partner	Buggery and attempted buggery (%) (n = 209)	Indecent assault (%) (n = 689)	Indecency with male aged 14+ (%) (n = 1580)
0–4	2.9	3.1	—
5–9	12.0	32.5	—
10–11	17.7	18.6	—
12–13	17.2	15.8	—
14–15	18.7	18.1	1.7
16–17	12.4	4.9	2.6
18–20	6.2	2.8	4.3
21–29	4.3	2.9	27.6
30+	6.7	1.3	63.8

are more severe and consent becomes less relevant, is 14. In both cases, the age reflects the average age of puberty. Ages of victims of heterosexual and homosexual offences are shown in Tables 13.4 and 13.5.

RELATIONSHIP BETWEEN SEX OFFENCES AND OTHER CRIMES: RECIDIVISM

As mentioned earlier, there is a marked association between sexual offences and other types of offence. The extent of this is shown in Table 13.6. Sex offenders as a group have a relatively low rate of recidivism for sexual offences. Christiansen et al (1965) followed up 2934 male sex offenders 24 years after their initial conviction and found an overall rate of recidivism of 10% for sex offences. The rate for first offenders was 7% and for those with previous convictions, 23%. Thus the legal process appears to have a deterrent effect on most offenders, leaving a few who show fairly high recidivism rates. In most studies, recidivism has been highest for indecent exposure and offences against children (Qualls 1978).

Table 13.6 Proportion of convicted adults with previous convictions (Walmsley & White 1979)

Offence	For a sexual offence	For any offence
Rape and attempted rape	22%	73%
Incest	12%	58%
Buggery or attempted buggery	43%	70%
USI with girls under 13	21%	62%

USI = unlawful sexual intercourse.

The recidivism for non-sexual offences amongst sex offenders tends to be generally high. Soothill (1980) reported a 22-year follow-up of 86 rapists convicted in England in 1951. By the end of the follow-up period, 6% had been re-convicted for rape and 49% for other offences. In a more recent cohort, Soothill and his colleagues found general recidivism to be highest in aggressive offenders and lowest amongst incest offenders. They also compared a group of rapists convicted in 1961 with a group of men acquitted of rape in the same year. They found that further convictions for both sexual and non-sexual offences were very similar in the two groups, leading them to suggest that the rules of evidence are loaded in favour of the defendant in rape cases.

THE RELATIONSHIP BETWEEN PORNOGRAPHY AND CRIME

Pornography is verbal or visual material, depicting sexual anatomy or activity, which is primarily intended to elicit sexual arousal. It may be related to crime in a number of ways. The production and circulation of pornography may transgress the law. Those who produce and distribute pornography may be involved in other criminal activities. Crimes may be committed as a consequence of exposure to pornography, or conversely, may be less likely to occur as a result of such exposure (Kutchinsky 1983). It is the two latter associations which have caused the greatest controversy. In the early 1970s the US Commission on Obscenity and Pornography published nine volumes of technical reports of a variety of studies. The overall conclusion was that it was difficult to demonstrate that pornography had any substantial effect on the occurrence of sexual crimes. (It is probably fair to say that for many of the studies it was inherently unlikely that the question would be answered in any case.) In 1979 the British Committee on Obscenity and Film Censorship (Williams committee) reviewed the evidence available and reached broadly similar conclusions. Since the US reports were published there had been a noticeable increase in the availability of child pornography which caused much concern.

It has been suggested that the greater availability of aggressive pornography has contributed to the increase in rape and sexual assault. Kutchinsky (1985) argues against this; the increase in rape was obvious well before the dramatic increase in pornography following its legalisation. And in West Germany the incidence of rape remained stable in the years following that legalisation. It is also noteworthy that in Denmark the legalisation of pornography was followed by a *decline* in the number of sexual offences against children, most marked between 1965 and 1973, the years when the availability of pornography was increasing most rapidly. Whilst one cannot conclude from this association that the decline in such crimes was a *result* of the availability of pornography, it is virtually out of the question that the pornography caused an increase in sexual crimes against children. Not everyone agrees with Kutchinsky's interpretation of the evidence, notably Court (1976) and Giglio (1985), though Kutchinsky (1985) presents a well argued rebuttal of their case.

There is a worrying discontinuity between the decreasing trends reported by Kutchinsky for sexual crimes against children in Denmark and the apparent major increase in child sexual abuse, at least in Britain and the USA. It is true that this apparent explosion is not yet evident in the British crime statistics, though this may change over the next few years. But one is bound to wonder whether the much greater use of video pornography that has accompanied the home video boom may have contributed to an increase in child sexual abuse within the family. Unfortunately that will not be an easy question to answer.

THE SEXUAL OFFENDER AND HIS VICTIM

In attempting to understand why people commit sexual offences and the effects that these offences have on their victims, we find the precise legal categories relatively unhelpful. There may be more in common between a rapist and a man convicted of indecent assault because he forced a woman to have oral sex with him, than between the second man and another man convicted of indecent assault because he interfered sexually but non-violently with a girl of 10. We will therefore consider sexual offenders and their victims under the following headings:

1. Rape and other forms of sexual violence.
2. Child sexual abuse and paedophilia.
3. Incest.
4. Indecent exposure and exhibitionism.
5. Voyeurism.
6. Other homosexual offences (i.e. those not included in categories 1 or 2).
7. Prostitution.

Throughout we must keep in mind the strong association between sexual offending and other types of criminal behaviour and also the need to consider motives or determinants other than the obviously sexual ones.

RAPE AND OTHER FORMS OF SEXUAL ASSAULT

Sexual assault is predominantly heterosexual. Buggery with violence or with the threat of it is perhaps closest to the male homosexual version of rape. However, the proportions of cases of buggery or attempted buggery which are truly non-consensual is small (Gebhard et al 1965; Walmsley & White 1979). Homosexual rape may be common in many male prisons. Davis (1970) gave a disturbing account of this aspect of the Philadelphia prison system, concluding that prison rape was 'epidemic', usually involving young, relatively weak prisoners. He saw this behaviour more as a means of asserting masculinity and power than of gaining sexual pleasure. The rape victim would not only be humiliated, he would also be looked upon as feminine. Brownmiller (1975) gave other evidence of this kind. Homosexual assaults between women sometimes occur (0.2% of cases of indecent assault on females in the UK in 1973 were by women; Walmsley & White 1979). They may also occur occasionally in women's prisons (Brownmiller 1975), though most homosexuality in women's institutions probably serves a rather different function to that in men's (Ward & Kassebaum 1964).

Rape of men by women remains a matter of legal controversy. In an American murder case, a male homosexual, accused of killing a woman, claimed that he had been raped by her, was terrified and feared for his own life. Sarrel, who gave evidence in this case, has reported other comparable cases (Sarrel & Masters 1982). But the overwhelming majority of rapes and sexual assaults involve females as the victims and we will concentrate on this type of offence. (Katz & Mazur (1979) provide comprehensive review of the rape literature.)

In the majority of cases, only one assailant is involved, but multiple or group rapes are common. In a British study, one in five rape victims and 40% of those convicted were involved in multiple or gang rapes (Walmsley

& White 1979). In Amir's American study (1971), 43% of victims and 71% of rapists were so involved. Other studies have shown variable but always significant proportions (Katz & Mazur 1979). It is possible that group rape is more prevalent in the USA, particularly in the large cities.

The ages of British rape victims are shown in Table 13.4. According to Katz & Mazur's review, there may be more victims in the young adult age groups in the USA. Group rape is also more likely to involve adolescent girls rather than children or adult women and to be carried out by boys in their teens or early 20s.

The proportion of rape which involves physical violence, whilst varying from study to study, is always high — around 80%. In about 20%, the violence is extreme. Injuries to the face are common and about 25% experience some genital trauma, though permanent physical disability appears to be unusual. Physical violence is more common with adult women and least common with children. It is more likely with group than with single rapes, with rapists who are strangers, who have been drinking alcohol or who have found themselves impotent during the assault. In the various American studies, somewhere between a quarter and a half of rapists use a weapon to threaten the victim, most commonly a knife. Death as a consequence of rape appears to be rare (Katz & Mazur 1979). Vaginal intercourse usually occurs, but according to Holmstrom & Burgess (1980) forced fellatio (22%) and breast manipulation or injury (12%) are relatively common and a wide variety of other sexual or excretory acts, such as anal intercourse or urinating on the victim, occasionally occur.

Holmstrom & Burgess (1980) concluded that there are four principal 'meanings' of the sexual assault:

1. The experience of power and control over the victim;
2. The expression of anger or hatred;
3. With group or pair rape, the male camaraderie experienced by the rapists;
4. The sexual experience, which in the view of Holmstrom & Burgess is never the dominant theme.

We will return to these issues further when considering the determinants of rape behaviour and the relationships between sexuality, aggression and dominance.

An important dimension of rape is the relationship between the rapist and his victim. Was the rapist a complete stranger, a casual acquaintance, or a friend or relative of the victim? The proportions of the British cases in these three categories were 50, 27 and 23% respectively (Walmsley & White 1979). In American studies, the proportion of rapists who are complete strangers appears to be higher but is related to the age of the victim. The majority of children and adolescents know the offenders, whereas the large majority of adult victims are raped by complete strangers (Katz & Mazur

1979). Chappell & Singer (1977) found that compared with Philadelphia, New York rapists were more likely to be older, to be a stranger to the victim and to rape alone rather than in groups. The previous relationship between rapist and victim has an important bearing on the acceptability of the victim's evidence, the likelihood of conviction and the severity of the sentence, as discussed earlier. It has been suggested that for these reasons, rape involving friends or relatives is less likely to be reported as it is less likely to be believed or lead to a conviction.

Characteristics of the rapist

The convicted rapist is predominantly a young man. In a British study, 40% were aged 17 to 20, and 19% aged 21–24 years. When children under 12 are assaulted, the offender is likely to be older and most teenage victims are raped by youths of a similar age (Walmsley & White 1979). He tends to come from the lower socioeconomic groups. In an English study Wright (1980) found 75% of rapists to be unskilled working-class men and only 2% were professional/managerial. In the USA, black and Spanish American men are over-represented (Katz & Mazur 1979). Evidence of the intelligence of rapists is inconclusive; it is not clear that they differ from other criminal groups in this respect (Vera et al 1979). Sexual assaults are often proceded by excess alcohol consumption.

As yet, no clear picture of the personality of the typical rapist has emerged and it is important to remember that characteristics of those involved in *reported* rape may differ significantly from those involved in unreported incidents (Howells 1984).

Levin & Stava (1987) have reviewed the literature on the personality of sex offenders. They stress the methodological short-comings of most of the research. With clearer definition of types of offence or precipitants some relevant personality types may start to emerge.

The majority of rapists are not married, presumably because they tend to be young. Those in Gebhard et al's (1965) study, being older, were more often married, though frequently with marital problems. However, we know very little about the wives of these men — an area of potentially great importance in understanding rape and its possible prevention.

West et al (1978) studied in depth a small group of rapists in a Canadian penitentiary. They concluded: 'The man who has an urge to rape is often the man who feels at a disadvantage with women. He doubts his attractiveness as a mate, he fears exploitation, he doubts his sexual proficiency or he is afraid of being cheated and so becomes demanding and jealous'. In his attack on women, he confirms their inferiority and reasserts his masculinity.

Gibbens et al (1977) divided rapists into three groups:

1. Those who raped or attempted to rape girls under 14 (30%);

2. Aggressive rapists amongst whom the rape seemed only a part of a general cycle of aggression (20%);
3. Others, with few or no records of offences (50%).

They did not give their reasons for categorising in this way and their third, largest category was extremely heterogeneous. They concluded that the rapist tends less often to be psychiatrically disordered or to have a previous record of sexual offences than other sexual offenders. Ellis & Brancale (1956) had earlier maintained that rapists tend to be sexually and psychiatrically normal individuals whose offence is a part of a general anti-social pattern.

Kanin (1985) compared a group of 71 college students who admitted to having raped girls they had dated with a control group of students of similar age. The rapists were substantially more experienced sexually than the controls, with a much higher frequency of sexual outlets with female partners. Kanin concluded that the high level of sexual success combined with an exploitative attitude to sexual relationships resulted in greater frustration when confronted with a non-compliant partner. This study illustrates well the overlap between criminal rape and the much more common socially endorsed exploitative sexuality.

Russell (1982) described the USA as a 'rape supportive culture'. Burt (1980) found that more than a half of an American sample agreed with the statement 'a woman who goes to the home or apartment of a man on the first date implies she is willing to have sex'. Howells et al (1984) found that British men who held stereotyped views about women's roles were more likely to blame the victim for the assault.

There are many men with aggressive and criminal tendencies; only a proportion of them rape. There are many men with doubts about their masculinity; very few of them rape. It is probably unwise to look for a stereotype of the typical rapist. An alternative view is to see most men as potential rapists, or the rapist as a relatively normal male who, as a result of socially learned attitudes to women, is likely to rape in certain circumstances. Some feminist writers take this view. Brownmiller (1975) presents an appalling catalogue of rape carried out in war conditions by men, most of whom presumably would not rape in normal circumstances. Probably no particular nationality is free from blame in this respect, though some may be more culpable than others. The most ghastly example of recent times was the mass rape of Bengali women during the Bangladesh war of independence. Accounts of rape by both American and South Vietnamese soldiers during the Vietnam war also make gruesome reading. The dehumanising effect of war obviously plays an important part and Brownmiller gives a convincing account of how much of this rape is an extension of the violence of war in which women become the particular victims. It may be those soldiers who have the least reason to feel proud as a result of the more conventional violence who assert their masculinity in this way (Brownmiller 1975).

Characteristics of the rape victim

Most rape victims are teenagers or young adult women, though no age group is immune. In the USA, 60% of rape victims as compared with 10% of the population are black. Rape victims tend to come from the lower socioeconomic groups, as do most rapists, probably indicating that the female most at risk is the one living in the same area or local community as the would-be rapist. However no woman, whatever her socioeconomic status, can regard herself as entirely safe. The characteristics of the typical rape victim are in fact very similar to those of the typical victim of non-sexual violence, except that the latter is more often male.

Evidence of sexual experience of rape victims prior to the assault is inconclusive. Whereas most recent studies show the majority of adolescent victims to be sexually experienced, there are no appropriately controlled data to indicate whether they are more so than would be expected by chance, and yet this is relevant to one of the most controversial issues concerning rape — victim precipitation. In cases of rape by a complete stranger, or where there is clear evidence of premeditation, the victim is unlikely to be considered in any way responsible. But in those cases where rape occurs between friends or casual acquaintances, the victim is likely to find herself under suspicion or held to be responsible to a greater or lesser extent. This underlies much of the humiliation that rape victims experience after reporting the rape, as discussed earlier. Thus if a girl allows herself to get involved in limited love-making but refuses to go 'all the way', she may have difficulty in having her charge of rape taken seriously. This remarkable fact stems from an almost universal attitude about male/female sexuality — that if a female allows a male to become sexually aroused in her presence, there comes a time when his arousal goes beyond the point of control and he can no longer be held responsible for his actions. Such a belief is by no means of recent origin. As Bullough (1976) commented about prevailing social attitudes in the past, 'the safest thing for a woman to do was to keep a careful check on her sexuality or to deny it in public, since if she did not she was seen as inviting rape or encouraging adultery'. The continuation of this belief is exemplified in the idea that if a young woman dresses in a sexually provocative way, she is 'asking for it' or 'deserves what she gets'.

The problem for the woman is further compounded by the social signifi-cance of being raped which prevails to a greater or lesser extent in most cultures. The raped woman is seen as 'defiled', 'spoiled', a reflection of her 'property status' that was discussed in Chapter 4. One of the most awful aspects of the mass rape of Bengali women was the stigmatisation they suffered, not only from society at large but in particular from their husbands, who were likely to disown them. By tradition, no Muslim husband takes back a wife who has been touched by another man, even if she is subdued by force. The Bangladesh government attempted to counter this trend by declaring that the rape victims were 'national heroines', but with little effect (Brownmiller 1975). Such reactions are less likely in Christian countries but do occur (Katz & Mazur 1979).

The universality and long-standing nature of these attitudes may tempt one to believe that they are inevitable because of our biological natures. But apart from the fact that there is no physiological basis to account for the assumed sex difference in sexual control, the implications that this value system has for the nature of male/female relationships are profound, and extend far beyond the problem of rape. The woman is seen as the responsible person and 'the property to be taken' at one and the same time. This is an issue which crops up time and time again in couples with sexual problems, where the woman is unable to feel safe enough to let herself go sexually (see Chapter 8). But more important, in societies where such abdication of interpersonal responsibility is more or less institutionalised, one should not be surprised to find other examples of man's inhumanity to man as well as to woman.

As we discussed earlier, many women are reluctant to reveal that they have been raped. In some instances they are frightened of reprisals from the rapist, but more often fear the stigmatisation that follows and being put on trial themselves in order to convince people that they were not responsible for the assault. This is a unique position for any victim of crime to find him- or herself in.

One of the more outstanding legal issues concerns marital rape. At the present time, the English law on this matter dates from the 17th century. 'The husband cannot be guilty of rape committed by himself upon his lawful wife, for by their mutual matrimonial consent and contract, the wife his given up herself in this kind unto her husband which she cannot retract'. The husband however can be charged with assault if he inflicts injury upon her. The Criminal Law Revision Committee in its working paper on sexual offences (CLRC 1980) addressed this problem. In an interesting discussion, the Committee showed itself to be divided in its opinion. There was agreement on the inherent complexity of the problem and the inevitable difficulty in weighing up evidence. However, those who preferred to leave the law unchanged in this respect expressed reasons which once again revealed disturbing attitudes towards male/female relationships. They expressed concern, no doubt sincere, for the continuation of the family unit and the fear that recourse to the law of rape could precipitate an irreconcilable breakdown in marriage. 'The type of questions which investigating police officers would have to ask would be likely to be greatly resented by husbands and their families. The family ties would be severed and the wife with children would have to cope with her emotional, social and financial problems as best she could and possibly the children might resent what she has done to their father. Nearly all breakdowns of marriage cause problems. A breakdown brought by a wife who had sought the protection of the criminal law of rape would be particularly painful'. This remarkable statement which attributes responsibility for the consequences of legal proceedings to the woman without giving her the choice whether to accept them, appears to deny the inherent violence and degradation of rape, whether it be of one's wife or not, confusing it with the sexual needs of men. The impact on the marriage seen as a consequence of the legal process pales into insignificance against the damaging consequences of the rape itself, and yet women, it would seem, are to be encouraged to tolerate such behaviour. Marital rape is an extension of marital violence, from which, in spite of the law, wives still find difficulty in gaining protection. And yet there is much more at stake than the rights and well-being of these women, important though they are. Violence and irresponsibility in the home are some of the most important, if not *the* most important reinforcers of violence in our society. As long as we, as a society, turn a blind eye to the violent behaviour of men within their homes, we should not be surprised to find those men and their children acting violently outside their homes.

To be fair to the Criminal Law Revision Committee, who presented their views in an honest and open way, it should be noted that the majority view was for a change in the law so that married men are not legally exempt from the charge of raping their wives. But they advocated the safeguard that prosecution would only proceed with the agreement of the Director of Public Prosecutions. Whether this arrangement would be a satisfactory solution remains a matter for debate, but at least a need for change has been acknowledge.

The reactions of the rape victim

A further aspect of evidence in rape cases is the reaction of the woman to the rape. If she screams, actually resists, or is seen to be physically injured, her story is more likely to be believed. Probably the over-riding emotional experience for most victims is 'a fear of death' (Katz & Mazur 1979). In those circumstances, one should expect a variety of reactions, not necessarily rational. Burnett et al (1985) found that a woman who normally harboured high anxiety about death would be less likely to put up physical resistance to rape. Clearly, for many women rape or the threat of rape is a threat to life. Also, many women show minimal physical resistance because of an understandable fear that by doing so they are more likely to be hurt or disfigured. Such relative passivity leads some rapists to conclude that the women were consenting, a form of deceit which becomes more understandable when prevailing social attitudes about female passivity and masochism are taken into account. Some women try to flatter or help the rapist in the hope that this will diffuse his aggression. In such cases the man may believe them to the extent of trying to arrange another meeting (West et al 1978) or of raping someone else (Gibbens et al 1977). It is nevertheless difficult for a woman to know how best to react, even assuming she is in a position to choose. Some rapists are likely to be discouraged by the act of resistance whilst others may be further aroused by it.

Rape is an exceedingly traumatic experience for most women. Hence it is not surprising that substantial psychological after-effects commonly occur. The initial reaction, as with most acute crises, is very variable; some women react with extreme distress and disorganisation, others with remarkable calmness. At varying times after this initial phase, however, more long-term reactions are likely. Anxiety and an inability to feel safe are common, often taking a form of phobic avoidance of the setting in which the rape occurred (Katz & Mazur 1979). A depressive reaction is also common and may be quite severe. In a study of 34 rape victims, 23% were moderately and 21% severely depressed as measured on the Beck depression inventory (Frank et al 1979). In a large study of 178 victims and 50 controls, 51% of the victims reported depressive symptoms compared with 8% of the controls. Many of the victims were experiencing depression several years after the assault (Becker et al 1984). Sexual problems are also common. Becker et al (1986) found sexual problems in 59% of survivors of sexual assault compared with 17% in a control group. Whilst for most women these psychological reactions will eventually subside, in some they may continue for years.

There has been disagreement about the relevance of the circumstances of the rape to the psychological after-effects. In one report it was concluded that the 'stranger' rape was the most traumatic whereas, in another, victims who were raped by persons known to them were seen to face more difficulties. Frank et al (1980) found no association between the circumstances of the rape and the psychological reactions, except that those who suffered physical injury or who were threatened by a weapon reported less problems in their post-rape relationship with their families, presumably because their rape was taken more seriously.

Becker et al (1984) found depression to be more common in women whose rape had involved a threatening weapon, suggesting that the life-threatening quality of the rape experience, and the associated feeling of no control over one's own life, are of particular importance in causing post-assault depression.

The possible determinants of rape

So far, we have emphasised the importance of power and hostility in rape. There is a tendency to see these two factors as sufficient explanation and to minimise the sexual aspect. 'Rape is not the aggressive expression of sexuality. It is sexual expression of aggression' (Groth, New York Times, 5 February 1980). It is important to get the sexual aspect into perspective.

What is the relationship between aggression and sexuality? It is commonly assumed that the two are closely linked in both animals and humans. Yet a brief look at the available evidence reveals confusion. Much of this stems from variable meanings of the term 'aggression'. Hinde (1974) points out that it is sometimes used to include all forms of assertiveness, even intellectual achievement. He draws a distinction, however, between establishing dominance or territorial rights and attacking another animal in such a way as to risk injuring it. He prefers to restrict the term 'aggression' to this latter type of behaviour. Such aggressive behaviour may lead to or be used to establish dominance, but there are other ways of achieving that particular goal. Bandura (1973) distinguishes between 'instrumental' aggression, which is used to achieve some particular goal and 'expressive' aggression which is primarily a manifestation of an emotional state.

But aggressive behaviour is a function of the interaction between the animal's internal state and environmental factors and as such, its determinants are complex, varied and not always easy to identify. For our present purposes, we certainly need to acknowledge and attempt to understand the role of the accompanying emotion. Thus the infliction of pain or minor injury may be an expression of anger or hostility or alternatively some other emotional state such as sexual excitement. In Chapter 2 we discussed the frequency with which painful stimuli are used during sexual excitement, with no indication in such cases that they are intended to express anger or assert dominance. Thus we have dominance (or power), anger and inflicted pain as three variables with complex inter-relationships. This complexity is further compounded in humans by the effect of language on social learning. Words such as 'fuck' and 'screw' are used to indicate both sexual and aggressive acts.

In Chapter 8, we stressed the importance of anger or resentment as a cause of sexual problems. Hinde (1974) states that amongst animals 'while aggressive and fleeing responses are often closely interwoven with the sexual ones, they interfere with mating rather than promote it'. Yet there is other evidence to suggest that aggressive behaviour, as defined by Hinde, may facilitate sexual arousal in certain circumstances. We thus have to allow for a variable relationship between aggression and sexuality, which can be summarised under three headings (see p. 130):

1. The physiological effect of anger; in certain circumstances the non-specific arousing effect of anger may facilitate arousal responses to sexual stimuli and vice versa.
2. The consequences of autonomic conditioning; the coexistence of anger and sexual response may result in sexual responses becoming conditioned to anger-provoking stimuli.
3. The psychological significance of the coexistence of anger and sexual response; thus in certain circumstances:
   a. either the occurrence of sexual behaviour or the withholding of it could be used to express anger and psychologically hurt the partner;
   b. the existence of anger may be incompatible with certain sexual responses (e.g. the tender, empathic touching of one's partner) but compatible with others (e.g. inflicting pain);
   c. anger may arise as a reaction to sexual failure.

How does the rapist fit into this scheme? First, he may use the *physical* dominance of the rape act as a way of asserting his *psychological* dominance and reinforcing his masculinity. Here the sexuality of the behaviour validates this function if one believes that it is masculine to dominate or conquer one's sexual partner. Whereas it would also boost one's masculinity to dominate physically another male of comparable strength without any sexuality being involved, it would not do so to dominate a woman physically unless the act was sexual. This all stems from our preconceived ideas about male/female stereotypes.

Secondly, he may use his victim as a substitute for some other woman, or as a representative of women in general for whom he has developed some hatred. Once again, simply to humiliate or physically hurt them would be less acceptable and in certain respects 'unmanly' (i.e. attacking a defenceless woman) but by using the sexual mode it becomes masculine behaviour. The justificatory role of sex in this respect is twofold; first, because it indicates a 'normal' male response and also because it involves 'sexual excitement', in which state the male is assumed to be relieved of his normal responsibilities.

Thirdly, the violence and or the illegal aspect of rape may have, as a result of autonomic conditioning, a sexually arousing effect. In such circumstances, the anticipation of a sexual attack would lead to an increase of sexual arousal. It is of some importance to establish the relevance of such a mechanism because the motivating effect of sexual excitement and the elimination of that motive following orgasm may be a crucial factor in understanding the rapist's behaviour.

Gebhard et al (1965) found that amongst the various groups of sex offenders, it was those involved in sexual assaults who were most likely to report arousal from sadomasochistic stimuli, to use fantasies during masturbation or to have dreams of a sadomasochistic nature. Up to 20% in each of the aggresssor groups came into this category.

In recent years increasing attention has been paid to the measurement of erectile response to various kinds of erotic stimuli as a way of distinguishing between different types of offender. Abel et al (1977) devised the rape index, which is the degree of erectile response to depictions of rape divided by the response to scenes of consensual sex. They demonstrated that the rape index discriminated between rapists and non-rapists. This finding was replicated by Barbaree et al (1979) and Quinsey et al (1981). Abel and his colleagues (1980) made a further interesting observation. They asked their rapists and their normal controls to suppress sexual responses to stimuli of both rape and non-sexual aggression. Rapists were incapable of suppressing their sexual responses to rape stimuli, in contrast to the non-rapists who could. Even more striking was their response to the non-sexual aggressive stimuli. Neither the rapists nor the controls showed much sexual response to these stimuli until they were actually asked to suppress their responses, when the rapists showed a paradoxical increase in response. This led Abel and his colleagues to suggest: 'Two psychological factors may lead the rapist to rape. First, through some learning process, he is more aroused to thoughts and fantasies of rape than the non-rapist. Second, as he attempts to inhibit his arousal to rape . . . it increases above its previous level'; in other words, a truly vicious spiral. We must be cautious in generalising from these intriguing findings, however. Murphy et al (1984) were unable to replicate them. And other studies have demonstrated the importance of situational factors — especially instructions — on how subjects, both normal and rapists, respond in such laboratory conditions. Thus Quinsey et al (1981) found that the responses of normal controls to rape stimuli were increased if they were told beforehand that such responses were common in normal men. Malamuth & Donnerstein (1982) found that normal subjects showed high arousal to rape scenes if it was apparent that the female victim was involuntarily sexually aroused. They also found considerable variability amongst normal males in their likelihood of being aroused by such scenes. They related this responsiveness to what they called 'rape proclivity' — which is a high self-rating of likelihood of raping 'if you could be assured of not being caught and punished'. About 35% of males report such likelihood on this measure, and those with high 'rape proclivity' show erectile responses to rape stimuli which are indistinguishable from those of actual rapists (Malamuth 1981).

Thus there are several reasons for being cautions about reading too much into a single measure of this kind, as Howells (1984) has stressed in his useful review. There are two key questions: Why do some men (perhaps many but certainly not all) seem to be capable of arousal and response to depictions of rape? Why do some of these men commit rape whilst others do not? Certainly we should hesitate before making predictions about the likelihood of re-offending on the basis of single psychophysiological tests such as these.

The possibility that there are different types of rapists remains a key issue. Abel and his colleagues distinguish between the 'true sexual deviant' rapist and the 'sexually normal' criminal rapist, emphasising the essentially sexual nature of the first type of behaviour, and the more antisocial aggressive quality of the second. Recently this group (Abel et al 1987) have reported that some rapists are 'true paraphiliacs', i.e. their histories reveal urges to rape beginning at an early age, similar to the history of other paraphiliacs, and some show a variety of paraphiliac tendencies apart from rape, e.g. voyeurism, sadism, exhibitionism. Whilst these observations are of interest, I am not happy with their use of the concept of 'paraphilia', particularly with its strong implications of psychopathology, i.e. certain types of sexual preference are forms of mental disorder in their own right. This is reminiscent of the 19th century vogue for defining varieties of 'mania' e.g. kleptomania, pyromania; an approach which did nothing to help our understanding of such behaviour. It is not therefore surprising that attempts to include rape or a tendency to rape as a mental disorder in diagnostic classificatory systems (e.g. DSM III R) have met with strong opposition from those who fear that as a consequence rapists will be treated as sick rather than criminal. The inclusion of a category of 'paraphiliac rapist' in the DSM III classification has been defended on the grounds that if it is not included it would not be possible to provide insurance-funded treatment to such individuals. It is however a disturbing nonsense to have administrative constraints of a health care system determining how we conceptualise important forms of abnormal or antisocial behaviour. Rape is a form of sexual assault. The determinants of such behaviour will be many and various. Some rapists will be mentally ill; they should be diagnosed on the basis of their mental illness, not this particular expression of it. In Britain sexual deviancy is specifically excluded from the definition of mental disorder in both the Scottish and English Mental Health Acts of 1983.

Nevertheless, Abel's group and others working in the field have usefully underlined the need to understand *both* the sexual *and* the aggressive components of rape. It is simplistic and unhelpful to view rape in general as *either* one *or* the other.

At various points in this book I have commented on the peculiar conditionability of sexual response and the repercussions that may follow. Rape is probably another important example of such a repercussion. However we cannot escape the importance of social determinants. The initial link between violence and sexuality that may lead to such conditioned responsiveness derives in most cases from the social setting. Let us therefore consider next the cross-cultural evidence.

Cross-cultural aspects of rape

If the social setting is important in determining the likelihood of rape then it is pertinent to consider to what extent rape reflects the cultural background in a society. We have already commented on the contrast between the USA and Europe; what of more primitive societies? Broude & Greene's (1980) analysis of cross-cultural codes of 65 societies found 15% in which men were typically hostile in their sexual advances, sexual overtures were rough or aggressive and not solicited or desired by the women. The Gusii of south-western Kenya, described by Le Vine (1959), provided a classic example of a culture in which sex was embedded in violence. A warlike form of marital sexuality was the norm. The wife was expected to put up a struggle and there was certainly no tenderness. The unmarried male, on the other hand, was highly likely to rape women from other clans. Of 34 societies in Broude & Greene's analysis they found 14 (41%) in which rape was common and 8 (24%) in which it was virtually absent.

Sanday (1981) analysed 156 societies and concluded that 47% were rape-free and 18% rape-prone. According to Sanday rape-prone cultures characteristically promoted male/female antagonism, and used rape as a mechanism of social control and to enhance male dominance. Rape-free societies showed sexual equality; women were highly valued and there were generally low levels of interpersonal violence. The three variables which correlated most highly with rape were 'degree of interpersonal violence' (r = 0.47); an 'ideology of male toughness' (r = 0.42) and 'low female decision-making' (r = 0.33). Gray (1984) found negative correlations across cultures between frequency of rape and the typical degree of the wife's power within marriage, though this did not reach statistical significance.

It seems likely that whilst the status of women in society will have a bearing on the likelihood of rape, the association will be confounded in complex societies such as ours. Thus in more sexually liberal societies the proportion of rapes *reported* may be higher (Jaffee & Straus 1987).

CHILD SEXUAL ABUSE, PAEDOPHILIA AND INCEST

At the time of writing a fierce public debate on this issue is in progress. The storm broke in Britain in June 1987 following a dramatic increase in the number of children in Cleveland being taken into care on the grounds of sexual abuse. This change appeared to follow the arrival in Cleveland of a paediatrician with a special interest in the subject. The resulting furore stemmed from the accusation that many children were being taken from their parents peremptorily by the social services, on the recommendation of hospital doctors, often, it has been claimed, when there was no clear evidence that the parents were responsible or even that sexual abuse had definitely occurred. This led to a government inquiry.

This storm has been building for some time. In the USA concern about child sexual abuse has been growing at a faster rate than in the UK, with evidence (e.g. from California) that sexual abuse is as common as non-sexual physical abuse. Concern to track down and prosecute the perpetrators has at times put civil liberties at risk, such is the level of feeling about such crimes. In Britain public awareness of the problems was increased when a popular television personality, Esther Rantzen, presented a programme on the topic to launch a telephone answering service for children experiencing abuse. This Childline received 60 000 calls in the first 3 days. Admittedly many callers were adults wanting to talk about sexual abuse during their own childhood. But it was also striking how many children called, determined that their identity should not be revealed.

I and many other sex therapists have been amazed in recent years by the increase in the number of patients who are describing sexual abuse, particularly incest, during their childhood. Most of us working in the field are genuinely confused by what is going on. Has there been a dramatic increase in child sexual abuse? Has it always been at a high level which is now being revealed because it is easier for victims to talk about it? Or is there some form of hysteria affecting our society, seeing problems where they do not exist, or at least attributing much more severe consequences to such childhood experiences than is in fact the case? It is timely to recall that Freud in his earlier writings reported his impression that many of his patients had been sexually abused as children. Subsequently, and to some extent in response to social pressure, he changed his interpretation of such reports and attributed them to fantasised wish fulfilment, fuelling much of his elaborate theory of Oedipal feelings and castration fear. Were his original assumptions correct, only to be buried by the massive weight of psychoanalytic orthodoxy ever since? This time we must get it right, though at the moment it doesn't look as though it is going to be easy.

It is therefore imperative that we strive to consider the issues dispassionately. So far a great deal of the debate has been ruled by passion. One set of myths gives ground to another. From the Freudian notion of children revealing their Oedipal fantasies we move to the common assertion that children *never* lie about sexual abuse. From the idea of sexual wish fulfilment we move to the belief that children *never* enjoy sexual experiences with adults. Somewhere between these views must lie the truth.

The current crisis in Cleveland starkly displays the two unacceptable faces of the problem; first, the inescapable fact that adults, including parents, do sexually abuse children, sometimes to a horrifying extent; secondly, the strength of emotional reaction to *any* incident of child sexual abuse. By law, any sexual behaviour between adult and child is an offence, no doubt rightly so. But no category of offender is so strongly reviled as this, regardless of the severity of the offence, which varies considerably. Any such offender in prison usually requires special protection from his fellow prisoners. Such strong feelings occur outside prison also, and the possibility has to be faced that some people are unjustly accused. Also important is the possibility that the emotionally charged methods of dealing with such cases might cause as much or even more harm to the child than the sexual abuse itself. Caught in between these two manifestations of the problem we find the social services, who, it would seem from their exposure in the media, stagger from one crisis to another, accused of acting either too late or too early, the scapegoats for a social problem that runs deep.

Sexual violence of any kind is abhorrent and such violence against children especially so. But the extent of the feelings about child sexual abuse cannot be explained only in terms of violence. Exploitation and betrayal of trust are clearly important, and, as we shall see, may be the most damaging for many victims in the long term. But there is perhaps a third factor that contributes to the emotional turmoil, and which we need to take into account; the difficulty many adults have in coming to terms with the sexuality of children. Much current writing on the subject sees the child as sexually indifferent, whereas children are sexual beings with their own sexual feelings and concerns, albeit less powerful than those that will affect them when they reach adolescence. The fact that children may be sexually aware does not in any sense justify their sexual exploitation by adults; in no way can a child be held responsible for what happens in such situations.

But such awareness does have a bearing on how the child will react to such experiences and on the probable long-term ill effects, and is therefore relevant to how we help children after such abuse. One of the ironies of the current situation is that we may now start to see more substantial research into normal childhood sexuality. As discussed in Chapter 3, such research has always been difficult in the past, mainly because of resistance to it from the adult world and the tendency to accuse such researchers of being themselves child molesters in disguise. Friedrich (1987) has recently shown in a study of 160 sexually abused children that an increase in sexual behaviour such as masturbation and sexual preoccupations tends to follow the experience of sexual abuse. It is clearly important to put these behavioural disturbances into perspective with a better understanding of normal childhood sexuality.

In our attempts to understand this behaviour we need to keep two aspects of the problem in mind. First, the likely motive of the adult perpetrator and second, the nature of the preceding relationship between the adult and the child.

For motivation, we can start by drawing parallels with rape of adult victims. To what extent is sexual assault of children a sexually motivated act or rather an expression of anger or dominance? This crucial question has not been adequately addressed. The issue is often blurred by terminology. This is reflected in the law, as we have already seen. Any incident involving physical contact of a sexual kind with a child is called 'assault' (although paradoxically, consensual coitus with a young girl is called 'unlawful sexual intercourse'). And this is regardless of whether force or even persuasion has been used. And it is not just the law that blurs what seems to be an important distinction. Katz & Mazur (1979), for example, in their generally admirable review, use the term 'assault' to describe all incidents in which children are sexually involved with adults, including genital exhibition and verbal approaches. One can make a strong case that any such incident is never justifiable, and that children should be protected from sexual approaches by adults, in which case the term 'sexual abuse' is appropriate. But whether the incident will *necessarily* be harmful to the child is arguable and in any case depends on a variety of factors, some of which involve the reactions of others to the event after it has happened.

We do appear to be witnessing a disturbing increase in the number of cases of general child abuse, including sexual abuse, which are being brought to the attention of the social services or police. For some reason this is not being reflected in the criminal statistics (see Fig. 13.4 and see p. 676 for reference to Danish statistics). An exception is the offence of 'gross indecency with a child'. This usually non-indictable offence led to convictions or cautions in 35 cases in 1971, 50 in 1976, 247 in 1981 and 328 in 1985. A national survey of the number of children registered by local authorities as in danger of abuse showed a sharp increase of 22% in 1987, including a sharp increase in the number of cases of sexual

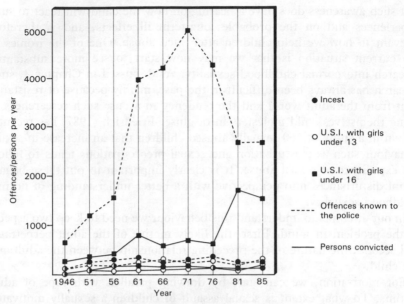

Fig. 13.4 Incidence of incest and unlawful sexual intercourse (U.S.I.) with girls aged under 13 and under 16 from 1946–1985. Offences known and persons convicted. (Criminal Statistics for England and Wales 1985)

abuse (Guardian, 7 July 1987). We must therefore take seriously the possibility that in many cases of sexual abuse, particularly those involving very young children, the same factors may be involved that lead to non-sexual physical abuse, and that the sexual component may be of secondary importance in determining the behaviour. One source of relevant evidence is a study by Mrazek et al (1981). A total of 1072 cases had been seen by a selected group of 1599 police surgeons, paediatricians, child psychiatrists and general practitioners. The cases were placed in one of three categories:

1. Type I: battered children whose injuries were primarily in the genital area;
2. Type II: children who had experienced attempted or actual intercourse or other inappropriate genital contact with an adult;
3. Type III: children who had been inappropriately involved with an adult in other kinds of sexual activity (e.g. coerced into taking part in pornographic photography).

Four per cent of cases were categorised as type I, 69% as type II and 16% as type III. However about 10% of the cases in types II and III involved physical injury.

In those cases where sexual motives are important, we will need to distinguish between the indiscriminate use of children for sexual purposes because they are available and more easily coerced than adults and the specific sexual preference for children, so-called paedophilia.

When we turn to the relationship between child and offender we have to address the issue of incest, the special significance of the incest taboo and the repercussions that follow from sexual interaction between family members. We will find that in general the emotional and developmental consequences of child sexual abuse are more profound when a parent or parent-substitute is involved, or when the special dynamics of the family group become affected. Incest is a crucially important and complex issue and we must give it special consideration.

The prevalence of child sexual abuse

How common are sexual relationships between adults and children? Tables 13.4 and 13.5 show the ages of victims of indictable sexual offences. This age distribution is broadly similar to those found in other studies (Katz & Mazur 1979). However, as with adult rape, the large majority of sexual incidents involving children are probably not reported (see below). As will be seen from Tables 13.4 and 13.5, the ratio of offences against girls to those against boys is approximately 2:1, similar to that found in an earlier study by Gibbens & Prince (1963). It is possible that boys are less likely to report these childhood incidents. If so, that may be because they are more likely to participate actively or that, for other reasons, the incidents generate more guilt or stigma. There is evidence that girls are less likely to report incidents in which they have been actively involved, and less likely to report the more severe incidents, even if they had not consented (Katz & Mazur 1979).

In the Kinsey survey 24% of women reported prepubertal sexual experiences with post-pubertal males (systematic questions were not asked of their male subjects; Gebhard & Johnson 1979). In a survey of college students, Landis (1956) found 30% of the males and 35% of the females had had such experiences during childhood. Four more recent American studies show considerable discrepancies in prevalence rates. Finkelhor (1979), in a non-representative sample of university students in New England, found 19% of women and 9% of men reporting sexual abuse during their childhood. In a later more representative study of parents, asked by questionnaire about their own childhood, the figures were 15% of women and 6% of men (Finkelhor 1984).

In possibly the most methodologically sound study to date, Russell (1983; see p. 204) interviewed a probability sample of 930 married women. Using a broad definition of sexual abuse (i.e. including non-contact abuse such as genital exposure and verbal solicitation) 48% had had such experiences by the age of 14 and 54% by 18. For contact abuse, 12% had experienced at least one such experience involving a family member before the age of 14, and 16% before the age of 18. The percentages for extrafamilial abuse were 20 and 31% respectively. Thus, combining intra- and extrafamilial situations, 28% before the age of 14 and 38% before the age of 18 were affected. *Only 2% of intrafamilial and 6% of extrafamilial incidents were reported to the police.* In a further California study, Wyatt (1985) found 62% reporting some form of abuse before the age of 18, with 47% experiencing contact abuse.

In a survey of Dutch university students, 13% of males and 18% of females reported childhood experiences of sexual abuse (Brongersma 1979). In 1984 MORI (Market and Opinion Research International, unpublished data) carried out a survey of a probability sample of 2019 adults in Britain. The interviewer made the following definitional statement to each subject: 'A child (any one under 16 years) is sexually abused when another person, who is sexually mature, involves the child in any activity which the person expects to lead to their own sexual arousal. This might involve intercourse, touching, exposure of the sexual organs, showing pornographic material or talking about things in an erotic way'. The subject was then asked if he or she had had any such experience before the age of 16: 12% of women and 8% of men said 'yes'. Non-contact abuse was more common than the contact variety, especially for the females.

Wyatt & Peters (1986a,b) have considered the possible explanations for these very different prevalence rates and pointed out a number of definitional and procedural factors. They concluded that the use of face-to-face interviewing produced higher rates, though it is not entirely clear to what extent this increases the validity of the rates. As they point out, 'Many women . . . tend to have experiences that they do not define as abuse, due to their own attributions regarding victimisation or their own perceptions of the definitions of the type of experience appropriate to the study'. Presumably we must also assume that investigators might also vary in what they regard as abuse. Russell and Wyatt's figures were also slightly inflated by taking an upper age of 18 (compared with 17 in Finkelhor's studies) and by the inclusion of abuse by peers, though they only included such cases where the experience was unwanted.

Characteristics of the offenders

At least 90% of adults who sexually abuse children are men (Finkelhor 1982).

In the Kinsey study 75% of the adults were aged 20 or over, the large majority under 40. Nearly 70% of these men were strangers, 12% family members. By contrast, 75% of the incidents reported by Finkelhor (1980) involved an older person known to the child. It was less likely to be a family member in the case of boys. Russell's (1983) extrafamilial incidents involved strangers (15%), acquaintances (40%) and friends of the family (14%). In Wyatt's (1985) study 45% of incidents involved strangers, 17% family members (four incidents out of 305 involved the father). In the MORI survey in Britain, 13% of perpetrators were family members.

Offenders against children are a mixed group. Mentally handicapped men are not infrequently involved and psychotics, drunks and elderly men in the early stages of a dementing process occasionally so (Gebhard et al 1965). A proportion of them will be men or teenage boys who are relatively indiscriminate about their sexual partners. This would particularly apply to those involving girls aged 12 and above. As mentioned earlier, below the age of 12 (or 14 for boys), and more particularly before the age of puberty, the offender is more likely to be substantially older than the child. Most have a particular interest in children, the so-called paedophile, who will be considered further below. Close relatives may not be paedophiliac even when they abuse young children; we will consider this more closely when discussing incest.

Type of sexual activity involved

As is seen in Tables 13.4 and 13.5, the large majority of *reported* incidents in which physical contact with children occurs do not involve coitus or buggery. Of the indictable offences in 1973, 89% of those involving girls under 13 and 82% of boys under 14 were called 'indecent assault'. Similar proportions were reported by Gebhard et al (1965) who found that with girls the commonest activity was genital touching (52%) and with boys genital touching (45%) and oral–genital contact (38%). In the majority it was the man touching the child; in a small proportion, both took an active part. In Wyatt's (1985) study of females the commonest type of contact abuse was 'being fondled' (39% of incidents); 17% involved intercourse and 10% attempted intercourse. In the MORI survey the commonest incident was non-contact, mainly genital exposure (50% of females and 23% of males). Genital touching was more common for males (29%) than females (14%). As it is unusual for women to abuse children sexually it follows that most abuse of boys is homosexual (Finkelhor 1984).

Recently it has been suggested that buggery may be particularly common when small children are being abused, and that with small girls anal penetration is more likely than vaginal (Hobbs & Wynne 1986). This has led to emphasis on clinical examination of the anal sphincter which is causing much controversy at the present time. Hobbs & Wynne, however, stress the importance of the child's verbal history in combination with the physical examination.

The paedophiliac offender

What characterises the man who is sexually attracted to prepubertal children? Most of our evidence is based on studies of convicted offenders. Probably the majority of paedophiles are never convicted; they are either extremely cautious or they confine their attentions to those children who are clearly seeking such encounters. In one American study of practising paedophiles who were interviewed, only 1% had ever been arrested

(Rossman 1979). One should therefore be cautious in generalising from those who are convicted.

Paedophiles cover a broad age range. Those convicted tend to be older than other sex offenders. The median age at first conviction in the Kinsey Institute study was 34.5 years for heterosexual and 30.2 years for homosexual offenders (Gebhard et al 1965). The majority prefer either female or male children; a small proportion are interested in both boys and girls. The Paedophile Information Exchange (PIE), an organisation of British paedophiles, surveyed its members and found that they were most attracted to girls aged 8–11 and boys aged 11–15 (O'Carroll 1980). It has been pointed out that this coincides with the age when childhood sexuality is most noticeable. Girls in particular enter a sexually quiescent period after this late childhood phase of activity (see Chapter 3).

The majority of paedophiles marry at some stage. Gebhard et al (1965) found in their group that marital breakdown and re-marriage were common but more happy marriages were reported than in most other groups of offenders. Other studies, however, have emphasised the problems paedophiles have in establishing satisfactory adult relationships, possibly encouraging their resort to relationships with children (Mohr et al 1964; Pacht & Cowden 1974). A number of studies of the personalities of paedophiles have been reported but they are inconsistent in their findings, partly due to methodological weaknesses (Levin & Stava 1987).

Ingram (1979) interviewed 11 men who had been sexually involved with boys. They reported strikingly similar backgrounds, with poor relations with their mothers and detached or fearful relationships with their fathers. They had had unhappy childhoods, deprived of love and with unrewarding contacts with their peer groups. Ingram concluded that this facilitated their tendencies to love emotionally deprived children. In this particular study, nearly all sexual incidents involved men who were well known to the boys, more than 80% in the role of teacher or youth leader. Ingram emphasised the extent to which many of these men were generally fond of boys, devoting much of their time to the welfare of children. There is no doubt that some paedophiles are of this kind. O'Carroll (1980) gives further examples. But it is also possible that in some cases time is spent helping children in order to gain sexual access to them; paedophiles presumably vary in their moral scruples as do other groups.

Determinants of paedophilia

The one thing that paedophiles clearly have in common is their sexual attraction to children. In other respects, they are a heterogeneous group and once again we should allow for a variety of causative factors. Preference for children may not be exclusive, though most commonly paedophiles are either sexually disinterested in adults or unable to succeed in sexual relationships with them. In some cases, called by Gebhard and his colleagues the sociosexually underdeveloped, the man enters adulthood inexperienced, inept or threatened as far as sex with his own age group is concerned, and one can see that a child partner would be less threatening and hence a more attractive proposition.

In some instances, the paedophilia is a continuation of a childhood pattern that originally was successful; the paedophile sticks with the type of partner he had success with in the past, rather than developing more mature relationships. In some instances, the paedophile may have sustained unduly close relationships with his mother, which then make a sexual relationship with another woman too threatening (as in the case of Wilfred Johnson, described by Parker (1969)), or has married a woman with whom his relationship is more like that between child and parent than between two adults. But in general we must remain uncertain why paedophiliac preferences develop and become apparently fixed. As yet, no adequate aetiological explanation has been put forward that would account for more than a small proportion of the cases.

On considering the evidence summarised here, it is difficult to avoid the conclusion that in many cases the social reaction against the paedophile and the severity of the sentences imposed on him by the courts are out of proportion to the gravity of his offence. This is important for two reasons. First, because the offender may be treated unjustly and secondly because the impact of the offence on the child is likely to be seriously compounded by the furore that follows it. At the same time, it is difficult to view child–adult sexuality as desirable or even acceptable, in spite of the case put forward by paedophiles themselves (O'Carroll 1980) or others asserting the 'sexual rights of the child' (Constantine 1979). Sexual violence toward children should be avoided in the same way as other forms of violence. As we shall see in the next section sexual exploitation by family members has a special significance and the capacity for long-term harm to the child is considerable. Other types of sexual interaction are probably best seen as an undesirable nuisance, mainly because a child is being exploited by an adult for his own sexual ends, and betrayed in the process by someone who should be in a position of responsibility. The rights of children are frequently abused, but one important right is to feel confidence in the responsibility that adults show towards them. But for the most part we should be prepared to see the average paedophile as someone more to be pitied for his inability to sustain a rewarding adult relationship than to be reviled.

INCEST

The taboo against incest is so universal it has generated a great deal of debate and speculation. And yet we remain largely uncertain about its origins. With the current concern with child sexual abuse no doubt this debate will gain a fresh impetus.

The precise forms of kinships for which sexual activity is proscribed vary from culture to culture. The taboo against mother–son incest is more or less universal; with father–daughter and brother–sister relationships there are exceptions. The strength of the taboos and the sanctions associated with them also vary considerably across cultures (Fox 1967). In some instances royalty has been exempt to allow them to maintain the sanctity of royal blood. Ancient Egypt and the Inca aristocracy are well known examples from the past. Restrictions on sexual relationships beyond the nuclear family vary enormously, reflecting the extent to which rules of descent are matrilineal or patrilineal. It is important to distinguish between rules concerning incest and those govering marriage, or exogamy. If a relationship is deemed incestuous then it will not be considered marriageable. But a man, whilst not allowed to marry his grandmother, his father's, son's, grandfather's or grandson's wife, his wife's mother, daughter, grandmother or granddaughter, is not legally prohibited in our society from having sex with them (Honoré 1978).

The various theories that have been put forward to account for the incest taboo can be considered under two headings — social and biological. Levi-Strauss (1969) is one of the main proponents of social determination. He sees the incest taboo as an important step in the socialisation of the human primate by which he retains his 'own' (i.e. his daughters) as something to exchange with others, the primal basis of social structure. As Fox (1980) points out, Levi-Strauss's explanation is better suited to explain exogamy than incest avoidance. A man could presumably have sex with his daughter and still be in a position to 'exchange' her in his dealings with others. Implicit in this kind of theory is the assumption that taboos are necessary to control a behaviour which would otherwise be likely to occur. This view was central to Freud's theory. But the contrasting and more biological explanation was that put forward by Westermark in his A Short History of Marriage (Westermark 1926). He suggested that there was a marked lack of erotic feeling between people who lived closely together from childhood, leading to little or no inclination for incestuous behaviour. This view was attacked by Freud and Sir James Frazer in the 1920s and lost favour until recently, when two interesting sources of evidence emerged to support it (see p. 249): that children brought up together in Israeli kibbutzim are most unlikely to fall in love and marry one another (Shepher 1971) and the strange custom in Taiwan of marrying children to each other when they are as young as 3 years, a pattern associated with a high incidence of sexual difficulty and marital breakdown in adulthood (Wolf 1970). But why, it is often asked, is there a need for an incest taboo if there is no inclination to behave incestuously? As Westermark himself cogently argued in his rebuttal of Freud and Frazer's criticism, one does not only have laws forbidding behaviour that we are *all* inclined to commit. In other words there is no need for incest taboos for most of us but there is for some. But the issue is much more complex than that. Fox (1980) attempts to reconcile these two apparently conflicting theoretical models, i.e. the need to control behaviour by taboo and the lack of inclination towards such behaviour that results from childhood propinquity. He points out how cultures vary considerably in the degree of propinquity that exists between opposite-sex siblings during childhood. He describes some societies where the degree of segregation between brother and sister may actually mystify and hence enhance the erotic potential of the incestuous relationship — certainly very different to the typical kibbutzim experience of boys and girls. Other evidence of the varying degree of segregation of the sexes during childhood and adolescence was considered in Chapter 4. It should however be stressed, rather more than Fox did, that this argument relates to brother–sister, but rather less well to parent–child incest. It is not necessarily irrelevant, however. As we shall see, the likelihood of incest involving a stepfather is substantially greater than that involving a father, who will have lived in relatively close proximity with the child since the child's birth.

Perhaps the most important part of Fox's analysis is his consideration of the cross-species comparative evidence, particularly from primates. It is striking how little attention has been paid to the comparative evidence by those seeking explanations of the incest taboo. Levi-Strauss (1969) saw incest taboo, or more precisely exogamy, as one of the attributes that distinguish humans from other animals. 'The important point on which human marriage and animal mating differs is that man became the exogamous animal. The exogamic rule, that we should find mates outside one's own social unit, is at the basis of all human social organisation'. This assertion was obviously made in ignorance of animal behaviour. Bischof (1975) has reviewed the comparative evidence of incest avoidance and found it to be widespread, though manifested in a variety of ways, and possibly serving a variety of purposes.

As far as primates are concerned a distinction needs first to be made between the different social structures and mating strategies, i.e. the promiscuous, multi-male pattern (e.g. chimpanzee); polygamous (e.g. gorilla); monogamous (e.g. gibbon) and solitary (e.g. orang-utan). Incest avoidance can be observed in all of these situations. The monogamous pattern is of interest. The gibbon lives in family groups consisting of a monogamous parental pair and their young. But the group only survives one generation as the father drives the sons away when they reach maturity, and the mother the daughters. A similar pattern is seen in monogamous marmosets, though it is common for three or four sets of offspring to be retained within the family group. The onset of puberty may be delayed in such circumstances and those reaching reproductive maturity either leave or are driven away from the family group.

Fox (1980) points out that in all the various primate mating strategies, the established senior males aim to monopolise the females, and the young or unsuccessful males are excluded. With the baboon, which Fox suggests provides the best primate model for early hominid social groups, the powerful males each collect a harem of females, but move around together with the other families to form a troop. Obviously there are more females than males in these troops; the remaining males, the young and less powerful, remain on the fringe of the troop in all male groups. Occasionally, one of these males will be able to take over a harem from a ageing senior, or manage to start one on his own. Fox draws a parallel between this primate model and the primitive human system that Freud (1918) described in Totem and Taboo, emphasising the crucial significance of the competition between the older (father) male and the younger males in the all-male group. He proposes that the determinants of exogamy and the incest taboos evolved from this basis. This is an interesting idea, though it places the emphasis on the male–male rivalry. In the monogamous primate with its family group, we see female–female rivalry expressed by the mother driving the daughter away as soon as there is any evidence of father–daughter sexual interaction. Perhaps the incest taboo against mother–son sex, which is certainly the most universal in human societies, derives from the male–male rivalry model, whereas the taboo against father–daughter sex, which is less strong in many cultures, derives from the family group model. And perhaps the propinquity mechanism of Westermark is most relevant to sibling incest. This of course is all very speculative, but it is certainly appropriate to take the primate evidence into account.

The other biological mechanism that has often been cited is the genetic disadvantage of inbreeding (Austin 1980). Few authorities now see this as of crucial importance in explaining incest avoidance. Inbreeding can be genetically advantageous, as many animal breeders will tell you. The high nobility of the Incas is said to have been maintained by brother–sister matings for 14 generations without any deformity or impairment. In the presence of genetic defects, inbreeding obviously has disastrous consequences.

We will not pursue further this intriguing but complex theoretical discussion in our attempt to understand incest in modern society. There is however one further general point that needs to be made. The need for a taboo is more easily understood in situations where the child has reached or is approaching sexual maturity. Incestuous behaviour between adult and young child may be of a different order and requires different explanations.

Legal aspects of incest

In English law, a man commits incest if he has or attempts to have sexual intercourse (i.e. vaginal intercourse) with a female he knows to be his daughter, sister, half-sister, granddaughter or mother. If the female involved is over 16, she also commits an offence (Freeman 1979).

In Scotland, the law against incest dates from 1567 and the offence was punishable by death until 1887. In England and Wales, incest (between parent and child, brother and sister) has only been a criminal offence since 1908. In the past it was punished by the ecclesiastical courts. From the early or mid 19th century until the 1908 Act, it was probably dealth with as rape or unlawful sexual intercourse. Some legal systems today, such as the French, Dutch and Belgian, do not have a specific crime of incest (Freeman 1979).

The prevalence of incest

The incidence of incest cases known to the police is shown in Figure 13.4. The majority (65%) of cases involve girls aged 10 to 15 (see Table 13.4). The type of relationship is shown in Table 13.7. Almost half of the liaisons involving paternal incest in Table 13.7 lasted for a year and only a quarter consisted of isolated incidents. By contrast, the majority of the sibling cases were isolated incidents.

Table 13.7 Type of relationship in incest cases for 1973 (Walmsley & White 1979)

	Percentage of total convicted	Person convicted
Grandpaternal	1	1 grandfather
Paternal	72	91 fathers, 2 daughters
Sibling	24	30 brothers, 1 sister
Maternal	3	2 sons, 2 mothers
Total		124 males, 5 females

We get some idea of the prevalence of incestuous relationships, whether reported or not, from the surveys described previously. In Finkelhor's study (1980), whereas 75% of incidents involved an older person known to the child, in 6% it was the father or stepfather. Some 15% of females and 10% of males reported some type of sexual experience involving a sibling, most commonly genital touching and fondling. In Russell's (1983) study 44 (4.7%) of 930 women had an incestuous relationship with their fathers. For 27 it was the biological father, for 15 the stepfather, 1 the foster and 1 the adoptive father. A total of 4.9% had sexual involvement with an uncle, 2% with a brother, 0.9% (8 women) with a grandfather, 0.3% (3 women) with a sister and 1 woman with her mother. It is noteworthy that in terms of the seriousness of the abuse, the stepfathers were the worst offenders. In Wyatt's (1985) study, 4 incidents out of 305 involved the father.

Finkelhor (1980) estimated that some form of father–daughter sexual interaction might occur in about 1.5% of families, though coitus would seldom be involved. (It is important to distinguish between the legal definition of incest given above and the psychosocial meaning which emphasises the relationship rather than the precise sexual act involved.)

The incest offender

No clear picture of the characteristics of the incest offender emerges from the literature. Weinberg (1976) suggested three categories:

1. The endogamic man who confines his social and sexual interest within his family.
2. The indiscriminately promiscuous personality.
3. The paedophiliac, who may be interested in young children apart from his own.

He did not present any evidence of the relative frequency of these types. Gebhard et al (1965) drew some distinction between those who offended against children (i.e. under 12 years of age) and those against adults, usually their teenage daughters, aged 17–18. The first type was described as a 'rather ineffectual, non-aggressive dependent sort of man who drinks heavily, works sporadically and is preoccupied with sexual matters'. The other type was less preoccupied sexually and generally more inhibited. He was described as 'conservative, moralistic, restrained, religiously devout, traditional and uneducated'. He sounds comparable in some respects to the men in Weinberg's endogamic group.

The more recent literature on incest shows a striking contrast in the emphasis placed on the family. As Finkelhor (1982) points out, the recent increased awareness of child sexual abuse within the family has been largely the result of child protection agencies and the women's movement. The former have tended to emphasise the family unit, both as a cause of the problem and as something that should be kept together if at all possible. Those in the women's movement have tended to concentrate on the male perpetrator, seeing child sexual abuse as an extension of the sexual exploitation of women by men, and seeking the removal and usually punishment of the male offender. Two accounts exemplifying these two contrasting viewpoints are those of Porter (1984) and Ash (1984). Porter edited a working party report sponsored by the Ciba Foundation. This is very much based on the family approach and rather surprisingly, more attention is paid to the characteristics of the mother of the incest victim than of the father or perpetrator. Ash's account is very much in the feminist mould, and strongly criticises the tendency to blame the mother who, it is stated, can seldom be seen to hold any responsibility for what happened, the man always being the culprit. Neither view seems to me to be sufficiently balanced. Clearly the family is likely to be important. It is also of interest that women who have been sexually abused themselves during childhood are more likely to have children who are sexually abused.

Incest families studied have often been crisis-ridden and characterised by discord, lax sexual morality and illegitimate births. The sexual relationship of the parents is often unsatisfactory. The number of children tends to be higher than average and the mother is away from home more than usual, often because of ill health (Ash 1984).

Furniss (1985) has described two types of sexually abusive family. In one the sexual abuse serves to avoid open conflict between the parents (the conflict-avoiding family). The mother, it is suggested, sets the rules for emotional relationships and the pattern of communication about sexual and emotional matters. In the second type more open parental conflict exists; the mother provides little support to the children and a child is 'sacrificed' to stop the conflict leading to family breakdown (the conflict-regulating family). The emphasis placed on the mother in both these descriptions is noteworthy.

Victims of child sexual abuse — extrafamilial involvement

Numerous studies have shown that children who are sexually involved with adults have disturbed family backgrounds: broken homes, inadequate parents, child neglect, illegitimacy and generally poor relationships amongst family members (Katz & Mazur 1979). It is therefore widely believed that these factors predispose the child to sexual exploitation. It is unlikely to be as simple as that. Certainly children deprived of love, or otherwise emotionally insecure, may be attracted to the apparently (and sometimes genuinely) loving relationships that paedophiles offer them. Burton (1968) compared a group of 41 children who had been sexually involved with adults with a comparison group of their age mates. They were assessed approximately 2 years after the offence. They were mainly distinguished from their controls by their tendency to seek affection. This had apparently been commented on by their teachers, who were unaware of their histories, as well as being evident in the psychological test results. This could of course be a consequence of the experience, but alternatively may have contributed to the incident in the first place. Also children from disturbed backgrounds may be more prone to sexual 'acting out', with less parental supervision and more exposure to at-risk situations.

However, the emotional status and the family background may well have a bearing on which cases are reported. There is little doubt that the consequences of reporting these incidents to the police can have traumatic effects on the child, both because of the emotional impact of the legal procedure, and in those cases where the child was gaining something from the relationship, from the emotional confusion that results. It is therefore likely that in well integrated and supportive families, parents will protect their child from further trauma by not reporting the incident, particularly if the offender is not seen as vicious. The disturbed family will not only find it more difficult to cope with such a crisis without outside support, but may also project their own guilt in their reactions to the episode, and their determination to punish the offender at all costs.

Finkelhor (1980) assessed factors which might increase the likelihood of child sexual abuse. Several of these involved the family. They included:

1. Low income family.

2. Social isolation of the child.
3. Presence of a stepfather (though it was not necessarily the stepfather who abused).
4. Conservative 'family' values held by the father.
5. Little physical affection shown by the father.
6. Absent mother.
7. Detached mother.
8. Mother never finished high school.
9. Mother with punitive attitudes towards sexual matters.

Finkelhor combined these variables to form a sex abuse risk factor scale. In his subjects with none of these risk factors, sexual abuse was almost non-existent. If five or more factors were present, two-thirds of the subjects had suffered abuse. This is a potentially important approach, though these findings clearly require careful replication before they could form the basis for intervention.

What are the effects on the children of these extrafamilial incidents? The majority show some acute disturbance, expressed as anxiety, behavioural problems such as truancy, bed-wetting or sometimes depression. But a substantial minority, varying in size from study to study, seem relatively unaffected by the experience. In the Kinsey survey (Kinsey et al 1953) nearly 80% of women with experience of childhood abuse said they were upset or frightened at the time. 'A small proportion had been seriously disturbed, but in most instances the reported fright was nearer the level that children will show when they see insects, spiders or other objects against which they have been adversely conditioned'. There was only one clearcut case of serious injury amongst 4441 women interviewed. For about 10% the experience was to some extent positive (Kinsey et al 1953). Forcible rape, or other types of violence, are more likely to produce adverse reactions, though possibly less predictably or severely than is the case with adult rape victims (Katz & Mazur 1979). Disturbances in the child's family are common. The reactions of the parents, particularly the mother, may be crucial. 'When parental support was complete with loving and consistent concern, the child was most apt to recover' (Katz & Mazur 1979). However, it is also likely that in such families the vulnerability of the child was less to start with.

The question of consent in such cases is a highly controversial issue. It is of course reasonable to assume that consent of a child in no way reduces the culpability of the adult involved. But it does have an effect on sentencing and it may also be relevant to the longer-term effects on the child. In those cases which come before the courts, it is usually difficult to establish the extent to which the child consented, particularly when below the age of 10. Walmsley & White (1979) concluded that with victims of indecent assault, about one-fifth of girls aged 10 to 12, one-third of girls aged 13 to 15, about one-fifth of boys aged 10 to 13 and about two-fifths of boys aged 14 to 15 consented. In Gebhard et al's study (1965), 16% of the girls under 12 and 86% of girls aged 12 to 15 were said to be 'encouraging' to the offender, whilst the percentages for the boys were 52% for the under 12s and 70% for those aged 12 to 15. These figures were based on evidence in the records; the percentages were, needless to say, higher according to the offenders themselves. It is perfectly possible that a child could be encouraging yet end up being frightened or disturbed by the experience. But we should also accept the possibility that in a proportion of cases the child gains some emotional reward from the experience. As we shall see, this is probably less likely when the abuser is a family member.

Victims of incest and intrafamilial sexual abuse

The peculiar difficulties that follow sexual abuse of a child by a family member, and which place the child in a seemingly impossible position, have been well described by Summit (1983) and I will refer extensively to his paper. He uses the term 'child sexual abuse accommodation syndrome' to describe a reaction 'which allows for the immediate survival of the child within the family but which tends to isolate the child from eventual acceptance, credibility or empathy within the larger society'. There are five components to this syndrome:

1. *Secrecy*. The child, following abuse, is readily caught in a web of secrecy. 'You musn't tell anyone or . . .' and a variety of alarming consequences may be spelt out, including the perpetrator being sent to prison, the family breaking up, the mother being heartbroken etc. The need for secrecy makes it clear that what has happened is *bad*, whilst the maintenance of secrecy seems to be the only safe escape route to follow.
2. *Helplessness*. The need for secrecy plus the natural tendency for a child to be influenced by an adult in a position of authority results in a sense of helplessness and the likelihood of acquiescence to further and continuing sexual abuse. 'The child has no choice but to submit quietly and to keep the secret . . . The threat of loss of love and loss of family is more frightening to the child than any threat of violence'. The resulting feeling of having allowed the abuse to occur then leads to self-condemnation and self-hate.
3. *Entrapment and accommodation*. Once the child becomes entrapped in this helpless situation, accommodation to the continuing abuse may result in a variety of maladaptive or pathological patterns of survival which may lead to long-term behavioural and personality problems. These include pathological dependency, self-punishment, self-mutilation, 'selective restructuring of reality and multiple personalities'. It is difficult for a child to accept the conclusion that a parent is ruthless and self-centred — 'this is tantamount to abandonment'. The only acceptable conclusion for the child is to believe that she has provoked the painful encounter. The potential for distortion of reality and self reproach in such a situation is well described by Summit: 'She may fight with both

parents but her greatest rage is likely to focus on her mother whom she blames for driving the father into her bed'. A child in these circumstances is given the power to destroy the family and hence the responsibility for holding it together — a demand which reinforces the sense of entrapment.

4. *Delayed, conflicted and unconvincing disclosure*. Disclosure either doesn't occur at all or often at a much later date when the child is locked in destructive battle with one or other parent which results from the chronic tension and unresolved resentment. Frequently therefore the child makes the disclosure at the time when she is least likely to be believed. According to Summit, most mothers are unaware of ongoing sexual abuse in the family. Faced with the child's disclosure there is an understandable tendency in many mothers to believe the father — 'to accept the alternative means annihilation of the family and a large piece of her own identity'.

5. *Retraction*. 'Whatever a child says about sexual abuse, she is likely to reverse it. . . In the chaotic aftermath of disclosure the child discovers that the threats underlying the secrecy are true'. The split in the family looms large, she may be disowned by other family members — and perhaps most unjust of all, she is the one most likely to be removed from the home, the father left unscathed because of the difficulties of mounting sufficient evidence against him. Summit has cogently warned of the dangers of our current scene in which discovery and disclosure are facilitated but the protection of the child against 'the secondary assaults of an inconsistent intervention system' is lacking. The rejection of the child's pleas for help may be the most traumatic aspect of the whole experience. It is not surprising that faced with the cataclysmic consequences of disclosure the child ends up retracting her complaint.

Summit's account is a persuasive description of the helplessness of the child's situation and the tendency for the adult world to collude in putting the child in the wrong at a time when help and understanding are urgently required. Perhaps we should be cautious about accepting this analysis too uncritically. But the case for taking Summit's analysis very seriously is strong, at least until or unless we have good evidence for not doing so. If injustice is to be avoided the priority should surely be with the child.

We should not however be unduly alarmist about the consequences of intrafamilial sexual abuse of a child. It is probable that many individuals have such experiences and escape significant long-term harm. Frenken (1987) has drawn a comparison between incest victims who seek professional help and those uncovered in community surveys such as Russell's (1983). Those seeking help are likely to have experienced much more frequent abuse over a longer period of time, for it to have started before they were 8 years old, to have occurred in families where there was general emotional neglect and where in addition to the sexual abuse the mother used the victim for her own material and emotional needs. It is important, as Frenken pointed out, not to generalise from cases seen in a clinical context to all those incidents that occur in the community. But a relatively high incidence of incest has been found in studies of delinquent girls and in one study 75% of prostitutes had been the victims of incest (Katz & Mazur 1979).

There are certainly no grounds for complacency. All the evidence points to the uncovering of a problem of major proportions, leaving us with the need to explain what has been happening. Finkelhor (1982) has suggested a number of factors that might contribute to this apparent epidemic. Divorce and re-marriage may be having both good and bad effects. Good, if children can escape from a chronically tense family situation in which abuse may be more likely, but bad if this leads to emotional neglect and social isolation. There is also the added factor of the stepfather who may enter a family group which includes girls close to puberty or adolescence and where there is not the safeguard of Westermark's propinquity mechanism that operates when the father has lived with the daughter since her birth. The erosion of traditional sexual norms has to be taken into account, and the recent increase in the viewing of pornographic videos in the home may turn out to be of importance. Finkelhor wonders whether the higher expectations of sexual relationships that women now have may be threatening to some men, who seek reassurance with less threatening children. He asks why child sexual abuse is largely perpetrated by men, and suggests that men may be more inclined to use sex as a means of gaining affection, and of bolstering their gender identity. He also makes the interesting suggestion that a child is a less discrepant sexual object for a man than for a woman.

But it is also probable that we are seeing an epidemic of disclosure by people who previously would have carried their secret with them to the grave. If we accept Summit's analysis it is not difficult to see how many people, after long periods of non-disclosure, may be permitted to disclose by their awareness from the media of the large number of others who have gone through the same type of experience.

It has been suggested recently that the law of incest should be changed. The National Council for Civil Liberties (NCCL 1976), in their evidence to the Criminal Law Revision Committee (CLRC), recommended that the crime of incest should be abolished. They believed the law as it governs assault and intercourse with minors would provide adequate protection, as is the case in some other countries in Europe. The British Medical Association and Royal College of Psychiatrists, on the other hand, advise maintaining the legal status quo on the grounds of greater genetic risks associated with incest (CLRC 1980). The CLRC discussed the various arguments in their report but found themselves divided, principally on whether to recommend a minimum age of say 18 or even 21, above which incest would not be a criminal offence (CLRC 1980). I hold the view, argued elsewhere (Bancroft 1978) that the existing law is justified as a legal reinforcement of the social taboo against incest. This taboo, in my view, is important principally in order to ensure a family environment in which childhood and adolescent sexuality can be expressed as an important part of sexual development, without being exploited. A parallel can be drawn with the taboo against doctor–patient sex; this taboo, backed up with professional if not legal sanctions, enhances the security of the professional relationship and facilitates the expression of sexual feelings and anxieties which may be necessary for therapeutic benefit. Children in the family should be protected in this similar but special way — hence the importance of the concept of incest.

However, the legal process that follows the breaking of this law may be inappropriate. In England and Wales, the Director of Public Prosecutions has to give his consent to any prosecution for incest and this may be a sufficient safeguard. But consideration should be given to providing some alternative form of sanction that would give social agencies the authority they need in dealing with such families whilst avoiding as far as possible the destructive effect of the usual legal process on the family and its individual members.

INDECENT EXPOSURE AND EXHIBITIONISM

Although indecent exposure is widely recognised throughout Europe, Britain is the only country to allocate this behaviour to a separate offence category. Most countries include it under some broad heading, such as offences against public morality. Comparative statistics are therefore difficult. There is reason to believe, however, that this behaviour is uncommon outside western Europe and the USA, and particularly uncommon in African countries (Rooth 1973b).

The number of convictions for indecent exposure for 3 separate years in England and Wales are shown in Table 13.2. Rooth (1972) has examined the conviction rates up to 1969 in more detail. Since 1948, there was a gradual upward trend, most marked between 1954 and 1964. The numbers in different age groups over this time period are shown in Table 13.8. The large majority of offenders are aged over 21 but the number of convictions in this age group has changed little in proportional terms, whereas the incidence in males aged 21 and under has more than doubled. Rooth links this to the general increase in juvenile delinquency over this period.

Gebhard et al (1965) found an early onset of the behaviour in most of

Table 13.8 Mean number of convictions for indecent exposure per year by age (Rooth 1972)

	14–17	17–21	21+	Total (over 14)
1948–1957	126 (6%)	185 (8%)	1887 (86%)	2198 (100%)
1960–1969	233 (9%)	356 (14%)	1953 (77%)	2542 (100%)
1970	253 (9%)	501 (18%)	2085 (73%)	2839 (100%)

their subjects. The majority of indecent exposers are only charged once; the court appearance seems to have a strong deterrent effect. However, the chance of re-conviction increases markedly with a second conviction, particularly for men previously convicted for non-sexual offences. In the Cambridge study (Radzinowicz 1957) the overall recidivism rate was 18.6% over 4 years. Forty per cent of re-convictions occurred within the first year after conviction. Convictions tend to become less frequent after the age of 40 (Rooth 1971).

Radzinowicz (1957) estimated that at least 80% of people convicted of indecent exposures are exhibitionists, i.e. people for whom genital display to members of the opposite sex is an end in itself. The remainder have a variety of other reasons for exposing themselves. Gebhard et al (1965) found that after the exhibitionist, the commonest offenders were those who exposed themselves when drunk for no very clear reason, except possibly disorganised solicitation, drunken humour or an expression of hostility. These men usually deny that they intended to expose. The third most common type was the mentally defective who exposes in the belief or hope that the female will be sexually excited; it is thus a form of sexual approach or solicitation.

The exhibitionist group is difficult to classify further (Rooth 1971). However, there are a number of variables which are probably crucial in understanding the different types of exhibitionism:

1. *The age of the victim.* A minority of exhibitionists expose persistently to prepubertal girls and in some of them this behaviour may lead on eventually to more direct sexual contact with children (Rooth 1973a). The commonest age of victim is at, or around, puberty.
2. *The nature of the act.* The exposure may be clearly sexual, associated with an erect penis, sexual excitement and masturbation either during the exposure or shortly afterwards. In some cases, the penis is flaccid and there is no obvious sexual arousal. The reaction of the female is often important and an exhibitionist may go on exposing until he produces the desired response. Rooth (1971) describes a typical example of an ideal exposure as 'one of dominance and mastery. The exhibitionist, usually timid and unassertive with women, suddenly challenges one with his penis, briefly occupies her full attention and conjures up in her some powerful emotion such as fear and disgust, or sexual curiosity and arousal. . . He experiences a moment of intense involvement in a situation in which he is in control. The reaction that he most dislikes is indifference'.
3. *The frequency of exposing behaviour.* In some exhibitionists, urges to expose occur occasionally, possibly at times of crisis or emotional distress. In between these episodes, exposure holds no particular appeal. For others, the idea of exposing is always sexually stimulating and may feature in masturbation fantasies. Such men experience the urge to

expose frequently. For them the behaviour has become a well established form of sexual stimulation which they may find difficult to control.

4. *Risk-taking.* Some exhibitionists are careful to avoid being caught or recognised. Others appear to behave in a way to *ensure* that they are caught. They may, for example, repeatedly expose from their car, so that their car registration number leads readily to their arrest.

Exhibitionists show a fairly normal range of intelligence and social class, though there is some evidence that they are underachievers. Although Rooth (1971) gives a vivid description of the personality and family background of exhibitionists, his comments are mainly based on clinical impression.

More systematic studies of the psychopathology and personality of this group generally find them within the normal range, though there is some suggestion that there may be two types — those who expose in response to stress, and those for whom it is a persistent, compulsive pattern of behaviour (Levin & Stava 1987).

The determinants of exhibitionism

Of the various common types of sexual offence, exhibitionism is probably the most difficult to understand. Once again, we are faced with the problem of distinguishing between sexual and non-sexual determinants. In certain circumstances, genital display does have a simple sexual significance. It is the most common form of sexual interaction amongst children (see Chapter 2) and may precede sexual activity between adults. With the exception of exposure by the mentally handicapped, the characteristics and circumstances of most of these acts do not suggest that they are aimed at establishing further sexual contact with the 'victim'. The theme of mastery and insult, which is much more noticeable, suggests that this is genital display as an expression of hostility. Such display is common amongst many species of primates, especially the males. It may therefore represent a primitive form of communication, though it remains a mystery why it should be expressed in a small proportion of men in this somewhat compulsive fashion.

As with sexual assault, the picture is further complicated by the sexualisation of the behaviour that occurs in a proportion of cases. Whether this is secondary conditioning of a sexual response to a behaviour which was initially non-sexual in its origins, or whether the act was primarily sexual, is not clear. But when the sexualisation is established then the behaviour is likely to be more persistent.

Other secondary determinants stem from the social consequences of the act. Not only is the offender likely to be punished, but his wife and family will probably feel humiliated. In many cases, one is struck by the apparent need of the exhibitionist to provoke these reactions. In such cases, one wonders to what extent the behaviour is reinforced by its being criminalised. If exhibitionism was no longer regarded as an offence, would that particular variety be more or less likely to occur? It will be interesting to see what happens in those countries such as Denmark where the behaviour has been decriminalised.

Certainly for the vast majority of exhibitionists, their behaviour should be seen as harmless, if unseemly and transiently unpleasant for the 'victim'. A substantial number of women must have witnessed such acts. Gittelson et al (1978) found that 44% of a group of nurses had had this experience, usually in their early teens. Though their initial reactions were often unpleasant, any continuing reaction seemed to be unusual.

Voyeurism. As an offence, voyeurism does not have a special category, but comes under the heading of 'breach of the peace', or if a number of victims are involved, 'being a public nuisance'. Hence the statistics of this type of offence are difficult to come by. Voyeurism, or scopophilia as it is sometimes called, is of theoretical interest beyond its forensic implications. First, there is a tendency in most people to look at sexually interesting scenes. In some, looking is preferred to actually participating, presumably because real contact is too threatening for one reason or another. This voyeuristic element is sometimes revealed in people's fantasies, in which they look at other people rather than participate themselves. This is often an important clue to their basic sexual problem. It has been suggested that as voyeurism is the opposite of exhibitionism, the two behaviours usually coexist (Rosen 1979) but there is no evidence to support this view.

Unfortunately, there is very little information about the characteristics of voyeurs, or 'peeping toms' as the offenders are often called. Gebhard et al (1965) interviewed a series of 56 'peepers' in their study of sex offenders. The average age at first conviction for this offence was 23.8 years. Relatively few were married, compared with other types of offender. Perhaps most important was the tendency for many of them to be sociosexually under-developed, having had less experience than is usual for their age, being shy with females and having marked feelings of inferiority.

Typically the voyeur peeps at a stranger, usually from outside the building. Voyeurs normally take care not to be seen. Occasionally they enter a building in order to peep, or alternatively they peep in the course of pursuing some other crime, such as burglary. Occasionally they draw attention to themselves, e.g. by tapping on the window. Gebhard and his colleagues believe that it is the peeper who enters buildings and draws attention to himself who is most likely to progress from peeping to sexual assault. But for the majority, assault is unlikely.

The most obvious explanation for this type of behaviour is that it provides a form of sexual stimulus without the threat of sexual contact or rejection. The peeper usually masturbates whilst peeping, and is likely to be easily aroused by looking at women. Hence the pattern becomes sexualised. It can thus be seen as an extension of the general tendency to look in those who are too frightened to participate. But other factors are presumably involved. The risk and its associated excitement may be a further incentive. For those who draw attention to themselves, the fear that their behaviour induces in the victim may indicate that expression of hostility or, as with the exhibitionist, the momentary feeling of power may be a determinant. In this respect, peeping has something in common with the obscene telephone call, an exploitation of modern technology which is probably on the increase. Whereas the sexuality of the telephone call may be a sufficient determinant in some cases, the hostile and sadistic element seems common and may be a further example of the expression of 'power through sex' that has recurred throughout this chapter.

HOMOSEXUAL OFFENCES

We have already stressed that homosexual offences are predominantly consensual and rarely involve violence. For the most part, the law is concerned with discouraging homosexual behaviour rather than protecting the individuals involved in it. Although below the age of 16, consent is regarded as irrelevant and any homosexual activity is considered an assault, we have the additional proscription of any homosexual behaviour involving males less than 21 years of age. The usual justification for this is that it affords protection for young males at what may be regarded as a crucial stage of their sexual development between 16 and 21. The Criminal Law Revision Committee (CLRC 1980), in their report, recommended that the minimum age for male homosexual acts should be 18 'in order to protect those young men between 16 and 18 whose sexual orientation has not yet become firmly settled'. They were also of the opinion that there was no comparable group of girls between 16 and 18 needing protection in this way.

Even if we accept that the active discouragement of homosexual development is desirable, the use of the law in this way is in my view based on a very doubtful assumption about sexual development and its determinants. It would seem most unlikely that for this age group, when sexual interest and arousability are probably close to maximum, the advantages of legal proscription would outweigh the disadvantages to sexual development. For those who have no doubts about their heterosexual preferences, the legal protection is not required. For those who do, the further anxiety and guilt engendered by the law are more likely to result in unhappy homosexuality than happy heterosexuality (see Chapter 2 for further discussion of the development of sexual preferences).

But apart from the legal consequences of these anomalies of the age of consent, we also have to consider homosexual acts that are offences because they occur in public. Here, there are two rather different aspects to consider: first, the fact that the law discriminates against the homosexual act in various ways, e.g. using a more restricted definition of privacy, a wider meaning of importuning and more restrictions against procuring than is the case with heterosexuality; secondly, as has been discussed repeatedly in this chapter, sexual offences may not simply be determined by sexual needs. In spite of the more restrictive law against homosexuality, it is still very much a small minority of homosexual acts that come to the attention of the police. It thus remains of interest why some people get caught, whilst the majority do not.

The depersonalisation of much of male homosexuality is one factor. There has been a degree of casual, impersonal sexual contact far greater than that in the heterosexual world (outside prostitution). Such contacts are often sought in non-private but anonymous places such as public toilets. In some areas, particularly outside large cities, such places may be the only contact points known to the homosexual. But for some, such places allow them to retain anonymity either for fear of public disclosure or fear of personal intimacy. If such men were prepared to seek their partners in established homosexual settings (e.g. gay clubs or discos) they would run much less risk of trouble with the law, but would be much more likely to be identified as gay. This may be particularly important for those who are trying to maintain a heterosexual front or marriage. Humphreys (1970), in his study of men frequenting public lavatories, found that a high proportion of them were married. It is probably this aspect of homosexual behaviour which will show the most dramatic changes as a result of the AIDS epidemic, and it would not be surprising if this was reflected in a reduction in the number of offences in this category.

An additional factor is the added excitement that comes from taking risks. Whether this incentive is more likely in homosexuals than heterosexuals is difficult to say, but it does appear to be a factor amongst some homosexual offenders. In Schofield's study (1965) in which men imprisoned for homosexual offences were compared with homosexual psychiatric patients and normal homosexuals, half of the offender group stated that they gained an extra thrill from knowing that they were breaking the law. This is probably linked with a more general tendency to criminal behaviour. Nearly half of the men in Schofield's study convicted for importuning or homosexual acts in public places also had convictions for non-sexual offences. This subgroup therefore shows some of the general anti-social tendencies together with evidence of disturbed backgrounds and relative socioeconomic deprivation found in other sex offender groups. For the remainder, they are rather the victims of a discriminatory legal system.

A further factor influencing who gets convicted is the attitude of the police. We have already mentioned the substantial increase in the number of convictions for gross indecency between adult males which followed the change in the law and which probably reflected a greater tendency for the police to make arrests or to press charges. Apart from this, there is reason to believe that certain types of homosexuals are more likely to be arrested, in particular those who show evidence of effeminacy or patterns of behaviour or dress identified as homosexual (Gebhard et al 1965; Schofield 1965).

Gebhard and his colleagues made the interesting point that it is the male who provides sexual stimulation for other males who is most likely to be arrested. The man who takes the active role in anal intercourse or who is the recipient of oral stimulation may well be released with a severe caution. The man who brings another man to orgasm is considered the 'real' homosexual. In a similar way, many men participating in a homosexual act do not regard themselves as really homosexual because they do not attempt to bring the other man to orgasm. The beneficiary in such cases is seen as more of a sexual opportunist. This attitude is probably widespread, reflecting the particular rejection of the effeminate homosexual mentioned in Chapter 6. It is also reminiscent of attitudes in ancient times when medical writers were more likely to regard the person who persistently took the passive role in anal intercourse as pathological, the active partner as debauched (von Schrenck-Notzing 1895).

As, in the majority of homosexual acts, stimulation is reciprocated, the choice of person to arrest may depend on the moment when the police officer intervenes. On the other hand, for the man who is clearly labelled as homosexual and effeminate by the police, the process of arrest may involve minimum evidence of importuning. Entrapment of such individuals by police officers masquerading as homosexuals is far from unusual. In Gebhard's series, one-fifth of the men were involved in unequivocal entrapment.

Amongst those who are charged with homosexual acts in relatively private places, there is a notable tendency to confess or to plead guilty. In Gebhard's series, more than three-quarters confessed fully. Schofield describes a number of cases where confessions were given with surprising and often ill-judged readiness. In many cases, this may reflect a lack of understanding of one's legal rights. In others it may stem from a desire to minimise publicity. But in some of these men, there may be a degree of guilt which encourages them to be caught and accept punishment.

HELPING THE VICTIMS OF SEXUAL OFFENCES

THE VICTIM OF RAPE

Rape and other forms of sexual assault are often life-threatening incidents during which aggression, humiliation, sexual abuse and frequently physical trauma and pain have been experienced. The immediate reaction to rape is therefore a form of post-traumatic crisis, sharing many features in common with other forms of crisis, but having in addition some characteristics of its own. Burgess & Holmstrom (1974) called this the 'rape trauma syndrome'.

The victim of rape is likely to require help at three stages: firstly, immediately following the rape; secondly, in the aftermath, during the next few days and weeks, and thirdly, coping with long-term consequences.

Immediately following the rape

Two types of support are required at this stage. Various procedures need to be gone through once the rape has been reported to the police, and are more to do with investigating the offence and finding the offender than with helping the victim. As discussed earlier, these procedures can be handled very insensitively by police and police doctors, adding substantially to the trauma. The victim clearly needs support whilst going through these procedures, and various ways in which the police could help were considered earlier and have been described by Chambers & Millar (1983). A chapter by O'Reilly (1984), who for many years led the Sex Crimes Analysis Unit in New York City, should be required reading for any police officer involved with rape victims. It is an admirable combination of compassion and common sense, with an understanding of the difficulties the police have to face in these circumstances.

The physical examination is a crucial part of the procedure, and whilst it is of some relevance to the victim's management, it is largely determined by the need for evidence. The doctor involved has considerable scope for making this part of the process more or less traumatic. A useful account of how to deal with the examination together with a description of the other practical procedures which are more or less obligatory (e.g. collecting specimens, blood tests for pregnancy, sexually transmitted disease, and prophylactic treatment for sexually transmitted infections) is given by Silverman & Apfel (1983).

Rape Crisis Centres often provide experienced women to accompany the victim to the police station or hospital to support her through this phase.

The aftermath

In helping the victim to cope with the aftermath of rape the general principles of crisis intervention apply. These have been described in detail elsewhere (Greenwood & Bancroft 1988) and will only be outlined here. Intervention may involve 'intensive care', when the person is so distressed or shocked that she is not able to look after herself, and for a short time at least others have to take over the responsibilities of her day-to-day living. A judgement whether this takeover of responsibility is necessary has to be made in each case. Implementing 'intensive care' usually means someone remaining with the victim until she has started to settle down. This type of care can be provided in hospital but more often it is arranged in the home of the victim, relative or friend. At this stage the woman may be in a state of mute shock, in which case some effort should be made to initiate more normal communication. Alternatively she may be uncontrollably agitated or distressed. The principal objective of intervention in such circumstances is to help her return to a less disorganised emotional state in which she can start to look usefully at what had happened, and also to ensure that she obtains a reasonable amount of sleep. In crisis states, lack of sleep simply adds to the individual's decompensation and inability to cope. Once the initial shock phase is beginning to pass, intervention can move into crisis counselling. The objectives are to deal appropriately with the emotional reaction and eventually, when the emotional state allows, to adopt problem-solving strategies to enable her to reorganise and re-enter normal living.

The crisis precipitated by rape is close to that produced by bereavement or loss (Hopkins & Thompson 1984), and once the initial shock phase is passed, the proper working through or mourning of this loss is a crucial part of recovery which can be greatly aided by sensitive counselling. As with other forms of loss there is a predictable sequence of reactions. After the shock, already described, comes denial, anger and guilt. Denial often shows itself as an assumption that the victim has got over the rape and is back to normal. Anger is usually an understandable fury towards the assailant, and sometimes at others. Guilt often shows itself as self-blame for having allowed the incident to happen. Each of these reactions must be acknowledged and dealt with.

The principal losses following rape are of trust (e.g. no longer able to trust men), freedom (no longer able to go out or stay at home alone) and, possibly most important, of identity (I am no longer the person I was). There is often a sense of being 'spoiled' by the rape, of no longer being as attractive or acceptable as a person or as an appropriate recipient of other people's love or affection. Often the woman feels that the incident has made her disgusting, so much so that she fears that the doctor who examines her will be offended by her defiled body. (This fear is not always ill-founded, as partners or spouses not infrequently reject someone who has been raped; see p. 680.)

The counsellor has several important tasks — firstly, to deal with the emotional reaction and sense of loss. As with other forms of bereavement, there is a crucial need for the victim to share her feelings with someone who can empathise. As with bereavement, relatives and friends often find this difficult to do, taking the view that 'the less said about it the better', which is usually their way of dealing with their own difficulties. In addition to sharing, acknowledging and validating the emotional experience, the counsellor can positively affirm various aspects of the victim's behaviour at the time of the rape — commending her for how she coped, how sensible or brave she was etc. (Silverman & Apfel 1983). The victim's assumptions about her culpability should be repeatedly and consistently challenged and resisted, the counsellor making it absolutely clear that there was no possible justification or excuse for the behaviour of the assailant. It is often necessary to consider how the victim should best deal with her anger. The inability to express her fury to the rapist can be intensely frustrating.

Although in the initial stages it is the post-traumatic aspect which is most important, the sexual implications of the assault should not be ignored. A high proportion of victims develop sexual problems following rape, and at an appropriate stage the sexual feelings and anxieties of the victim should be explored (Becker et al 1986).

A further important role for the counsellor is to work with the partner or family of the victim. They may be not only affected by feelings of guilt for having allowed it to happen, but also influenced by the common myths and prejudices surrounding rape. These can lead to negative feelings towards the victim, as already mentioned. Silverman & Apfel (1983) stress the importance of not being judgemental in such circumstances, but rather spending time with the relatives, apart from the victim, to help them come to terms with these feelings.

The counsellor should also be on the look-out for other post-rape problems which may require specialised help. Depression is a common feature and may only become apparent some time after the rape. The incident may bring to the surface pre-existing problems in the family or marriage which then require help in their own right.

Long-term consequences

It is not unusual for victims to experience adverse reactions years after the assault. Often this is because they did not adequately work through their feelings at the time (sometimes they told no one about it at the time). The unresolved feelings are then reactivated by some subsequent event — it may be the rape of a friend. Some delayed 'mourning' may then be required.

THE CHILD VICTIM OF SEXUAL ABUSE IN THE FAMILY

There are many parallels between the needs and problems of the adult rape victim and the child who has been sexually abused by an adult. In both, the initial disclosure is made much more difficult and traumatic by the need to establish evidence of legal significance. Whereas the interests of the allegedly abused child are acknowledged as having priority, there are nevertheless statutory requirements for involvement of the police, which do not apply in rape cases, as well as the need to protect other children who may become victims if the offender is not apprehended.

One point that has emerged from the current crisis over child sexual abuse in Britain is that there is widespread uncertainty and disagreement about how one should proceed. This is most obvious when identifying the existence of sexual abuse in the very young. Talking to young children about such highly charged topics is a very difficult task. Play techniques, which have been developed by child psychologists and psychiatrists for general use, are helpful. Recently, anatomically correct dolls have become available for the specific purpose of assessing the possibility of sexual abuse. They appear to be useful but there is a need for caution. It is one thing to use such projective techniques to aid clinical assessment; it is quite another matter to use evidence from such procedures in a court of law. Boat

& Everson (1987) videotaped 224 supposedly non-abused children playing with anatomically correct dolls in a standardised 'doll interview'. About 10% of these children used the dolls in sexually suggestive ways which might have been taken to indicate evidence of sexual abuse by other workers. Thus, although such responses are uncommon, and may be significant in a particular case, they cannot be taken as sufficient evidence that abuse has occurred.

Once sexual abuse has been established or suspected, the style of intervention varies according to the nature of the abuse. When children have been abused by strangers, there is a particular need to work with the family, as the reactions of family members, especially parents, may be important in determining whether the child suffers long-term consequences. The parents should be helped to deal with the child in a supportive way, encouraging open discussion of what happened rather than maintaining a collusive silence which serves to reinforce the 'badness' of what happened. Such incidents provide an opportunity for parents to have more open discussions of sexual matters which help to place the abuse incident into perspective whilst also having a generally beneficial educational effect.

When abuse involves an acquaintance, and even more a family member, intervention becomes much more problematic. There is likely to be a need for individual support for the child. It is of paramount importance to ensure that the child has *someone* who believes the story and who repeatedly affirms the child's fundamental innocence (whatever the circumstances) in a consistent fashion. It is not always possible to achieve that, especially in those cases where the abuse is denied by the adult, there is no corroborative evidence and the family closes ranks to prevent contact with the child. Clearly there is also likely to be a need for counselling and support for the parents (and for the perpetrator — see below). Many workers advocate family therapy and report success in keeping many families together which might otherwise disintegrate in such circumstances (e.g. Giarretto 1977). The Ciba working party on the subject (Porter 1984) made recommendations for family involvement, as well as guidelines for general management of such cases, based on the work of the NSPCC Special Unit and Family Centre in Northamptonshire.

It is probably fair to say, however, that this whole area of intervention is undergoing widespread and intense scrutiny and that (hopefully by the time the next edition of this book is due) a much clearer and less controversial picture of intervention will emerge.

HELPING THE ADULT WHO WAS SEXUALLY ABUSED DURING CHILDHOOD

This problem is presenting itself with increasing frequency to sex therapists and counsellors in a variety of settings. Given that many such subjects have suffered long-term effects because the problem was inadequately dealt with during childhood, or not dealt with at all, there is a commonsense assumption that one should belatedly try to work through the processes that should have been worked through years before. But it is not always clear how best to proceed. Whilst there seems to be no grounds for doubting the stories given by such adults, it is not always clear to what extent the childhood experience needs to be dealt with intensively, or whether it is being used as an alternative explanation for current problems which need attention. There is a need for systematic studies of such cases to give us more guidance about treatment.

The use of groups

The methods of intervention described so far have involved individual or family counselling methods. Groups are also being used widely, in particular for women who have been raped or who were sexually abused during childhood (e.g. Tsai & Wagner 1978). There are obvious advantages to the group format in this context; it can be particularly helpful to have a number of women with similar experiences who can share their feelings and validate each other's reactions. Once again we have little evidence of the efficacy of such groups, and of the possible pitfalls, and what sort of leadership is required, etc. But it is likely that such groups will provide the mainstay of support for most types of adult victims. Attempts are also being made to provide groups for the offenders (see below).

THE MANAGEMENT OF SEX OFFENDERS

There is little doubt that the most effective method of discouraging sexual offences is the threat of legal sanctions. The large majority of sex offenders are not re-convicted. There is nevertheless a small minority of recidivists who may present considerable problems both to themselves and to society. It is an unfortunate fact that the sex offender who is most likely to benefit from psychological treatment or counselling is also the one who is effectively controlled by the law. The recidivist usually presents a formidable treatment problem.

In addition, there is a major ethical problem involved in the treatment of sex offenders. It is essential, from the ethical point of view, to distinguish between social control, which is control of the offender for the benefit of society, and treatment aimed at helping the offender. The normal methods of social control, such as custodial sentences, are subject to the normal rigors of the legal process and are consequently not so problematic. There are, however, other methods of controlling behaviour, in particular the use of drugs and psychosurgery, which because of their medical connotations are used without the full protection of the legal process and are hence open to abuse.

Drugs that lower sexual drive can be used as part of genuine medical treatment and do have a place in that respect. But their use in the management of offenders, particularly those in custody, raises serious problems. In such circumstances, it is difficult, if not impossible, to ensure consent free from coercion. The offender may end up receiving social control without the safeguards that accompany the usual legal sanctions, justified on the grounds that it is 'medical treatment' and in the offender's own interest. Such use would be creating a most dangerous precedent. Quite apart from the rights of the sex offender, one can see how drugs could eventually be used for other types of offence, e.g. to control aggressive behaviour — the thin end of a particularly worrying medicopolitical wedge.

I hold the view very strongly that if such methods are to be used, they should only be used under the public scrutiny of the court, and not according to the personal judgement of a forensic physician or psychiatrist. Some attempt to safeguard against such a development was introduced in the 1983 Mental Health Acts, where, under Section 57, the administration of libido-reducing hormone preparations by means of surgical implant not only must receive formal consent of the offender but also the concurring opinion of a member of the Mental Health Act Commission.

With this major qualification about their use, let us therefore consider the effects of such drugs as well as psychosurgery before passing on to psychological methods of treatment and counselling.

Pharmacological reduction of sexual interest

In Chapter 2, we discussed the evidence for hormonal and biochemical determinants of human sexuality and concluded that sexual appetite or interest was androgen-dependent in the majority of males, whereas for other aspects of sexuality, such as erectile reponse, the role of androgens is less certain. It is thus feasible that unwanted sexual drive can be controlled by interfering with its hormonal basis. Whether such an approach is useful in managing the sex offender obviously depends on the extent to which his criminal behaviour is determined by his sexual drive. As we have seen throughout this chapter, this is not a straightforward matter. But in a proportion of cases, such an approach is likely to be effective.

Oestrogens have been used for this purpose for more than 25 years (Scott 1964). The precise mechanism of action has not been established but is probably a combination of an anti-gonadotrophic effect resulting in a reduction of circulating androgen levels, and some more direct anti-androgenic effect at the target organ. Oestrogens are unpleasant hormones for men to take, however. Nausea is common and gynaecomastia develops in the majority of cases. Malignant change in the resulting breast tissue and thrombotic complications elsewhere may occasionally occur. Progestagens have also been used in both males and females (Heller et al 1958; Kupperman 1963). Medroxyprogesterone is the preparation currently used in the USA (Walker 1978). Once again, the mechanism of action is not fully understood. There are undoubted anti-gonadotrophic effects leading to a marked reduction of circulating testosterone, but other progestational effects may also be involved. Side-effects are probably less troublesome than with oestrogens, but impairment of spermatogenesis may be a problem (Walker 1980). The preparation most in favour at the present time is cyproterone acetate, an anti-androgen which combines a specific blocking of androgen effects with an anti-gonadotrophic action. Its effectiveness in controlling a variety of sexual offence behaviour has been claimed (Davies 1974; Laschet & Laschet 1969). Although various tranquillisers have been used (Bartholomew 1968), a butyrophenone, benperidol, has been marketed as having specific libido-reducing effects (Sterkmans & Geerts 1966). The mechanism of action of such a drug is not known and the endocrine effects are not the same as those produced by cyproterone acetate or oestrogens (Murray et al 1975).

Almost all the evidence of the efficacy of these pharmacological agents is of an uncontrolled kind and therefore cannot be regarded as conclusive. In one controlled study, benperidol was found to be significantly more effective than chlorpromazine or placebo in reducing sexual interest, though the effect on sexual activity was not significant (Tennent et al 1974). In another controlled study, cyproterone acetate was found to be similar to ethinyloestradiol in short-term effects, both preparations producing a reduction in self-reported sexual interest and activity (Bancroft et al 1974). In neither study was there any reduction in erectile response to erotic films, although with cyproterone acetate, responses to erotic slides and to fantasies were reduced. Both studies involved 5 weeks of drug administration only and controlled evidence of more long-term effects is still lacking. None of these drugs is free from side-effects. Benperidol has sedative as well as extrapyramidal effects. Cyproterone acetate may cause temporary tiredness or depression, gynaecomastia in about 20% of cases and suppression of spermatogenesis which is probably reversible. Wincze et al (1986) have reported comparable effects with medroxyprogesterone acetate.

The use of drugs to control sexual offences is therefore still of uncertain value. This is of particular relevance when using them for social control, when it is necessary to be more certain of such effects before using drugs as an alternative to imprisonment. In addition, the potentially irreversible side-effects, such as gynaecomastia, pose major ethical problems when used in this context. A further problem is to ensure that the drugs are taken. Preparations of injectable oestrogen, medroxyprogesterone and a long-acting injectable form of cyproterone acetate are available.

The use of such drugs as part of genuine medical treatment is less problematic. They are then used at the request of the patient, who carries the responsibility for whether he takes them or not. Similarly, he can decide whether to run the risks of side-effects once they have been fully explained to him. Some individuals may find that the reduction of sexual interest is a considerable relief and drug administration can be combined with other psychological methods of treatment (Walker 1978).

Surgical methods of control

Far more controversial than pharmacological methods of control has been the use of irreversible surgical procedures, notably castration and psychosurgery. Castration has been advocated for the reason given above — the substantial reduction of androgens that results. Heim & Hursch (1979) have recently reviewed the principal follow-up studies of surgical castration for sexual offenders. Although in each study they looked at there was a proportion of men, ranging from 10 to 34%, who continued to be sexually active indefinitely after the operation, the majority in each study showed a rapid decline in sexual interest with others showing a more gradual decline. As discussed in Chapter 2, this is consistent with the evidence from men castrated for medical purposes; whereas sexual interest typically declines, the capacity for erection, if the circumstances are right, may continue. Heim & Hursch (1979) rightly point out the methodological problems in evaluating the outcome in such cases, most of which are comparable to those affecting uncontrolled drug studies. But they rather overstate the case when claiming that there is no scientific basis for the operation. They also object to the operation on ethical grounds and these should be quite sufficient. It is difficult to see how this operation, which is not only irreversible but also physically and psychologically mutilating, can be justified even in the face of unequivocal proof of its efficacy in reducing sexual offences.

Similar considerations apply to the use of psychosurgery to control sexual offenders. Stereotaxic hypothalamotomy, aimed at ablating the ventromedial nucleus on one side, has been advocated as a specific method of controlling unwanted sexual behaviour. Needless to say, a good scientific rationale of such a procedure has not been presented and the ethical objections are insurmountable (see p. 69). This approach, which has been largely confined to West Germany, has been most strongly criticised on both scientific and ethical grounds by Rieber & Sigusch (1979).

Psychological methods of treatment

Psychological treatment is less problematic from the ethical point of view. Change is only likely to occur if it is desired and actively sought by the offender. 'Brainwashing' or thought reform methods cannot be considered in the same category. Not only are their results uncertain, but they require total control of the individual's environment, combined with an ever-present fear of death — both continued for a long time (Bancroft 1974). Whilst it may be theoretically possible to arrange such conditions within penal institutions, they can hardly be regarded as methods of treatment.

It is of course possible to employ psychological principles to control behaviour within penal institutions without recourse to such extreme techniques. The use of systems of token reinforcement and withdrawal of privileges to encourage desirable behaviour and discourage the undesirable have been tried. They are of limited value in such settings, however, either resulting in countercontrol by the prisoners or change which is restricted to the prison environment and not generalised to life outside (Remington 1979).

The psychological methods that concern us here are of a very different kind. They depend on an appropriate therapist–client relationship of the type described in Chapter 10. This is of 'adult–adult' type, as between a teacher and his adult pupil; the responsibility for change must lie with the pupil, however much the teacher provides guidance. Unfortunately it is difficult to achieve such a relationship when the offender is either confined in prison or under pressure from the legal system to be compliant (Bancroft 1979). However, it is such a therapeutic relationship that is required if offenders are to be helped, at least on an individual basis.

Group therapy may have advantages within prison for these reasons (West et al 1978); participants will use other group members to reflect their own problems and confront them with their need to accept reponsibility for their actions. But here also lack of security and fear that one's release may be jeopardised will inhibit offenders from revealing all their fears and concerns.

Directive and behavioural methods of psychotherapy have gained favour in the treatment of the sexual offender. Whereas in the early stages of behaviour therapy there was a tendency to prescribe specific and rather limited techniques such as aversion therapy, there have been major changes in recent years and now a more broad-spectrum and flexible approach is advocated, designed to fit the needs of the individual case (Abel et al 1978). Before embarking on such treatment, it is therefore necessary to make a careful assessment of what Abel and his colleagues call the 'excesses and deficits'. In many respects these are similar in the different categories of sexual offenders, as will have become apparent in this chapter. Certain aspects are more specific to particular kinds of offence, such as the arousing effect of force or aggression on many rapists. The problem areas on which to focus in treatment and counselling can be considered under the following headings:

1. Problems in establishing satisfactory sexual relationships.
2. Problems in established relationships of a sexual or general kind.
3. Problems of lowered self-esteem, lack of assertiveness or lack of rewarding activities.
4. Inadequate sexual arousal to normal sexual stimuli.
5. Problems of self-control and inappropriate sexual arousal to deviant stimuli.

Whenever possible, it is desirable and more effective to take a constructive, positive approach to treatment, to help the individual build up or reinforce new and more adaptive behaviours rather than simply to eliminate old, undesirable ones. Sociosexual difficulties in establishing relationships can be tackled by means of social skills training on either a group or individual basis. The individual offender's methods of social interaction are analysed and fed back to him by means of video or audio recordings and appropriate comments. New ways of behaving are modelled and rehearsed. Methods of self-assertion are practised. Role playing of relevant social situations using female subjects is often used, and both non-verbal and verbal skills are considered (Pacht et al 1962; Abel et al 1978; Crawford & Allan 1979).

Individual counselling may have similar goals, particularly in offenders outside institutions. Thus specific target behaviours, such as limited approach to a particular sexual partner, may be agreed and the offender sent away to try them out. His attempts are then discussed with the therapist and possible reasons for failure considered and alternative approaches planned (Bancroft 1977).

In those men with established relationships, sexual problems are common and counselling with the couple, as described in Chapter 10, is often appropriate. The assumption is that if 'normal' sexuality becomes more rewarding, there will be less need for the anti-social forms of sex. The relevant problem in the relationship may not be sexual, however. A tendency for sex offenders, particularly exhibitionists and paedophiles, to marry rather dominant women has already been mentioned. General marital counselling aimed at altering the balance of power in the relationship may be beneficial.

General counselling or psychotherapy may also be helpful in those whose sexual offences are reflections of generally low self-esteem. In what ways can this individual re-organise his life to bolster his self-respect and provide greater personal rewards? Does he need special help with educational deficits? Would he benefit from some re-training, etc.?

Inadequate sexual responsiveness to appropriate stimuli may also be the focus of treatment, relevant to some individuals who have no current sexual partner. Exploration of sexual fantasies may be helpful, as discussed in Chapter 10. Systematic modification of fantasies during masturbation may be used (Bancroft 1974, 1977).

Most obvious as a goal of treatment is the improvement of self-control over anti-social sexual urges or, alternatively, a reduction in the strength of those urges. It is in this area of self-control that responsibility must be unequivocally placed with the offender. In both group and individual therapy, the open statement of a commitment to self-control can be helpful, making it more difficult for the offender to engage in self-deception. For this reason, periodic but regular contact between offender and therapist can be beneficial with little more involved than 'keeping an eye' on the offender and reiterating his commitment to self-control. At the same time, the thera-peutic relationship can be maintained and the channels of communication kept open so that they can be used at times of crisis.

There are also more direct methods of enhancing self-control. In those cases where offences occur in a specific situation, as at the end of a predict-able sequence of events, plans can be made to interrupt the sequence at an early stage and introduce some alternative, well rehearsed behaviour. Thus if an exhibitionist tends to visit a particular place to expose himself, an early point on the route to that place should be identified and linked clearly with an alternative response (e.g. whenever you find yourself walking up X road, stop at the telephone box and phone up the hospital, asking to speak to the therapist). Such an approach requires not only a predictable sequence of behaviour for it to be easily applied, but also a fair level of motivation. But there are cases which benefit from such tactics. Such self-management methods are described in more detail by Kanfer (1975).

Aversive techniques of one kind or another may still have a place in this respect. A stimulus that would typically provoke anti-social behaviour is associated, either in imagination or reality, with a noxious stimulus, such as an electric shock or an imagined traumatic event. This 'pairing' is carried out repeatedly, either in the presence of the therapist or by the subject on his own. Whereas the original rationale of such aversive techniques was based on principles of aversive learning or conditioning, there is no evidence that any clearcut classical or operant learning is involved, or if it is, that it is relevant to the change that follows (Bancroft 1974). Nor is it clear whether aversion leads directly to a reduction in the arousing prop-erties of deviant stimuli, or whether the greater control of behaviour that follows is based on some cognitive mediating process. It may be, for example, that recall of the aversive experience is effective in blocking the arousal that might otherwise occur. It could well be this mechanism that makes the threat or the past experience of legal sanctions effective in so many cases. The would-be offender, on the verge of offending, conjures up the thought of the legal consequences and this is sufficient to deter him from taking the action. Similarly, the person who has experienced aversion therapy may recall the aversive experiences in the same way, hence blocking or reducing sexual arousal that might otherwise occur. Because of this basic uncertainty about the underlying process of change, aversive techniques should be seen as empirical, and because of their associated ethical prob-lems, should be used cautiously. So far, no one has demonstrated clear superiority of aversive methods over other approaches in controlling unwanted behaviour. On the other hand, they can be seen as a potentially useful addition to the therapeutic range. Abel and his colleagues believe that they have a place in reducing that sexual arousability of the rapist to sexual aggression, which, as we have seen, may be particularly important in some rapists. But adequate controlled evidence supporting this view should be obtained before these methods are generally advocated.

As an alternative, the judicious use of libido-lowering drugs can be combined with these other counselling approaches. By reducing the strength of deviant urges, it may be more feasible for the sex offender to begin to build up a more appropriate repertoire of alternative behaviours. It is nevertheless important to ensure that the use of drugs, by suggesting a more medical type of treatment, does not undermine the offender's sense of responsibility for his own behaviour, or foster an attitude of passive dependence.

In general, the sexual offender who is not adequately controlled by legal sanctions poses a rather daunting prospect to the therapist. However, if the problems that result both for the offender himself and his victims are sufficiently serious, concentrated efforts to find effective ways of helping him should be made.

REFERENCES

Abel G G, Barlow D H, Blanchard E B, Guild D 1977 The components of the rapist's sexual arousal. Archives of General Psychiatry 34: 395–403

Abel G G, Blanchard E H, Becker J V 1978 An integrated treatment program for rapists. In: Rada R (ed) Clinical aspects of the rapist. Grune & Stratton, New York

Abel G G, Becker J V, Skinner L J 1980 Aggressive behavior and sex. Psychiatric clinics of North America 3: 133–151

Abel G G, Rouleau J-L, Coyne B J 1987 Are some rapists paraphiliacs? Paper presented at 13th Annual meeting of International Academy Sex Research, Tutzing, West Germany

Amir M 1971 Patterns in forcible rape. University Press, Chicago

Ash A 1984 Father–daughter sexual abuse: the abuse of paternal authority. Social Theory and Institutions, Bangor

Austin C R 1980 Constraints on sexual behaviour. In: Austin C R, Short R V (eds) Human sexuality. Cambridge University Press, Cambridge, pp 124–150

Bancroft J 1974 Deviant sexual behaviour: modification and assessment. Clarendon Press, Oxford

Bancroft J 1977 The behavioural approach to treatment. In: Money J, Musaph H (eds) Handbook of sexology. Excerpta Medica, Amsterdam

Bancroft J 1978 Commentary on Noble M, Mason J K Incest. Journal of Medical Ethics 4: 69–70

Bancroft J 1979 The nature of the patient–therapist relationship: its relevance to behaviour modification of offenders. British Journal of Criminology 19: 416–419

Bancroft J H J, Tennent T G, Loucas K, Cass J 1974 Control of deviant sexual behaviour by drugs: behavioural effects of oestrogens and anti-androgens. British Journal of Psychiatry 125: 310–315

Bandura A 1973 Aggression: a social learning analysis. Prentice-Hall, Englewood Cliffs, New Jersey

Barbaree H E, Marshall W L, Lanthier R D 1979 Deviant sexual arousal in rapists. Behaviour Research and Therapy 17: 215–222

Bartholomew A A 1968 A long acting phenothiazine as a possible agent to control deviant sexual behavior. American Journal of Psychiatry 124: 917–923

Becker J V, Skinner L J, Abel G G, Axelrod R, Treacy E C 1984 Depressive symptoms associated with sexual assault. Journal of Sexual and Marital Therapy 10: 185–192

Becker J V, Skinner L J, Abel G G, Cichon J 1986 Level of post assault sexual functioning in rape and incest victims. Archives of Sexual Behavior 15: 37–49

Bischof N 1975 The comparative ethology of incest avoidance. In: Fox R (ed) Biosocial anthropology. Malaby Press, London

Boat B W, Everson M D 1987 Research and issues in using anatomical dolls. Paper presented at 13th Annual meeting of International Academy Sex Research, Tutzing, West Germany

Brongersma 1979 The unknown paedophile. Unpublished manuscript cited in O'Carroll 1980
Broude G J, Greene S J 1980 Cross cultural codes on 20 sexual attitudes and practices. In: Barry III H, Schlegel A (eds) Cross cultural samples and codes. University of Pittsburgh Press, Pittsburgh pp 313–333
Brownmiller S 1975 Against our will. Men, women and rape. Simon Schuster, New York
Bullough V L 1976 Sexual variance in society and history. Wiley, New York
Burgess A W, Holmstrom L L 1974 Rape: victims of crisis. Robert J. Brady, Bowie
Burnett R C, Templer D I, Barker P C 1985 Personality variables and circumstances of sexual assault predictive of a women's resistance. Archives of Sexual Behavior 14: 183–188
Burt M R 1980 Cultural myths and supports for rape. Journal of Personality and Social Psychology 38: 217–230
Burton L 1968 Vulnerable children: three studies of children in conflict. Routledge & Kegan Paul, London
Chambers G, Millar A 1983 Investigating sexual assaults. HMSO, Edinburgh
Chambers G, Millar A 1986 Prosecuting sexual assaults. HMSO, Edinburgh
Chappell D, Singer S 1977 Rape in New York City: a study of materials in the police files and its meaning. In: Chappell D, Geis M, Geis G (eds) Forcible rape: the crime, the victim and the offender. Columbia University Press, New York
Christiansen K O, El Nielsen M, Le Maire L, Sturup G K 1965 Recidivism among sexual offenders. In: Scandinavian studies in criminology, vol I. Universites Forlaget, Oslo, pp 55–85
CLRC 1980 Working paper on sexual offence. HMSO, London
Commission on Obscenity and Pornography 1970 The report of the commission on obscenity and pornography, vols 1–7 US Government Printing Office, Washington, DC
Constantine L 1979 The sexual rights of children: implications of a radical perspective. In: Cook M, Wilson G (eds) Love and attraction. Pergamon, Oxford
Court J H 1976 Pornography and sex crimes: a re-evaluation in the light of recent trends around the world. International Journal of Criminology and Penology 5: 129–157
Crawford D A, Allen J V 1979 A social skills training programme with sex offenders. In: Cook M, Wilson G (eds) Love and attraction. Pergamon, Oxford, pp 503–508
Criminal Statistics for England and Wales 1985 HMSO, London
Davies T S 1974 Cyproterone acetate for male hypersexuality. Journal of International Medical Research 2: 159–163
Davis A J 1970 Sexual assaults in the Philadelphia prison system and sheriff's van. In: Shiloh A (ed) Studies in human sexual behavior: the American scene. Charles C. Thomas, Springfield, Illinois
Ellis A, Brancale R 1956 The psychology of sex offenders. Thomas, Springfield, Illinois
Finkelhor D 1979 Sexuality victimized children. Free Press, New York
Finkelhor D 1980 Sex among siblings: a survey on prevalence, variety and effects. Archives of Sexual Behavior 9: 171–194
Finkelhor D 1982 Sexual abuse — a sociological perspective. Child Abuse and Neglect 6: 95–102
Finkelhor D 1984 Child sexual abuse: new theory and research. Free Press, New York
Fox R 1967 Kinship and marriage. Penguin, London
Fox R 1980 The red lamp of incest. Hutchinson, London
Frank E, Turner S M, Duffy B 1979 Depressive symptoms in rape victims. Journal of Affective Disorders 1: 269–277
Frank E, Turner S M, Duffy B 1980 Initial response to rape: the impact of factors within the rape situation. Journal of Behavioural Assessment 2: 39–53
Freeman M D A 1979 The law and sexual deviation. In: Rosen I (ed) Sexual deviation. Oxford University Press, Oxford
Frenken J 1987 A typology of incest experiences in help-seeking former incest victims. Paper presented at 13th Annual meeting of International Academy Sex Research, Tutzing, West Germany
Frenken J, Doomen J 1984 Strafbare seksualiteit. Oprattingen en aanpak van politie, justitie en hulpverlening. Van Loghum Slaterus, Deventer
Freud S 1918 Totem and taboo. Norton, New York
Friedrich W N 1987 Consequences of sexual abuse in the context of normative sexual behavior in children. Paper presented at 13th Annual meeting of International Academy Sex Research, Tutzing, West Germany

Furniss T 1985 Conflict-avoiding and conflict regulating patterns in incest and child sexual abuse. Acta Paediopsychiatrica 50: 6

Gebhard P H, Johnson A B 1979 The Kinsey data: marginal tabulations of the 1938–1963 interviews conducted by the Institute for Sex Research. Saunders, Philadelphia

Gebhard P, Gagnon J, Pomeroy N, Christenson C 1965 Sex offenders. Harper Row, New York

Giarretto H 1977 Humanistic treatment of father–daughter incest. Child Abuse and Neglect 1: 411–476

Gibbens T C N, Prince J 1963 Child victims of sex offences. Institute for the Study and Treatment of Delinquency, London

Gibbens T C N, Way C, Soothill K L 1977 Behavioural types of rape. British Journal of Psychiatry 130: 32–42

Giglio E D 1985 Pornography in Denmark: a public policy model for the United States? Comparative Social Research 8: 281–300

Gittelson N L, Eacott S E, Mehta B M 1978 Victims of indecent exposure. British Journal of Psychiatry 132: 61–66

Gray J P 1984 The influence of female power in marriage on sexual behaviour and attitudes: a holocultural study. Archives of Sexual Behavior 13: 223–232

Greenwood J, Bancroft J 1988 Basic counselling and crisis intervention. In: Kendell R E, Zealley A (eds) Companion to psychiatric studies, 4th edn. Churchill Livingstone

Griffin T, Morris J 1987 Social trends no 17 HMSO, London

Heim N, Hursch C J 1979 Castration for sex offenders: treatment or punishment? A review and critique of recent European literature. Archives of Sexual Behavior 8: 281–304

Heller C G, Laidlaw W M, Harvey H T, Nelson D L 1958 Effects of progestational compounds on the reproductive processes of the human male. Annals of the New York Academy of Science 71: 649–665

Hinde R A 1974 Biological bases of human social behaviour. McGraw Hill, New York

Hindelang M J, Davis B J 1977 Forcible rape in the United States: a statistical profile. In: Chappell D, Geis M, Geis G (eds) Forcible rape: the crime, the victim and the offender. Columbia University Press, New York

Hobbs C J, Wynne J M 1986 Buggery in childhood — a common syndrome of child abuse. Lancet ii: 792–796

Holmstrom L L, Burgess A W 1980 Sexual behaviour of assailants during reported rapes. Archives of Sexual Behavior 9: 427–446

Honoré T 1978 Sex law. Duckworth, London

Hopkins J, Thompson E H 1984 Loss and mourning in victims of rape and sexual assault. In: Hopkins J (ed) Perspectives on rape and sexual assault. Harper & Row, London

Howells K 1984 Coercive sexual behaviour. In: Howells K (ed) The psychology of sexual diversity. Blackwell, Oxford

Howells K, Shaw F, Greasley M, Robertson J, Gloster D 1984 Perceptions of rape in a British sample: effects of relationship, victim status, sex and attitudes to women. British Journal of Social Psychology 23: 35–40

Humphreys R A L 1970 Tea room trade. Aldine, Chicago

Ingram M 1979 The participating victim: a study of sexual offences against prepubertal boys. In: Cook M, Wilson G (eds) Love and attraction. Pergamon, Oxford, pp 511–517

Jaffee D, Straus M A 1987 Sexual climate and reported rape: a state-level analysis. Archives of Sexual Behavior 16: 107–124

Kanfer F H 1975 Self-management methods. In: Kanfer F H, Goldstein A P (eds) Helping people change. Pergamon, New York, pp 309–355

Kanin E J 1985 Date rapists: differential sexual socialisation and relative deprivation. Archives of Sexual Behavior 14: 219–232

Katchadourian H A 1985 Fundamentals of human sexuality, 4th edn. Holt, Rinehart & Winston, New York, pp 111–134

Katz S, Mazur M A 1979 Understanding rape victims: a synthesis of research findings. Wiley, New York

Kinsey A C, Pomeroy W B, Martin C E, Gebhard P H 1953 Sexual behaviour in the human female. Saunders, Philadelphia

Koss M P, Oros C J 1982 Sexual experiences survey: a research instrument investigating sexual aggression and victimization. Journal of Consulting and Clinical Psychology 50: 455–457

Kupperman H S 1963 Human endocrinology. Davies, Philadelphia, p 397

Kutchinsky B 1983 Obscenity and pornography: behavioral aspects. In: Kadish S H et al Encyclopedia of crime and justice, vol 3. Free Press, pp 1077–1086

Kutchinsky B 1985 Pornography and its effects in Denmark and the United States. Comparative Social Research 8: 301–330

Landis J T 1956 Experiences of 500 children with adult sexual deviation. Psychiatric Quarterly (suppl) 30: 91–109

Laschet V, Laschet L 1969 Anti-androgens in the treatment of sexual deviations of men. Journal of Steroid Biochemistry 6: 821–826

Lemert E 1967 Human deviance, social problems and social control. New Jersey

Levin S M, Stava L 1987 Personality characteristics of sex offenders: a review. Archives of Sexual Behavior 16: 57–80

Le Vine R A 1959 Gusii sex offenses: a study in social control. American Anthropologist 61: 965–990

Levi-Strauss C 1969 The elementary structures of kinship. Beacon, Boston

Malamuth N M 1981 Rape proclivity among males. Journal of Social Issues 37: 138–157

Malamuth N M, Donnerstein E 1982 The effects of aggressive and pornographic mass media stimuli. In: Berkowitz L (ed) Advances in experimental social psychology, vol 15. Academic, New York

Mill J S 1859 On liberty. London

Mohr J W, Turner R E, Jerry M B 1964 Pedophilia and exhibitionism. University of Toronto Press, Toronto

Mrazek P B, Lynch M, Bentovim A 1981 Recognition of child sexual abuse in the United Kingdom. In: Mrazek P B, Kempe C H (eds) Sexually abused children and their families. Pergamon, Oxford

Murphy W D, Krisak J, Stalgaitis S, Anderson K 1984 The use of penile tumescence measures with incarcerated rapists: further validity issues. Archives of Sexual Behavior 13: 545–554

Murray M A F, Bancroft J H J, Anderson D C, Tennent T G, Carr P J 1975 Endocrine changes in male sexual deviants after treatment with anti-androgens, oestrogens or tranquillisers. Journal of Endocrinology 67: 179–188

NCCL 1976 Sexual offences; evidence to the Criminal Law Revision Committee. Report no 13. NCCL, London

O'Carroll T 1980 Paedophilia: the radical case. Peter Owen, London

O'Reilly H J 1984 Crisis intervention with victims of forcible rape: a police perspective. In: Hopkins J (ed) Perspectives on rape and sexual assault. Harper & Row, London

Pacht A R, Cowden J E 1974 An exploratory study of 500 sex offenders. Criminal Justice and Behavior 1: 13–20

Pacht A R, Halleck S L, Ehrmann J C 1962 Diagnosis and treatment of the sex offender: a 9 year study. American Journal of Psychiatry 118: 802–808

Parker T 1969 The twisting lane: some sex offenders. Hutchinson, London

Peters J J 1975 Social, legal and psychological effects of rape on the victim. Pennsylvania Medicine 78: 34–66

Porter R (ed) 1984 Child sexual abuse within the family. Ciba Foundation report. Tavistock, London

Qualls C B 1978 The prevention of sexual disorder: an overview. In: Qualls C B, Wincze S P, Barlow D H (eds) The prevention of sexual disorder. Plenum, New York

Quinsey V L, Chaplin T C, Varney G A 1981 A comparison of rapists and non-sex offenders' sexual preferences for mutually consenting sex, rape and physical abuse of women. Behavioral Assessment 3: 127–135

Radzinowicz L 1957 Sexual offences. MacMillan, London

Remington R E 1979 Behaviour modification in American penal institutions. British Journal of Criminology 19: 333–352

Rieber I, Sigusch V 1979 Psychosurgery in sex offenders and sexual deviants in West Germany. Archives of Sexual Behavior 8: 523–528

Rooth F G 1971 Indecent exposure and exhibitionism. British Journal of Hospital Medicine April: 521–533

Rooth F G 1972 Changes in the conviction rate for indecent exposure. British Journal of Psychiatry 121: 89–94

Rooth F G 1973 Exhibitionism, sexual violence and paedophilia. British Journal of Psychiatry 122: 705–710

Rooth F G 1973 Exhibitionism outside Europe and America. Archives of Sexual Behavior 2: 351–363

Rosen I 1979 Exhibitionism, scopophilia and voyeurism. In: Rosen I (ed) Sexual deviation. Oxford University Press, Oxford

Rossman G P 1979 Sexual experience between men and boys: exploring the pederast underground. Temple Smith, London

Russell D E H 1982 Rape in marriage. MacMillan, New York

Russell D E H 1983 The incidence and prevalence of intrafamilial and extrafamilial sexual abuse of female children. Child Abuse and Neglect 7: 133–146

Sanday P R 1981 The socio-cultural context of rape: a cross-cultural study. Journal of Social Issues 37: 5–27

Sarrel P, Masters W 1982 Sexual molestation of men by women. Archives of Sexual Behavior 11: 2

Schofield M 1965 Sociological aspects of homosexuality. A comparative study of three types of homosexuals. Longman, London

Scott P D 1964 Definition, classification, prognosis and treatment. In: Rosen I (ed) Pathology and treatment of sexual deviation. Oxford University Press, Oxford

Shepher J 1971 Mate selection among second generation kibbutz adolescents and adults: incest avoidance and negative imprinting. Archives of Sexual Behavior 1: 293–307

Silverman D C, Apfel R J 1983 Caring for the victims of rape. In: Nadelson C C, Marcotte D B (eds) Treatment interventions in human sexuality. Plenum, New York

Soothill K 1980 Sexual offenders — the value of long-term cohort studies. British Journal of Sexual Medicine 7: 36–42

Sterkmans P, Geerts F 1966 Is benperidol (RF504) the specific drug for the treatment of excessive and disinhibited sexual behaviour? Acta Neurologica et Psychiatrica Belgica 66: 1030–1040

Summit R C 1983 The child sexual abuse accommodation syndrome. Child Abuse and Neglect 7: 177–193

Tennent G, Bancroft J, Cass J 1974 The control of deviant sexual behavior by drugs: a double-blind controlled study of benperidol, chlorpromazine and placebo. Archives of Sexual Behavior 3: 261–271

Tsai M, Wagner N N 1978 Therapy groups for women sexually molested as children. Archives of Sexual Behavior 7: 417–428

Vera H, Barnard G W, Holzer C 1979 The intelligence of rapists: new data. Archives of Sexual Behavior 8: 375–378

von Schrenck-Notzing A 1895 The use of hypnosis in psychopathia sexualis with special reference to contrary sexual instinct. Translated by Chaddock C G 1956. Institute of Research, Hypnosis Publication Society, Julian Press, New York

Walker P A 1978 The role of antiandrogens in the treatment of sex offenders. In: Qualls C B, Wincze J P, Barlow D H (eds) The prevention of sexual disorders. Plenum, New York, pp 117–136

Walker P A 1980 Paper read at International Academy of Sex Research. Annual Meeting. Oct. 1980, Tucson

Walmsley R 1980 Prosecution rates, sentencing practice and maximum penalties for sexual offences. In: West D J (ed) Sex offenders in the criminal justice system. Cropwood Conference Series no 12, Cambridge

Walmsley R, White K 1979 Sexual offences, consent and sentencing. Home Office Research Study no 54. HMSO, London

Ward D A, Kassebaum G G 1964 Homosexuality: a mode of adaptation in a prison for women. Social Problems 12: 159–177

Weinberg S K 1976 Incest behaviour. Citadel, New York

West D J 1984 The victim's contributions to sexual offences. In: Hopkins J (ed) Perspectives on rape and sexual assault. Harper & Row, London

West D J, Roy C, Nichols F L 1978 Understanding sexual attacks. Heinemann, London

Westermark E 1926 A short history of marriage. MacMillan, New York

Williams Committee 1979 Report of the committee on obscenity and film censorship. Cmnd 7772. HMSO, London

Wincze J P, Bansal S, Malamud M 1986 Effects of medroxyprogesterone acetate on subjective arousal, arousal to erotic stimulation and nocturnal penile tumescence in male sex offenders. Archives of Sexual Behaviour 15: 293–306

Wolf A P 1970 Childhood association and sexual attraction: a further test of the Westermark hypothesis. American Anthropologist 72: 503–515

Wolfenden J 1957 Report on homosexual offences and prostitution. HMSO, London

Wright R 1980 The English rapist. New Society, 17th July

Wyatt G E 1985 The sexual abuse of Afro-American and white American women in childhood. Child Abuse and Neglect 9: 507–519

Wyatt G E, Peters S D 1986a Issues in the definition of child sexual abuse in prevalence research. Child Abuse and Neglect 10: 231–240

Wyatt G E, Peters S D 1986b Methodological considerations in research on the prevalence of child sexual abuse. Child Abuse and Neglect 10: 241–251

Index